Macleod's Clinical Examination

Edited by

Graham Douglas BSc(Hons) MBChB FRCPE
Consultant Physician
Aberdeen Royal Infirmary
Honorary Reader in Medicine
University of Aberdeen

Fiona Nicol BSc(Hons) MBBS FRCGP FRCPE
Formerly GP Principal and Trainer
Stockbridge Health Centre, Edinburgh
Honorary Clinical Senior Lecturer
University of Edinburgh

Colin Robertson BA(Hons) MBChB FRCPEd FRCPE FSAScot
Honorary Professor of Accident and Emergency Medicine
University of Edinburgh

Illustrations by
Robert Britton
Ethan Danielson

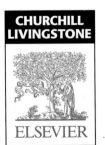

CHURCHILL
LIVINGSTONE

ELSEVIER

Thirteenth
edition

Edinburgh London New York Oxford Philadelphia St Louis Sydney Toronto 2013

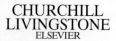

CHURCHILL
LIVINGSTONE
ELSEVIER

First edition 1964
Second edition 1967
Third edition 1973
Fourth edition 1976
Fifth edition 1979
Sixth edition 1983
Seventh edition 1986

Eighth edition 1990
Ninth edition 1995
Tenth edition 2000
Eleventh edition 2005
Twelfth edition 2009
Thirteenth edition 2013

ISBN 9780702047282
International ISBN 9780702047299

British Library Cataloguing in Publication Data
A catalogue record for this book is available from the British Library

Library of Congress Cataloging in Publication Data
A catalog record for this book is available from the Library of Congress

ELSEVIER your source for books, journals and multimedia in the health sciences

www.elsevierhealth.com

Working together to grow
libraries in developing countries

www.elsevier.com | www.bookaid.org | www.sabre.org

ELSEVIER   BOOK AID International   Sabre Foundation

The publisher's policy is to use paper manufactured from sustainable forests

Printed in China

Last digit is the print number: 10 9 8 7 6 5

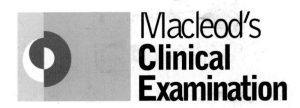

Macleod's
Clinical
Examination

John Macleod
(1915–2006)

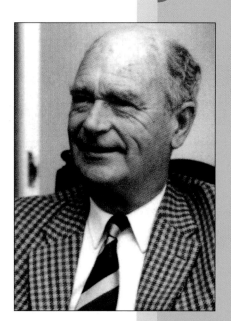

John Macleod was appointed consultant physician at the Western General Hospital, Edinburgh, in 1950. He had major interests in rheumatology and medical education. Medical students who attended his clinical teaching sessions remember him as an inspirational teacher with the ability to present complex problems with great clarity. He was invariably courteous to his patients and students alike. He had an uncanny knack of involving all students equally in clinical discussions and used praise rather than criticism. He paid great attention to the value of history taking and, from this, expected students to identify what particular aspects of the physical examination should help to narrow the diagnostic options.

His consultant colleagues at the Western welcomed the opportunity of contributing when he suggested writing a textbook on clinical examination. The book was first published in 1964 and John Macleod edited seven editions. With characteristic modesty he was very embarrassed when the eighth edition was renamed *Macleod's Clinical Examination*. This, however, was a small way of recognising his enormous contribution to medical education.

He possessed the essential quality of a successful editor – the skill of changing disparate contributions from individual contributors into a uniform style and format without causing offence; everybody accepted his authority. He avoided being dogmatic or condescending. He was generous in teaching others his editorial skills and these attributes were recognised when he was invited to edit *Davidson's Principles and Practice of Medicine*.

For Elsevier

Content Strategist: *Laurence Hunter*
Content Development Specialist: *Helen Leng*
Project Manager: *Louisa Talbott*
Designer/Design Direction: *Miles Hitchen*
Illustration Manager: *Jennifer Rose*

Preface

The skills of history taking and physical examination are central to the practice of clinical medicine. This book describes these and is intended primarily for medical undergraduates. It is also of value to primary care and postgraduate hospital doctors, particularly those studying for higher clinical examinations or returning to clinical practice. The book is also an essential reference for nurse practitioners and other paramedical staff who are involved in medical assessment of patients.

This edition has four sections: Section 1 details the principles of history taking and general examination; Section 2 covers symptoms and signs in individual system examinations; Section 3 reviews specific situations; and a new Section 4 deals with how to apply these techniques in an OSCE.

The text has been extensively revised and edited, with two new chapters on the frail elderly and the febrile adult. The number of illustrations has been increased and many have been updated. Line drawings illustrate surface anatomy and techniques of examination; over 330 photographs show normal and abnormal clinical appearances.

We recognise the current debate where some decry clinical examination because of the lack of evidence supporting many techniques. Where evidence exists, however, we highlight this in a new feature for this edition: evidence-based examination boxes (EBEs). We are convinced of the need to acquire and hone clinical examination skills to avoid unnecessary expensive and potentially harmful over-investigation. Nevertheless, there is a need to evaluate rigorously many clinical symptoms and signs. It is possible to open this book at almost any page and find a topic which cries out for evidence-based analysis. We continue to hope that the book will stimulate this enquiry and would encourage these responses and incorporate them in future editions.

This 13th edition of *Macleod's Clinical Examination* – full text, illustrations and videos – is available in an online version, as part of Elsevier's 'Student Consult' electronic library. It is closely integrated with *Davidson's Principles and Practice of Medicine*, and is best read in conjunction with that text.

G.D.
F.N.
C.R.
Edinburgh and Aberdeen
2013

Acknowledgements

We are very grateful to all the contributors and editors of previous editions; in particular, we owe an immeasurable debt to Dr John Munro for his teaching and wisdom.

We greatly appreciate the constructive suggestions and help that we have received from past and present students, colleagues and focus groups in the design and content of the book.

We are particularly grateful to the following medical students who undertook detailed reviews of the book and gave us a wealth of ideas to implement in this latest edition: Alessandro Aldera, University of Cape Town; Sabreen Ali, University of Sheffield; Bernard Ho, St George's University of London; Edward Tzu-Yu Huang, University of Birmingham; Emma Jackson, University of Manchester; Amit Kaura, University of Bristol; Brian Morrissey, University of Aberdeen; Neena Pankhania, University of Leicester; Tom Paterson, University of Glasgow; Christopher Roughley, University of Warwick; and Christopher Saunders, University of Edinburgh.

We wish to thank the many individuals who have provided advice and support: Jackie Fiddes for designing the manikins and for her computer skills; Steven Hill of the Department of Medical Illustration, University of Aberdeen; Jason Powell for his help with illustrations; Victoria Buchan for her help linking the examination videos with the online text; Helen Leng and Laurence Hunter at Elsevier.

G.D.
F.N.
C.R.

Picture and box credits

We are grateful to the following individuals and organisations for permission to reproduce the figures and boxes listed below:

Chapter 1

Fig. 1.1 WHO Guidelines on Hand Hygiene in Health Care First Global Patient Safety Challenge Clean Care is Safer Care http://www.who.int/gpsc/clean_hands_protection/en/ © World Health Organization 2009. All rights reserved. **Box 1.1** Courtesy of the General Medical Council (UK).

Chapter 2

Box 2.32 Trzepacz PT, Baker RW, The psychiatric mental status examination 1993 by permission of Oxford University Press USA. **Box 2.50** Hodkinson HM, Evaluation of a mental test score for assessment of mental impairment in the elderly Age and Ageing 1972 1(4): 233-8 by permission of Oxford University Press.

Chapter 3

Figs 3.19C and **3.28A–D** Forbes CD, Jackson WF. Color Atlas of Clinical Medicine. 3rd edn. Edinburgh: Mosby; 2003.

Chapter 5

Fig. 5.3 Currie G, Douglas G, eds. Flesh and Bones of Medicine. Edinburgh: Mosby; 2011.

Chapter 6

Figs 6.6D, 6.16A–D and **6.38A** Forbes CD, Jackson WF. Color Atlas of Clinical Medicine. 3rd edn. Edinburgh: Mosby; 2003. **Fig. 6.6E** Colledge NR, Walker BR, Ralston SH, eds. Davidson's Principles and Practice of Medicine. 21st edn. Edinburgh: Churchill Livingstone; 2010. **Fig. 6.8C** Haslett C, Chilvers ER, Boon NA, Colledge NR, eds, Davidson's Principles and Practice of Medicine, 19th edn. Edinburgh: Churchill Livingstone; 2002. **Box 6.19** Reproduced by kind permission of the British Hypertension Society.

Chapter 7

Fig. 7.24D Forbes CD, Jackson WF. Color Atlas of Clinical Medicine. 3rd edn. Edinburgh: Mosby; 2003. **Box 7.7** Reproduced from British Medical Journal Fletcher CM, Elmes PC, Fairbairn AS et al 2(5147):257 1959 with permission from BMJ Publishing Group Ltd. **Box 7.11** Reproduced from Murray W. Johns. A new method for measuring daytime sleepiness: the Epworth Sleepiness Scale, Sleep, 1991; 14(6): 540-545. ESS contact information and permission to use: MAPI Research Trust, Lyon, France. E-mail: PROinformation@mapi-trust.org Internet: www.mapi-trust.org. **Box 7.17** Reproduced from Thorax Lim WS 58(5):377 2002 with permission from BMJ Publishing Group Ltd. **Box 7.23** Reproduced from Wells PS, Anderson DR, Rodger M et al, 2000 Derivation of a Simple Clinical Model to Categorize Patients Probability of Pulmonary Embolism: Increasing the Models Utility with the SimpliRED D-dimer, Thromb Haemost 83(3) 416-420 with permission from Schattauer Publishers.

Chapter 8

Fig. 8.10 Reproduced by kind permission of Dr K W Heaton, Reader in Medicine at the University of Bristol. © 2000 Norgine Pharmaceuticals Ltd. **Figs 8.31A&B** and **8.32** Forbes CD, Jackson WF. Color Atlas of Clinical Medicine. 3rd edn. Edinburgh: Mosby; 2003. **Box 8.15** Reproduced by kind permission of the Rome Foundation. **Box 8.20** Reproduced from Journal of the British Society of Gastroenterology Rockall TA et al 38(3):316 1996 with permission from BMJ Publishing Group Ltd. **Box 8.34** Reproduced from Conn HO, Leevy CM, Vlahcevic ZR et al 1977 Comparison of lactulose and neomycin in the treatment of chronic portal-systemic encephalopathy. A double blind controlled trial, Gastroenterology 72(4): 573 with permission from Elsevier Inc. **Box 8.47** Reproduced from Pugh RNH, Murray-Lyon IM, Dawson JL et al Transection of the oesophagus for bleeding oesophageal varices British Journal of Surgery 646-649 1973 with permission from John Wiley and Sons.

Chapter 9

Fig. 9.12 Pitkin J, Peattie AB, Magowan BA. Obstetrics and Gynaecology: An Illustrated Colour Text. Edinburgh: Churchill Livingstone; 2003. **Box 9.4** Reproduced from Barry MJ, Fowler FJ Jr, O'Leary MP et al The American Urological Association symptom index for benign prostatic hyperplasia. The Measurement Committee of the American Urological Association. J Urol. 1992 148(5):1549-57. ESS contact information and permission to use: MAPI Research Trust, Lyon, France. E-mail: PROinformation@mapi-trust.org Internet: www.mapi-trust.org

Chapter 11

Fig. 11.15 Epstein O, Perkin GD, de Bono DP, Cookson J. Clinical Examination. 2nd edn. London: Mosby; 1997. **Box 11.18** Medical Research Council scale for muscle power. Aids to examination of the peripheral nervous system. Memorandum no 45 London Her Majesty's Stationery Office 1976 © Crown Copyright.

Chapter 12

Figs 12.15A&B Forbes CD, Jackson WF. Color Atlas of Clinical Medicine. 3rd edn. Edinburgh: Mosby; 2003. **Fig. 12.16** Nicholl D, ed. Clinical Neurology. Edinburgh: Churchill Livingstone; 2003. **Figs 12.27A–D** Epstein O, Perkin GD, de Bono DP, Cookson J. Clinical Examination. 2nd edn. London: Mosby; 1997.

Chapter 13

Fig. 13.20 Scully C, Oral and Maxillofacial Medicine. 2nd edn. Edinburgh: Churchill Livingstone; 2008. **Figs 13.21A** and **13.25B** Bull TR. Color Atlas of ENT Diagnosis. 3rd edn. London: Mosby-Wolfe; 1995.

Chapter 14

Fig. 14.2 Colledge NR, Walker BR, Ralston SH, eds. Davidson's Principles and Practice of Medicine. 21st edn. Edinburgh: Churchill Livingstone; 2010. **Fig. 14.9A** Forbes CD, Jackson WF. Color Atlas of Clinical Medicine. 3rd edn. Edinburgh: Mosby; 2003. **Box 14.3** Reproduced from Aletaha D, Neogi T, Silman AJ et al 2010 Rheumatoid arthritis classification criteria: an American College of Rheumatology/European League Against Rheumatism collaborative initiative, Arthritis & Rheumatism 2569-2581 with permission from John Wiley and Sons. **Box 14.13** Reproduced from Annals of the rheumatic diseases Beighton P, Solomon L, Soskolne CL 32(5): 413 1973 with permission from BMJ Publishing Group.

Chapter 15

Figs 15.7, 15.8, 15.11A&B and **15.12** Lissauer T, Clayden G. Illustrated Textbook of Paediatrics. 2nd edn. Edinburgh: Mosby; 2001. **Fig. 15.17** Child Growth Foundation. **Fig. 15.23** Courtesy of Dr Jack Beattie, Royal Hospital for Sick Children, Glasgow. **Box 15.4** Reproduced with permission of International Anesthesia Research Society from Current researches in anesthesia & analgesia Apgar V 32(4) 1953; permission conveyed through Copyright Clearance Center, Inc.

Chapter 16

Fig. 16.2 Reproduced from Clarifying Confusion: The Confusion Assessment Method: A New Method for Detection of Delirium Inouye SK, vanDyck CH, Alessi CA et al Annals of Internal Medicine 113 1990 with permission from the American College of Physicians. **Fig 16.3** Reproduced by kind permission of BAPEN.

Chapter 19

Fig. 19.9 Reproduced with the kind permission of the Resuscitation Council (UK). **Box 19.1** Adapted from Hillman K, Parr M, Flabouris A et al 2001 Redefining in-hospital resuscitation: the concept of the medical emergency team. Resuscitation 48(2): 105-110 with permission from Elsevier Ltd. **Box 19.14** Reproduced from The Lancet 304(7872), Teasdale G, Jennett B, Assessment of coma and impaired consciousness: a practical scale, 81–84, 1974 with permission from Elsevier Ltd.

How to get the most out of this book

The purpose of this book is to document and explain how to:

- Talk with a patient
- Take the history from a patient
- Examine a patient
- Formulate your findings into differential diagnoses
- Rank these in order of probability
- Use investigations to support or refute your differential diagnosis.

Initially, when you approach a section, we suggest that you glance through it quickly, looking at the headings and how it is laid out. This will help you to see in your mind's eye the framework to use.

Learn to speed-read. It is invaluable in medicine and in life generally. Most probably, the last lesson you had on reading was at primary school. Most people can dramatically improve their speed of reading and increase their comprehension by using and practising simple techniques.

Try making mind maps of the details to help you recall and retain the information as you progress through the chapter. Each of the systems chapters is laid out in the same order:

- Introduction and anatomy
- Symptoms and definitions
- The history: what questions to ask and how to follow them up
- The physical examination: what and how to examine
- Investigations: those done at the patient's side (near-patient tests); laboratory investigations; imaging; and invasive investigations.

Your purchase of the book entitles you to access the complete text online and to search using key words or using the index. You can view all the illustrations and use the hypertext-linked page cross-references to navigate quickly through the book.

Return to this book to refresh your technique if you have been away from a particular field for some time. It is surprising how quickly your technique deteriorates if you do not use it regularly. Practise at every available opportunity so that you become proficient at examination techniques and gain a full understanding of the range of normality.

Ask a senior colleague to review your examination technique regularly; there is no substitute for this and for regular practice. Listen also to what patients say – not only about themselves but also about other health professionals – and learn from these comments. You will pick up good and bad points that you will want to emulate or avoid.

Finally, enjoy your skills. After all, you are learning to be able to understand, diagnose and help people. For most of us, this is the reason we became doctors.

Boxes and tables

Boxes and tables are a popular way of presenting information and are particularly useful for revision. They are classified by the type of information they contain using the following symbols:

 Causes

 Clinical features

 Investigations

 EBE Evidence-based examination

 Other information

Evidence-based examination

Evidence-based examination applies the best available evidence from scientific method to clinical decision making and is an increasingly essential part of modern clinical practice. However, most clinical examination techniques have developed over generations of medical practice without rigorous scientific assessment. To highlight examples where there is evidence-based examination we have included 55 EBE boxes. The art of medicine depends on being able to combine scientific rigour with long-established techniques but this area needs to be re-evaluated and updated constantly as new information comes to light.

Examination sequences

Throughout the book there are outlines of techniques that you should follow when examining a patient. These are identified with a red heading 'Examination sequence'. The bullet-point list provides the exact order to undertake the examination.

To help your understanding of how to perform these techniques many of the examination sequences have been filmed and those marked with the symbol above can be viewed as part of the Student Consult online text.

Glasgow Coma Scale videos

The Glasgow Coma Scale (GCS) is the globally accepted standard means of assessing conscious state. It is validated and reliable. Included as part of the Student Consult website are two video demonstrations of how the Scale should be performed in clinical situations:

- using the GCS: how to perform the different elements of the GCS
- clinical scenarios: using the GCS in a clinical context.

As well as demonstrating correct techniques, the videos illustrate common pitfalls in using the GCS and give guidance on how to avoid these.

Video production team

Writer, narrator, director and producer

Mr Jacques Kerr

Nurses

Dr Sharon Mulhern
Mr Jacques Kerr

Patient

Stevie Allen

Production

Mirage Television Productions

For more information see www.practicalgcs.com

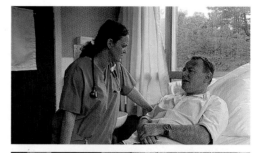

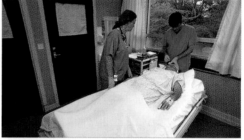

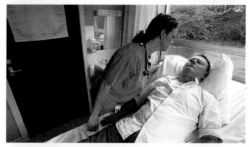

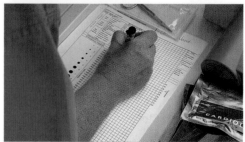

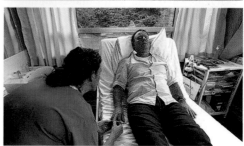

Clinical skills videos

By logging on to the Student Consult website you will have access to clinical examination videos, custom-made for this textbook. Filmed using qualified doctors, with hands-on guidance from the authorship team, and narrated by one of the editors, Professor Colin Robertson, these videos offer you the chance to watch trained professionals performing many of the examination routines described in the book. By helping you to memorise the essential examination steps required for each major system and by demonstrating the proper clinical technique, these videos should act as an important bridge between textbook learning and bedside teaching. The videos will be available for you to view again and again as your clinical skills develop and will prove invaluable as you prepare for your clinical OSCE examinations.

Each examination routine has a detailed explanatory narrative but for maximum benefit view the videos in conjunction with the book. To facilitate this, sections of the videos are also linked to the online text, thus allowing you to view the relevant examination sequences as you progress through each chapter.

Video contents

- Examination of the cardiovascular system
- Examination of the respiratory system
- Examination of the gastrointestinal system
- Examination of the neurological system
- Examination of the ear
- Examination of the musculoskeletal system
- Examination of the thyroid gland

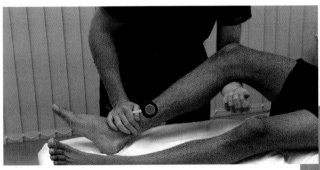

Video production team

Director and editor
Dr Iain Hennessey

Producer
Dr Alan Japp

Sound and narrator
Professor Colin Robertson
Dr Nick Morley

Clinical examiners
Dr Amy Robb
Dr Ben Waterson

Patients
Abby Cooke
Omar Ali

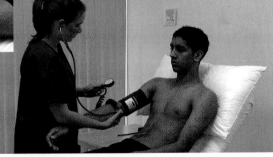

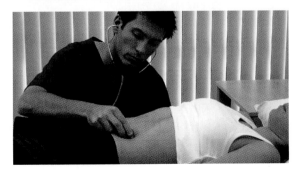

Contributors

Elaine Anderson MD FRCS(Ed)
Clinical Director, Breast and Plastics, NHS Lothian;
Consultant Breast Surgeon, Western General Hospital,
Edinburgh

John Bevan BSc(Hons) MBChB(Hons) MD FRCPE
Consultant Endocrinologist, Aberdeen Royal Infirmary;
Honorary Professor of Endocrinology, University of
Aberdeen

Andrew Bradbury BSc MB ChB(Hons) MD MBA FRCS(Ed)
Sampson Gamgee Professor of Vascular Surgery, and
Director of Quality Assurance and Enhancement,
College of Medical and Dental Sciences, University of
Birmingham; Consultant Vascular and Endovascular
Surgeon, Heart of England NHS Foundation Trust,
Birmingham

Gareth Clegg MB ChB BSc(Hons) MRCP PhD FCEM
Senior Clinical Lecturer, University of Edinburgh;
Honorary Consultant in Emergency Medicine, Royal
Infirmary of Edinburgh

Nicki Colledge BSc(Hons) FRCPE
Consultant Physician in Medicine for the Elderly,
Liberton Hospital and Royal Infirmary of Edinburgh;
Honorary Senior Lecturer, University of Edinburgh

Allan Cumming MBChB MD FRCPE
Dean of Students, College of Medicine and Veterinary
Medicine, University of Edinburgh

Richard Davenport DM FRCPE
Consultant Neurologist, Western General Hospital and
Royal Infirmary of Edinburgh; Honorary Senior
Lecturer, University of Edinburgh

Graham Devereux MA MD PhD FRCPE
Professor of Respiratory Medicine, University of
Aberdeen; Honorary Consultant Physician, Aberdeen
Royal Infirmary, Aberdeen

Graham Douglas BSc(Hons) MBChB FRCPE
Consultant Physician, Aberdeen Royal Infirmary;
Honorary Reader in Medicine, University of Aberdeen

Jamie Douglas BSc MedSci MBChB MRCGP
General Practitioner, Albion Medical Practice, Ashton
Under Lyne, Lancashire

Colin Duncan MD FRCOG
Senior Lecturer in Reproductive Medicine, Consultant
Gynaecologist, University of Edinburgh

Andrew Elder BSc MBChB FRCPE FRCPSG FRCP
Consultant in Acute Medicine for the Elderly and
Honorary Senior Lecturer, Western General Hospital,
Edinburgh and University of Edinburgh

Rebecca Ford MEd MRCP MRCS(Edin) FRCOphth
Consultant Ophthalmologist, Aberdeen Royal
Infirmary

David Gawkrodger DSc MD FRCP FRCPE
Consultant Dermatologist, Royal Hallamshire Hospital,
Sheffield; Honorary Professor of Dermatology,
University of Sheffield

Jane Gibson BSc(Hons) MD FRCPE FSCP(Hon)
Consultant Rheumatologist, Fife Rheumatic Diseases
Unit, NHS Fife, Kirkcaldy, Fife; Honorary Senior
Lecturer, University of St Andrews

Neil Grubb BSc(Hons) MBChB MRCP MD
Consultant Cardiologist and Electrophysiologist,
Edinburgh Heart Centre, Royal Infirmary of
Edinburgh; Honorary Senior Lecturer, University of
Edinburgh

Iain Hennessey MBChB(Hons) BSc(Hons) MRCS MMIS
Specialty Trainee in Paediatric Surgery, Alder Hey
Children's Hospital, Liverpool

James Huntley MA MCh DPhil FRCPE FRCS(Glas)
FRCS(Edin)(Tr&Orth)
Consultant Orthopaedic Surgeon, Royal Hospital for
Sick Children, Yorkhill; Honorary Clinical Associate
Professor, University of Glasgow

John Iredale DM FRCP FMedSci FRSE
Professor of Medicine, Director MRC Centre for
Inflammation Research, Dean of Clinical Medicine,
Queen's Medical Research Institute, University of
Edinburgh

Alan Japp MBChB(Hons) BSc(Hons) MRCP
Cardiology Registrar, Royal Infirmary of Edinburgh

Jacques Kerr BSc MB BS FRCS FCEM
Consultant in Emergency Medicine and Clinical Lead,
Department of Emergency Medicine, Borders General
Hospital, Melrose

Robert Laing MD FRCPE
Consultant Physician in Infectious Diseases, Aberdeen
Royal Infirmary; Honorary Clinical Senior Lecturer,
University of Aberdeen

Andrew Longmate MBChB FRCA FFICM
Consultant Anaesthetist, Forth Valley Royal Hospital,
Larbert, Stirlingshire

Elizabeth MacDonald FRCPE
Consultant Physician in Medicine of the Elderly,
Western General Hospital, Edinburgh

Alastair MacGilchrist MD FRCPE FRCPS(Glas)
Consultant Gastroenterologist/Hepatologist, Royal
Infirmary of Edinburgh

Hadi Manji MA MD FRCP
Consultant Neurologist and Honorary Senior Lecturer,
National Hospital for Neurology and Neurosurgery,
London

Nicholas Morley MA (Cantab) MBChB MRCSEd FRCR
Clinical Lecturer in Radiology, Edinburgh Cancer
Research UK Centre, University of Edinburgh

Dilip Nathwani MBChB FRCP(Ed;Glas;Lond) DTM&H
Consultant Physician and Honorary Professor of
Infection, Ninewells Hospital and Medical School,
Dundee

Fiona Nicol BSc(Hons) MBBS FRCGP FRCPE
Formerly GP Principal and Trainer, Stockbridge Health
Centre, Edinburgh; Honorary Clinical Senior Lecturer,
University of Edinburgh

Jane Norman MD FRCOG F Med Sci
Professor of Maternal and Fetal Health, Consultant
Obstetrician, University of Edinburgh

John Olson MD FRCPE FRCOphth
Consultant Ophthalmic Physician, Aberdeen Royal
Infirmary; Honorary Reader, University of Aberdeen

Paul O'Neill MD FRCP
Professor of Medical Education, University of
Manchester and Honorary Consultant Physician,
UHSM NHS Foundation Trust, Manchester

Rowan Parks MD FRCSI FRCS(Edin)
Professor of Surgical Sciences and Honorary
Consultant Surgeon, Royal Infirmary of Edinburgh

Stephen Payne MS FRCS FEB(Urol)
Consultant Urological Surgeon, Central Manchester
Foundation Trust, Manchester

Stephen Potts MA FRCPsych
Consultant Psychiatrist, Department of Psychological
Medicine, Royal Infirmary of Edinburgh: Honorary
Senior Clinical Lecturer, University of Edinburgh

Colin Robertson BA(Hons) MBChB FRCPE FRCSEd FSAScot
Honorary Professor of Accident and Emergency
Medicine, University of Edinburgh

Laura Robertson BMedSci(Hons) MBBS FRCA
Specialty trainee in Anaesthesia, Western Infirmary of
Glasgow

David Snadden MBChB MClSc MD FRCGP FRCPE CCFP
Professor of Family Practice and Executive Associate
Dean Education, Faculty of Medicine, University of
British Columbia, Canada

James C Spratt BSc MBChB MD FRCP FESC FACC
Consultant Cardiologist, Forth Valley Royal Hospital,
Larbert, Stirlingshire

Ben Stenson MD FRCPCH FRCPE
Consultant Neonatologist, Simpson Centre for
Reproductive Health, Royal Infirmary of Edinburgh;
Honorary Professor of Neonatology, University of
Edinburgh

Kum Ying Tham MBBS FRCS(Ed) MSc
Consultant, Emergency Department, Tan Tock Seng
Hospital; Assistant Dean, Lee Kong Chian School of
Medicine, Singapore

Steve Turner MBBS MD MRCP(UK) FRCPCH
Senior Clinical Lecturer in Child Health, University of
Aberdeen; Honorary Consultant Paediatrician, Royal
Hospital for Sick Children, Aberdeen

Janet Wilson MD FRCS(Ed) FRCS(Eng) FRCSLT(Hon)
Professor of Otolaryngology Head and Neck Surgery,
University of Newcastle; Honorary Consultant
Otolaryngologist, Freeman Hospital, Newcastle
upon Tyne

Advisory board

We are proud that *Macleod's Clinical Examination* is regularly consulted by a range of health professionals and at a variety of levels in their training. It is our wish that the content is regarded as accurate and appropriate by all our readers. To ensure this aim, this latest edition has benefited from detailed advice from an Advisory Board comprising students and junior doctors, as well as representatives from the nursing and ambulance professions, primary care and the academic community. Significant changes have resulted as a direct result of this invaluable input.

Macleod's international reputation has grown with each edition and as editors we receive and value the feedback from our global readership. To ensure we take full account of the variations of international curricula we have recruited representatives from key geographical areas to the Advisory Board whose detailed comments and critical appraisal have been of great help in shaping the content of this new edition.

We acknowledge the enthusiasm and support of all our Advisory Board members and thank them for contributing to this edition. We have listed their details at the time that they reviewed the book.

UK advisory board

Graeme Finnie, Medical Student, University of Aberdeen

Paul Gowens, Head of Clinical Governance and Quality, Scottish Ambulance Service, Dunfermline

Mike Greaves, Professor and Head of School of Medicine and Dentistry, University of Aberdeen

Chris Griffiths, Professor of Primary Care, Barts and The London School of Medicine and Dentistry, London

Kate Haslett, Specialty trainee in Oncology, Glasgow

Jayne Langran, Clinical Educator/Chest Pain Nurse Specialist, Coronary Care Unit, Raigmore Hospital, Inverness

Anthea Lints, Professor and Director of Postgraduate General Practice Education, South East Scotland Deanery, Edinburgh

Will Muirhead, Foundation Year 1 Doctor, Queen's Medical Centre, Nottingham

Sarah Richardson, Medical Student, University of Edinburgh

Laura Robertson, Specialty Registrar in Anaesthetics, Glasgow

Gordon Stewart, Professor, Department of Medicine, University College London

International advisory board

Wael Abdulrahman Almahmeed, Consultant Cardiologist and Head of the Division of Cardiology, Shaikh Khalifa Medical City, Abu Dhabi, United Arab Emirates

Maaret Castrén, Professor in Emergency Medicine, Department of Clinical Science and Education, Karolinska Institute, Stockholm, Sweden

Jyothi Mariam Idiculla, Associate Professor, Department of Internal Medicine, St John's Medical College, Bangalore, India

Shubhangi Kanitkar, Professor of Medicine, Dr D.Y. Patil Medical College and Hospital, Pune, India

Kar Neng Lai, Yu Chiu Kwong Chair of Medicine, Department of Medicine, University of Hong Kong, Hong Kong

Kum-Ying Tham, Consultant Emergency Physician, Tan Tock Seng Hospital and Clinical Associate Professor, Yong Loo Lin School of Medicine, National University of Singapore, Singapore

Contents

SECTION 3 EXAMINATION IN SPECIFIC SITUATIONS

SECTION 4 ASSESSING CLINICAL EXAMINATION TECHNIQUE

Colin Robertson
Fiona Nicol
Graham Douglas

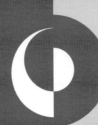

Approach to the patient

1

BEING A 'GOOD' DOCTOR

From your first day as a student you have professional obligations placed upon you by the public, the law and your colleagues which continue throughout your working life. Patients want more than merely intellectual and technical proficiency. To be a good doctor or nurse it is much easier if you genuinely like and are interested in people. Most patients want a doctor who listens to them and over 70 separate qualities have been listed as being important. Fundamentally, though, we all want doctors who:

- are knowledgeable
- respect people, healthy or ill, regardless of who they are
- support patients and their loved ones when and where needed
- always ask courteous questions, let people talk and listen to them carefully
- promote health as well as treat disease
- give unbiased advice, let people participate actively in all decisions related to their health and healthcare, assess each situation carefully and help whatever the situation
- use evidence as a tool, not as a determinant of practice
- humbly accept death as an important part of life; and help people make the best possible arrangements when death is close
- work cooperatively with other members of the healthcare team
- are proactive advocates for their patients, mentors for other health professionals and ready to learn from others, regardless of their age, role or status.

Doctors also need a balanced life and to care for themselves and their families. In short, we want doctors who are happy and healthy, caring and competent, and who care for people throughout their life.

One way to reconcile these expectations with your inexperience and incomplete knowledge or skills is to put yourself in the situation of the patient and/or relatives. Consider how you would wish to be cared for in the patient's situation, acknowledging that you are different and your preferences may not be the same. Most clinicians approach and care for patients differently once they have their own or a relative's experience as a patient. Doctors, nurses and everyone involved in healthcare have a profound influence on how patients experience illness and their sense of dignity. When you are dealing with patients, always consider your:

- **A: attitude** – how would I feel in this patient's situation?
- **B: behaviour** – always treat patients with kindness and respect
- **C: compassion** – recognise the human story that accompanies each illness
- **D: dialogue** – listen to and acknowledge the patient.

CONFIDENTIALITY AND CONSENT

As a student and as a doctor or nurse you will be given private and intimate information about patients and

1.1 The duties of a registered doctor

- The care of your patient is your first concern
- Protect and promote the health of patients and the public
- Provide a good standard of practice and care
  - Keep your professional knowledge and skills up to date
  - Recognise and work within the limits of your competence
  - Work with colleagues to serve your patients' interests best
- Treat patients as individuals and respect their dignity
  - Treat patients politely and considerately
  - Respect patient confidentiality
- Work in partnership with the patient
  - Listen to your patients and respond to their concerns and preferences
  - Give information in a way they can understand
  - Respect their right to reach decisions with you about their care
  - Support patients in caring for themselves to improve and maintain their health
- Be honest and open, and act with integrity
  - Act without delay if you have a good reason to believe that you or a colleague may be putting patients at risk
  - Never discriminate unfairly against patients or colleagues
  - Never abuse your patient's or the public's trust in you or the profession

Courtesy of the General Medical Council (UK).

their families. This information is confidential, even after a patient's death. This is a general rule, although its legal application varies between countries. In the UK, follow the guidelines issued by the General Medical Council (Box 1.1). There are exceptions to the general rules governing patient confidentiality, where failure to disclose information would put the patient or someone else at risk of death or serious harm, or where disclosure might assist in the prevention, detection or prosecution of a serious crime. If you find yourself in this situation, contact the senior doctor in charge of the patient's care immediately and inform him or her of the situation.

Take all reasonable steps to ensure that consultation and examination of a patient is private. Never discuss patients where you can be overheard or leave patients' records, either on paper or on screen, where they can be seen by other patients, unauthorised staff or the public. Always obtain consent or other valid authority before undertaking any examination or investigation, providing treatment or involving patients in teaching or research. Even where you have been given signed consent to disclose information about the patient, only disclose what is being asked for. If you have any doubts discuss your report with the patient so that he is clear about what information is going to a third party.

Clearly record your findings in the patient's case notes immediately after the consultation. These case notes are confidential and must be stored securely. They also constitute a legal document that could be used in a court of law. Keeping accurate and up-to-date case notes is an essential part of good patient care (p. 32). Remember that what you write may be seen by the patient, as in many countries, including the UK, patients can ask for and receive access to their medical records.

PERSONAL RESPONSIBILITIES

Always look after yourself and maintain your own health. Register with a general practitioner (GP). Do not self-diagnose and self-treat. If you know, or think that you might have, a serious condition you could pass on to patients, or if your judgement or performance could be affected by a condition or its treatment, consult your GP and be guided as to the need for secondary referral. Heed your doctor's advice regarding investigations, treatment and changes to your working practice. Protect yourself, your patients and your colleagues by being immunised against common but serious communicable diseases where vaccines are available, e.g. hepatitis B.

Your professional position is a privileged one; do not use it to establish or pursue a sexual or improper emotional relationship with a patient or someone close to the patient. Do not give medical care to anyone with whom you have a close personal relationship. Do not express your personal beliefs, including political, religious or moral ones, to your patients in ways that exploit their vulnerability or could cause them distress.

DRESS AND DEMEANOUR

The way you dress is important in establishing a successful patient–doctor relationship. Your dress style and demeanour should never make your patient or colleagues uncomfortable or distract them. Smart, sensitive and modest dress is appropriate; expressing your personality is not. Exposing your chest, midriff and legs may not only create offence but impede communication. Have short or three-quarter-length sleeves or roll long sleeves up, away from your wrists, before examining patients or carrying out procedures. This allows you to clean your hands effectively and reduces the risk of cross-infection. Tie back long hair and keep any jewellery simple and limited to allow effective hand washing. Some medical schools and hospitals require students and staff to wear white coats or 'scrubs' for reasons of professionalism, identification and as a barrier to infection. If this is the case, these must be clean and smart and you should always wear a name badge which can be read easily, i.e. not at your waist.

Whenever you see a patient or relative, introduce yourself fully and clearly. A friendly smile helps to put your patient at ease.

How you speak to, and address, a patient depends upon the patient's age, background and cultural environment. Many older patients prefer not to be called by their first name, and it is best to ask patients how they would prefer to be addressed.

COMMUNICATION SKILLS

A consultation is a meeting of two experts: you as the clinician and the patient as an expert on his own body and mind. Excellent communication skills allow you to identify a patient's problem rapidly and accurately and improve patient satisfaction (p. 7). Poor communication skills are associated with increased medicolegal

vulnerability and clinician burnout. Improve your skills by videoing yourself consulting with a patient (having obtained informed signed consent) and review this with a senior clinician using one of the many techniques developed for this. Continually seek to improve your communication skills. These will develop with experience but can always be improved.

Most doctors and nurses work in teams with colleagues in other professions. Working in teams does not change your personal accountability for your conduct and the care you provide. Try to act as a positive role model and motivate and inspire your colleagues. Always respect the skills and contributions of your colleagues and communicate effectively with them particularly when handing over care.

EXPECTATIONS AND RESPECT

The literary and media stereotypes of doctors frequently involve miraculous intuition, the confirmation of rare and brilliant diagnoses and the performance of dramatic life-saving interventions. Reality is different. Medicine often involves seeing and treating patients with common conditions and chronic diseases where we may only be able to provide palliation or simply bear witness to patients' suffering. The best doctors are humble and recognise that humans are infinitely more complex, demanding and fascinating than one can imagine. They understand that much so-called medical 'wisdom' is at best incomplete, and often simply wrong.

If a patient under your care has suffered harm or distress, act immediately to put matters right, if that is possible. Apologise and explain fully and promptly to the patient what has happened, and the likely effects. Patient complaints about their care or treatment are often the result of a breakdown in communication and they have a right to expect a prompt, open, constructive and honest response. Do not allow a patient's complaint to affect adversely the care or treatment you provide.

HAND WASHING AND CLEANLINESS

Transmission of microorganisms from the hands of healthcare workers is the main source of cross-infection

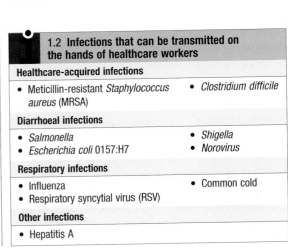

1.2 Infections that can be transmitted on the hands of healthcare workers	
Healthcare-acquired infections	
• Meticillin-resistant *Staphylococcus aureus* (MRSA)	• *Clostridium difficile*
Diarrhoeal infections	
• *Salmonella* • *Escherichia coli* 0157:H7	• *Shigella* • *Norovirus*
Respiratory infections	
• Influenza • Respiratory syncytial virus (RSV)	• Common cold
Other infections	
• Hepatitis A	

1

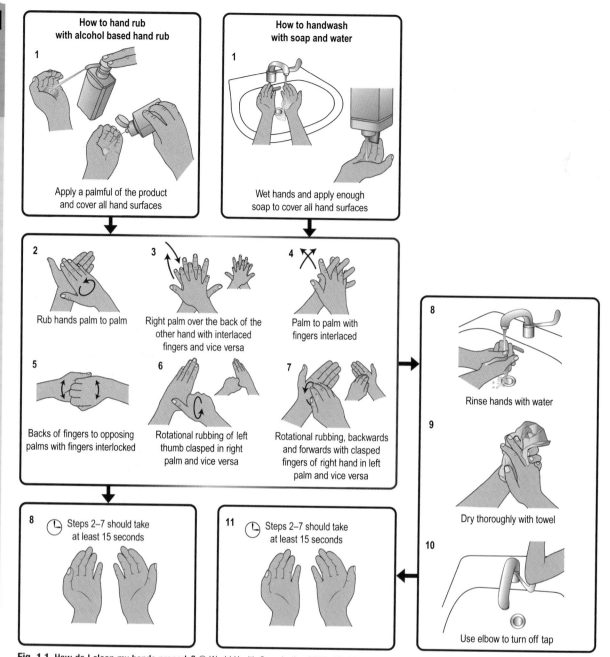

How to hand rub with alcohol based hand rub

1
Apply a palmful of the product and cover all hand surfaces

How to handwash with soap and water

1
Wet hands and apply enough soap to cover all hand surfaces

2
Rub hands palm to palm

3
Right palm over the back of the other hand with interlaced fingers and vice versa

4
Palm to palm with fingers interlaced

5
Backs of fingers to opposing palms with fingers interlocked

6
Rotational rubbing of left thumb clasped in right palm and vice versa

7
Rotational rubbing, backwards and forwards with clasped fingers of right hand in left palm and vice versa

8
Rinse hands with water

9
Dry thoroughly with towel

10
Use elbow to turn off tap

8
Steps 2–7 should take at least 15 seconds

11
Steps 2–7 should take at least 15 seconds

Fig. 1.1 How do I clean my hands properly? © World Health Organization 2009. All rights reserved.

in hospitals, primary care surgeries and nursing homes. Healthcare-acquired infections complicate up to 10% of hospital admissions and in the UK 5000 people die from them each year (Box 1.2).

Hand washing is the single most effective way to prevent the spread of infection. It is your responsibility to prevent the spread of infection and routinely wash your hands after every clinical examination. Do not be put off by lack of hand hygiene agents or facilities for hand washing, or being short of time.

- If your hands are visibly soiled, wash thoroughly with soap and water.

- If your hands are not obviously dirty, wash with soap and water or use an alcohol-based rub or gel.
- Always wear surgical gloves when you may be in contact with blood, mucous membranes or non-intact skin.

While washing with alcohol-based gels will remove most microorganisms, e.g. meticillin-resistant *Staphylococcus aureus* (MRSA), *Escherichia coli, Salmonella*, when dealing with patients with influenza, norovirus or *Clostridium difficile* infection, always clean hands with liquid soap and water (Fig. 1.1).

David Snadden
Robert Laing
Stephen Potts
Fiona Nicol
Nicki Colledge

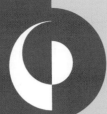

History taking

2

2

TALKING WITH PATIENTS

Think about the last time you visited your doctor. What prompted your visit? What arrangements did you have to make? Even a straightforward visit can be a big event. You have to make an appointment, work out what you are going to say and possibly arrange time off work or for child care. People visit doctors for many reasons (Box 2.1). They may have already spoken to family, friends or other health professionals, tried various remedies, and trawled the internet for information to explain their illness or problem. Most patients have some idea of what might be wrong with them and have worries or concerns they wish to discuss.

All patients seek explanation and meaning for their symptoms. You need to work out why the patient has come to see you, what he is most concerned about, and then agree with him the best course of action.

The first and major part of any consultation is talking with your patient. Communication is integral to clinical examination and is most important both at the start of the interview, to gather information, and at the end, to find common ground and engage your patient in his management.

PATIENT-CENTRED MEDICINE

Patient-centred medicine helps you understand your patient as a whole person. Good communication supports the building of trust between you and your patient and helps you provide clear and simple information (Boxes 2.2 and 2.3). It allows you to understand each other and agree goals together. Communication means much more than 'taking a history'; it is about involving your patients in their healthcare. Poor communication leads to misunderstanding, conflicting messages and patient dissatisfaction, and is the root cause of complaints and litigation. Over time you will develop your own consulting style; consultation frameworks are useful places to start (Box 2.4).

BEGINNING

Setting up

Preparation

Read your patient's records and any transfer or admission letters before you see your patient.

Where will you see your patient?

Choose a quiet, private space. This is often difficult in hospital, where privacy may be afforded only by curtains, which means no privacy at all. Always be sensitive

---

2.1 Reasons why people visit doctors

- They have reached their limits of tolerance
- They have reached their limits of anxiety
- They have problems of daily living presenting as symptoms
- For prevention
- For administrative reasons

2.2 Effective communication skills

Improve patient satisfaction

- Patients understand what is wrong
- They understand what they can do to help

Improve doctor satisfaction

- Patients are more likely to follow advice when they agree mutual goals with their doctor

Improve health by positive support and empathy

- Improve health outcomes
- Enhance the relationship between doctor and patient

Use time more effectively

- Active listening helps the doctor recognise what is wrong
- Active listening leads to fewer patient complaints

2.3 Tips for effective conversations

- Speak clearly and audibly
- Ask open questions to start with
- Don't interrupt your patient
- Try and appear unhurried
- Use silence to encourage explanations
- Do not use jargon or emotive words
- Find out about your patient as a person
- Clarify and summarise what you understand – you may need to do this more than once
- Make sure the story makes sense to you – keep seeking facts until it does
- Acknowledge emotions
- Seek ideas, concerns and expectations
- Negotiate mutual goals

2.4 Consulting with patients (BASICS)

Beginning

- Setting up
- Preparation
- Introduction

Active listening

- The patient's experience of his illness

Systematic enquiry

- Disease-oriented systematic enquiry

Information gathering

- Clinical examination

Context

- Understanding your patient as a person

Sharing

- Information
- Agreeing action and goals

to privacy and dignity. If your patient is in hospital but is mobile, use a side room or interview room. If there is no alternative to speaking to patients at their bedside, let them know that you understand your conversation may be overheard and give them permission not to answer sensitive questions about which they feel uncomfortable.

How long will you have?

Consultation length varies. In UK general practice the average length is 12 minutes. This is usually adequate, as the doctor may have seen the patient on several occasions and is familiar with the family and social background. In hospital 5–10 minutes may be adequate for returning outpatients, but for new and complex problems 30 minutes or more is usually needed. If you are a student, allow at least 30 minutes.

How will you sit?

Arrange seating in a non-confrontational way. If you use a desk, arrange the seats at the corner of the desk. This is less formal and helps communication (Fig. 2.1A). If you use a computer, make sure the screen and keyboard do not get in the way. Face your patient, not the screen (Fig. 2.1B). At a bedside, pull up a chair and sit level with your patient to see him easily and gain eye contact.

Non-verbal communication

First impressions are important. Your demeanour, attitude and dress influence your patient from the outset. Be professional in dress and behaviour (p. 3) and show concern for your patient's situation. Avoid interruptions such as the telephone (Fig. 2.1B).

Look for non-verbal cues such as distress and mood. Changes in your patient's demeanour and body

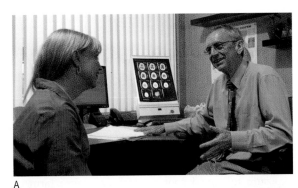

A

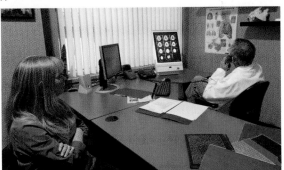

B

Fig. 2.1 Seating arrangements.

language during the consultation can be clues to difficulties that she cannot express verbally. If the patient's body language becomes 'closed' – that is, she may cross her arms and legs and break off eye contact – this may indicate discomfort (Fig. 2.1B).

Starting your consultation

Introduce yourself, and anyone else who is with you. Use your patient's and your own names to confirm identity. It may be appropriate to shake hands. If you are a student, inform the patient that you are in training; patients are usually eager to help. Write down facts that are easily forgotten, e.g. blood pressure readings or family tree, but writing notes should not interfere with the consultation.

Here are some ideas on how to get an interview going, though the words you use will change depending on the situation:

Good morning, Mrs Jones. I have got the right person, haven't I? I'm Mr Brown. I'm a fourth-year medical student. I've been asked to come and talk with you and examine you.

It might take me 20–30 minutes, if that's all right.

I see that you can't really get out of bed so we'll need to talk here. I'll pull the screens round. I'm sorry it's not very private. If I ask you a question that you don't want to answer in case other people overhear, then just say so.

I'll need to make a few notes so I don't forget anything important. Now, if I'm writing things down, it doesn't mean I'm not listening. I still will be.

Are you happy with all that?

Active listening

Hearing your patient's story about his illness experience is vital. Ask open questions to start with (see below). In the community, try 'How can I help you today?' or 'What has brought you along to see me today?'

Active listening means encouraging the patient to talk by looking interested, making encouraging comments or noises, e.g. 'Tell me a bit more' or 'Uhuh', and giving the impression that you have time for the patient. Active listening helps gather information and allows patients to tell their story in their own words. Clarify anything you do not understand. Tell patients what you think they have said and ask if your interpretation is correct (reflection).

The way you ask a question is important:

- *Open questions* encourage the patient to talk. They start with a word like 'where' or 'what', or a phrase like 'tell me more about …'. They are most useful initially when you are finding out what is going on and encouraging the patient to talk
- *Closed questions*, e.g. 'Have you had a cough today?' seek specific information as part of a systematic enquiry. They invite 'yes' or 'no' answers.

Both types of question have their place.

Can we start with you telling me what has happened to bring you into hospital? (*Opening*)

Well, I've been getting this funny feeling in my chest over the last few months. It's been getting worse and worse but it was really awful this morning. I got really breathless and felt someone was crushing me.

Can you tell me a bit more about the crushing feeling? (*Open questioning*)

Well, it was here, across my chest. It was sort of tight.

And did it go anywhere else? (*Clarifying*)

Well, maybe up here in my neck.

So, you had a tight pain in your chest this morning that went on a long time and you felt it in your neck? (*Summarising*)

You've had the pain for the last few months. Can you tell me more? (*Reflecting and open questioning*)

Well, it was the same but not that bad, though it's been getting worse recently.

OK. Can you remember when it first started? (*Clarifying*)

Oh, 3 or 4 months ago.

Does anything make it worse? (*Open questioning*)

Well, if I go up steps or up hills that can bring it on.

What do you do?

Stop and sometimes take my puffer.

Your what? (*Clarifying*)

This spray the doctor gave me to put in my mouth.

Can you show me it, please?

OK.

And what does it do? (*Clarifying*)

Well, it takes the pain away, but I get an awful headache with it.

So, for a few months you've had a tightness in your chest, which gets worse going up hills and upstairs and which goes away if you use your spray. Sometimes you feel the pain in your neck. But today it came on and lasted longer but felt the same. Have I got that right? (*Summarising*)

No, it was much worse this morning.

Once you have established what has happened, find out about your patient's ICE:

- **I**: Ideas on what is happening to him
- **C**: Concerns in terms of the impact on him
- **E**: Expectations of the illness and of you, the doctor.

Patients will have feelings and ideas about what has happened to them, and these may or may not be accurate. A patient with chest pain might think he has indigestion while you are considering angina. Ask: 'Do you have any thoughts about what might be happening to you?' A simple question like: 'What were you thinking I might do today?' can avoid unnecessary prescriptions or investigations. Modern medicine may be unable to 'cure' a problem, and the important issue is what you can do to help a patient to function.

Empathy

Being empathic helps your relationship with patients and improves their health outcomes (p. 2). What is empathy and how do you express it? Empathy is not sympathy, the expression of sorrow; it is much more. It is helping your patients feel that you understand what they are going through. Try to see the problem from their point of view and relate that to them.

Consider a young teacher who has recently had disfiguring facial surgery to remove a benign tumour from her upper jaw. Her wound has healed, but she has a drooping lower eyelid and significant facial swelling. She returns to work. Think how you would feel and imagine yourself in this situation. Express empathy through questions which show you can relate to your patient's experience.

So, are you all healed up from your operation now?

Yes, but I still have to put drops in my eye.

And what about the swelling under your eye?

That gets worse during the day, and sometimes by afternoon I can't see that well.

And how does that feel at work?

Well, it's really difficult. You know, with the kids and everything. It's all a bit awkward.

I can understand that that must make you feel pretty uncomfortable and awkward. That must be very difficult. How do you cope? Thinking about it makes me wonder if there are any other areas that are awkward for you, maybe in other aspects of your life, like the social side …

Understanding your patient's context

The context of our lives has a major influence on how we deal with illness. Finding out about your patient's context is crucial. It is far more than just a 'social history'. You should understand your patients' personal constraints and supports, including where they live, who they live with, where they work, who they work with, what they actually do, their cultural and religious beliefs, and their relationships and past experience. It is about your patient as a person. It may not be appropriate to explore these sensitive areas with everyone, or on an initial consultation, but they are important in any long-term doctor–patient relationship. Understanding the whole person modifies the information you give and the way you give it, the treatment you advise and the drugs you use.

Enquire about your patient's job and explore in some depth what this job entails, as this may have a bearing on the illness. A single job description can cover many tasks, e.g. engineer, so find out what your patient actually does, whether there are any stresses involved, and if there are any relationships at work that affect him, for example, a bullying boss or a harassing colleague.

In the following dialogue, Patient A is under stress and Patient B may be suffering the consequences of exposure to fungal spores which can cause farmer's lung. However, their initial answer to the first question is the same.

Doctor: So, tell me what your job is.

Patients A and B: I work on a farm.

Doctor: Yes, but what do you actually do?

Patient A: Well, I own the farm and mostly do the book work and buying and selling of animals.

Patient B: I'm a labourer on the farm.

Doctor: So, what are you doing at the moment?

Patient A: It's been a terrible year with the drought. The yields are down and I'm trying to get another loan from the bank manager.

Patient B: Well, just now we work in the barn first thing in the mornings, cleaning up and then laying feed for the cattle. It's very mouldy this year. After that, we're in the fields doing the early ploughing.

Find out about your patient's home circumstances. Try asking, 'Is there anyone at home with you?' or 'Is there anyone that can help?' and be equally tactful enquiring about relationships and the home environment. If a 15-year-old newly diagnosed diabetic is about to go home, ask about the home circumstances: who is at home and are the relationships supportive? Different arrangements should be made for a patient in a stable home whose mother is a healthcare worker compared to one from a deprived background, who has a lone parent and poor relationships.

Patients' beliefs influence healthcare. Religious and cultural beliefs affect how they cope with a disability or a dying relative, and whether they will accept certain treatments. Be sensitive to, and tolerant of, these issues.

Sometimes the consultation also gives you an opportunity to bring up issues around preventive activities, and a chance to address risk factors and lifestyle challenges. Examples include smoking cessation, dealing with obesity and drug or alcohol dependency, or illnesses that run in the family.

Sharing information and agreeing goals

Clarify and summarise what you say. Use words that the patient will understand and tailor the explanation to your patient.

Explain what you have found and what you think this means. Give important information first and check what has been understood. Provide the information in small chunks and warn the patient how many important things are coming: for example, 'There are two important things I want to discuss with you. The first is …'.

Use simple language and ensure your patient understands the treatment options and likely prognosis. What you say should be accurate and unambiguous, and the information should be given sensitively. Imagine yourself in the patient's position and your response. There is no place for being abrupt or for brutal honesty.

Engaging your patient

Make sure patients are involved in any decisions. Share your ideas with them, make suggestions and encourage them to contribute their thoughts. Be sensitive to your patients' body language. If they seem unclear about something or disagree with you, reflect this back to them. Use phrases like 'Are you comfortable with what I'm saying?' or 'Is there anything that I've said that isn't clear to you or has maybe confused you?' Whenever possible help decision making by giving written information to take home or by suggesting other sources of information: for example, self-help groups or the internet. Check they have understood you and discuss any investigations or treatment you think might be needed, including risks or side-effects (Box 2.3).

In this way, you will be able to negotiate a mutually agreed plan. For example, a patient with cancer may have the choice of surgery or radiotherapy. By involving him and discussing the pros and cons of treatments, you will enable the patient to reach a decision that you both understand and agree with. The patient will have to live with the consequences of the treatment, which will be much easier to accept if he has chosen the treatment himself.

Try to agree realistic goals. These might be areas that your patient needs to work on. For example, if the patient is trying to stop smoking, then you may set goals together that involve when he is going to stop, what help he will need, e.g. support groups, nicotine replacement therapy or both, how he will identify risky situations, e.g. socialising, and handle these to avoid being tempted to have a cigarette.

Finally, arrange for follow-up if necessary or give the patient some idea about when to return. This depends on how the patient is feeling and on any treatment you have suggested. End a complex discussion by briefly summarising what you have agreed, or ask your patient to summarise for you (Box 2.4).

DIFFICULT SITUATIONS

Your patient has communication difficulties

If your patient does not speak your language, or has hearing or speech difficulties such as dysphasia or dysarthria, follow the principles of good communication, but in addition you can do the following:

- Use an interpreter, but remember to address the patient, not the interpreter.
- Write things down for your patient if he can read.
- Employ lip reading or sign language.
- Involve someone who is used to communicating with your patient.

Your patient has cognitive difficulties

Be alert for early signs of dementia. You may have to rely on help from relatives or carers. If you do suspect this, use a memory or mental status test (Ch. 16).

Sensitive situations

Doctors sometimes need to ask personal or sensitive questions and examine intimate parts. If you are talking to a patient who may have a sexually transmitted disease, broach the subject sensitively. Indicate that you are going to ask questions in this area, and make sure the conversation is entirely private. Here are some examples of questions that might work.

Because of what you're telling me, I need to ask you some rather personal questions. Is that OK?

Can you tell me if you've had any casual relationships recently?

Are you worried that you might have picked anything up – I mean, in a sexual way?

You've told me that you think you're at risk. Can I ask if you have a regular sexual partner?

Follow this up with: 'Is your partner male or female?' If there is no regular partner, ask how many sexual partners there have been in the past year and how many have been male and how many female.

Ask permission sensitively if you need to examine intimate areas. This is most likely for examination of the breasts, genitals or rectum, but may apply in some circumstances or cultures whenever you need to touch the patient. First warn your patient; then seek permission to carry out an examination, explaining what you need to do. Always offer a chaperone, even if you are of the same gender as the patient. Record the chaperone's name and position. If patients decline the offer, respect their wishes and record this in the notes.

Give clear instructions about what clothes they need to remove. If necessary, reschedule an intimate examination until sufficient time, appropriate facilities or a chaperone are available.

Your patient is emotional

Ill people feel vulnerable and may become angry or distressed. Exploring their reasons for the emotion often defuses the situation. Recognise that your patient is angry or sad and ask him to explain why. Use phrases such as, 'You seem angry about something' or 'Is there something that is upsetting you?' Recognise your patient's emotion, show empathy and understanding, encourage him to talk and offer what explanations you can.

Talkative patients or those who want to deal with a lot of things at once may respond to: 'I only have a short time left with you, so what's the most important thing we need to deal with now?' If patients have a long list of complaints, suggest: 'Of the six things you've raised today, I can only deal with two, so tell me which are the most important to you and we'll deal with the rest next time.'

Set professional boundaries if your patient becomes overly familiar: 'Well, it would be inappropriate for me to discuss my personal issues with you. I'm here to help you so let's focus on your problem.'

Cultural sensitivity

Patients from a culture that is not your own may have different social rules (Box 2.5). Ideas around eye contact, touch and personal space may be different. In some western cultures, it is normal to maintain eye contact for long periods; in most of the world, however, this is seen as confrontational or rude. Shaking hands with the opposite sex is strictly forbidden in certain cultures. Death may be dealt with differently in terms of what the family expectations of physicians may be, who will expect to have information shared with them and what rites will be followed. Appreciate and accept differences in your patients' cultures and beliefs. When in doubt, ask them. This lets them know that you are aware of, and sensitive to, these issues.

Third-party information

Confidentiality is your first priority (p. 2). You may need to obtain information about your patient from someone else: usually a relative and sometimes a friend or carer.

2.5 Transcultural awareness

- Use appropriate eye contact
- Use appropriate hand gestures
- Respect personal space
- Consider physical contact between sexes, e.g. shaking hands
- Be sensitive to cultures and beliefs surrounding illness
- Ask yourself what should happen as death approaches?
- Ask yourself what should happen after death?

2.6 Talking to patients by telephone

- Listen actively and take a detailed history
- Frequently clarify and paraphrase to ensure that the messages got across in both directions
- Listen for cues (such as pace, pauses, change in voice intonation)
- Offer opportunities to ask questions
- Offer patient education
- Safety net – make sure the patient knows what to do if things don't improve
- Document carefully
- As the assessment is based solely on the history, and the management plan cannot be reinforced with non-verbal cues, being systematic in covering all issues is especially important

Ask your patient's permission and have the patient present to maintain confidentiality. If the patient cannot communicate, you will have to rely on family and carers to understand what has happened to the patient. Third parties may approach you without your patient's knowledge. Find out who they are, what their relationship to the patient is, and whether your patient knows the third party is talking to you. Tell third parties that you can listen to them but cannot divulge any clinical information without the patient's express permission. They may tell you about sensitive matters, such as mental illness, sexual abuse, or drug or alcohol addiction. This information needs to be sensitively explored with your patient to confirm the truth.

Telephone consultation

Consulting with patients using the telephone brings specific challenges as there are no visual cues to changes in body language or demeanour. The principles of good communication apply, but it is even more important to listen actively to your patient and frequently check your mutual understanding. Do not make assumptions or jump to diagnoses. Much of clinical medicine relies on direct observation and your intuition as a physician, so err on the side of caution when deciding whether to see a patient or not (Box 2.6).

Breaking bad news

Breaking bad news is one of the most difficult communication tasks you will face. Follow the principles of good communication. Speak to your patient in a quiet private environment. Ask patients who else they would like to be present – this may be a relative or partner – and offer a nurse or counsellor. Then find out how much

2.7 Framework for breaking bad news: SPIKES

Setting

- Privacy
- People
- You, be calm and attentive

Perception

- What your patient already knows

Invitation

- What does the patient want to know?

Knowledge

- Warn the patient that you have bad news

Empathy

- Acknowledge and address the patient's emotions

Summary and strategy

- The patient knows and agrees what the next steps are

2.8 Examples of terms used by patients that should be clarified

- Allergy
- Angina
- Arthritis
- Diarrhoea
- Dizziness
- Eczema
- Fits
- Heart attack
- Migraine
- Pleurisy
- Vertigo

they know and how much they want to know. Share the information you have. Plan in advance what you need to share, and prioritise so that the important information, which may include a diagnosis and the next steps in planning, do not get lost in a lot of detail. Respond to their feelings, as they may be upset or bewildered, and ensure that they understand and agree on the next steps (Box 2.7).

GATHERING INFORMATION

The presenting complaint

Diagnosis

Experienced clinicians make a diagnosis by recognising patterns of symptoms. With experience you will refine your questions according to the presenting complaint; you should then have a list of possible diagnoses (a differential diagnosis), before you examine the patient.

Ensure that patients tell you the problem in their own words and record this. Use your knowledge to direct your questioning. Clarify what they mean by any term they use. Some terms need to be explored (Box 2.8). Each answer increases or decreases the probability of a particular diagnosis, and excludes others.

In the following example, the patient is a 65-year-old male smoker. His age and smoking status increase the probability of certain diagnoses related to smoking. A cough for 2 months increases the likelihood of lung cancer and chronic obstructive pulmonary disease (COPD). Chest pain does not exclude COPD since he could have pulled a muscle on coughing, but the pain may be pleuritic from infection or thromboembolism. In turn, infection could be caused by obstruction of an airway by lung cancer. Haemoptysis lasting 2 months dramatically increases the chance of lung cancer. If the patient also has weight loss, the positive predictive value of all these answers is very high for lung cancer. This will focus your examination and investigation plan.

What is your main problem? (*Open question*)

> *I've had a cough that I just can't seem to get rid of. It started after I'd been ill with flu about 2 months ago. I thought it would get better but it hasn't and it's driving me mad.*

Can you please tell me more about the cough?
(*Open question*)

> *Well, it's bad all the time. I cough and cough, and bring up some phlegm. I can't sleep at night sometimes and I wake up feeling rough because I've slept so poorly. Sometimes I get pains in my chest because I've been coughing so much.*

Follow up by asking key questions to clarify the cough.

Can you tell me about the pains? (*Open question*)

> *Well, they're here on my side when I cough.*

Does anything else bring on the pains? (*Open and prompting question*)

> *Taking a deep breath.*

Follow this up by asking key questions about the pain (see Box 2.10).

What colour is the phlegm? (*Closed question, focusing on the symptom offered*)

> *Clear.*

Have you ever coughed up any blood? (*Closed question*)

> *Yes, sometimes.*

How often? (*Closed question*)

> *Oh, most days.*

How much? (*Closed question, clarifying the symptom*)

> *Just streaks, but sometimes a bit more.*

Do you ever get wheezy or feel short of breath with your cough?

> *A bit.*

How has your weight been? (*Open question, seeking additional confirmation of serious pathology*)

> *I've lost about 6 kilos.*

What sort of pathology does the patient have?

Think about which pathological process may account for the symptoms. Diseases are either congenital or acquired, and there are only certain pathological processes that cause acquired disease. The onset, progression, timescale and associated symptoms of the presenting complaint may guide you to the likely pathology (Box 2.9).

2.9 Deciding on the type of pathology

Type of pathology	Onset of symptoms	Progression of symptoms	Associated symptoms/pattern of symptoms
Infection	Usually hours	Usually fairly rapid over hours or days	Fevers, localising symptoms, e.g. pleuritic pain and cough
Inflammation	Often quite sudden	Weeks or months	Localising symptoms of variable severity, often coming and going
Metabolic	Very variable	Hours to months	Steadily progressive in severity with no remission
Malignant	Gradual	Weeks to months	Weight loss, fatigue
Toxic	Abrupt	Rapid	Dramatic onset of symptoms; vomiting often a feature
Trauma	Abrupt	Little change from onset	Diagnosis usually clear from history
Vascular	Sudden	Hours	Rapid development of associated physical signs
Degenerative	Gradual	Months to years	Gradual worsening interspersed with periods of more acute deterioration

What about physical signs?

Some diseases have no physical signs, e.g. migraine or angina. Other conditions almost always produce physical signs, e.g. fractured neck of femur or stroke. The absence of physical signs may simply reflect the early stage of a disease while some diseases have few or no signs, e.g. Addison's disease. Experience should help you to rank the reliability of signs to support your diagnosis, e.g. the patient with a history suggesting a transient ischaemic attack may have a carotid bruit but its absence would not exclude this diagnosis. However, a moderately breathless patient with suspected asthma is likely to have wheeze on chest auscultation. If there is no, or minimal, wheeze and the patient has an elevated jugular venous pressure (Ch. 6) with peripheral oedema and inspiratory crackles on inspiration, heart failure with pulmonary oedema is likely. You should have a clear differential diagnosis before examining the patient. Always reconsider your diagnosis if you do not find an expected physical sign or find an unexpected one.

Pain

The characteristics of pain suggest the likely cause. Explore these to make a differential diagnosis. Use the SOCRATES approach (Box 2.10), the principles of which can also be helpful for other symptoms, including dizziness or shortness of breath.

Associated symptoms

Any severe pain can produce nausea, sweating and faintness from the vagal and sympathetic response but some associated symptoms suggest a particular underlying cause; e.g. visual disturbance may precede migraine; palpitation (suggesting an arrhythmia) might occur with angina. Pain disturbing sleep suggests a physical cause.

Effects on lifestyle

Ask 'How do you cope with the pain?' This helps you to gain insight into the patient's coping strategies (ICE:

2.10 Characteristics of pain (SOCRATES)

Site

- Somatic pain, often well localised, e.g. sprained ankle
- Visceral pain, more diffuse, e.g. angina pectoris

Onset

- Speed of onset and any associated circumstances

Character

- Described by adjectives, e.g. sharp/dull, burning/tingling, boring/stabbing, crushing/tugging, preferably using the patient's own description rather than offering suggestions

Radiation

- Through local extension
- Referred by a shared neuronal pathway to a distant unaffected site, e.g. diaphragmatic pain at the shoulder tip via the phrenic nerve (C_3, C_4)

Associated symptoms

- Visual aura accompanying migraine with aura
- Numbness in the leg with back pain suggesting nerve root irritation

Timing (duration, course, pattern)

- Since onset
- Episodic or continuous
  - If episodic, duration and frequency of attacks
  - If continuous, any changes in severity

Exacerbating and relieving factors

- Circumstances in which pain is provoked or exacerbated, e.g. food
- Specific activities or postures, and any avoidance measures that have been taken to prevent onset
- Effects of specific activities or postures, including effects of medication and alternative medical approaches

Severity

- Difficult to assess, as so subjective
- Sometimes helpful to compare with other common pains, e.g. toothache
- Variation by day or night, during the week or month, e.g. relating to the menstrual cycle

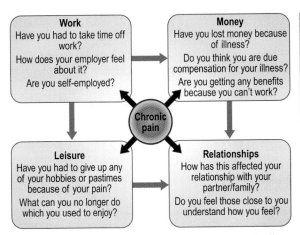

Work
Have you had to take time off work?
How does your employer feel about it?
Are you self-employed?

Money
Have you lost money because of illness?
Do you think you are due compensation for your illness?
Are you getting any benefits because you can't work?

Chronic pain

Leisure
Have you had to give up any of your hobbies or pastimes because of your pain?
What can you no longer do which you used to enjoy?

Relationships
How has this affected your relationship with your partner/family?
Do you feel those close to you understand how you feel?

Fig. 2.2 The effects of chronic pain: questions you might ask. Note that pain affects several areas of a patient's life but that these are interlinked.

2.11 Pain threshold

Increased

- Exercise
- Analgesia
- Positive mental attitude
- Personality

Decreased

- Sleep deprivation
- Depression
- Financial and personal worries
- Anxiety and fear about the cause
- Past experience

---

p. 8). Areas to consider in relation to chronic pain are shown in Figure 2.2.

Attitudes to illness

Many symptoms, such as pain and fatigue, are subjective and patients with identical conditions can present with dramatically different histories.

- Pain threshold and tolerance: these vary between patients and also in the same person in different circumstances. Patients vary in their willingness to speak about their discomfort (Box 2.11).
- Past experience: personal and family experience influence the response to symptoms. A family history of sudden death from heart disease may affect how a person interprets chest pain.
- Gains: most illness brings some gains to the patient. These vary from attention from family and friends to financial allowances and avoiding work or stress. Patients may not be conscious of these but sometimes deliberately exaggerate symptoms (p. 27).

Examples of questions that can be used to ask about common symptoms are shown in Box 2.12.

Past history

Past medical history may be relevant to the presenting complaint: e.g. previous migraine in a patient with

---

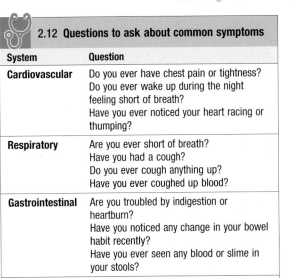

2.12 Questions to ask about common symptoms

System	Question
Cardiovascular	Do you ever have chest pain or tightness? Do you ever wake up during the night feeling short of breath? Have you ever noticed your heart racing or thumping?
Respiratory	Are you ever short of breath? Have you had a cough? Do you ever cough anything up? Have you ever coughed up blood?
Gastrointestinal	Are you troubled by indigestion or heartburn? Have you noticed any change in your bowel habit recently? Have you ever seen any blood or slime in your stools?
Genitourinary	Do you ever have pain or difficulty passing urine? Do you have to get up at night to pass urine? If so, how often? Have you noticed any dribbling at the end of passing urine? Have your periods been quite regular?
Musculoskeletal	Do you have any pain, stiffness or swelling in your joints? Do you have any difficulty walking or dressing?
Endocrine	Do you tend to feel the heat or cold more than you used to? Have you been feeling thirstier or drinking more than usual?
Neurological	Have you ever had any fits, faints or blackouts? Have you noticed any numbness, weakness or clumsiness in your arms or legs?

2.13 Past history

- Have you had any serious illness that brought you to see your doctor?
- Have you had to take time off work because of ill health?
- Have you had any operations?
- Have you attended any hospital clinics?
- Have you ever been in hospital? If so, why was that?

---

headache; haematemesis and multiple minor injuries in a patient with suspected alcohol abuse.

Ask open questions initially but move to closed questions to obtain relevant, meaningful information (Box 2.13).

Drug history

Ask about prescribed drugs and other medications, including over-the-counter remedies, herbal and homeopathic remedies, laxatives, analgesics and vitamin/mineral supplements. Note the name of each drug, dose,

2.14 Example of a drug history

Drug	Dose	Duration	Indication	Side-effects, patient concerns
Aspirin	75 mg daily	5 years	Started after myocardial infarction	Indigestion
Atenolol	50 mg daily	5 years	Started after myocardial infarction	Causes cold hands (? compliance)
Cocodamol (paracetamol + codeine)	Up to 8 tablets daily	4 weeks	Back pain	Causes constipation
Salbutamol MDI	2 puffs as necessary	6 months	Asthma	Palpitation, agitation

dosage regimen and duration of treatment, along with any significant adverse effects. Clarify, if necessary, with the general practitioner (GP). For patients being prescribed drugs for addiction, e g. methadone, ask the dispensing community pharmacy to stop dispensing for the duration of the hospital admission (Box 2.14).

Compliance, concordance and adherence

Half of all patients do not take prescribed medicines as directed. Patients who take their medication as prescribed are said to be compliant. Concordance implies that the patient and doctor have negotiated and reached an agreement on management, and adherence with therapy is likely (though not guaranteed) to improve.

Ask patients to describe how and when they take their medication. Check to see if they know the names of the drugs and what they are for. Give them permission to admit that they do not take all their medicines by saying: 'That must be difficult to remember'.

Drug allergies/reactions

Ask if your patient has ever had an allergic reaction to medication, especially before prescribing an antibiotic (particularly a penicillin or vaccine). Clarify exactly what patients mean by allergy. Drug allergies are over-reported by patients: only 1 in 7 who report a rash with penicillin will have a positive penicillin skin test. Note other allergies, such as foodstuffs or pollen. Record true allergies prominently in the patient's case records, drug chart and computer notes. If the patient has had a severe or life-threatening allergic reaction advise him to wear an alert necklace or bracelet (Fig. 3.3).

Family history

Start with open questions, such as: 'Are there any illnesses that run in your family?' Follow up the presenting complaint, e.g. 'Is there any history of heart disease in your family?' Many illnesses are associated with a positive family history but are not due to a single-gene disorder (Box 2.15).

Document illness in first-degree relatives, i.e. parents, siblings and children. If you suspect an inherited disorder such as haemophilia, go back three generations for details of racial origins and consanguinity (Fig. 2.3). Note whether your patient or any close relative has been adopted. Record the health of other household members,

2.15 Examples of single-gene inherited disorders

Autosomal dominant	
• Adult polycystic kidney disease	• Myotonic dystrophy
• Huntington's disease	• Neurofibromatosis

Autosomal recessive	
• Cystic fibrosis	• Alpha-thalassaemia
• Sickle cell anaemia	• Alpha-1-antitrypsin deficiency

X-linked	
• Duchenne muscular dystrophy	• Haemophilia A
	• Fragile X syndrome

since this may suggest environmental risks to the patient's health.

Social history

The social history helps you to understand the context of the patient's life and possible relevant factors (Box 2.16). Focus on the relevant issues; for example, ask an elderly woman with a hip fracture if she lives alone, whether she has any friends or relatives nearby, what support services she receives and how well suited her house is for someone with poor mobility.

The patient's illness may affect others such as a relative for whom the patient cares; but there may be no one at home to look after the patient because, although she is married, her husband works abroad. Successful discharge from hospital to the community requires these problems to be addressed.

Lifestyle

Exercise

Does your patient undertake sports or regular exercise? What is it, how often does he do it and how strenuous is it? Has the patient modified the exercise because of illness?

Diet

Does your patient have any dietary restrictions and how has he decided on these? Some patients believe that they have a food intolerance and may follow rigid exclusion diets with no medical evidence. Ask about

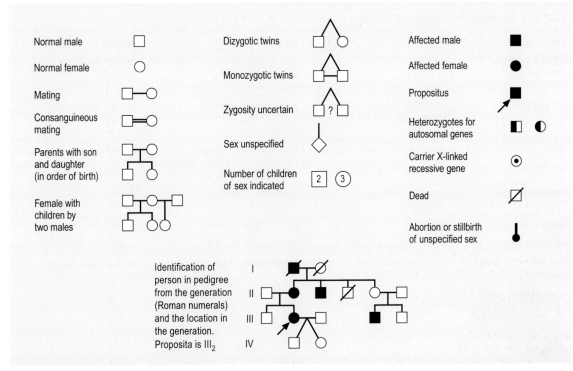

Fig. 2.3 Symbols used in constructing a pedigree chart, with an example.

2.16 The social history	
Upbringing	**Problems**
• Birth injury or complications • Early parental attachments and disruptions • Schooling, academic achievements or difficulties • Further or higher education and training • Behaviour problems	• Partner's health, occupation and attitude to patient's illness • Who else is at home? Any problems, e.g. health, violence, bereavement? • Any trouble with the police?
Home life	**House**
• Emotional, physical or sexual abuse* • Experiences of death and illness • Interest and attitude of parents	• Type of home, size, owned or rented • Details of home, including stairs, toilets, heating, cooking facilities, neighbours
Occupation	**Community support**
• Current and previous (clarify exactly what a job entails) • Exposure to hazards, e.g. chemicals, asbestos, foreign travel, accidents and compensation claims • Unemployment: reason and duration • Attitude to job	• Social services involvement, e.g. home help, meals on wheels • Attitude to needing help
	Sexual history*
Finance	
• Circumstances, including debts • Benefits from social security	**Leisure activities**
	• Hobbies and pastimes • Pets
Relationships and domestic circumstances	**Exercise**
• Married or long-term partner • Quality of relationship	• What, where and when?
	Substance misuse*
*only ask if relevant to the history	

2.17 Examples of occupational disorders

Occupation	Factor	Disorder	Presents
Shipyard workers, boilermen	Asbestos	Pleural plaques Asbestosis Mesothelioma	Over 20 years later
Dairy farmers	*Leptospira hadjo* Fungus spores on mouldy hay	Lymphocytic meningitis Farmer's lung (hypersensitivity pneumonitis)	Within 1 week Within 4–18 hours
Divers	Surfacing from depth too quickly	Decompression sickness Central nervous system, skin, bone and joint symptoms	Immediately and up to 1 week
Industrial workers	Chemical exposure, e.g. chromium	Dermatitis on hands	Variable
Bakery workers	Flour dust	Occupational asthma	Variable
Healthcare workers	Cuts, needlestick injuries	HIV, hepatitis B and C	Incubation period >3 months
Work involving noisy machinery	Excessive noise	Sensorineural hearing loss	Develops over months

HIV, human immunodeficiency virus.

2.18 Incubation periods of travel-related infections

Disease	Incubation period	Travel to presentation	Usual symptoms
Falciparum malaria	8–25 days	Up to 6 weeks	Fever
Vivax malaria	8–27 days	Up to 1 year	Fever
Typhoid fever	10–14 days	Up to 3 weeks	Fever, headache
Dengue fever	3–15 days	Up to 3 weeks	Fever, headache
Schistosomiasis	2–63 days	Up to 10 weeks	Itch, fever, haematuria, abdominal discomfort
Hepatitis A	28–42 days	Up to 6 weeks	Jaundice
HIV infection	12–26 weeks	Up to ?12 years	Weight loss, pneumonia

HIV, human immunodeficiency virus.

the frequency and times of meals and the types of foods eaten.

Occupational history

Work profoundly influences health, while unemployment is associated with increased morbidity and mortality. Some occupations are associated with particular illnesses (Box 2.17).

Take a full occupational history from all patients. 'Tell me about all the jobs you have done in your working life.' Clarify what the patient does at work, in particular, any chemical or dust exposure (p. 8). Symptoms that improve over the weekend or during holidays suggest an occupational disorder. Hobbies may also be relevant, e.g. psittacosis pneumonia or hypersensitivity pneumonitis in those who keep birds.

Travel history

Returning travellers commonly present with illness. They risk unusual or tropical infections, and air travel itself increases certain conditions, e.g. middle-ear problems or deep vein thrombosis. The incubation period is helpful in deciding on the likelihood of an illness (Box 2.18).

List the countries visited and the dates they were there. Enquire about the type of accommodation used and the activities undertaken, including sexual contacts. Note any travel vaccination or malarial prophylaxis taken.

Sexual history

Only take a full sexual history if this is appropriate (p. 221). Ask questions sensitively and objectively. Signal your intentions: 'As part of your medical history, I need to ask you some questions about your relationships. Is this all right?' (Box 2.19).

Smoking

Ask if your patient has ever smoked; if so, find out for how long, what form (cigarettes, cigars, pipe,

2.19 Taking a sexual history

- Are you currently in a relationship?
- How long have you been with your partner?
- Is it a sexual relationship?
- Have you had any (other) sexual partners in the last 12 months?
- How many were male? How many female?
- When did you last have sex with:
  - your partner?
  - anyone else?
- Do you use barrier contraception – sometimes, always or never?
- Have you ever had a sexually transmitted infection?
- Are you concerned about any sexual issues?

2.20 Calculating pack years of smoking

A 'pack year' is smoking 20 cigarettes a day (1 pack) for one year

$$\frac{\text{Number of cigarettes smoked per day} \times \text{Number of years smoking}}{20}$$

For example, a smoker of 15 cigarettes a day who has smoked for 40 years would have smoked:

$$\frac{15 \times 40}{20} = 30 \text{ pack years}$$

2.21 An alcohol history

- Quantity and type of drink
- Daily/weekly pattern (especially binge drinking and morning drinking)
- Usual place of drinking
- Alone or accompanied
- Purpose
- Amount of money spent on alcohol
- Attitudes to alcohol

2

2.22 Calculating units of alcohol

Method 1

Standard measure (1 unit) =	1 small glass of wine
	1 half-pint of beer
	1 short of spirits

Method 2

| Standard measure (1 unit) = | 25 ml of 40% alcohol |
| | = 10 ml ethanol |

x% proof = x units of alcohol per litre

Examples

1 litre of 40% proof spirits contains 400 ml ethanol or 40 units
  750 ml (standard bottle) contains 30 units alcohol
1 litre of 4% beer contains 40 ml ethanol or 4 units
  500 ml can contains 2 units of alcohol
Alternatively, use an online calculator, e.g. http://www.drinkaware.co.uk/how-many-units.html.

chewed) and how much. For smokers, use 'pack years' (Box 2.20) to estimate the risk of tobacco-related health problems (Fig. 2.4) (p. 145). Most patients with COPD have tobacco consumption >20 pack years. If appropriate, enquire about other substances smoked, e.g. cannabis, heroin. Don't forget to ask non-smokers about their exposure to environmental tobacco smoke (passive smoking).

Alcohol

Try asking: 'Do you ever drink any alcohol?' Use open questions, giving permission for patients to tell you, and do not judge them. Follow up with closed questions covering:

- what?
- when?
- how much? (Box 2.21).

Other useful questions are:

- When did you last have a drink?
- What's the most you ever drink?

The number of units of alcohol consumed each week can be calculated in two ways (Box 2.22).

Alcohol problems

- Hazardous drinking is the regular consumption of more than:
  - 24 g of pure ethanol (3 units) per day for men
  - 14 g of pure ethanol (2 units) per day for women.

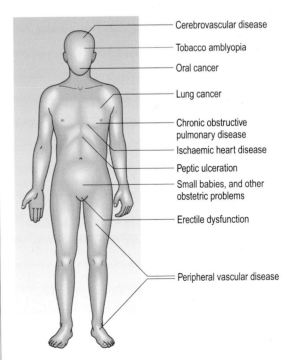

Cerebrovascular disease
Tobacco amblyopia
Oral cancer
Lung cancer
Chronic obstructive pulmonary disease
Ischaemic heart disease
Peptic ulceration
Small babies, and other obstetric problems
Erectile dysfunction
Peripheral vascular disease

Fig. 2.4 Tobacco-related disorders.

2.23 Features of alcohol dependence

- A strong, often overpowering, desire to take alcohol
- Inability to control starting or stopping drinking and the amount that is drunk
- Tolerance, where increased doses are needed to achieve the effects originally produced by lower doses
- Withdrawal state when drinking is stopped or reduced, including tremor, sweating, rapid heart rate, anxiety, insomnia and occasionally seizures, disorientation or hallucinations (delirium tremens). It is relieved by more alcohol
- Neglect of other pleasures and interests
- Continuing to drink in spite of being aware of the harmful consequences

 2.24 The CAGE questionnaire

- **C**ut down: Have you ever felt you should cut down on your drinking?
- **A**nnoyed: Have people annoyed you by criticising your drinking?
- **G**uilty: Have you ever felt bad or guilty about your drinking?
- **E**ver: Do you ever have a drink first thing in the morning to steady you or help a hangover (an eye opener)?

Positive answers to two or more questions suggest problem drinking; confirm this by asking about the maximum taken.

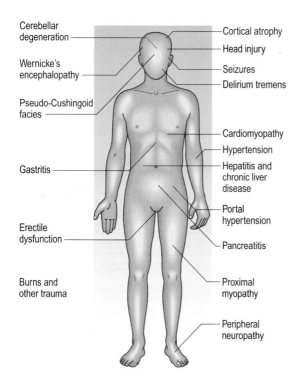

Fig. 2.5 Alcohol-related disorders.

Labels: Cerebellar degeneration · Wernicke's encephalopathy · Pseudo-Cushingoid facies · Gastritis · Erectile dysfunction · Burns and other trauma · Cortical atrophy · Head injury · Seizures · Delirium tremens · Cardiomyopathy · Hypertension · Hepatitis and chronic liver disease · Portal hypertension · Pancreatitis · Proximal myopathy · Peripheral neuropathy

- Binge drinking, involving a large amount of alcohol causing acute intoxication, is more likely to cause problems than if the same amount is consumed over 4 or 5 days. Everyone should have at least 2 days per week when they drink no alcohol.
- Harmful drinking results in physical or mental health damage or disruption to social circumstances.
- Alcohol dependence is when alcohol use takes a higher priority over other behaviours that previously had greater value (Box 2.23).

Identifying alcohol problems early is important because of the health risks to patients and their families (Fig. 2.5). It can be difficult and screening tests can help. The CAGE questionnaire is easy to remember and will identify heavy drinkers but is not very sensitive (Box 2.24). The fast alcohol screening test (FAST) questionnaire is more sensitive but more complex (Box 2.25).

Non-prescribed drug use

Ask all patients who may be using drugs about their use of non-prescribed drugs. In Britain about 30% of the adult population has used illegal or non-prescribed drugs (mainly cannabis) at some time (Boxes 2.26 and 2.27).

Systematic enquiry

Systematic enquiry uncovers symptoms that may have been forgotten. Ask: 'Is there anything else you would like to tell me about?' Until you are experienced, run through with every patient all of the symptoms in Box 2.28. Follow up any positive response by asking questions to increase or decrease the probability of certain diseases.

Some examples of targeted systematic enquiry are as follows:

- The smoker with weight loss: are there any respiratory symptoms, e.g. unresolving chest infection or haemoptysis to suggest lung cancer?
- The patient with recurrent mouth ulcers: do any alimentary symptoms suggest Crohn's disease or coeliac disease?
- The patient with palpitation: are there any endocrine symptoms to suggest thyrotoxicosis or is there a family history of thyroid disease? Is the patient anxious or drinking too much coffee?
- If a patient smells of alcohol, ask about related symptoms, such as numbness in the feet due to alcoholic neuropathy.

Putting it all together

With all the relevant information assembled, you should have a list of differential diagnoses. Before you examine the patient:

- Briefly summarise what the patient has told you.
- Reflect this back to the patient. This allows patients to correct anything you have misunderstood and add anything they have forgotten.
- Gain the patient's permission to examine him.

2.25 The fast alcohol screening test (FAST) questionnaire

For the following questions please circle the answer that best applies

1 drink = 1/2 pint of beer or 1 glass of wine or 1 single measure of spirits

1. Men: How often do you have eight or more drinks on one occasion?
    Women: How often do you have six or more drinks on one occasion?
    - Never (0)
    - Less than monthly (1)
    - Monthly (2)
    - Weekly (3)
    - Daily or almost daily (4)

2. How often during the last year have you been unable to remember what happened the night before because you had been drinking?
    - Never (0)
    - Less than monthly (1)
    - Monthly (2)
    - Weekly (3)
    - Daily or almost daily (4)

3. How often during the last year have you failed to do what was normally expected of you because of drinking?
    - Never (0)
    - Less than monthly (1)
    - Monthly (2)
    - Weekly (3)
    - Daily or almost daily (4)

4. In the last year has a relative or friend, or a doctor or other health worker been concerned about your drinking or suggested you cut down?
    - Never (0)
    - Yes, on one occasion (2)
    - Yes, on more than one occasion (4)

Scoring FAST

First stage

If the answer to question 1 is *Never*, then the patient is probably not misusing alcohol

If the answer is Weekly or Daily or Almost daily, then the patient is a hazardous, harmful or dependent drinker

50% of people are classified using this one question

Second stage

Only use these questions if the answer is *Less than monthly* or *Monthly*

Score questions 1–3: 0, 1, 2, 3, 4

Score question 4: 0, 2, 4

Minimum score is 0

Maximum score is 16

Score for hazardous drinking is 3 or more

2.26 Non-prescribed drug history

- What drugs are you taking?
- How often and how much?
- How long have you been taking drugs?
- Any periods of abstinence? If so, when and why did you start using drugs again?
- What symptoms do you have if you cannot get drugs?
- Do you ever inject? If so, where do you get the needles and syringes?
- Do you ever share needles, syringes or other drug paraphernalia?
- Do you see your drug use as a problem?
- Do you want to make changes in your life or change the way you use drugs?
- Have you been checked for blood-borne viruses?

2.27 Complications of drug misuse

Infections

- Hepatitis B and C
- Soft-tissue infection and abscesses
- Necrotising fasciitis
- Septic pulmonary thromboembolism
- Lung abscesses
- Aspiration pneumonia
- HIV
- Endocarditis
- Tetanus
- Wound botulism
- Sexually transmitted disease: many work in the sex industry to finance their habit

Injury

- Thrombophlebitis and deep vein thrombosis
- Skin ulceration
- Arterial injury and occlusion

Overdose

- Rhabdomyolysis and renal failure
- Respiratory failure

Chaotic lifestyle leading to

- Poor nutrition
- Poor dental hygiene
- Failure to care for dependants
- Debt
- Crime
- Prison

2.28 Systematic enquiry: cardinal symptoms

General health

- Well-being
- Appetite
- Weight change
- Energy
- Sleep
- Mood

Cardiovascular system

- Chest pain on exertion (angina)
- Breathlessness:
  - Lying flat (orthopnoea)
  - At night (paroxysmal nocturnal dyspnoea)
  - On minimal exertion – record how much
- Palpitation
- Pain in legs on walking (claudication)
- Ankle swelling

Respiratory system

- Shortness of breath (exercise tolerance)
- Cough
- Wheeze
- Sputum production (colour, amount)
- Blood in sputum (haemoptysis)
- Chest pain (due to inspiration or coughing)

Gastrointestinal system

- Mouth (oral ulcers, dental problems)
- Difficulty swallowing (dysphagia – distinguish from pain on swallowing, i.e. odynophagia)
- Nausea and vomiting
- Vomiting blood (haematemesis)
- Indigestion
- Heartburn
- Abdominal pain
- Change in bowel habit
- Change in colour of stools (pale, dark, tarry black, fresh blood)

Genitourinary system

- Pain passing urine (dysuria)
- Frequency passing urine (at night, nocturia)
- Blood in the urine (haematuria)
- Libido
- Incontinence (stress and urge)
- Sexual partners – unprotected intercourse

Men

If appropriate:
- Prostatic symptoms, including difficulty starting – hesitancy
  - Poor stream or flow
  - Terminal dribbling
- Urethral discharge
- Erectile difficulties

Women

- Last menstrual period (consider pregnancy)
- Timing and regularity of periods
- Length of periods
- Abnormal bleeding
- Vaginal discharge
- Contraception
- If appropriate:
  - Pain during intercourse (dyspareunia)

Nervous system

- Headaches
- Dizziness (vertigo or lightheaded)
- Faints
- Fits
- Altered sensation
- Weakness
- Visual disturbance
- Hearing problems (deafness, tinnitus)
- Memory and concentration changes

Musculoskeletal system

- Joint pain, stiffness or swelling
- Mobility
- Falls

Endocrine system

- Heat or cold intolerance
- Change in sweating
- Excessive thirst (polydipsia)

Other

- Bleeding or bruising
- Skin rash

THE PSYCHIATRIC HISTORY

Mental disorders are very common, frequently coexist with physical disorders, and cause much mortality and morbidity. Psychiatric assessment has four elements:

- history
- mental state examination (MSE)
- selective physical examination
- collateral information.

THE HISTORY

The distinction between symptoms and signs is less clear in psychiatry than the rest of medicine. The psychiatric interview, which covers both, has three purposes:

- to obtain a history (Boxes 2.29 and 2.30)
  – symptoms
- to assess the present mental state – signs
- to establish rapport to help further management.

Sensitive topics

In some settings, and for some subjects, use particular skill and tact to obtain answers and to maintain rapport. This applies particularly to:

- sexual issues, e.g. sexual dysfunction, gender identity
- major traumatic experiences, e.g. rape, childhood sexual abuse, witnessing a death
- illicit drug use
- crime
- suicidal or homicidal ideas
- non-clinical settings, e.g. police stations, prisons.

2.29 Content of a psychiatric history

- Referral source
- Reason for referral
- History of presenting complaint(s)
- Systematic enquiry into other relevant problems and symptoms
- Past medical/psychiatric history
- Prescribed and non-prescribed medication
- Substance use: illegal drugs, alcohol, tobacco, caffeine
- Family history (including psychiatric disorders)
- Personal history

2.30 Personal history

- Childhood development
- Losses and experiences
- Education
- Occupation(s)
- Financial circumstances
- Relationships
- Partner(s) and children
- Housing
- Leisure activities
- Hobbies and interests
- Forensic history (trouble with the police and courts)

You should develop good rapport at the first interview, and consolidate it before raising a sensitive topic, though sometimes you have to cover such material without delay. In these cases, tell the patient about the nature of and reason for your sensitive enquiries (Box 2.31).

The uncooperative patient

Adapt your assessment when a patient is mute, agitated, hostile or otherwise uncooperative, and place greater reliance on observation and collateral information. The safety of the patient, other patients, staff and yourself is paramount so you may only be able to make a partial assessment of agitated or hostile patients.

Mental state examination

The MSE systematically evaluates the patient's mental condition at the time of interview (Box 2.32). The aim is to establish signs of disorder that, with the history, enable you to make, suggest or exclude a diagnosis. While making specific enquiries, you should observe, evaluate, and draw inferences in the light of the history. This is daunting, but with good teaching, practice and experience you will learn the skills.

MSE involves:

- observation of the patient
- incorporation of relevant elements of the history
- specific questions exploring various mental phenomena
- short tests of cognitive function.

The focus is determined by the history and potential diagnoses. For example, detailed cognitive assessment in an elderly patient presenting with confusion is crucial; similarly, carefully evaluate mood and suicide risk when the presenting problem is depression.

2.31 Sensitive topics: what to ask

- You said a few minutes ago that sometimes you wish you had died in your sleep. I need to ask you a bit more about that thought. Have you ever considered doing something that would make that happen?
- You've just told me that you feel your life isn't worth living. Do you ever think in the same way about your children's lives?
- You indicated that something terrible happened to you when you were a child. Do you want to tell me more about that now?

2.32 Elements of the Mental State Examination (MSE)

- Appearance
- Behaviour
- Speech
- Mood
- Thought form
- Thought content
- Perceptions
- Cognition
- Insight
- Risk assessment

2.33 Behaviour: definitions

Term	Definition
Agitation	A combination of psychic anxiety and excessive, purposeless motor activity
Compulsion	An unnecessary, purposeless action that the patient is unable to resist performing repeatedly
Disinhibition	Loss of control over normal social behaviour
Motor retardation	Decreased motor activity, usually a combination of fewer and slower movements
Posturing	The maintenance of bizarre gait or limb positions for no valid reason

2.34 Speech: definitions

Term	Definition
Clang associations	Thoughts connected by having a similar sound rather than by meaning
Mutism	Absence of speech without impaired consciousness
Neologism	An invented word, or a new meaning for an established word
Pressure of speech	Rapid, excessive, continuous speech (due to pressure of thought)
Word salad	Meaningless string of words, often with loss of grammatical construction
Echolalia	Senseless repetition of the interviewer's words.

Appearance

Observe:
- general elements, e.g. attire, signs of self-neglect
- facial expression
- scars, tattoos, features of injury and/or self-injury
- signs of physical disease, e.g. spider naevi (chronic alcoholic liver disease), exophthalmos (thyrotoxicosis).

Behaviour

Observe:
- cooperation, rapport, eye contact
- social behaviour, e.g. aggression, disinhibition
- overactivity, e.g. agitation, compulsions
- underactivity, e.g. stupor, motor retardation
- abnormal activity, e.g. posturing, involuntary movements (Box 2.33).

Speech

Observe:
- articulation, e.g. stammering, dysarthria
- quantity, e.g. mutism, garrulousness

2.35 Mood: definitions

Term	Definition
Blunting	Loss of normal emotional sensitivity to experiences
Catastrophic reaction	An extreme emotional and behavioural overreaction to a trivial stimulus
Flattening	Loss of the range of normal emotional responses
Incongruity	A mismatch between the emotional expression and the associated thought
Lability	Superficial, rapidly changing and poorly controlled emotions

2.36 Mood: what to ask

- How has your mood been lately?
- Have you noticed any change in your emotions recently?
- Has your family commented recently on your mood?
- Do you still enjoy things that normally give you pleasure?

- rate, e.g. pressured, slowed
- volume, e.g. whispering, shouting
- tone and quality, e.g. accent, emotionality
- fluency, e.g. staccato, monotonous
- abnormal language, e.g. neologisms, dysphasia, clanging (Box 2.34).

Mood

This is the pervasive emotional state. Affect is the observable expression of emotions, which is more variable over time. A useful analogy is to think of a patient's mood as a climate, with affect as the current weather.

Assess mood objectively by observation, and subjectively from the history and specific enquiries (Boxes 2.35 and 2.36). Disturbance of mood is the most important feature of depression, mania and anxiety, but mood changes commonly occur in other mental disorders such as schizophrenia and dementia.

Abnormalities of mood consist of:
- problematic pervasive mood, e.g. depressed, elated, anxious, fearful, angry, suspicious, irritable, perplexed
- abnormal range, e.g. flattened, expanded
- abnormal reactivity, e.g. blunted, labile, catastrophic
- inappropriateness, e.g. incongruous to circumstances.

Thought form

Loosening of associations is sometimes termed formal thought disorder, and is a core feature of schizophrenia. Subjectively, patients may report having difficulty thinking clearly. Hypomania is characterised by pressure of thoughts and flights of ideas. With depression these processes are slowed and impoverished; this is also characteristic of dementia (Box 2.37).

2.37 Thought form: definitions

Term	Definition
Circumstantiality	Trivia and digressions impairing the flow but not direction of thought
Concrete thinking	Inability to think abstractly
Flight of ideas	Rapid shifts from one idea to another, retaining sequencing
Loosening of associations	Logical sequence of ideas impaired Subtypes include knight's move thinking, derailment, thought blocking and, in its extreme form, word salad
Perseveration	Inability to shift from one idea to the next
Pressure of thought	Increased rate and quantity of thoughts

2.38 Thought content: definitions

Term	Definition
Hypochondriasis	Unjustified belief of suffering from a particular disease in spite of appropriate examination and reassurance
Morbid thinking	Depressive ideas, e.g. themes of guilt, burden, unworthiness, failure, blame, death, suicide
Phobia	A senseless avoidance of a situation, object or activity stemming from a belief that has caused an irrational fear
Preoccupation	Beliefs that are not inherently abnormal but which have come to dominate the patient's thinking
Ruminations	Repetitive, intrusive, senseless thoughts or preoccupations
Obsessions	Ruminations which persists despite resistance.

Elements of thought form are:
- rate, e.g. pressure of thought, retardation (slowing)
- flow, e.g. flights of ideas, circumstantiality, perseveration
- sequencing, e.g. loosening of associations
- abstract thinking, e.g. concrete thought.

Record examples of speech from the history to show how a person thinks and expresses thoughts.

Thought content

This is assessed from the history and specific enquiries (Box 2.38). Note thought content from what the patient has discussed during history taking and then explore it by further questioning. It is divided into preoccupations, ruminations and abnormal beliefs:
- Preoccupations are common in normal and abnormal mood states: an anxious person worries about physical illness, or the morbid thoughts of depression.

2.39 Thought content: what to ask

- What have your main worries been recently?
- What has been on your mind lately?
- Do you have any particular thoughts you keep coming back to?

2.40 Abnormal beliefs: definitions

Term	Definition
Delusion	An abnormal belief, held with total conviction, which is maintained in spite of proof or logical argument to the contrary and is not shared by others from the same culture
Delusional perception	A delusion which arises fully formed from the false interpretation of a real perception, e.g. a traffic light turning green confirms that aliens have landed on the rooftop
Magical thinking	An irrational belief that certain actions and outcomes are linked, often culturally determined by folklore or custom, e.g. fingers crossed for good luck
Overvalued ideas	Beliefs that are held, valued, expressed and acted on beyond the norm for the culture to which the person belongs
Thought broadcasting	The belief that the patient's thoughts are heard by others
Thought insertion	The belief that thoughts are being placed in the patient's head from outside
Thought withdrawal	The belief that thoughts are being removed from the patient's head

- Ruminations are preoccupations which are abnormal because they are so repetitive or groundless. They occur in hypochondriasis and obsessional disorders (Box 2.39).
- Abnormal beliefs fall into two categories: those that are not diagnostic of mental illness, e.g. overvalued ideas, superstitions, magical thinking, and those that invariably signify mental illness, i.e. delusions. The main difference is that delusions either lack a cultural basis for understanding the belief or have been derived from abnormal processes.

Overvalued ideas are beliefs of great personal significance that are abnormal because of their effects on a person's behaviour or well-being. For example, patients with anorexia nervosa may still believe they are fat when they are seriously underweight. They respond to beliefs about their body image rather than their weight (Box 2.40).

Delusional beliefs matter greatly to the person, resulting in powerful emotional and important behavioural consequences: they are always of clinical significance. They are classified by their content, such as:
- paranoid
- religious
- grandiose
- hypochondriacal
- guilt

2.41 Abnormal beliefs: what to ask

- Have there been times when you've thought something strange is going on?
- Do you ever think you're being followed or watched?
- Do you ever feel other people can interfere with your thoughts or actions?

2.42 Perceptions: definitions

Term	Definition
Depersonalisation	A subjective experience of feeling unreal
Derealisation	A subjective experience that the surrounding environment is unreal
Hallucination	A false perception arising without a valid stimulus from the external world
Illusion	A false perception that is an understandable misinterpretation of a real stimulus in the external world
Pseudohallucination	A false perception which is perceived as part of one's internal experience

- love
- jealousy
- infestation
- thought interference
- control.

Bizarre delusions are easy to recognise, but not all delusions are weird ideas: a man convinced that his partner is unfaithful may or may not be deluded. Even if a partner were unfaithful, it would still amount to a delusional jealousy if the belief were held without evidence or for some unaccountable reason, such as finding a dead bird in the garden.

Delusions can sometimes be understood as the patient's way of trying to make sense of his experience. Their content often gives a clue that may help type the underlying illness, e.g. delusions of guilt suggest severe depression whereas grandiose delusions typify mania (Box 2.41). Some delusions are characteristic of schizophrenia, most notably a delusional perception or primary delusion. These include 'passivity phenomena': the belief that thoughts, feelings or acts are no longer controlled by the person's free will.

Perceptions

Assess perceptions using the history and specific enquiries backed up by observation (Box 2.42). People normally distinguish easily between their inner and outer worlds and know what is real and what reality feels like. This can occasionally be disrupted so that normal perceptions become unfamiliar while abnormal perceptions seem real. These anomalies fall into several categories:

- depersonalisation, derealisation
- altered perceptions: sensory distortions, illusions
- false perceptions: hallucinations, pseudohallucinations.

Depersonalisation and derealisation are associated with severe tiredness and intense anxiety, but also occur in most types of mental illness. With altered perceptions

2.43 Perceptions: what to ask

- Do you ever hear voices when nobody is talking?
- What do they say?
- Where do they come from?
- Have you had any visions?
- Have you ever felt that you were not real or that the world around you wasn't real?

there is a real external object but its subjective perception has been distorted. Sensory distortions, such as unpleasant amplification of light (photophobia) or sound (hyperacusis), can occur in physical diseases, but are also common in anxiety states and drug intoxication or withdrawal. Diminution of perceptions, including pain, can occur in depression and schizophrenia.

Illusions commonly occur among people with established impairment of vision or hearing. They are also found in predisposed patients subjected to sensory deprivation, notably after dark in a patient with clouding of consciousness.

True hallucinations arise without external stimuli; they usually indicate severe mental illness, but can occur naturally when going to sleep (hypnagogic) or waking up (hypnopompic). Hallucinations can be:

- auditory
- visual
- olfactory
- gustatory
- tactile.

Any form of hallucination can occur in any severe mental disorder. The most common are auditory and visual hallucinations, the former are associated with schizophrenia, the latter with delirium. Some auditory hallucinations are characteristic of schizophrenia, e.g. voices discussing the patient in the third person, or giving a running commentary on the person's activities.

Pseudohallucinations are common. The key distinction from a true hallucination is that these phenomena occur within the patient, rather than arising externally. They have an 'as if' quality, and lack the vividness and reality of true hallucinations. Consequently, the affected person is not usually distressed by them; and does not normally feel the need to respond, as happens with true hallucinations (Box 2.43).

Cognition

This is assessed from the history and observation; evaluate any deficit using standard tests. Use the history, observation, MSE and rating scales (see below) together to diagnose and distinguish between the 'three Ds' (dementia, delirium and depression) which are common in the elderly and hospital patients.

Core cognitive functions include (Box 2.44):

- level of consciousness
- orientation
- memory
- attention and concentration
- intelligence.

Mental disorders are rarely associated with a reduced level of (or clouded) consciousness, except delirium (which is both a physical and a mental disorder), where it is common.

2.44 Cognition: definitions

Term	Definition
Clouding of consciousness	A reduced level of consciousness observed as drowsiness (coma in extreme cases)
Confabulation	Plausible but false memories that cover memory gaps

2.45 Insight: definitions

Term	Definition
Insight	Recognising that abnormal mental experiences are in fact abnormal Accepting that these abnormalities amount to a mental illness Accepting the need for treatment

2.46 Insight: what to ask

- Do you think anything is wrong with you?
- What do you think is the matter with you?
- If you are ill, what do you think needs to happen to make you better?

Orientation is a key aspect of cognition, being particularly sensitive to impairment. Disorientation is the hallmark of the 'organic mental state' found in delirium and dementia. Abnormalities may be evident during the interview. Check the patient's knowledge of the current time and date, recognition of where he is (place) and identification of familiar people (person).

Memory function is divided into:

- Registration: test by asking the patient to repeat the names of three unrelated objects e.g. apple, table, penny; any mistake is significant. Alternatively, slowly and clearly say several random single digits, e.g. 6, 3, 5, 9, 1, 4, 7. Then ask the patient to repeat them. A person with normal function can repeat at least five digits.
- Short-term memory: test by giving the patient some new information; once this has registered, check retention after 5 minutes (with a distracting task in between). Do the same with the names of three objects; any error is significant. Alternatively, use a six-item name and address, e.g. Mr David Green, 25 Sharp Street. More than one error indicates impairment.
- Long-term memory is assessed mainly from the personal history that the patient provides. Gaps and mistakes are often obvious, but some patients confabulate (fill in gaps in their memory with unconsciously fabricated facts) so check the account with a family member if possible. Failing long-term memory is characteristic of dementia, although this store of knowledge can be remarkably intact in the presence of severe impairment of other cognitive functions. Confabulation is a core feature of Korsakoff's syndrome, a complication of chronic alcoholism.

Impaired attention and concentration occur in many mental disorders and are not diagnostic. Impaired attention is observed as increased distractibility, with the patient responding inappropriately to extraneous stimuli which may be real, e.g. a noise outside the room, or unreal, e.g. auditory hallucinations. Concentration is the patient's ability to stick with a mental task. It is tested by using simple, repetitive sequences, such as asking the patient to repeat the months of the year in reverse or to do the 'serial 7s' test, in which 7 is subtracted from 100, then from 93, then 86, etc. Note the finishing point, the number of errors and the time taken.

Estimate intelligence clinically from a combination of the history of educational attainment and occupations, and at interview from vocabulary, general knowledge, abstract thought, foresight and understanding. If in doubt as to whether the patient has a learning disability, or if there is a discrepancy between the history and presentation, a psychologist should formally test IQ.

Insight is the degree to which a patient agrees that he is ill and in need of treatment. Insight matters, since absent or incomplete insight leads to non-compliance (Boxes 2.45 and 2.46).

Risk assessment

Risk assessment is a crucial part of every psychiatric assessment. Consider:

- The person(s) at risk.

Usually the patient, but others at risk are likely to be family, or, less commonly, specific individuals (neighbours, celebrities) or members of specific groups (defined by age, ethnicity, occupation, etc.).

- Nature of the risk:

There may be direct risk to life and limb (as in suicide, self-harm or violence to others) or indirect risk to health (through refusal of treatment for physical or mental illness) or welfare (through inability to provide basic care – food, warmth, shelter, hygiene – for oneself or one's dependants).

Evaluate risk in all psychiatric assessments (Box 2.47), but in depth when the:

- presentation includes acts or threats of self-harm or reports of command hallucinations
- past history includes self-harm or violent behaviour
- social circumstances show a recent, significant loss
- mental disorder is strongly associated with risk, e.g. depression or a paranoid state.

Screening questions for mental illnesses

A psychiatric diagnosis is made by identifying particular clusters of symptoms and mental state changes in the patient. Cover certain areas routinely when you suspect a particular mental illness (Box 2.48). No single question clinches the diagnosis for any specific type of mental disorder, but some features are closely associated with particular mental illnesses, e.g:

- passivity phenomena and schizophrenia
- re-experiencing an ordeal and post-traumatic stress disorder
- phobia of normal weight and anorexia nervosa.

2.47 Risk assessment: what to ask

Suicide/self-harm

- How do you feel about the future?
- Have you thought about ending your life?
- Have you made plans to end your life?
- Have you attempted to end your life?

Homicide/harm to others

- Are there people you know who would be better off dead?
- Have you thought about harming anyone else?
- Have you been told to harm anyone else?

 2.48 Screening questions for mental illnesses

When you suspect an anxiety disorder

- What physical symptoms have you been experiencing?
- How relaxed have you been feeling recently?
- Have there been any particular concerns or worries on your mind recently?

When you suspect a depressive disorder

- How has your mood been recently?
- Are you still enjoying things the way you used to?
- How do you view the future just now?

When you suspect schizophrenia

- Have you any beliefs that you think other people might find odd?
- Have you had any unusual experiences recently?
- Have you had any difficulty controlling your thinking?
- Have you heard people's voices when there's no one around? (Where do you think the voices come from? What do they say?)

However, these features may occur in other mental disorders.

Some symptoms are non-specific but important. They include:

- sleep disturbance
- impaired concentration
- anxiety.

THE PHYSICAL EXAMINATION

Physical and mental disorders are associated, so always consider the physical dimension in any patient presenting with a psychiatric complaint. The patient's age, health and mode of presentation will determine the extent of physical assessment required. Usually, general observation, coupled with basic cardiovascular and neurological examination, is adequate.

Collateral history

This is important, especially when the patient:

- has a severe learning disability or confusional state
- has a mental disorder that prevents effective communication
- is very disturbed or uncooperative.

Sources of third-party information include family and other carers, as well as past and present GPs and other

 2.49 Personality disorder

Definition

Patterns of experience and behaviour which are:
- Pathological (i.e. outwith social norms)
- Problematic (for the patient and/or others)
- Pervasive (affecting most or all areas of a patient's life)
- Persistent (adolescent onset, enduring throughout adult life and resistant to treatment)

 2.50 The Abbreviated Mental Test

Each question scores 1 mark; a score of 8/10 or less indicates confusion
- Age
- Date of birth
- Time (to the nearest hour)
- Year
- Hospital name
- Recognition of two people, e.g. doctor, nurse
- Recall address
- Dates of First World War (or other significant event)
- Name of the monarch (or prime minister, president as appropriate)
- Count backwards from 20 to 1

health professionals. Previous psychiatric assessments are valuable when considering a diagnosis of personality disorder, as this depends on information about behaviour patterns over time rather than details of the current presentation (Box 2.49).

Psychiatric rating scales

Most of these were developed in research studies to assist diagnosis, or to measure change in severity of illness. Some require special training; all should be used sensibly. In general, scales are too inflexible and limited in scope to replace a well-conducted standard psychiatric interview, but they can be useful adjuncts for screening, measuring response to treatment or focusing on particular areas. In routine practice, scales are most widely used to assess cognitive function when an organic brain disorder is suspected. They include:

- Abbreviated Mental Test (AMT): takes <5 minutes (Box 2.50)
- Mini Mental State Examination (MMSE): takes 5–10 minutes.

Well-known instruments assessing areas other than cognition include:

- general morbidity:
  - General Health Questionnaire (GHQ)
- mood disorder:
  - Hospital Anxiety and Depression Scale (HADS)
  - Beck Depression Inventory (BDI)
- alcohol:
  - CAGE questionnaire (Box 2.24)
  - FAST questionnaire (Box 2.25).

MEDICALLY UNEXPLAINED SYMPTOMS (MUS)

Symptoms are not synonymous with disease but are subjective experiences that may arise from many sources (Box 2.51). There is a major distinction between disease and illness. Disease is a cluster of symptoms resulting from demonstrable pathological processes, e.g. coronary artery disease. Illness (or disorder) is a cluster of symptoms where there may be no demonstrable pathological process despite clearly impaired function, e.g. anxiety.

When symptoms impair a patient's normal function, do not fit characteristic patterns of disease and persist without any abnormalities on examination and investigation, they are called 'functional' or 'medically unexplained'. More than 30% of patients attending their GP have MUS (with similar proportions in secondary care, where disease prevalence is much greater) (Fig. 2.6). MUS cause similar levels of disability to those resulting from disease and are often associated with significant emotional distress. If such patients are not managed effectively, fruitless investigations and harm from unnecessary drugs or procedures may result. The approach to such patients is important and may differ between specialists.

MUS raise strong feelings in patients and doctors. Patients may feel they are not believed, or that their symptoms are being dismissed as 'all in the mind'. Doctors may feel their competence is being questioned.

A dualistic model of mind and body as separate entities is too simplistic and clinically unhelpful. If you think of physical disorders as 'real' and MUS as 'not real' because they arise from emotional distress or psychiatric disorder your patients will soon detect this and react accordingly. Symptoms result from complex interactions between biological, social and psychological factors; each component is unique to the individual. Many people with severe diseases cope with their symptoms, function remarkably well and work in full-time jobs. Others, with apparently modest symptoms, cannot function effectively. There may be little correlation between symptom severity, disease processes, social functioning and response to treatment. Patients with a proven disease may not improve symptomatically with treatment. For example, therapy for *Helicobacter pylori*-associated gastritis in a patient with a peptic ulcer may cure the ulcer but not the dyspeptic symptoms. We should understand our patients as individuals and help them to cope with the distress that their symptoms provoke.

Symptoms and definitions

Many terms are used to describe MUS and most specialities have a name for the common ones they see (Box 2.52). These include symptom labels (low back pain), symptom syndromes (chronic fatigue syndrome, irritable bowel syndrome), non-diagnoses (MUS, functional), psychological causes (psychosomatic), psychological processes (somatisation), psychiatric diagnoses (conversion disorder) and malingering (fictitious symptoms simulated for material gain).

Patients with multiple symptoms are more likely to have MUS. In general, the more symptoms a patient has, the greater the likelihood of psychiatric illness or distress, e.g. anxiety and depression. Certain symptoms are more likely to be MUS and are not accompanied by any

2.51 Examples of factors influencing symptoms

Factors	Example
Pathological	Chest pain from coronary artery disease
Physiological	Tremor
Psychological	Paraesthesia from hyperventilation
Behavioural	Weakness from excess bed rest
External	Compensation and the welfare state

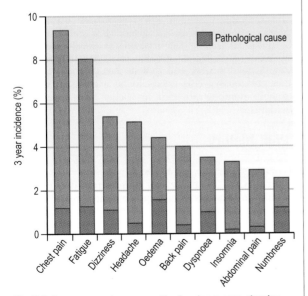

Fig. 2.6 Common symptoms presenting in primary care, showing the percentage with an underlying pathological cause.

2.52 Examples of medically unexplained symptoms and 'functional' syndromes in the medical specialities

Neurology	Functional weakness, tension headache, non-epileptic attacks, hemisensory symptoms
Gastroenterology	Irritable bowel syndrome, non-ulcer dyspepsia, chronic abdominal pain
Gynaecology	Chronic pelvic pain, urethral syndrome
Ear, nose and throat	Functional dysphonia, globus
Cardiology	Atypical chest pain, unexplained palpitation, non-cardiac chest pain
Rheumatology	Fibromyalgia
Infectious disease	(Postviral) chronic fatigue syndrome
Immunology/allergy	Multiple chemical sensitivity syndrome

2.53 Symptoms and their relationship to physical disease	
Sometimes	**Infrequently**
Chest pain	Fatigue
Breathlessness	Back pain
Syncope	Headache
Abdominal pain	Dizziness

EBE   2.54 Risk factor for medically unexplained symptoms (MUS)

Women who have experienced parental illness or lack of care during childhood are predisposed to MUS.

Craig TKJ, Cox AD, Klein K. Intergenerational transmission of somatization behaviour: a study of chronic somatisers and their children. Psychol Med 2002;32:805–816.

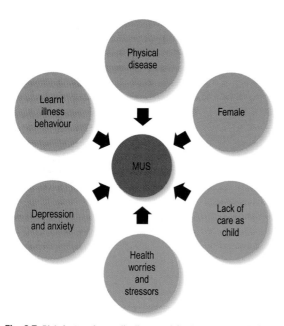

Fig. 2.7 Risk factors for medically unexplained symptoms (MUS).

of the usual features that suggest serious physical disease. Some symptoms are particularly unlikely to be associated with significant disease (Box 2.53).

Causes

Certain factors increase the risk of MUS (Fig. 2.7 and Box 2.54).

History

MUS are so common that primary care physicians become adept at spotting this from the history. Making

EBE   2.55 Misdiagnosis and conversion disorder

24% of people diagnosed with conversion disorder develop an illness that could have explained their presenting symptoms.

Stone J, Smyth R, Carson A et al. Systematic review of misdiagnosis of conversion symptoms and 'hysteria'. BMJ 2005;331:989.

a positive diagnosis from the history and confirming this by negative findings on physical examination allow reassurance and an explanation tailored to the patient.

Presenting complaint

Keep an open mind when talking with all patients; remember that patients with MUS may also have or develop disease. Always take a full history and perform a full clinical examination. Patients will feel that you are taking them seriously and you are less likely to miss any serious physical disease (Box 2.55).

Accept all symptoms at face value and find out about all of them. Explore exacerbating and relieving factors. Find out when it all started; try asking 'when did you last feel well?'

Patients' beliefs in their illness matter; what do they think is wrong? Why have they come now and what do they hope you can do for them? How disabling are their symptoms? What do the symptoms now prevent them from doing? Find out what a typical day is like.

What has happened to them with previous doctors? Patients may complain about previous doctors or certain treatments they have been offered. Allowing a patient to express dissatisfaction shows that you are interested, and helps you avoid suggesting management options the patient is likely to reject. However, recognise that you are only being shown one side of a complicated situation. Maintain a professional approach, ensuring that you do not get drawn into criticising other healthcare providers or their actions.

Often, there are inconsistencies in the history which you should explore and highlight for the patient, e.g. a patient with severe disabling chest pain without angiographic evidence of coronary artery disease may still firmly believe he has angina. His records show that this is not the case and that he has clearly been told this previously. This needs to be explored with him to help demonstrate that his belief is not based on evidence.

Past history

Whenever possible, get all the previous notes, or at least summaries of them. Review these carefully, including childhood illnesses. This can be time-consuming but worth the effort.

Social history

Note any welfare benefits where money is being received for disability, or legal cases where financial compensation may be pending.

Psychiatric history

Leave this until last. To gain the patient's trust you should be empathic and non-judgemental. Patients will then gain confidence that you are not going to use their emotional symptoms 'against them'. Patients are acutely sensitive to questions that suggest they are making things up so frame your questions carefully in terms of their symptoms. Ask 'Do your symptoms ever make you feel down or frustrated?' rather than 'Do you ever feel depressed?'

Do not ask about a history of abuse at a first consultation unless the patient volunteers the information. If the abuse was in the past, do not feel that you have to do anything other than bear witness to the patient's past suffering and acknowledge it. Patients need to feel in control as their past experience has been about being in someone else's power. Follow local guidelines for any current abuse that may be revealed.

Physical examination

The physical assessment begins as soon as you see the patient in the waiting room and ends when the patient leaves the consulting room. Watch carefully for inconsistent signs, though this does not tell you if symptoms are consciously or unconsciously produced. The symptoms dictate the clinical features that you should look for. Usually there are no physical signs of disease but some non-pathological signs are associated with MUS. These do not exclude disease so interpret them with caution. The history has often suggested the diagnosis and so you are seeking to exclude any unexpected physical findings that warrant further investigation as well as to demonstrate to patients that you are taking them seriously, e.g. in irritable bowel syndrome you may find evidence of bloating and some tenderness but otherwise the gastrointestinal examination will be normal (Ch. 8).

Any signs you find may vary between examinations but overall the examination is commonly normal.

Investigation

The main objective of investigation is to reassure the physician and the patient. Routine, standard investigations and management to exclude all physical illness are costly, unhelpful, risk side-effects and do not achieve the longer-term reassurance of patients. Before proceeding with any investigation, discuss the likelihood and significance of a normal test result with the patient. The effect of diagnostic testing will depend on what the patient thinks a normal result means. Patients are more likely to be satisfied when your explanation makes sense to them, removes blame and helps generate ideas about how they can manage their symptoms.

PUTTING IT ALL TOGETHER

Positively identify patients with MUS early by recognising the possibility as you listen to their complaints. Some

2.56 Common functional syndromes

In all cases, physical examination and investigation fail to reveal an underlying physical cause and symptoms should have lasted more than 3 months in those marked with an asterisk.

Chronic fatigue syndrome	Persistent fatigue
Irritable bowel syndrome	Abdominal pain, altered bowel habit (diarrhoea or constipation), and abdominal bloating
Chronic pain syndrome	*Persistent pain in one or more parts of the body sometimes following injury but which outlasts the original trauma
Fibromyalgia	*Pain in the axial skeleton with trigger points (tender areas in the muscles)
Chronic back pain	*Pain, muscle tension, or stiffness localised below the costal margin and above the inferior gluteal folds, with or without leg pain
Urethral syndrome	Recurrent dysuria and urinary frequency but absence of significant bacteriuria

2.57 Examples of possible patients' concerns for common-functional disorders

Symptoms	Patient's concern	Common diagnosis
Tired all the time Abdominal pain – relieved by defecation Bloating Low back pain Rabbit pellet stools	Bowel cancer	Irritable bowel syndrome
Band-like headache Coming on during the day Not relieved by analgesics	Brain tumour	Tension headache
Sharp intermittent left-sided chest pain	Heart attack	Musculoskeletal chest pain and anxiety

symptoms are more likely to be medically unexplained than others (Box 2.56). Work with your patient's ideas and together plan a way forward that avoids unnecessary investigations and treatment (Box 2.57). In 75% of primary care patients with no abnormality on physical examination, symptoms are self-limiting. Reviewing the patient may be more appropriate than performing costly and potentially confusing investigations.

2

2

DOCUMENTING THE FINDINGS: THE CASE NOTES

The case notes, or records, are the written record of a patient's medical condition. They include your initial findings, proposed investigations and plan of management, together with information about the patient's progress. Information is recorded for each episode of illness over time and shared by all the healthcare staff caring for a patient. Notes should therefore be accurate, legible, dated and signed. Primary care records contain the whole story of a patient's health rather than discrete episodes of hospital care, and follow the patient if he changes practices (Box 2.58).

You may write notes while talking with a patient, but do not let this interrupt the discussion and maintain as much eye contact as possible. Active listening is difficult if you are writing, so make brief notes to remind yourself of the important points, and only write up the full history and physical findings when the examination is completed. Only record objective findings. Never make any judgemental or flippant remarks.

Although structured proformas for recording history and examination findings are used in many hospitals, it is not necessary to record every detail in every patient. Only record negative findings if they are relevant. For example, in a patient with breathlessness, the negative details of the respiratory enquiry are important but negative responses to the gastrointestinal enquiry can be condensed to a single entry of 'none'. You may use abbreviations but they should not be obscure or ambiguous (Fig. 2.8). The prefix '°' is often used to signify 'no': for example, '° tenderness'. Use diagrams to show the site and size of superficial injuries or wounds, and for the abdomen to illustrate the position of tenderness, masses or scars (Fig. 8.12). Record injuries accurately; you may be asked to give legal evidence from the notes many months later (Box 2.59).

Unitary or 'multidisciplinary' notes allow the whole team to record their findings in one document rather than each keeping separate case records. Unitary records can be cumbersome but encourage shared care, avoid duplication and make it easy to access information.

Computer records

Records may be held on paper or online. Computers allow easy access to medical and prescribing information during the consultation. All electronic data should be stored securely, accessible only to relevant staff and password-protected. Paperless general practices hold all patient information on computer and this can be downloaded on to laptops for domiciliary use. Some patients carry Smart cards holding their entire medical record.

Confidentiality

The case record is confidential and constitutes a legal document that may be used in a court of law. You cannot share details with anyone who is not involved in a patient's care, unless the patient gives fully informed written consent. This includes insurance companies, lawyers, the police and research workers. You may only

2.58 Information in the case record

- History and examination findings
- Investigations and results
- Management plan
- Assessments by other health professionals, e.g. dieticians, health visitors
- Information and education provided to patients and their relatives
- Correspondence about the patient
- Patient's progress
- Advance directives or 'living wills'
- Contact details for next of kin

2.59 Describing wounds

Position

- Where on the body, including which aspect of a limb

Size and orientation

- e.g. 5 cm × 3 mm vertical scratch

Appearance

- e.g. colour, shape

Type of lesion

- Abrasion: loss of the outer skin due to impact with a rough surface
- Scratch: linear abrasion due to drawing of a sharp point over the skin
- Bruise: bleeding within the tissues beneath the skin
- Laceration: tearing of the skin due to blunt trauma; ragged edges
- Incised wound: cut or gash; sharp edges
- Penetrating wound: breaches full skin thickness; depth is greater than length

break confidence if a patient poses a risk to himself or other members of the public.

In the UK, patients have the right to receive a copy of their paper case record and to see any personal information held on computer, including their medical records. Remember this when you make your notes or record information about third parties, particularly in cases of sexual abuse. Some patients already hold their own records, usually when antenatal or diabetic care is shared between hospital and community. You can stop patients seeing a part of their record if you think it would seriously harm their physical or mental health or that of any other individual.

Writing letters

Letters must be written when referring a patient to a specialist, and to the GP following an outpatient consultation or hospital admission. The hospital discharge letter (or summary) is structured in a standard format, which can be adapted for referral and outpatient letters.

The text should be brief; concentrate on the main issues but include any unexpected findings or complications and relevant investigation results. Include the reason for referral as well as the diagnosis, along with full details of the patient's past history and current medication. Ensure copies of letters are sent to the patient's GP and any other specialist involved in the patient's care.

Most letters are dictated and typed, although structured computerised letters may also be used. When dictating, remember the following:

- State your name and the date of dictation.
- State the patient's name and date of birth.
- State other important dates, e.g. the patient's attendance at an outpatient appointment, or hospital admission.
- Speak slowly and clearly. Spell out unusual medical terms.
- Say 'full stop' at the end of a sentence and 'new paragraph' as required, and include any details of punctuation required. Use paragraph headings as in Box 2.60.

2.60 Discharge letter headings

- Diagnosis
  - Primary or active
  - Inactive: list comorbidities or previous illnesses
- Procedures or operations
- History (include important social factors)
- Examination
- Investigations: only give detailed results if abnormal
- Clinical progress: brief description of course during hospital stay
- Social arrangements where relevant
- Drugs on discharge, including doses and duration of course
- Follow-up arrangements
- Information given to patients (and relatives)

In many hospitals, voice-activated recognition is now in use and instructions for this may vary from the above. Letters are always easier to dictate when you have just seen the patient rather than several days later.

2

Date : 03.08.13
Time : 14.00

MARY BROWN aged 78
32 Tartan Cresc.
Edinburgh
DOB 12.09.35

Emergency admission to CCU via GP: Dr Wells, High St., Edinburgh

History from patient

PC Chest pain   2 hours
     Breathlessness   1 hour
     Dizziness   30 mins

HPC
Severe pain 'like a band around chest' while watching TV which has now lasted 2 hours despite using GTN, aspirin and diltiazem.
Radiates to jaw and inner aspect of L arm.
Has gradually become breathless over the last hour and dizzy in last 30 minutes.

First began 6 months ago: episode of lower retrosternal chest pain after walking about 1/2 mile uphill:
- no associated palpitation or SOB.
Two further episodes over the next 3 months.

3 months ago: increasing frequency of pain
- now brought on by walking 200 yards on the flat or climbing 1 flight of stairs
- worse after heavy meals
- other features of pain as before.

2 months ago: visited GP who diagnosed angina. Prescribed GTN which gave effective relief.

1 week ago: three episodes of chest pain at rest, all immediately relieved by GTN.
°Blackouts °pain in calves on exertion.

PH			
Tonsillectomy	1952	Hospital X	
Perforated peptic ulcer	1977	Hospital Y	
COPD	Since 1990	General practitioner	

°MI, °DM, °J, °HBP, °Stroke, °RF, °TB

DH	DOSE	FREQUENCY	DURATION
Salbutamol inhaler	2 puffs	As necessary	3 years
Zopiclone	7.5mg	At night	6 months
Senokot (self medication)	2 tabs	2–3 times per week	10 years
GTN spray	1 puff	As required	2 months
Aspirin	75mg	Once daily	2 months
No allergies			

FH

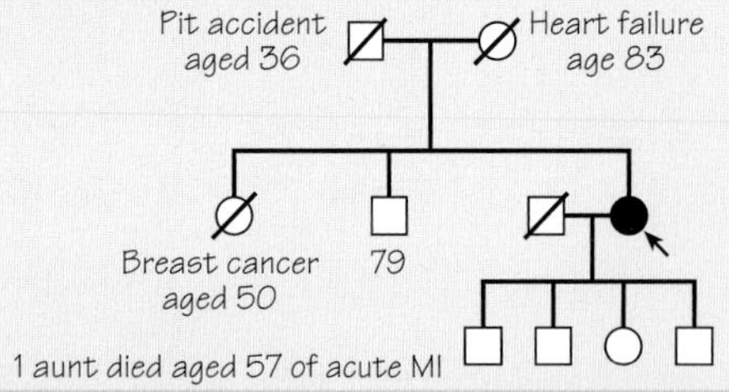

Pit accident aged 36 — Heart failure age 83
Breast cancer aged 50   79
1 aunt died aged 57 of acute MI

1

Fig. 2.8 Case notes: example.

Demographic Details

Always record
- The patient's name and address, date of birth and age
- Any national health identification number such as CHI in the UK
- Source of referral e.g. from Emergency Department or General Practitioner
- GP's name and address
- Source of history e.g. patient, relative, carer
- Date and time of examination

Presenting Complaint (PC)

State the major problem in one or two of the patient's own words (or give a brief list), followed by the duration of each. Do not use medical terminology.

History of Presenting Complaint (HPC)

Describe the onset, nature and course of each symptom.
Paraphrase the patient's account and condense it if necessary.
Omit irrelevant details.
Put particularly telling comments in inverted commas.
Include other parts of the history if relevant, such as the smoking history in patients with cardiac or respiratory presentations, or family history in disorders with a possible genetic trait such as hypercholesterolaemia or diabetes.
Correct grammar is not necessary.
GTN – glyceryl trinitrate
SOB – short of breath

Past History (PH)

Tabulate in chronological order.
Include important negatives, e.g. in a patient with chest pain ask about previous myocardial infarction, angina, hypertension or diabetes mellitus and record whether these are present or absent. Jaundice is important because it may pose a risk to healthcare workers if due to hepatitis B or C.

COPD – Chronic obstructive pulmonary disease
   MI – Myocardial infarction
  DM – Diabetes mellitus
    J – Jaundice
 HBP – Hypertension
  RF – Rheumatic fever

Drug History (DH)

Tabulate these and include any allergies particularly to drugs.
Record any previous adverse drug reactions prominently on the front of the notes as well as inside.

Family History (FH)

Record the age and current health or the causes of or the ages at death of the patient's parents, siblings and children.
Use the symbols shown in Fig. 2.3 to construct a pedigree chart.

Fig. 2.8 (Continued)

SH

Retired cleaner.
Widow for 3 years. Lives alone in sheltered housing.
Smoked 20/day from age 19.
Teetotal.
HH once a week for cleaning and shopping. Daughter nearby visits regularly.

SE

CVS: See above.

RS: Long-standing cough most days with white sputum on rising in morning only. °Haemoptysis.
Wheezy in cold weather.

GI: Weight steady.
Nil else of note.

GUS: PARA 1 + 0. °PMB, °urinary symptoms

CNS: Nil of note.

MSS: Occasional pain and stiffness in right knee on exertion for 5 years.

ES: Nil of note.

O/E

Anxious, frail, cachectic lady.
Weight 45 kg. Height 1.25 m
2 cm craggy mass in upper, outer quadrant L breast. Fixed to underlying tissues.
<u>Patient unaware of this</u>
1 cm node in apex of left axilla.
°Pallor, °cyanosis, °jaundice, °clubbing.

CVS

P90 reg, small volume, normal character.
BP 140/80 JVP + 3 cms normal character, °oedema, AB 5ICS MCL, °thrills.
HS I + II + 2/6 ESM at LLSE °radiation.
°Bruits.
PP:

	Radial	Brachial	Carotid	Femoral	Popliteal	Post. Tibial	Dorsalis pedis
R	+	+	+	+	+/-	+/-	+/-
L	+	+	+	+	+	+	+

(Normal +, Reduced +/-, Absent -)

RS

Trachea central. Reduced cricosternal distance and intercostal indrawing on inspiration.
Expansion reduced but symmetrical.
PN resonant.
BS vesicular and quiet.
VR normal and symmetrical.

2

Fig. 2.8 (Continued)

Social History (SH)
Occupation
Marital status
Living circumstances; type of housing and with whom
Smoking
Alcohol
Illicit drug use (if appropriate)
Social support in the frail or disabled

HH – home help

Systematic Enquiry (SE)
Document positive responses that do not feature in the HPC.

CVS – Cardiovascular system
RS – Respiratory system
GI – Gastrointestinal system
GUS – Genito-urinary system
PMB – Postmenopausal bleeding
CNS – Central nervous system
MSS – Musculoskeletal system
ES – Endocrine system

General / On examination (OE)
Physical appearance e.g. frail, drowsy, breathless
Mental state e.g. anxious, distressed, confused
Undernourished, cachectic, obese
Abnormal smells e.g. ketones, alcohol, uraemia, fetor hepaticus
Record height, weight and waist circumference
Skin e.g. cyanosis, pallor, jaundice, any specific lesions or rashes
Breasts, normal or describe any mass
Hands; finger clubbing, or abnormalities of skin and nails
Lymph nodes; characteristics and site

Cardiovascular System (CVS)
Pulse (P) rate, rhythm, character and volume
Blood pressure (BP)
Jugular venous pressure (JVP) height and character
Presence or absence of ankle oedema
Apex beat (AB) position, character, presence of thrills
Heart sounds (HS) any added sounds, murmurs and grade
Peripheral pulses (PP) and bruits

5ICS – 5th intercostal space
MCL – Mid clavicular line
ESM – Ejection systolic murmur
LLSE – Lower left sternal edge

Respiratory System (RS)
Any chest wall deformity
Trachea central or deviated
Signs of hyperinflation
Expansion and its symmetry
Percussion note (PN) and site of any abnormality
Breath sounds (BS), any added sounds and site of abnormality
Vocal resonance (VR) and site of abnormality

Fig. 2.8 (Continued)

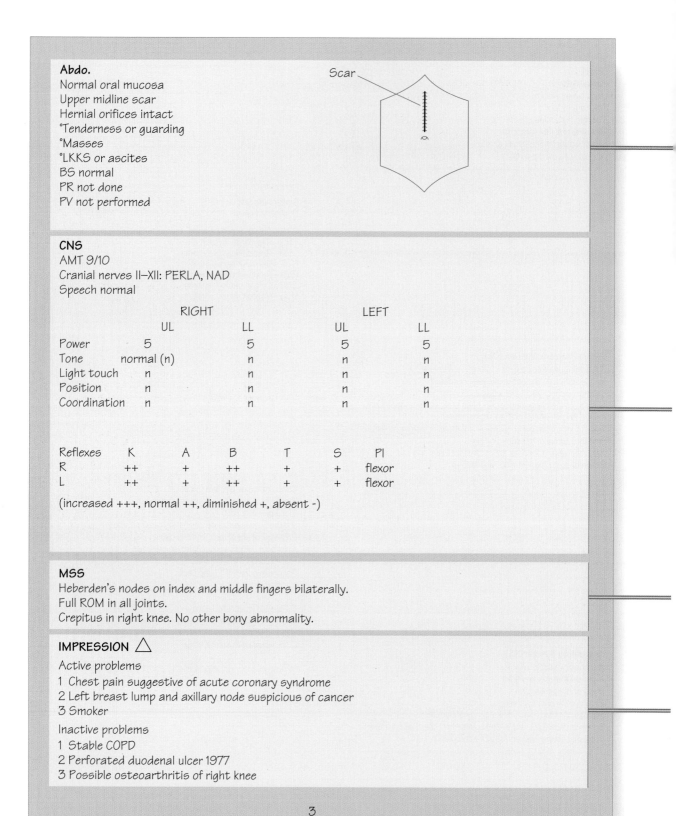

Abdo.
Normal oral mucosa
Upper midline scar
Hernial orifices intact
°Tenderness or guarding
°Masses
°LKKS or ascites
BS normal
PR not done
PV not performed

Scar

CNS
AMT 9/10
Cranial nerves II–XII: PERLA, NAD
Speech normal

| | RIGHT | | LEFT | |
	UL	LL	UL	LL
Power	5	5	5	5
Tone	normal (n)	n	n	n
Light touch	n	n	n	n
Position	n	n	n	n
Coordination	n	n	n	n

Reflexes	K	A	B	T	S	Pl
R	++	+	++	+	+	flexor
L	++	+	++	+	+	flexor

(increased +++, normal ++, diminished +, absent -)

MSS
Heberden's nodes on index and middle fingers bilaterally.
Full ROM in all joints.
Crepitus in right knee. No other bony abnormality.

IMPRESSION △

Active problems
1 Chest pain suggestive of acute coronary syndrome
2 Left breast lump and axillary node suspicious of cancer
3 Smoker

Inactive problems
1 Stable COPD
2 Perforated duodenal ulcer 1977
3 Possible osteoarthritis of right knee

3

Fig. 2.8 (Continued)

Abdominal System (AS)
Mouth
 Any abnormality – own teeth or dentures
Abdomen
 Scars and site
 Shape, distended or scaphoid
 Hernial orifices
 Tenderness and guarding and site of this
 Masses and description of these
 Enlargement of liver, kidneys or spleen (shorten to LKKS)
 Ascites if present
 Bowel sounds (BS); presence and character
 Rectal examination (PR) record whether or not it was
 performed and your findings. It should not be done in patients
 with cardiac disease as this may provoke an arrhythmia.
 In women; vaginal examination (VE) is only carried
 out if relevant
 In men; external genitalia

Central Nervous System (CNS)
In older patients, record the abbreviated mental test (AMT) score
In impaired consciousness, head injury or possible raised
intracranial pressure record the Glasgow Coma Scale (GCS)

Abnormal speech
Cranial nerves; record abnormalities only
Fundoscopy
Tabulate the remaining examination
If it is relevant record the presence or absence of tremor, gait,
abnormality, fasciculation, dyspraxia, two point discrimination,
stereognosis or sensory neglect.

PERLA – Pupils equal and react to light and accommodation
 NAD – No abnormality detected
 UL – Upper limb
 LL – Lower limb
 K – Knee
 A – Ankle
 B – Biceps
 T – Triceps
 S – Supinator
 Pl – Plantar

Musculoskeletal System (MSS)
Gait if abnormal
Muscle or soft tissue changes
Swelling, colour, heat, tenderness
Deformities in the bones or joints
Limitation of ranges of movements (ROM) in any affected joint

Clinical Diagnosis or Impression
Record your conclusions and the most likely diagnoses in order
of probability.
In patients with multiple pathology make a problem list so the key
issues are seen immediately.

△ Diagnosis

Fig. 2.8 (Continued)

Plan

ECG performed on admission shows sinus rhythm and deep ST depression in leads II, III and aVF

Troponin at 12 hours
Repeat ECG in 1 hour
Chest X-ray
Full blood count
Urea and electrolytes, glucose

Oxygen and cardiac monitor
IV morphine and metoclopramide
Aspirin and clopidogrel
Low molecular weight heparin
Continue aspirin and diltiazem
Discuss beta-blocker with consultant in view of COPD
Advice to stop smoking

When stable
1 Review anti-anginal management
2 Referral for mammography and fine needle aspiration of breast lump
3 Spirometry and assessment of inhaler technique

Information given

Diagnosis and treatment explained to patient and daughter
N.B. Breast lump not mentioned at this stage until discussed with senior staff

A. Doctor (signed)
A. DOCTOR   (Date and Time) capitals

Progress notes

3.8.13
1800 Ward Round – Dr Consultant

No further chest pain

O/E
P70 BP 100/70
JVP not elevated, °oedema
HS I + II and ESM as above
Chest clear
Breast lump noted

ECG at 4 hours – resolution of inferior ST changes

Impression

Acute coronary syndrome – no ST segment elevation

Plan

Await troponin
Continue LMW heparin
Check lipid profile
For echocardiography in view of murmur then consider ACE inhibitor
Spirometry and assessment of inhaler technique

Consultant to discuss finding of breast lump
with patient and daughter

A. Doctor (signed)
A. DOCTOR   (Date and Time) capitals

4

Fig. 2.8 (Continued)

Plan
- List the investigations required. When a result is already available, for example of an electrocardiograph, record it.
- Record any immediate management instigated
- If uncertain about an investigation or treatment, precede with a '?' and discuss with a more senior member of staff

Information given
Document what you have told the patient and any other family member. It is also important to document any diagnosis that you have not discussed.
If the patient voices any concerns or fears, document these too.

Progress Notes
Follow the same structure with these additions
- Changes in the patient's symptoms
- Examination findings
- Results of new investigations
- Clinical impression of the patient's progress
- Plans for further management, particularly drug changes.

Make progress notes regularly depending on the speed of change in the patient's condition; in an intensive therapy setting, this may be several times a day but, in a stable situation, daily or alternate days.
Date, time and sign all entries.
Record any unexpected change in the patient's condition as well as routine progress notes.

Fig. 2.8 (Continued)

Graham Douglas
John Bevan

The general examination

3

3

THE SETTING FOR A PHYSICAL EXAMINATION

Privacy is essential when you examine a patient. Pulling the curtains around the bed in a ward obscures vision but not sound. Talk quietly but ensure good communication, which may be difficult with deaf or elderly patients (Ch. 2). The room should be warm and well lit. Subtle abnormalities of complexion such as mild jaundice are easier to detect in natural light. The height of the examination couch or bed should be adjustable, with a step to enable patients to get on to it easily. An adjustable backrest is essential, particularly for breathless patients who cannot lie flat.

Seek permission and sensitively, but adequately, expose the areas of the body to be examined; cover the rest of the patient with a blanket or sheet to ensure that he or she does not become cold. Avoid unnecessary exposure and embarrassment. A female patient will appreciate the opportunity to replace her bra after her chest examination before you examine her abdomen. Tactfully ask relatives to leave the room before the physical examination. Sometimes it is appropriate for a relative to remain if the patient is very apprehensive, if you need a translator or if the patient requests it. Parents should always be present when you examine children (Ch. 15).

Always offer a chaperone for any intimate examination to prevent misunderstandings and to provide support and encouragement for the patient (Ch. 2). Record the chaperone's name and presence. If patients decline the offer, respect their wishes and record this in the notes.

Collect together all the equipment you need before starting the examination (Box 3.1).

SEQUENCE FOR PERFORMING A PHYSICAL EXAMINATION

Keep an open mind as you talk with the patient and formulate a differential diagnosis. You may miss the correct diagnosis if you are unduly swayed by early clues in the history, overvalue recent or memorable cases or lean too heavily towards diagnoses that seem to match a pattern. Examine the patient, looking for signs that will confirm or refute your diagnoses.

With experience, you will develop your own style and sequence of physical examination (Box 3.2). There is no single correct way of performing a physical examination. A regular routine reduces errors of omission.

The sequence of examination is:

- Inspection
- Palpation
- Percussion
- Auscultation (Fig. 3.1).

Learn to integrate these smoothly into each component of the physical examination.

FIRST IMPRESSIONS

The physical examination starts as soon as you see the patient. Assess patients' general demeanour and external appearance, and watch how they rise from their chair and walk into the room.

Gait and posture

Observe the patient as he walks towards you. The gait may suggest an important neurological or musculoskeletal disorder or provide clues to the patient's emotions and overall function. Disorders of gait occur because of pain, fixed or immobile joints, muscle weakness or abnormal limb control (Fig. 3.2). If the patient is in bed, look at his posture.

3.1 Equipment required for a full examination

- Stethoscope
- Pen torch
- Measuring tape
- Ophthalmoscope
- Otoscope
- Sphygmomanometer
- Tendon hammer
- Tuning fork
- Cotton wool
- Disposable Neurotips
- Wooden spatula
- Thermometer
- Magnifying glass
- Accurate weighing scales and a height-measuring device (preferably a Harpenden stadiometer)
- Disposable gloves may be required
- Facilities for obtaining blood samples and urinalysis

3.2 A personal system for performing a physical examination

- Handshake and introduction
- Note general appearances while talking:
  - Does the patient look well?
  - Any immediate and obvious clues, e.g. obesity, plethora, breathlessness
  - Complexion
- Hands and radial pulse
- Face
- Mouth and ears
- Neck
- Thorax
  - Breasts
  - Heart
  - Lungs
- Abdomen
- Lower limbs
  - Oedema
  - Circulation
  - Locomotor function and neurology
- Upper limbs
  - Movement and neurology
- Cranial nerves, including fundoscopy
- Blood pressure
- Temperature
- Height and weight
- Urinalysis

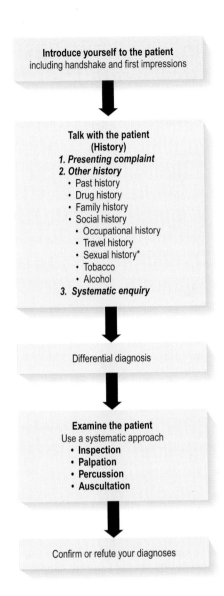

* if appropriate

Fig. 3.1 Overall plan of clinical assessment.

3.3 Information from a handshake

Features	Diagnosis
Cold, sweaty hands	Anxiety
Cold, dry hands	Raynaud's phenomenon
Hot, sweaty hands	Hyperthyroidism
Large, fleshy, sweaty hands	Acromegaly
Dry, coarse skin	Regular water exposure Manual occupation Hypothyroidism
Delayed relaxation of grip	Myotonic dystrophy
Deformed hands/fingers	Trauma Rheumatoid arthritis Dupuytren's contracture

3.4 Abnormal facial expressions

Features	Diagnosis
Poverty of expression	Parkinsonism
Startled expression	Hyperthyroidism
Apathy, with poverty of expression and poor eye contact	Depression
Apathy, with pale and puffy skin	Hypothyroidism
Lugubrious expression with bilateral ptosis	Myotonic dystrophy
Agitated expression	Anxiety Hyperthyroidism Hypomania

The handshake

Introduce yourself and shake hands. This may provide diagnostic clues (Box 3.3). Greet your patient in a friendly but professional manner. Note if his right hand works; in patients with a right hemiparesis you may need to shake his left hand. Avoid too firm a grip, particularly in patients with arthritis.

Facial expression and general demeanour

Ask yourself:
• 'Does this patient look well?'
Facial expression and eye-to-eye contact reflect physical and psychological well-being (Box 3.4), but in some cultures direct eye-to-eye contact is impolite. Patients who deliberately self-harm may cover their face with their hands or bedclothes and be reluctant to communicate. Actively recognise the features of anxiety, fear, anger or grief, and explore the reasons for these. Some patients conceal anxieties and depression with inappropriate cheerfulness.

Clothing

Clothing gives clues about personality, state of mind and social circumstances. Young people wearing dirty clothes may have problems with alcohol or drug addiction, or be making a personal statement. Unkempt elderly patients with faecal or urinary soiling may be unable to look after themselves because of physical disease, immobility, dementia or other mental illness. Anorectic patients wear baggy clothing to cover weight loss. Consider blood-borne viral infections, e.g. hepatitis B or C, in patients with tattoos. A MedicAlert bracelet (Fig. 3.3) or necklace highlights important medical conditions and treatments.

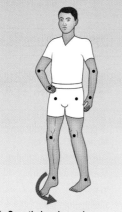

A) Spastic hemiparesis
One arm held immobile and close to the side with elbow, wrist and fingers flexed. Leg extended with plantar flexion of the foot. On walking, the foot is dragged, scraping the toe in a circle (circumduction). Caused by upper motor neurone lesion, stroke.

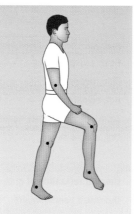

B) Steppage gait
Foot is dragged or lifted high and slapped onto the floor. Unable to walk on the heels. Caused by foot drop owing to lower motor neurone lesion.

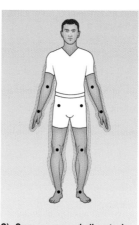

C) Sensory or cerebellar ataxia
Gait is unsteady and wide based. Feet are thrown forward and outward and brought down on the heels.
In sensory ataxia, the patient watches the ground. With eyes closed, he cannot stand steadily (positive Romberg sign).
In cerebellar ataxia, turns are difficult and patients cannot stand steadily with feet together whether eyes open or closed. Caused by polyneuropathy or posterior column damage, e.g. syphilis.

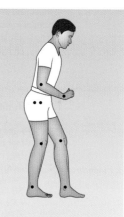

D) Parkinsonian gait
Posture is stooped with head and neck forwards. Arms are flexed at elbows and wrists. Little arm swing. Steps are short and shuffling and patient is slow in getting started (festinant gait). Caused by lesion in the basal ganglia.

Fig. 3.2 Abnormalities of gait.

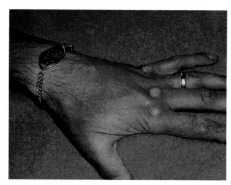

Fig. 3.3 MedicAlert bracelet.

Complexion

Facial colour depends on oxyhaemoglobin, reduced haemoglobin, melanin and carotene. Unusual skin colours are due to abnormal pigments, e.g. the sallow yellow-brownish tinge in chronic kidney disease. A bluish tinge is produced by abnormal haemoglobins, e.g. sulphaemoglobin or methaemoglobin, or by drugs, e.g. dapsone. Some drug metabolites cause striking abnormal coloration of the skin, particularly in areas exposed to light, e.g. mepacrine (yellow), amiodarone (bluish-grey) and phenothiazines (slate-grey) (Fig. 3.4).

Haemoglobin

Untanned European skin is pink due to the red pigment oxyhaemoglobin in the superficial capillary–venous plexuses. A pale complexion may be misleading but can suggest anaemia (Box 3.5). The pallor of anaemia is best seen in the mucous membranes of the conjunctivae, lips and tongue and in the nail beds (Fig. 3.5). Angular stomatitis (Fig. 3.19B) and koilonychia (spoon-shaped) nails (Fig. 4.15F) can be features of iron deficiency anaemia. Ask about dyspepsia, change in bowel habit and heavy menstrual periods if you are investigating anaemia.

Pallor from vasoconstriction occurs during a faint or from fear. Vasodilatation may produce a pink complexion, even in anaemia. Perimenopausal women may have transient pink flushing, particularly of the face, due to vasodilatation, which may be accompanied by sweating. Facial plethora is caused by raised haemoglobin concentration with elevated haematocrit (polycythaemia) (Box 3.6). Blue sclerae are a sensitive indicator of iron deficiency anaemia.

Cyanosis

Cyanosis is a blue discoloration of the skin and mucous membranes that occurs when the absolute concentration of deoxygenated haemoglobin is increased (Box 3.7). It can be difficult to detect, particularly in black and Asian patients.

3

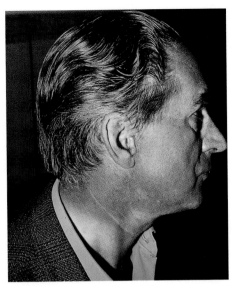
Fig. 3.4 Phenothiazine-induced pigmentation.

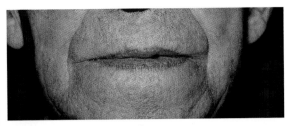
Fig. 3.6 Central cyanosis of the lips.

3.6 Types of polycythaemia

Primary

- Polycythaemia rubra vera

Secondary

- Hypoxia
  - Chronic lung disease
  - Cyanotic congenital heart disease
  - Altitude
- Excess erythropoietin
  - Adult polycystic kidney disease
  - Renal cancer
  - Ovarian cancer

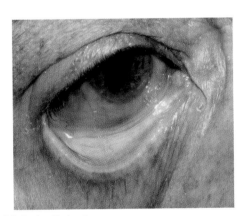
Fig. 3.5 Conjunctival pallor.

EBE 3.7 Central cyanosis

The minimum arterial level of deoxyhaemoglobin required to detect central cyanosis is 2.38 g/dl. The mean value for detection is 3.48 ± 0.55 g/dl.

Barnett HB, Holland JG, Josenhans WT. When does central cyanosis become detectable? Clin Invest Med 1982;5:39–43.
McGee S. Evidence based physical diagnosis, 2nd edn. St Louis, MO: Saunders, Elsevier, 2007, p. 86.

Central cyanosis

This is seen at the lips and tongue (Fig. 3.6). It corresponds to an arterial oxygen saturation (SpO_2) of <90% and usually indicates underlying cardiac or pulmonary disease. Anaemic or hypovolaemic patients rarely have central cyanosis because severe hypoxia is required to produce the necessary concentration of deoxygenated haemoglobin. Conversely patients with polycythaemia can become cyanosed at normal arterial oxygen saturation.

Peripheral cyanosis

This occurs in the hands, feet or ears, usually when they are cold. In healthy people it occurs in cold conditions when prolonged peripheral capillary flow allows greater oxygen extraction and hence increased levels of deoxyhaemoglobin. In combination with central cyanosis, it is most often seen with poor peripheral circulation due to shock, heart failure, vascular disease and venous obstruction, e.g. deep vein thrombosis.

3.5 Types of anaemia

Microcytic (MCV < 80 fl)

- Chronic blood loss
- Iron deficiency
- Anaemia of chronic disease
- Thalassaemia
- Sideroblastic anaemia

Macrocytic (MCV > 96 fl)

- Megaloblastic marrow due to vitamin B_{12} or folate deficiency
- Excess alcohol
- Haemolytic disorders
- Liver disease
- Hypothyroidism

Normocytic (MCV 80–96 fl)

- Acute blood loss
- Anaemia of chronic disease
- Chronic kidney disease
- Connective tissue disorders
- Marrow infiltration

MCV, mean corpuscular volume.

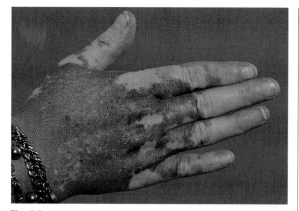

Fig. 3.7 Vitiligo.

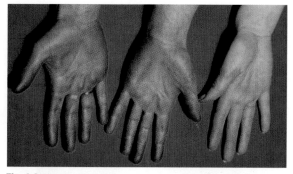

Fig. 3.8 Hypercarotenaemia.

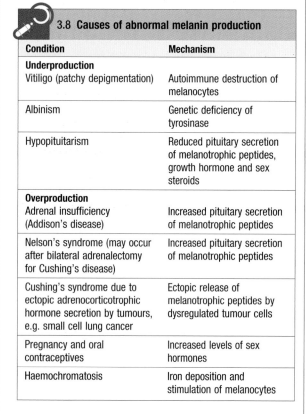

3.8 Causes of abnormal melanin production

Condition	Mechanism
Underproduction	
Vitiligo (patchy depigmentation)	Autoimmune destruction of melanocytes
Albinism	Genetic deficiency of tyrosinase
Hypopituitarism	Reduced pituitary secretion of melanotrophic peptides, growth hormone and sex steroids
Overproduction	
Adrenal insufficiency (Addison's disease)	Increased pituitary secretion of melanotrophic peptides
Nelson's syndrome (may occur after bilateral adrenalectomy for Cushing's disease)	Increased pituitary secretion of melanotrophic peptides
Cushing's syndrome due to ectopic adrenocorticotrophic hormone secretion by tumours, e.g. small cell lung cancer	Ectopic release of melanotrophic peptides by dysregulated tumour cells
Pregnancy and oral contraceptives	Increased levels of sex hormones
Haemochromatosis	Iron deposition and stimulation of melanocytes

Melanin

Skin colour is greatly influenced by the deposition of melanin (Box 3.8).

Vitiligo

This chronic condition produces bilateral symmetrical depigmentation, commonly of the face, neck and extensor aspects of the limbs, resulting in irregular pale patches of skin. It is associated with autoimmune diseases, e.g. diabetes mellitus, thyroid and adrenal disorders, and pernicious anaemia (Fig. 3.7).

Albinism

This is an inherited disorder in which patients have little or no melanin in their skin or hair. The amount of

EBE 3.9 Jaundice

Clinical detection of jaundice depends upon the level of serum bilirubin, ambient lighting and colour perception of the examining clinician: 70–80% of observers will detect jaundice if levels are 43–51 umol/L, 83% at 171 umol/L and 96% if levels are >256 umol/L.

Hung OL, Kwan NS, Cole AE et al. Evaluation of the physician's ability to recognise the presence or absence of anaemia, fever and jaundice. Acad. Emerg. Med. 2000: 7; 146–156
Ruiz MA, Saab S, Rickman LS. The clinical detection of scleral icterus: Observations of multiple examiners. Mil. Med. 1997: 162; 560–563

pigment in the iris varies; some individuals have reddish eyes, but most have blue.

Overproduction of melanin

This can be due to excess of the pituitary hormone, adrenocorticotrophic hormone, as in adrenal insufficiency. It produces brown pigmentation, particularly in skin creases, recent scars, sites overlying bony prominences, areas exposed to pressure, e.g. belts and bra straps, and the mucous membranes of the lips and mouth, where it results in muddy brown patches (Fig. 5.17A–C).

Pregnancy and oral contraceptives

These may produce chloasma (blotchy pigmentation of the face). Pregnancy increases pigmentation of the areolae, axillae, genital skin and linea alba (producing a dark line in the midline of the lower abdomen-linea nigra).

Carotene

Hypercarotenaemia occurs in people who eat large amounts of raw carrots and tomatoes, and in hypothyroidism. A yellowish discoloration is seen on the face, palms and soles, but not the sclerae, and this distinguishes it from jaundice (Fig. 3.8).

Bilirubin

Jaundice is detectable when serum bilirubin concentration is elevated and the sclerae, mucous membranes and skin become yellow (Fig. 8.8 and Box 3.9). In longstanding jaundice a green colour develops in the sclerae and skin due to biliverdin. Patients with pernicious anaemia have a lemon-yellow complexion due to a combination of mild jaundice and anaemia.

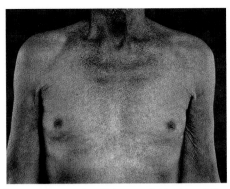

Fig. 3.9 Haemochromatosis with increased skin pigmentation.

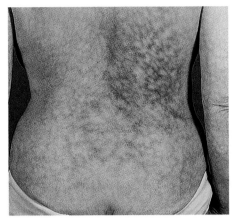

Fig. 3.10 Erythema ab igne.

Iron

Haemochromatosis increases skin pigmentation due to iron deposition and increased melanin production (Fig. 3.9). Iron deposition in the pancreas causes diabetes mellitus and the combination with skin pigmentation is called 'bronzed diabetes'.

Haemosiderin, a haemoglobin breakdown product, is deposited in the skin of the lower legs following extravasation of blood into subcutaneous tissues from venous insufficiency. Local deposition of haemosiderin (erythema ab igne or 'granny's tartan') occurs with heat damage to the skin from sitting too close to a fire or from applying local heat, such as a hot water bottle, to the site of pain (Fig. 3.10).

Easy bruising

Approximately 20% of patients complain they bruise easily (Fig. 3.24). It is more common in the elderly because of increased skin and subcutaneous tissue fragility and a greater likelihood of increased episodes of minor trauma. A lifelong tendency suggests an inherited disorder whereas recent onset suggests an acquired disorder. Enquire if there are other family members with a similar problem (bleeding disorder), what drugs the patient is receiving, e.g. anticoagulants, corticosteroids and ask about recurrent nose bleeds (epistaxis) and heavy menstrual periods (menorrhagia).

Odours

Everybody has a natural smell, produced by bacteria acting on apocrine sweat; this may be altered by antiperspirants, deodorants and perfume. Excessive sweating and poor personal hygiene increase body odour and may be compounded by dirty or soiled clothing and stale urine. Excessive body odour occurs in:

- extreme old age or infirmity
- major mental illness
- alcohol or drug misuse
- physical disability preventing normal hygiene
- severe learning difficulties.

Tobacco's characteristic lingering smell pervades skin, hair and clothing. Marijuana (cannabis) can also be identified by smell. The smell of alcohol on a patient's breath, particularly in the morning, may suggest an alcohol problem.

Halitosis (bad breath) is caused by decomposing food wedged between the teeth, gingivitis, stomatitis, atrophic rhinitis and tumours of the nasal passages.

Other characteristic odours include:

- fetor hepaticus: stale 'mousy' smell of the volatile amine, dimethylsulphide, in patients with liver failure
- ketones: a sweet smell (like nail varnish remover) due to acetone in diabetic ketoacidosis or starvation
- uraemic fetor: fishy or ammoniacal smell on the breath in uraemia
- putrid or fetid smell of chronic anaerobic suppuration due to bronchiectasis or lung abscess
- foul-smelling belching in patients with gastric outlet obstruction
- strong faecal smell in patients with gastrocolic fistula.

Spot diagnoses

Many disorders have characteristic facial features (Fig. 3.11). Osteogenesis imperfecta is an autosomal dominant condition causing fragile and brittle bones in which the sclerae are blue due to abnormal collagen formation. In systemic sclerosis the skin is thickened and tight, causing loss of the normal wrinkles and skin folds, 'beaking' of the nose, and narrowing and puckering of the mouth. Hereditary haemorrhagic telangiectasia is an autosomal dominant condition associated with small dilated capillaries or terminal arteries (telangiectasia) on the lips and tongue. Dystrophia myotonica is an autosomal dominant condition with characteristic features of frontal balding, bilateral ptosis and delayed relaxation of grip after a handshake.

Major chromosomal abnormalities

There are several genetic or chromosomal syndromes that you should easily recognise on first contact with the patient.

Down's syndrome (trisomy 21 – 47XX/XY + 21)

Down's syndrome is characterised by typical physical features, including short stature, a small head with flat

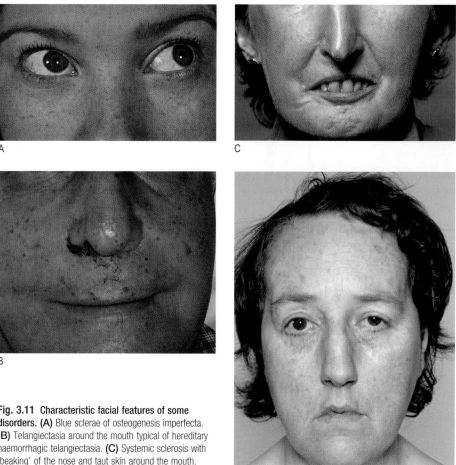

Fig. 3.11 Characteristic facial features of some disorders. (A) Blue sclerae of osteogenesis imperfecta. **(B)** Telangiectasia around the mouth typical of hereditary haemorrhagic telangiectasia. **(C)** Systemic sclerosis with 'beaking' of the nose and taut skin around the mouth. **(D)** Dystrophia myotonica with frontal balding and bilateral ptosis.

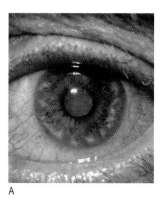

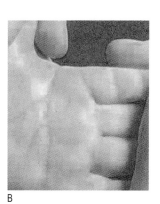

Fig. 3.12 Down's syndrome. (A) Brushfield's spots: grey-white areas of depigmentation in the iris. **(B)** Single palmar crease.

occiput, upslanting palpebral fissures, epicanthic folds, a small nose with a poorly developed bridge and small ears. Grey-white areas of depigmentation are seen in the iris (Brushfield's spots; Fig. 3.12A). The hands are broad with a single palmar crease (Fig. 3.12B), the fingers are short and the little finger is curved.

Turner's syndrome (45XO)

Turner's syndrome is due to loss of a sex chromosome. It occurs in 1:2500 live female births and is a cause of delayed puberty in girls. Typical features include short stature, webbing of the neck, small chin, low-set ears, low hairline, short fourth finger, increased carrying angle at the elbows and widely spaced nipples ('shield-like chest').

Achondroplasia

This is an autosomal dominant disease of cartilage caused by mutation of the fibroblast growth factor gene. Although the trunk is of normal length, the limbs are

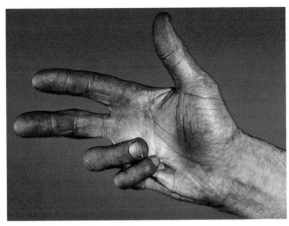

Fig. 3.13 Dupuytren's contracture.

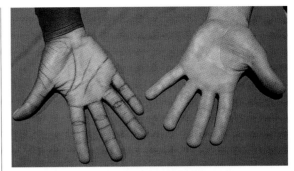

Fig. 3.14 **Normal palms.** African (left) and European (right).

3

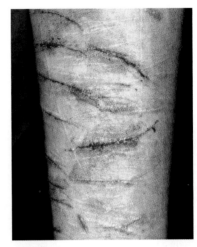

Fig. 3.15 **Self-cutting.**

very short and broad. The vault of the skull is enlarged, the face is small and the bridge of the nose is flat.

THE HANDS

Examination sequence

- Inspect the dorsal and then palmar aspects of both hands.
- Note changes in the:
  - skin
  - nails
  - soft tissues (evidence of muscle wasting)
  - tendons
  - joints.
- Feel the temperature.

Abnormal findings

Deformity

Deformity may be diagnostic: for example, the flexed hand and arm of hemiplegia or radial nerve palsy, and ulnar deviation at the metacarpophalangeal joints in longstanding rheumatoid arthritis (Fig. 14.34). Dupuytren's contracture is a thickening of the palmar fascia causing fixed flexion deformity and usually affecting the little and ring fingers (Fig. 3.13). Arachnodactyly (long thin fingers) are typical of Marfan's syndrome (Fig. 3.28B). Trauma is the most common cause of hand deformity.

Colour

Look for cyanosis in the nail bed and tobacco staining of the fingers (Fig. 7.8). Examine the skin creases for pigmentation, although pigmentation is normal in many non-European races (Fig. 3.14).

Temperature

In a cool climate the temperature of the patient's hand is a good guide to peripheral perfusion. In chronic obstructive pulmonary disease, the hands may be cyanosed due to reduced arterial oxygen saturation but warm due to vasodilatation from elevated arterial carbon dioxide levels. In heart failure the hands are often cold and cyanosed because of vasoconstriction in response to a low cardiac output. If they are warm, heart failure may be due to a high-output state, such as hyperthyroidism.

Skin

The dorsum of the hand is smooth and hairless in children and in adult hypogonadism. Manual work may produce specific callosities due to pressure at characteristic sites. Disuse results in soft, smooth skin, as seen on the soles of the feet in bed-bound patients.

Look at the flexor surfaces of the wrists and forearms. Note any venepuncture marks of intravenous drug use and linear (usually transverse), multiple wounds or scars from deliberate self-harm (Figs 3.15 and 3.16). Look carefully at the fingernails, which can provide useful diagnostic clues (Fig. 4.15).

Finger clubbing

Clubbing is painless soft-tissue swelling of the terminal phalanges. The enlargement increases convexity of the nail. It may be produced by growth factors from

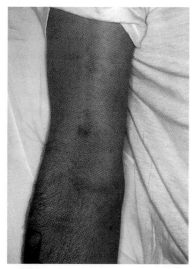

Fig. 3.16 The linear marks of intravenous injection at the right elbow.

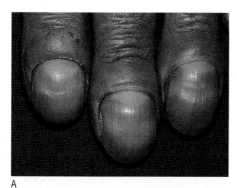

A

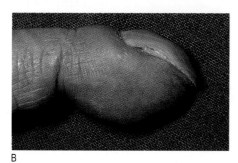

B

Fig. 3.17 Clubbing. (A) Anterior view. **(B)** Lateral view.

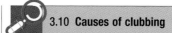

3.10 Causes of clubbing

Congenital or familial (5–10%)
Acquired
Thoracic (~70%)
Lung cancer
Chronic suppurative conditions
Bronchiectasis
Lung abscess
Empyema
Cystic fibrosis
Mesothelioma
Fibroma
Pulmonary fibrosis
Cardiovascular
Cyanotic congenital heart disease
Infective endocarditis
Arteriovenous shunts and aneurysms
Gastrointestinal
Cirrhosis
Inflammatory bowel disease
Coeliac disease
Others
Thyrotoxicosis (thyroid acropatchy)

Examination sequence

- Look across the nail bed from the side of each finger. Observe the distal phalanges, nail and nail bed.
- Measure the anteroposterior distance (the interphalangeal depth) at the level of the distal interphalangeal joint (Fig. 3.18A). Repeat at the level of the nail bed (Fig. 3.18B).
- Measure the nail bed angle (Fig. 3.18B).
- Place the nails of corresponding fingers back to back and look for a visible gap between the nail beds – Schamroth's window sign (Fig. 3.18C).
- Place your thumbs under the pulp of the distal phalanx and use your index fingers alternately to see if you can feel movement of the nail on the nail bed. This is fluctuation. (Fig. 3.18A).

Abnormal findings

Finger clubbing is present if:

- the interphalangeal depth ratio (*B/A* in Fig. 3.18B) is >1
- the normal nail-fold angle (CBA upper digit) is <180° while in clubbing this (DBA lower digit) is >190° (Fig. 3.18B)
- Schamroth's window sign is absent (Fig. 3.18C).

Increased nail bed fluctuation may be present, but its presence is subjective and less discriminatory than the above features.

Joints

Arthritis frequently involves the small joints of the hands. Rheumatoid arthritis typically affects metacarpophalangeal and proximal interphalangeal joints (Fig. 14.34), and osteoarthritis and psoriatic arthropathy affect the distal interphalangeal joints (Fig. 14.12).

megakaryocytes and platelets lodged in nail bed capillaries stimulating vascular connective tissue (Fig. 3.17).

It is an important sign of major diseases, although it may be congenital (Box 3.10). It usually takes weeks or months to develop, and may disappear if the underlying condition is cured. Clubbing usually affects the fingers symmetrically, but may involve the toes. Unilateral clubbing can be caused by proximal vascular conditions, e.g. arteriovenous shunts for dialysis. Autoimmune hyperthyroidism may be associated with thyroid acropachy – clubbing which is more pronounced on the radial side of the hand (Fig. 5.3C).

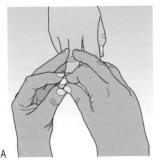
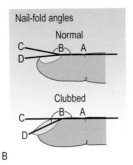
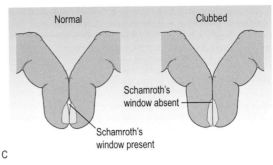

Fig. 3.18 Examining for finger clubbing. (A) Testing for fluctuation of the nail bed. **(B)** Nail fold angles. **(C)** Schamroth's window sign.

3

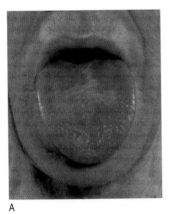
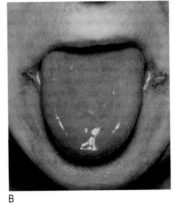
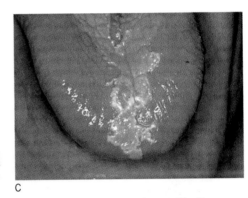

Fig. 3.19 The tongue as a diagnostic aid. (A) Large tongue (macroglossia) of acromegaly. **(B)** Smooth red tongue and angular stomatitis of iron deficiency. **(C)** Leukoplakia.

Muscles

Small muscle wasting of the hands is common in rheumatoid arthritis, producing 'dorsal guttering' of the hands. In carpal tunnel syndrome, median nerve compression leads to wasting of the thenar muscles (Fig. 14.29), and cervical spondylosis with nerve root entrapment causes small muscle wasting.

THE TONGUE

Examination sequence

- Ask the patient to put out his tongue.
- Look at the size, shape, movements, colour and surface (Fig. 3.19).

Normal findings

Tongue furring is normal and common in heavy smokers

Geographic tongue describes red rings and lines which change over days or weeks on the surface of the tongue. It is usually not significant but can be due to riboflavin (vitamin B$_2$) deficiency

Abnormal findings

- Tremor can be due to anxiety, thyrotoxicosis, delirium tremens or parkinsonism.

- Fasciculation (irregular ripples or twitching of the tongue) occurs in lower motor neurone disorders, e.g. motor neurone disease.
- Macroglossia (enlargement of the tongue) may occur in acromegaly, amyloidosis or tumour infiltration.
- White patches that may be scraped off the tongue are due to the fungal yeast, *Candida* (oral thrush). Common causes include inhaled steroids, immune deficiency, e.g. HIV and terminal illness.
- Glossitis is a smooth reddened tongue due to atrophy of the papillae. It is common in alcoholics, in nutritional deficiencies of iron, folate and vitamin B$_{12}$, and in 30% of patients with coeliac disease. Glossitis may cause a burning sensation over the tongue but usually a painful tongue is a symptom of anxiety or depression.
- Leukoplakia is a thickened white patch that cannot be scraped off the tongue. It may be premalignant.

LUMPS OR SWELLINGS

Patients often present with a lump they have just found. This does not necessarily mean that it has developed recently. Ask about any changes since they noticed it and whether there are any associated features, e.g. pain, tenderness or colour change. During examination you may find a lump the patient is unaware of.

Size

Accurately measure the size of any lump (preferably using callipers), so that with time you can detect significant change.

Position

The origin of some lumps may be obvious, e.g. in the breast, thyroid or parotid gland; in other sites, e.g. the abdomen, this is less clear. Multiple lumps may occur in neurofibromatosis (Fig. 3.20A), skin metastases, lipomatosis and lymphomas.

Attachments

Lymphatic obstruction causes fixation of the skin with fine dimpling at the opening of hair follicles that resembles orange peel (peau d'orange) (Fig. 10.6).

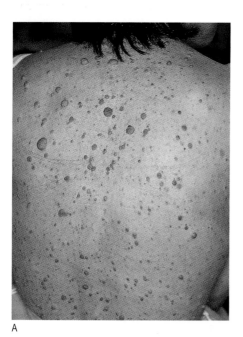

A

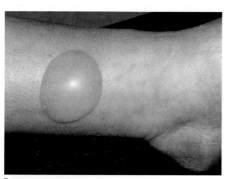

B

Fig. 3.20 Lumps and swellings. (A) Neurofibromatosis. **(B)** Blister on leg.

This is common in malignant disease when attachment to deeper structures, e.g. underlying muscle, may occur.

Consistency

The consistency of a lump can vary from soft to 'stony' hard. Very hard swellings are usually malignant, calcified or dense fibrous tissue. Fluctuation indicates the presence of fluid, e.g. abscess, cyst, blister or soft encapsulated tumours, e.g. lipoma.

Edge

The edge or margin may be well delineated or ill defined, regular or irregular, sharp or rounded. The margins of enlarged organs, e.g. thyroid gland, liver, spleen or kidney, can usually be defined more clearly than those of inflammatory or malignant masses. An indefinite margin suggests infiltrating malignancy, in contrast to the clearly defined edge of a benign tumour.

Surface and shape

The surface and shape of a swelling can be characteristic. In the abdomen examples include an enlarged spleen or liver, a distended bladder or the fundus of the uterus in pregnancy. The surface may be smooth or irregular, e.g. the surface of the liver is smooth in acute hepatitis but is often nodular in metastatic disease.

Pulsations, thrills and bruits

Arterial swellings (aneurysms) and highly vascular tumours are pulsatile (they move in time with the arterial pulse). Other swellings may transmit pulsation if they lie over a major blood vessel. If the blood flow through a lump is increased, a systolic murmur (bruit) may be auscultated and, if loud enough, a thrill may be palpable. Bruits are also heard over arterial aneurysms and arteriovenous malformations.

Inflammation

Redness, tenderness and warmth suggest inflammation.
- Redness (erythema): the skin over acute inflammatory lesions is usually red due to vasodilatation. In haematomas the pigment from extravasated blood may produce the range of colours in a bruise (ecchymosis).
- Tenderness: inflammatory lumps, e.g. boil or abscess, are usually tender or painful, while non-inflamed swellings are not: lipomas, skin metastases and neurofibromas are characteristically painless.
- Warmth: inflammatory lumps and some tumours, especially if rapidly growing, may feel warm due to increased blood flow.

Transillumination

In a darkened room, press the lighted end of a pen torch on to one side of the swelling. A cystic swelling, e.g. testicular hydrocoele, will light up if the fluid is translucent, providing the covering tissues are not too thick (Fig. 15.9 and Box 3.11).

Examination sequence

■ Inspect the lump, noting any change in colour or texture of the overlying skin.
■ Define the site and shape of the lump.
■ Measure its size and record the findings diagrammatically.
■ Gently palpate for tenderness or change in skin temperature.
■ Feel the lump for a few seconds to determine if it is pulsatile.
■ Assess the consistency, surface texture and margins of the lump.
■ Try to pick up an overlying fold of skin to assess whether the lump is fixed to the skin.
■ Try to move the lump in different planes relative to the surrounding tissues to see if it is fixed to deeper structures.
■ Compress the lump on one side; see and feel if a bulge occurs on the opposite side (fluctuation). Confirm the fluctuation in two

planes. Fluctuation usually indicates that the lump contains fluid, although some soft lipomas can feel fluctuant.
■ Auscultate for vascular bruits.
■ Transilluminate.

3.11 Features to note in any lump or swelling (SPACESPIT)	
• **S**ize	• **P**ulsation, thrills and bruits
• **P**osition	• **I**nflammation
• **A**ttachments	• Redness
• **C**onsistency	• Tenderness
• **E**dge	• Warmth
• **S**urface and shape	• **T**ransillumination

THE LYMPH NODES

Lymph nodes may be palpable in normal people, especially in the submandibular, axilla and groin regions (Fig. 3.21). Distinguish between normal and pathological nodes. Pathological lymphadenopathy may be local or generalised, and is of diagnostic and prognostic significance in the staging of lymphoproliferative and other malignancies.

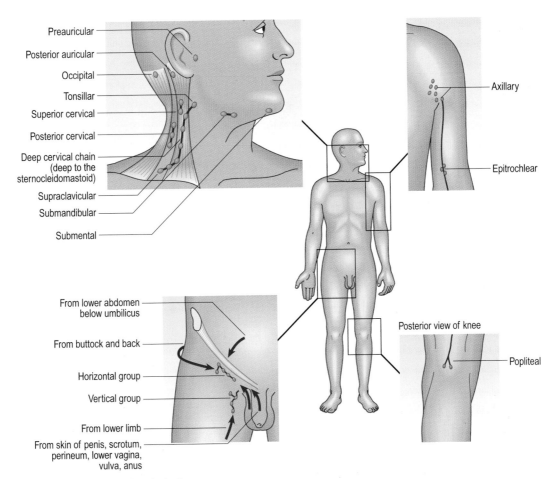

Preauricular
Posterior auricular
Occipital
Tonsillar
Superior cervical
Posterior cervical
Deep cervical chain (deep to the sternocleidomastoid)
Supraclavicular
Submandibular
Submental

Axillary
Epitrochlear

From lower abdomen below umbilicus
From buttock and back
Horizontal group
Vertical group
From lower limb
From skin of penis, scrotum, perineum, lower vagina, vulva, anus

Posterior view of knee
Popliteal

Fig. 3.21 Distribution of palpable lymph glands.

Size

Normal nodes in adults are <0.5 cm in diameter.

Attachments

Lymph nodes fixed to deep structures or skin suggest malignancy.

Consistency

Normal nodes feel soft. In Hodgkin's disease they are characteristically 'rubbery', in tuberculosis they may be 'matted', and in metastatic cancer they feel hard.

Tenderness

Acute viral or bacterial infection, including infectious mononucleosis, dental sepsis and tonsillitis, causes tender, variably enlarged lymph nodes.

Examination sequence

General principles
- Inspect for visible lymphadenopathy.
- Palpate one side at a time using the fingers of each hand in turn.

- Compare with the nodes on the contralateral side.
- Assess:
  - site
  - size.
- Determine whether the node is fixed to:
  - surrounding and deep structures
  - skin.
- Check consistency.
- Check for tenderness.

Cervical nodes
- Examine the cervical and axillary nodes with the patient sitting.
- From behind, examine the submental, submandibular, preauricular, tonsillar, supraclavicular and deep cervical nodes in the anterior triangle of the neck (Fig. 3.22A).
- Palpate for the scalene nodes by placing your index finger between the sternocleidomastoid muscle and clavicle. Ask the patient to tilt his head to the same side and press firmly down towards the first rib (Fig. 3.22B).
- From the front of the patient, palpate the posterior triangles, up the back of the neck and the posterior auricular and occipital nodes (Fig. 3.22C).

Axillary nodes
- From the patient's front or side, palpate the right axilla with your left hand and vice versa (Fig. 3.23A).
- Gently place your fingertips into the apex of the axilla and then draw them downwards, feeling the medial, anterior and posterior axillary walls in turn.

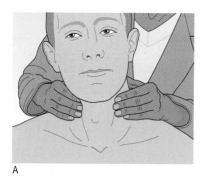
A

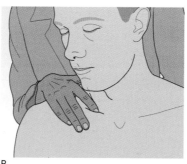
B

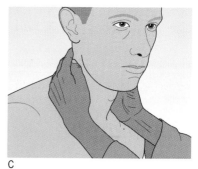
C

Fig. 3.22 Palpation of the cervical glands. (A) Examine the glands of the anterior triangle from behind, using both hands. **(B)** Examine for the scalene nodes from behind with your index finger in the angle between the sternocleidomastoid muscle and the clavicle. **(C)** Examine glands in the posterior triangle from the front.

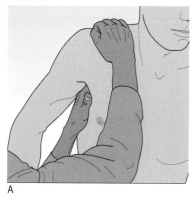
A

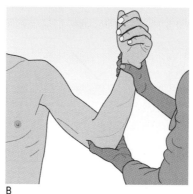
B

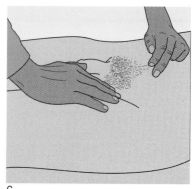
C

Fig. 3.23 Palpation of the axillary, epitrochlear and inguinal glands. (A) Examination for right axillary lymphadenopathy. **(B)** Examination of the left epitrochlear glands. **(C)** Examination of the left inguinal glands.

Epitrochlear nodes

- Support the patient's right wrist with your left hand, hold his partially flexed elbow with your right hand and use your thumb to feel for the epitrochlear node. Examine the left epitrochlear node with your left thumb (Fig. 3.23B).

Inguinal nodes

- Examine for the inguinal and popliteal nodes with the patient lying down.
- Palpate over the horizontal chain, which lies just below the inguinal ligament, and then over the vertical chain along the line of the saphenous vein (Fig. 3.23C).

Abnormal findings

If you find localised lymphadenopathy, examine the areas which drain to that site. Infection commonly causes lymphadenitis (localised tender lymphadenopathy); e.g. in acute tonsillitis the submandibular nodes are involved. If the lymphadenopathy is non-tender, look for a malignant cause, tuberculosis or features of HIV infection. Generalised lymphadenopathy occurs in a number of conditions (Box 3.12). Examine for enlargement of the liver and spleen, and for other haematological features, such as purpura (bruising under the skin), which can be large (ecchymoses) or pinpoint (petechiae; Fig. 3.24).

3.12 Important common causes of lymphadenopathy

Generalised

- Viral: Epstein–Barr virus (glandular fever or Burkitt's lymphoma), cytomegalovirus, human immunodeficiency virus
- Bacterial: brucellosis, syphilis
- Protozoal: toxoplasmosis
- Malignancy: lymphoma, acute or chronic lymphocytic leukaemia
- Inflammatory: rheumatoid arthritis, systemic lupus erythematosus, sarcoidosis

Localised

- Infective: acute or chronic, bacterial or viral
- Malignancy: lymphoma

WEIGHT AND HEIGHT

Weight is an important indicator of general health and nutrition. Serial weight measurements are useful in monitoring acutely ill patients and those with chronic disease. Serial height is helpful in monitoring growth in children and osteoporotic vertebral collapse in the elderly.

Record the body mass index (BMI), rather than weight alone, as it is independent of the patient's height. BMI is calculated from the formula: $weight/height^2$ (using metric units, kg/m^2). Obesity is defined by BMI and race (Box 3.13).

BMI, however, does not describe body fat distribution and excess intra-abdominal fat is an independent predictor of hypertension, insulin resistance, type 2 diabetes mellitus and coronary artery disease. Waist circumference correlates better with visceral fat and indirectly measures central adiposity. Health risk is increased when waist circumference exceeds 94 cm (37 inches) for men and 80 cm (32 inches) for women. Waist:hip ratio is strongly related to risk of coronary artery disease. 'Pear shape' and a waist:hip ratio of ≤0.8 in females or <0.9 in males have a good prognosis, whereas 'apple-shaped' subjects with a greater waist:hip ratio have an increased risk of coronary artery disease and the 'metabolic syndrome' (Fig. 3.25).

3.13 The relationship between body mass index (BMI), nutritional status and ethnic group

	BMI non-Asian	BMI Asian
Severe malnutrition	<16	<16
Underweight	<18.5	<18.5
Normal	18.5–24.9	18.5–22.9
Overweight	25–29.9	23–24.9
Obese	30–39.9	25–29.9
Morbidly obese	≥40	≥30

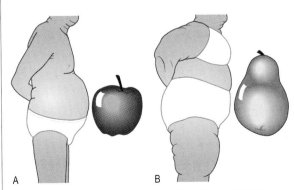

A   B

Fig. 3.25 Abdominal obesity and generalised obesity. (A) Abdominal obesity (apple shape). **(B)** Generalised obesity, where fat deposition is mainly on the hips and thighs (pear shape).

Fig. 3.24 Petechiae.

Examination sequence

- Note any abnormalities in stature or body proportions,
- Measure height using a vertical scale with a rigid, adjustable arm piece. In the serial assessment of growth in children and teenagers, measure height to the nearest millimetre using a calibrated stadiometer (Fig. 15.20).
- The patient should stand erect and be weighed in his indoor clothing without shoes. Calculate and record BMI.
- Look for abnormal fat distribution.
- Measure the waist with the patient standing at the level equidistant between the costal margin and iliac crest. The measurement should record the maximum diameter, so measure over any abdominal fat and not under it.
- Look for any evidence of malnutrition or specific vitamin deficiencies.

Nutritional status

Illness may produce profound changes in an individual's nutritional requirements, appetite and ability to eat. Malnutrition delays recovery from illness and surgery, and delays wound healing. Record BMI initially and repeat this at least weekly in an acute setting, and monthly in outpatients or in the community, to monitor nutritional status.

Vitamin deficiencies

Vitamins are organic substances that have key roles in certain metabolic pathways. They are fat-soluble (vitamins A, D, E and K) or water-soluble (vitamins of the B-complex group and vitamin C).

Vitamin deficiencies occur in older people and alcoholic patients, and are common in developing countries. Folate (vitamin B_9) deficiency is usually due to poor intake and causes macrocytic anaemia and glossitis. Vitamin B_{12} deficiency is usually caused by the autoimmune disorder pernicious anaemia but can occur in vegans, small-bowel overgrowth, or ileal disease or resection. Vitamin C deficiency (scurvy) is less common and produces extensive bruising, particularly in the elderly living alone without access to fresh fruit and vegetables (Fig. 3.26). Those with alcohol dependency may eat poorly and also become deficient in vitamin B_1 (thiamine). Small-bowel malabsorption and liver and biliary tract disease can lead to deficiency of fat-soluble vitamins (Box 3.14).

Abnormal findings

Obesity

Obesity is a major worldwide health problem, largely as a result of changes in lifestyle. It is caused by excess calorie intake associated with inadequate exercise. Rarely, it is secondary to hypothyroidism, Cushing's syndrome, Prader–Willi syndrome or drugs (Box 3.15). It is associated with hypertension, hyperlipidaemia, type 2 diabetes mellitus, gallbladder disease and sleep apnoea (Fig. 3.27). Increased BMI is associated with several malignancies, particularly oesophageal and

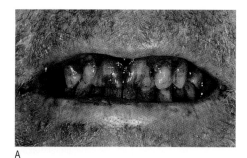

A

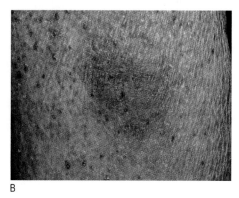

B

Fig. 3.26 Scurvy. (A) Bleeding gums. **(B)** Bruising and perifollicular haemorrhages.

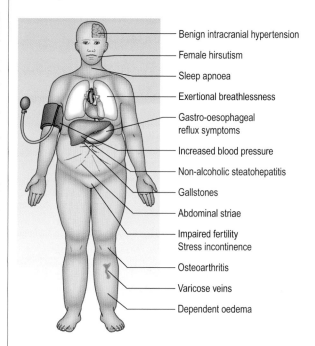

- Benign intracranial hypertension
- Female hirsutism
- Sleep apnoea
- Exertional breathlessness
- Gastro-oesophageal reflux symptoms
- Increased blood pressure
- Non-alcoholic steatohepatitis
- Gallstones
- Abdominal striae
- Impaired fertility Stress incontinence
- Osteoarthritis
- Varicose veins
- Dependent oedema

Fig. 3.27 Complications of obesity.

renal cancer in both sexes, thyroid and colon cancer in men and endometrial and gallbladder cancer in women. Obesity reduces life expectancy by about 7 years, about the same as a lifetime of heavy smoking.

Weight loss

Weight loss is important and may be due to:
- reduced food intake from a poor appetite (anorexia)

3.14 Vitamins and deficiencies

Vitamin	Source	Deficiency
Fat-soluble		
Vitamin A (retinol)	Liver, milk, butter, cheese, fish oils	Xerophthalmia – night blindness Keratomalacia
Vitamin D (cholecalciferol)	Manufactured in skin under influence of sunlight	Rickets in children Osteomalacia
Vitamin E (α-tocopherol)	Vegetables, seed oils	Haemolytic anaemia Ataxia
Vitamin K	Green vegetables, dairy products	Bleeding disorder
Water-soluble		
Vitamin B_1 (thiamine)	Cereals, grains, beans, pork	Beri-beri – neuropathy (dry) or heart failure (wet) Wernicke–Korsakoff syndrome
Vitamin B_2 (riboflavin)	Milk	Glossitis, stomatitis
Vitamin B_3 (nicotinic acid)	Meat, cereals	Pellagra – dermatitis, diarrhoea and dementia
Vitamin B_6 (pyridoxine)	Meat, fish, potatoes, bananas	Polyneuropathy
Biotin	Liver, egg yolk, cereals, yeast	Dermatitis, alopecia, paraesthesiae
Folate (vitamin B_9)	Green vegetables	Megaloblastic anaemia
Vitamin B_{12} (cobalamin)	Animal products	Megaloblastic anaemia Neurological disorders
Vitamin C (ascorbic acid)	Fresh fruit and vegetables	Scurvy – extensive bleeding, bruising and perifollicular haemorrhages

3.15 Drugs associated with weight gain

Class	Examples
Anticonvulsants	Sodium valproate, phenytoin, gabapentin
Antidepressants	Citalopram, mirtazapine
Antipsychotics	Chlorpromazine, risperidone, olanzapine, lithium
Beta-blockers	Atenolol
Oral corticosteroids	Prednisolone, dexamethasone
Migraine prophylaxis	Pizotifen
Sulphonylureas/ hypoglycaemic agents	Gliclazide, pioglitazone
Insulin	All formulations
Protease inhibitors for HIV infection	Indinavir, ritonavir, lopinavir

- malabsorption or loss of nutrients, e.g. in prolonged diarrhoea
- metastatic cancer, e.g. of the lung, breast or gastrointestinal tract
- serious and prolonged infection, e.g. tuberculosis
- untreated advanced HIV infection
- chronic inflammation, e.g. inflammatory bowel disease.

In most of these systemic disorders, weight loss is associated with anorexia. Occasionally, weight loss is associated with a normal or increased appetite (thyrotoxicosis, coeliac disease or type 1 diabetes mellitus). The patient's complaint of weight loss does not always correlate with true weight loss. Temporary weight loss is most commonly associated with anxiety, depression or a deliberate attempt to lose weight.

Malnutrition and starvation are major problems worldwide, even in the developed world. Malnutrition is found in up to 40% of UK hospital admissions, particularly the elderly, usually due to poverty or illness. Weight loss due to malnutrition also occurs in anorexia nervosa, alcohol abuse and drug addiction.

Short stature

Short stature is usually familial, so ask about the height of the patient's parents and siblings (p. 366). Any significant childhood illness will reduce the rate of growth and may limit final height. Identify causes of short stature from associated features. Other disorders, such as renal tubular acidosis, intestinal malabsorption and hypothyroidism, may be less obvious in young people and delay the diagnosis. Loss of height is part of normal ageing but is accentuated by compression fractures of the spine due to osteoporosis, particularly in women. In postmenopausal women loss of >5 cm height is an indication to investigate for osteoporosis.

Tall stature

Tall stature is less common than short stature and is usually familial. Most individuals with heights above the 95th centile are not abnormal so ask about the height of close relatives. Abnormal causes of increased height include:

- Marfan's syndrome
- hypogonadism
- pituitary gigantism.

In Marfan's syndrome, the limbs are long in relation to the length of the trunk, and the arm span exceeds height

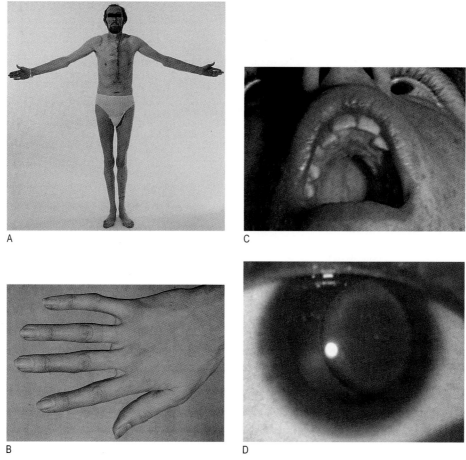

A

C

B

D

Fig. 3.28 Marfan's syndrome, an autosomal dominant condition. (A) Tall stature and reduced upper segment to lower segment ratio (note surgery for aortic dissection). **(B)** Long fingers. **(C)** High-arched palate. **(D)** Dislocation of the lens in the eye.

(Fig. 3.28A). Additional features include long slender fingers (arachnodactyly) (Fig. 3.28B), narrow feet, a high-arched palate (Fig. 3.28C), upward dislocation of the lenses of the eyes (Fig. 3.28D), cardiovascular abnormalities such as mitral valve prolapse, and dilatation of the aortic root with aortic regurgitation.

During puberty, the epiphyses close in response to stimulation from the sex hormones, so in some patients with hypogonadism the limbs continue to grow for longer than usual.

Pituitary gigantism is a very rare cause of tall stature due to excessive growth hormone secretion before epiphyseal fusion has occurred.

HYDRATION

In adults 60–65% of body mass is water. A male weighing 70 kg has 42 litres of water, of which two-thirds is intracellular (28 litres), 12% interstitial fluid (9.4 litres) and the remainder circulating blood plasma (4.6 litres). Women have a smaller percentage of total body water than men, although they may have cyclical fluctuations in weight due to perimenstrual fluid retention.

Dehydration

It is easy to underestimate the severity of dehydration. Assess hydration in all patients, especially those with excess fluid loss, e.g. vomiting, diarrhoea, sweating, burns and polyuria, and when ambient temperature is raised. If you know the patient's usual weight, useful information is obtained by weighing him.

Tachycardia is a common feature. Loss of skin turgor occurs in severe dehydration but adults can lose 4–6 litres before the skin becomes dry and loose. Blood pressure may be low and postural hypotension may indicate intravascular volume depletion. A dry tongue is an unreliable indicator of dehydration since it often occurs in mouth breathing.

Oedema

Oedema is tissue swelling due to an increase in interstitial fluid. The capillary wall separates the interstitial fluid and plasma compartments. The distribution of water between the vascular and interstitial spaces is determined by the balance between hydrostatic pressure forcing water out of the capillary, and colloid osmotic (oncotic) pressure, drawing fluid into the vascular space (Starling's forces). Oncotic pressure depends largely on circulating protein concentration, particularly serum albumin.

Oedema can be generalised, localised or postural.

The cardinal sign of subcutaneous oedema is pitting of superficial tissues. Pitting on pressure may not be demonstrable until body weight has increased by 10–15%. Day-to-day alterations in body weight are usually the most reliable index of changes in body water.

Hypothyroidism is characterised by mucinous infiltration of tissues (myxoedema). In contrast to oedema, myxoedema and chronic lymphoedema do not pit on pressure.

Generalised oedema

There are two principal causes of generalised oedema (Box 3.16):

- fluid overload
- hypoproteinaemia.

Distinguish them by assessing the jugular venous pressure (p. 114). The jugular venous pressure is usually elevated in fluid overload but not in hypoproteinaemia (Box 3.17).

Fluid overload

Fluid overload may be due to heart failure or renal disease, or be iatrogenic (result from medical intervention).

- Heart failure causes oedema in the following ways:
  - Renal underperfusion activates the renin–angiotensin–aldosterone system (secondary hyperaldosteronism) and releases vasopressin, leading to salt and water retention.
  - Renal blood flow is reduced, causing increased salt and water reabsorption.
  - When the patient lies flat, blood redistributes from the legs into the torso, increasing venous return to the heart. In the failing heart this results in increased end-diastolic pressure within the left ventricle, leading to pulmonary oedema. The patient therefore experiences orthopnoea (breathlessness on lying flat).

- Renal disease, e.g. acute glomerulonephritis, may reduce urine volume, with increased circulating and extracellular fluid volume and increased tubular reabsorption of sodium.
- Iatrogenic causes include excess fluid replacement, especially intravenously, producing fluid overload.

Hypoproteinaemia

Hypoproteinaemia, particularly hypoalbuminaemia, reduces oncotic pressure and encourages fluid to move to the interstitial space, causing oedema.

3.16 Causes of oedema

Low plasma oncotic pressure

Low serum albumin due to:
- Increased loss – nephrotic syndrome
- Decreased synthesis – chronic liver disease
- Malabsorption – protein-losing enteropathy, e.g. Crohn's disease and coeliac disease
- Malnutrition – kwashiorkor

Increased hydrostatic pressure

High venous pressure/obstruction due to:
- Deep vein thrombosis
- Venous insufficiency
- Pregnancy
- Pelvic tumour
- Heart failure
- Intravascular volume expansion, e.g. excess intravenous fluid, renal failure

Increased capillary permeability

- Local – soft-tissue infection/inflammation
- Systemic – severe septicaemia
- Drugs, e.g. calcium channel blockers
- Acute allergy

Lymphatic obstruction (lymphoedema) – non-pitting

- Malignant infiltration
- Congenital abnormality – Milroy's disease
- Radiation injury
- Elephantiasis – tropical (filarial) worm infestation

3.17 Features suggesting different causes of oedema

Heart failure	Hypoproteinaemia	DVT or ruptured Baker's cyst*	Lymphoedema	Fat
Pitting	Pitting	Pitting	Non-pitting	Non-pitting
JVP raised	JVP not raised	Warm	Not worse at the end of the day	Spares the feet
Gallop rhythm (third heart sound)		Calf tenderness		Patient obese

*On examination is not possible to distinguish a deep venous thrombosis (DVT) from a ruptured Baker's cyst.
JVP, jugular venous pressure.

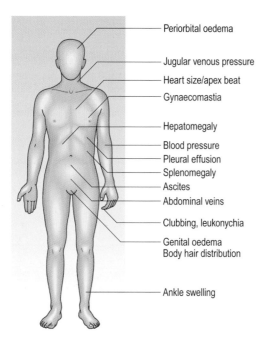

- Periorbital oedema
- Jugular venous pressure
- Heart size/apex beat
- Gynaecomastia
- Hepatomegaly
- Blood pressure
- Pleural effusion
- Splenomegaly
- Ascites
- Abdominal veins
- Clubbing, leukonychia
- Genital oedema
  Body hair distribution
- Ankle swelling

Fig. 3.29 Features to look for in oedema.

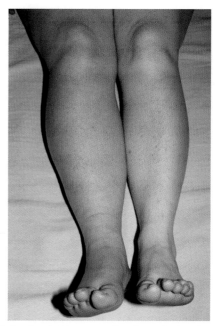

Fig. 3.30 Swollen right leg, suggesting deep vein thrombosis or inflammation, e.g. soft-tissue infection or ruptured Baker's cyst.

Nephrotic syndrome causes heavy proteinuria and most patients with a hepatic cause will have features of chronic liver disease (Fig. 8.11).

The distribution of generalised oedema (Fig. 3.29) is determined by gravity. In semirecumbent patients it is usually found in the ankles, backs of the thighs and the lumbosacral area. If the patient lies flat, it may involve the face and hands, as in nephrotic syndrome.

Localised oedema

This may be caused by venous, lymphatic, inflammatory or allergic disorders.

Venous causes

Increased venous pressure increases hydrostatic pressure within capillaries, producing oedema in the area drained by that vein. Venous causes include deep vein thrombosis, external pressure from a tumour or pregnancy, or venous valvular incompetence from previous thrombosis or surgery. Conditions which impair the normal muscle pumping action, e.g. hemiparesis and forced immobility, increase venous pressure by impairing venous return. As a result oedema may occur in immobile, bed-ridden patients, in a paralysed limb, or in a healthy person sitting for long periods, e.g. during travel (Fig. 3.30).

Lymphatic causes

Normally, interstitial fluid returns to the central circulation via the lymphatic system. Any cause of impaired lymphatic flow, e.g. intraluminal or extraluminal obstruction, may produce localised oedema (lymphoedema) (Fig. 3.31). If the condition persists, fibrous tissues proliferate in the interstitial space and the affected area becomes hard and no longer pits on pressure. In the UK, the commonest cause of leg lymphoedema is

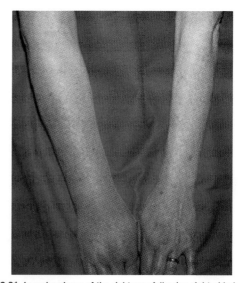

Fig. 3.31 Lymphoedema of the right arm following right-sided mastectomy and radiotherapy.

congenital hypoplasia of leg lymphatics (Milroy's disease), and in the arm after radical mastectomy and/or irradiation for breast cancer. Lymphoedema is common in some tropical countries because of lymphatic obstruction by filarial worms (elephantiasis).

Inflammatory causes

Any cause of tissue inflammation, including infection or injury, liberates mediators, e.g. histamine, bradykinin and cytokines, which cause vasodilatation and increase capillary permeability. Inflammatory oedema is accompanied by the other features of inflammation (redness, tenderness and warmth) and is therefore painful.

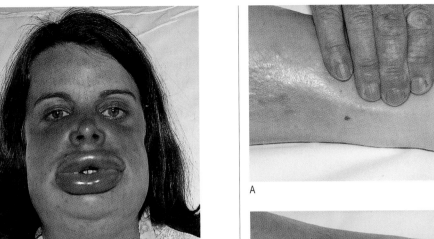

Fig. 3.32 Angio-oedema following a wasp sting.

Allergic causes

Increased capillary permeability occurs in acute allergic conditions. The affected area is usually red and pruritic (itchy) because of local release of histamine and other inflammatory mediators but, in contrast to inflammation, is not painful.

Angio-oedema is a specific form of allergic oedema affecting the face, lips and mouth (Fig. 3.32). Swelling may develop rapidly and may be life-threatening if the upper airway is involved.

Postural oedema

This is due to failure of muscle movement and is common in the lower limbs of inactive patients.

Examination sequence

- Apply firm pressure with your fingers or thumb for at least 15 seconds (Fig. 3.33). Pitting may persist for several minutes until it is obliterated by the slow return of the displaced fluid.
- Assess the state of hydration by looking for sunken orbits and dry mucous membranes. Gently pinch a fold of skin on the neck or anterior chest wall, hold it for a few seconds and then release. Well-hydrated skin springs back into position immediately, in severe dehydration skin subsides abnormally slowly.
- Record weight and urine output.
- Record the pulse rate and supine/erect blood pressures. Look for tachycardia >100 bpm and postural hypotension (a fall >20 mmHg in systolic pressure on standing).
- Check for oedema in the ankles and legs. In bed-bound patients, check for sacral oedema.
- Examine the jugular venous pressure (p. 114).

TEMPERATURE

The 'normal' oral or ear temperature is 37°C but may range between 35.8°C and 37.2°C (98–99°F) (Box 17.2). There is a circadian variation, with the lowest readings

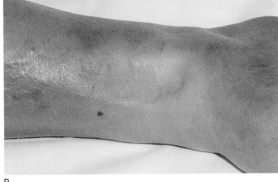

A

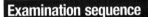

B

Fig. 3.33 Demonstration of pitting oedema.

3.18 Clinical features of hypothermia

Core temperature	Clinical features
36°C	Increased metabolic rate, vasoconstriction
35°C (hypothermia)	Shivering maximal, impaired judgement
34°C	Uncooperative
33°C	Depressed conscious level
28–32°C (severe hypothermia)	Progressive depression of conscious level, muscle stiffness Failure of vasoconstrictor response and shivering Bradycardia, hypotension, J waves present on electrocardiogram, risk of arrhythmias
28°C	Coma, patient may appear dead, absent pupillary and tendon reflexes Spontaneous ventricular fibrillation
20°C	Asystole/profound bradyarrhythmias

occurring in the early morning. Rectal temperature is about 0.5°C higher than oral. The axilla is an unreliable site for measuring temperature. Use a digital thermometer under the tongue, or in the rectum or the external auditory meatus. Mercury thermometers have been replaced by electronic devices, which are safer and more accurate (Fig. 3.34).

3

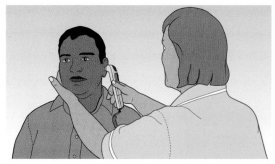

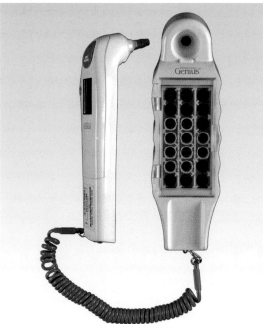

Fig. 3.34 Electronic thermometer.

Fever

Fever is an increase in body temperature usually caused by a cellular response to infection, immunological disturbance or malignancy (Ch. 17).

Hypothermia

Hypothermia is a core temperature <35°C and is easily missed unless rectal temperature is measured. As body temperature falls, conscious level is progressively impaired. Altered consciousness is common with core temperatures <28°C (Box 3.18), and may mimic death (Box 20.2). If you suspect hypothermia, measure temperature at more than one site, e.g. external auditory meatus and rectum.

Hypothermia occurs in:

- elderly immobile patients living alone, particularly during the winter
- water immersion and near-drowning
- prolonged unconsciousness in low ambient temperatures, especially combined with alcohol intoxication (which causes peripheral vasodilatation), drug overdosage, stroke or head injury
- severe hypothyroidism.

David Gawkrodger

The skin, hair and nails

4

EXAMINATION OF THE SKIN, HAIR AND NAILS

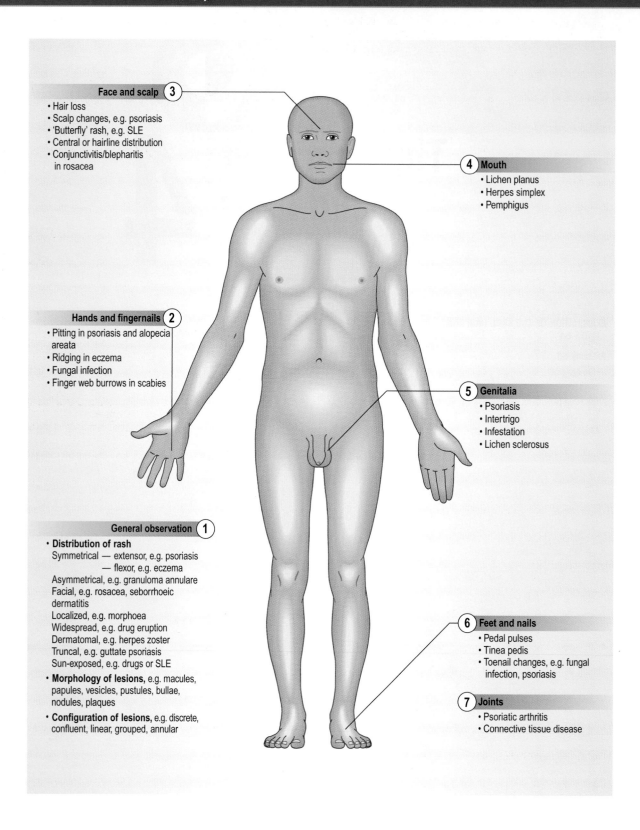

Face and scalp ③
- Hair loss
- Scalp changes, e.g. psoriasis
- 'Butterfly' rash, e.g. SLE
- Central or hairline distribution
- Conjunctivitis/blepharitis
  in rosacea

Mouth ④
- Lichen planus
- Herpes simplex
- Pemphigus

Hands and fingernails ②
- Pitting in psoriasis and alopecia
  areata
- Ridging in eczema
- Fungal infection
- Finger web burrows in scabies

Genitalia ⑤
- Psoriasis
- Intertrigo
- Infestation
- Lichen sclerosus

General observation ①
- **Distribution of rash**
  Symmetrical — extensor, e.g. psoriasis
            — flexor, e.g. eczema
  Asymmetrical, e.g. granuloma annulare
  Facial, e.g. rosacea, seborrhoeic
  dermatitis
  Localized, e.g. morphoea
  Widespread, e.g. drug eruption
  Dermatomal, e.g. herpes zoster
  Truncal, e.g. guttate psoriasis
  Sun-exposed, e.g. drugs or SLE
- **Morphology of lesions,** e.g. macules,
  papules, vesicles, pustules, bullae,
  nodules, plaques
- **Configuration of lesions,** e.g. discrete,
  confluent, linear, grouped, annular

Feet and nails ⑥
- Pedal pulses
- Tinea pedis
- Toenail changes, e.g. fungal
  infection, psoriasis

Joints ⑦
- Psoriatic arthritis
- Connective tissue disease

ANATOMY

The skin is the largest organ in the body, making up 16% of body weight. It protects the body from external factors and keeps the internal organs intact (Fig. 4.1 and Box 4.1).

Skin has three layers:

- epidermis
- dermis
- subcutis.

The epidermis is stratified squamous epithelium with four layers (basal, prickle, granular and horny), representing the stages of keratin maturation. The main cell, the keratinocyte, produces keratin. Keratinocytes lose their nuclei in the granular layer and, as flat plates, form the horny layer. Melanocytes (5–10% of the cell population) originate from the neural crest. They synthesise melanin and are most numerous on the face and other exposed sites. Langerhans cells are dendritic, immunologically active antigen-presenting cells that form a network throughout the epidermis.

The dermis is a supportive connective tissue matrix containing specialised structures. It is thin (0.6 mm) on the eyelids and thicker (3 mm or more) on the back, palms and soles. It contains fibroblasts, dendritic cells, mast cells, macrophages and lymphocytes. Collagen fibres make up 70% of the dermis and give strength and toughness. Elastin fibres provide the skin with elasticity. Glycosaminoglycans form a semisolid matrix that allows some movement of dermal structures, such as hair follicles, sweat glands, blood and lymphatic vessels, and nerves.

The subcutis is a loose layer of connective tissue and fat of variable thickness (up to 3 cm thick on the abdomen).

The hair and nails are specialised epidermal structures.

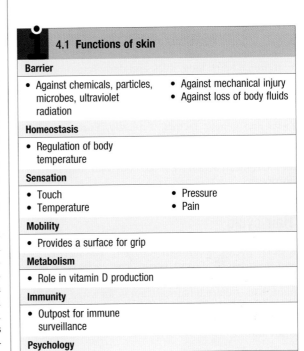

4.1 Functions of skin

Barrier

- Against chemicals, particles, microbes, ultraviolet radiation
- Against mechanical injury
- Against loss of body fluids

Homeostasis

- Regulation of body temperature

Sensation

- Touch
- Temperature
- Pressure
- Pain

Mobility

- Provides a surface for grip

Metabolism

- Role in vitamin D production

Immunity

- Outpost for immune surveillance

Psychology

- Sexual attraction
- Self-image

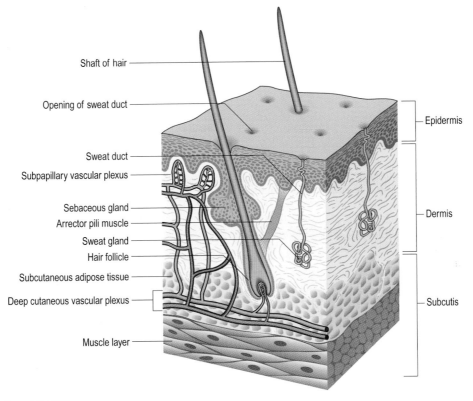

Shaft of hair
Opening of sweat duct
Sweat duct
Subpapillary vascular plexus
Sebaceous gland
Arrector pili muscle
Sweat gland
Hair follicle
Subcutaneous adipose tissue
Deep cutaneous vascular plexus
Muscle layer

Epidermis
Dermis
Subcutis

Fig. 4.1 Structure of the skin.

Hair has a protective and sexual function and hairs cover the surface of the skin, except for the glabrous skin of the palms and soles, the glans penis and the vulval introitus. The follicle density is greatest on the face. The hair shaft has an outer cuticle enclosing a cortex of packed keratinocytes.

There are three types of hair:

- lanugo: fine and long; found in the fetus
- vellus hairs: short, fine and light in colour; cover most body surfaces
- terminal hairs: long, thick and dark; found on the scalp, eyebrows, eyelashes, pubic, axillary and beard areas.

Amount and type of hair vary and are influenced by racial and genetic factors. Typically, Europeans have straight hair, black Africans have curly hair and East Asians have sparse facial and body hair. People from the Mediterranean area have more body hair than northern Europeans.

Hair cycle

Regular cycles of growth (anagen), resting (telogen) and shedding (catagen) occur. The cycle lasts up to 5 years for scalp hair, but less for eyebrow, axillary and pubic hair. Adjacent hairs are not in the same phase but illness or childbirth can synchronise the hair cycle and cause an alarming loss of large amounts of hair (telogen effluvium).

Puberty

Body hair develops with sexual maturity, with wide normal variation in its pattern (Fig. 15.19). At puberty, androgens induce vellus hairs of the pubic region to develop into terminal hairs. Gonadotrophins are not involved in this process, so patients with gonadotrophin deficiency have pubic hair but no other pubertal development. Axillary hair appears 2 years after pubic hair and coincides with the onset of facial hair in boys (p. 368).

Nails

The nail is a plate of hardened, densely packed keratin protecting the finger tip. It facilitates grasp and tactile sensitivity in the finger pulp (Fig. 4.2). The nail matrix contains dividing cells that mature, keratinise and move forward to form the nail plate, which in the finger is 0.3–0.5 mm thick and grows at 0.1 mm/24 hours (Fig. 4.2). Toenails grow more slowly. Adjacent dermal capillaries produce the pink colour of the nail; the white lunula is the visible distal part of the matrix.

Symptoms and definitions

Symptoms include:

- a rash
- itch (pruritus) and sleep disturbance (Box 4.2)
- a growth or lump
- discharge, crusting and smell
- scales falling from the skin or scalp
- disfigurement and psychological distress

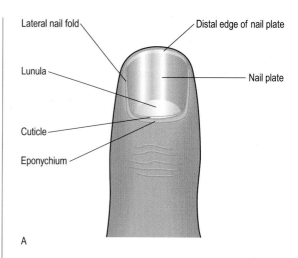

A

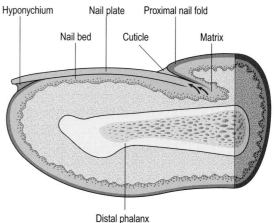

B

Fig. 4.2 Structure of the nail.

4.2 Causes of severe pruritus	
Condition	**Look for:**
Scabies	Burrows on hands or feet
Dermatitis herpetiformis	Small blisters on extensor sites
Urticaria	Intermittent wheals on limbs or trunk
Eczema	Scaly, crusted, excoriated or lichenified patches
Insect bites	Linear or grouped patterns of recent onset
Lichen planus	Typical purplish papules on wrists
Generalised itch	If no rash, check blood tests for renal, haematological or hepatic diseases

- inability to work or pursue leisure activities, e.g. swimming.

Rashes

The distribution on the body, morphology (shape) of individual lesions and their grouping (configuration)

4.3 Some examples of skin lesions and systemic disease		
Skin lesions	**Associations**	**Ask about**
Erythema nodosum	Sarcoidosis, tuberculosis, poststreptococcal infection, connective tissue diseases, drugs	Cough and sputum, breathlessness, sore throat, drugs
Pyoderma gangrenosum	Ulcerative colitis, rheumatoid arthritis, leukaemia	Rectal bleeding, joint symptoms
Dermatitis herpetiformis	Gluten enteropathy	Family history, change in bowel habit
Generalised purpura	Idiopathic thrombocytopenic purpura and other haematological disorders	Family history, haematuria, fever and weight loss
Dermatitis artefacta	Personality disorders	Stresses or anxieties

4

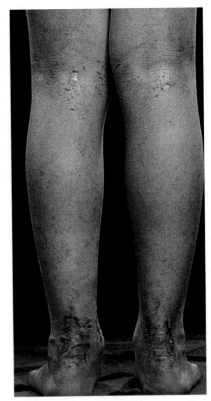

Fig. 4.3 Distribution: flexural. Atopic eczema in the popliteal fossae and ankles.

can be diagnostic. The history of a lesion and systemic features can also be helpful.

Distribution patterns

- Symmetrical or universal eruptions suggest systemic or constitutional causes.
- Asymmetrical rashes that spread from one focus are more likely to be due to fungal, bacterial or viral infection (Box 4.3).

The time and evolution of the spread and change in morphology help diagnosis.

- An itchy rash typically involving the flexures of the popliteal fossa, antecubital fossa, neck and face occurs in atopic eczema (Fig. 4.3).
- Extensor plaques on elbows and knees, the scalp and the sacrum suggest psoriasis (Fig. 4.4).
- Facial:
  - Seborrhoeic dermatitis, an inflammatory reaction to a yeast, *Malassezia*, that forms part of normal skin flora, affects the forehead, nasolabial folds and scalp.
  - Acne vulgaris produces comedones (blackheads), pustules and cysts and also affects the chest and back. Rosacea causes telangiectasia together with the above features.
  - Sun damage and malignant tumours, such as basal cell cancer, are relatively common (Fig. 4.5).
  - Psoriasis is uncommon.
- Truncal:
  - Guttate psoriasis, following a streptococcal throat infection
  - Pityriasis rosea, which usually starts with one lesion, the 'herald patch'
  - Tinea versicolor, caused by *Pityrosporum* yeast
  - Urticaria, producing itchy wheals that clear within 24 hours (Fig. 4.5E).

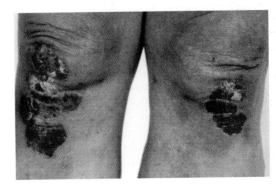

Fig. 4.4 Distribution: extensor. Psoriasis on the knees.

- Peripheral:
  - Wrist lesions suggest lichen planus (Fig. 4.6). Look at the buccal mucosa for the white lacy lesions of Wickham's striae to confirm this.
  - Lower leg lesions include necrobiosis lipoidica (associated with diabetes mellitus and occasionally rheumatoid arthritis: Fig. 4.5F), erythema nodosum (due to sarcoidosis or poststreptococcal infection) and vasculitis caused by circulating immune complexes damaging dermal blood vessels (Fig. 4.5G).
  - Hands or feet can be affected by fungal infection, typically 'athlete's foot' (caused by *Trichophyton*) (Fig. 4.5H).

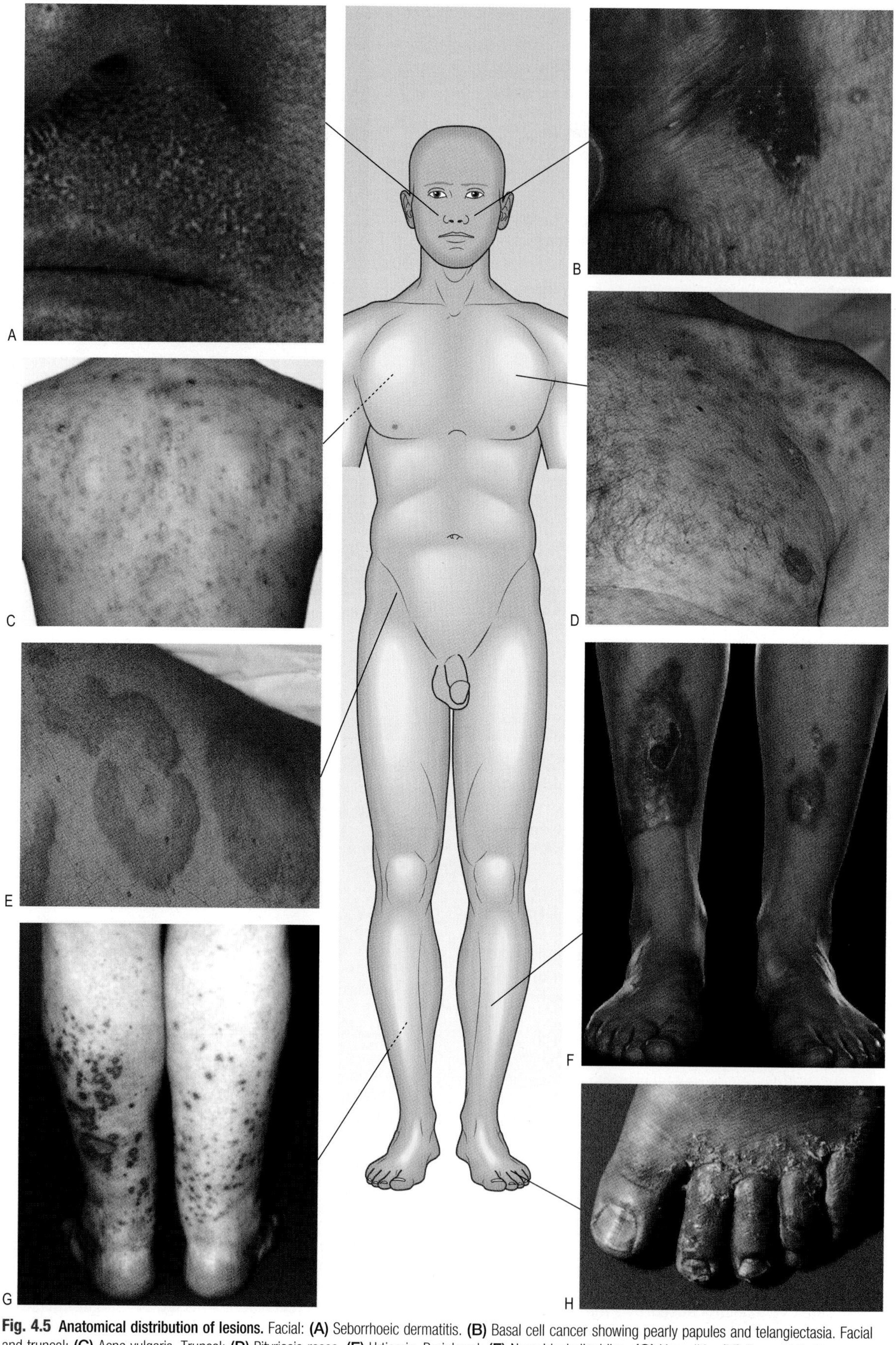

4

Fig. 4.5 Anatomical distribution of lesions. Facial: **(A)** Seborrhoeic dermatitis. **(B)** Basal cell cancer showing pearly papules and telangiectasia. Facial and truncal: **(C)** Acne vulgaris. Truncal: **(D)** Pityriasis rosea. **(E)** Urticaria. Peripheral: **(F)** Necrobiosis lipoidica. **(G)** Vasculitis. **(H)** Fungal infection.

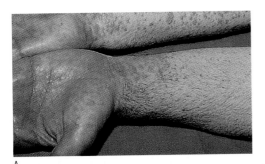

A

B

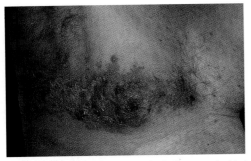

C

Fig. 4.6 Diagnostic sequence, lichen planus. (A) Discrete flat-topped papules on the wrist. **(B)** Wickham's striae visible on close inspection. **(C)** White lacy network of striae on buccal mucosa.

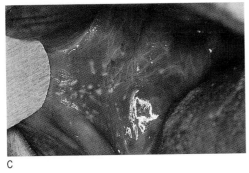

Fig. 4.7 Distribution: dermatomal. This distribution suggests shingles.

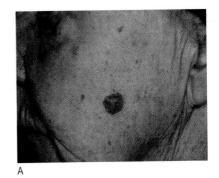

A

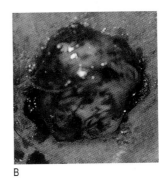

B

Fig. 4.8 Nodule. (A) Seborrhoeic wart. **(B)** Squamous cell cancer.

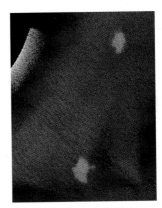

Fig. 4.9 Macule. Macules can be pigmented (a freckle), erythematous (haemangioma) or hypopigmented, as shown here in vitiligo.

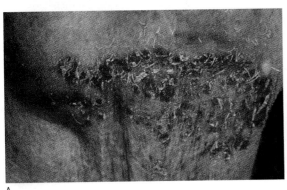

A

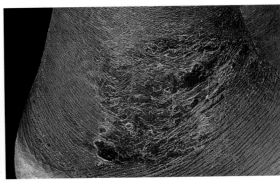

B

Fig. 4.10 Plaque. (A) Lupus vulgaris (tuberculosis of the skin). **(B)** Tuberculoid leprosy.

4.4 Terms used to describe skin lesions

Term	Definition	Term	Definition
Abscess	A localised collection of pus	Milium	A small white cyst that contains keratin
Atrophy	Loss of epidermis, dermis or both, thin, translucent and wrinkled skin, visible blood vessels	Nodule	A solid elevation of skin >5 mm in diameter
Bulla	A fluid-filled blister >5 mm in diameter	Papilloma	A nipple-like projection from the surface of the skin
Burrow	A tunnel in epidermis caused by a parasite, e.g. *Acarus* in scabies	Papule	A solid elevation of skin <5 mm in diameter
Callus	Local hyperplasia of horny layer on palm or sole, due to pressure	Petechia	A haemorrhagic punctate spot 1–2 mm in diameter
Comedo	A plug of sebum and keratin wedged in a dilated pilosebaceous orifice on the face	Plaque	A palpable elevation of skin >2 cm diameter and <5 mm in height
Crust	Dried exudate, e.g. serum, blood or pus, on the skin surface	Purpura	Extravasation of blood resulting in redness of skin or mucous membranes
Cyst	A nodule consisting of an epithelial-lined cavity filled with fluid or semisolid material	Pustule	A visible collection of pus in a blister
Ecchymosis	A macular red or purple haemorrhage, >2 mm in diameter, in skin or mucous membrane	Scale	Accumulation of easily detached fragments of thickened keratin
Erosion	A superficial break in the epidermis, not extending into dermis, heals without scarring	Scar	Replacement of normal tissue by fibrous connective tissue at the site of an injury
Erythema	Redness of the skin due to vascular dilatation	Stria	Atrophic linear band in skin, white, pink or purple, from connective tissue changes
Excoriation	A superficial abrasion, often linear, due to scratching	Telangiectasia	Dilated dermal blood vessels resulting in a visible lesion
Fissure	A linear split in epidermis, often just extending into dermis	Ulcer	A circumscribed area of skin loss extending into the dermis
Freckle	A macular area showing increased pigment formation by melanocytes	Vesicle	A clear, fluid-filled blister <5 mm in diameter
Lichenification	Chronic thickening of skin with increased skin markings, from rubbing or scratching	Wheal	A transitory, compressible papule or plaque of dermal oedema, red or white, indicating urticaria
Macule	A localised area of colour or textural change in the skin		

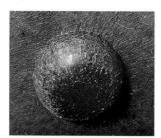

Fig. 4.11 Bulla from an insect bite.

- Sun-exposed, on the face (sparing areas beneath the eyes and lower lip), the V of the neck or the posterior neck and exposed areas of the arms and legs. Causes include connective tissue diseases, e.g. systemic lupus erythematosus (SLE), photosensitising drugs, e.g. thiazide diuretics or non-steroidal anti-inflammatory drugs, cutaneous porphyrias or a primary sun sensitivity condition, e.g. polymorphic light eruption or a photosensitive eczema.
- Dermatomal, e.g. herpes zoster (shingles) (Fig. 4.7).

Morphology is the shape and pattern of the skin lesions (Box 4.4 and Figs 4.8–4.11). Lesions may be:

- Monomorphic (all have the same appearance), as in guttate psoriasis
- Pleomorphic (of differing appearance), as in chickenpox.

Configuration is the pattern in which lesions are arranged and include linear, grouped, annular (in a ring), or the Koebner phenomenon (an eruption in an area of local trauma) (Fig. 4.12). Secondary changes of crusting, erosion and excoriation complicate primary lesions.

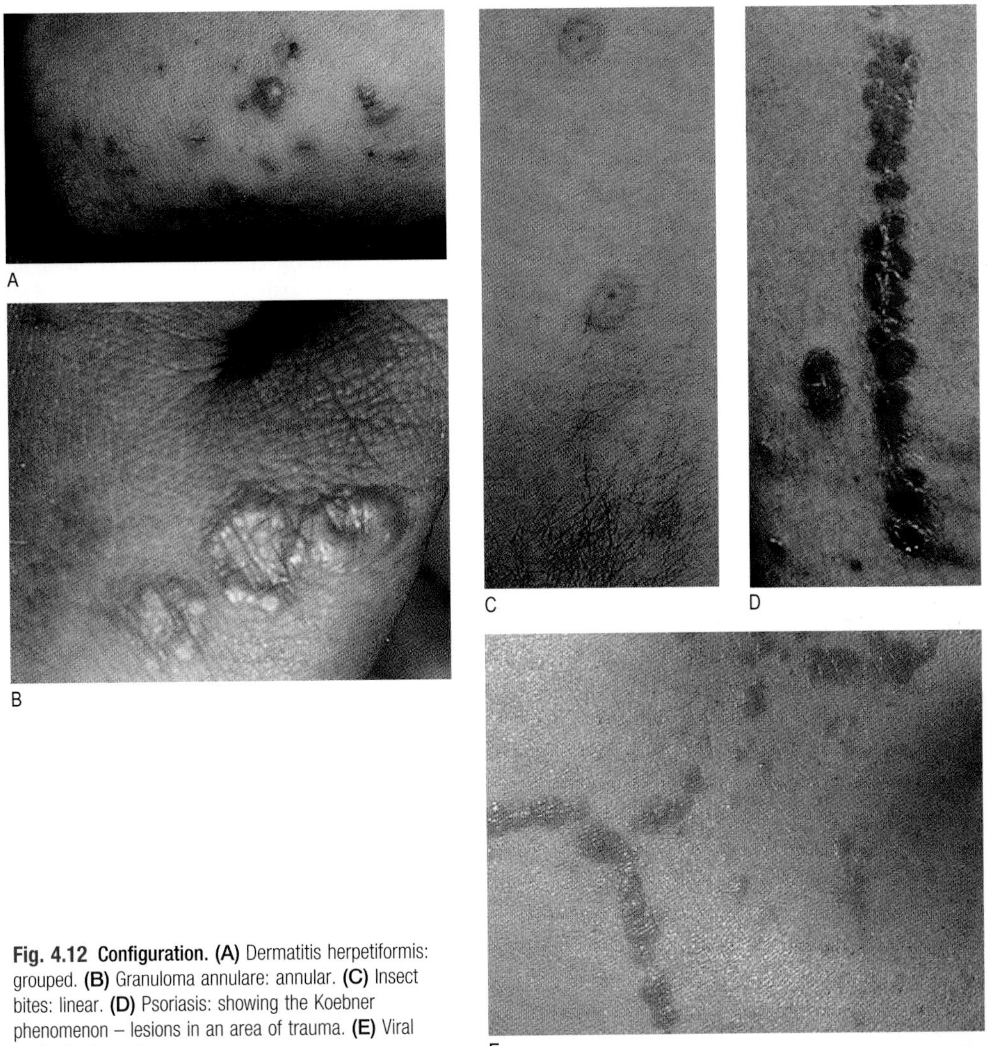

4

Fig. 4.12 **Configuration. (A)** Dermatitis herpetiformis: grouped. **(B)** Granuloma annulare: annular. **(C)** Insect bites: linear. **(D)** Psoriasis: showing the Koebner phenomenon – lesions in an area of trauma. **(E)** Viral warts: Koebner phenomenon.

Duration

Actinic keratoses (Fig. 4.13) are typically present for several years and slowly increase in number. Basal cell cancers commonly develop over 1–2 years and may show ulceration. Squamous cell cancers form more rapidly over weeks or months.

Associated features

In a patient with a hand eruption, look for skin lesions elsewhere, e.g. atopic eczema affecting the antecubital or popliteal fossae or psoriasis on the elbows, knees or scalp, and for burrows of scabies between the fingers or genitalia. The vulva and penis can be affected by psoriasis but only rarely by eczema. Asymmetrical arthritis of large joints and of distal interphalangeal joints is found in up to 30% of patients with psoriasis (Fig. 14.3B).

Common patterns of hair disease

Hair loss (alopecia) can be total or partial (Fig. 4.14):
- Diffuse alopecia. In common male-pattern hair loss terminal scalp hairs undergo miniaturisation to

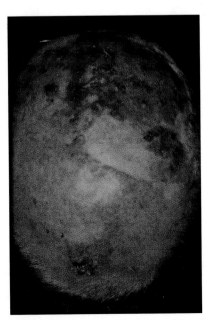

Fig. 4.13 **Actinic keratoses on the scalp.** A skin graft from the removal of a previous squamous cell carcinoma is evident.

vellus hairs. This ageing phenomenon is strongly inherited and depends on androgens. Age-related hair loss in women is more diffuse. Non-scarring diffuse hair loss occurs in hypothyroidism, hypopituitarism and iron deficiency, connective tissue diseases, e.g. SLE, postpartum or postmenopausal or may be drug-induced, e.g. cytotoxic agents.

- Localised non-scarring alopecia. In alopecia areata there is circumscribed loss of scalp, beard or eyebrow hair. Alopecia areata may involve the whole scalp (alopecia totalis) or all body hair. (alopecia universalis). Localised hair loss can be caused by fungal infection, hair pulling, traction from braiding and secondary syphilis.

- Scarring alopecia. Burns, severe infections, e.g. herpes zoster, lichen planus and SLE, may permanently scar the scalp with permanent hair loss.
- Loss of secondary sexual hair. In old age, cirrhosis and hypopituitarism, axillary and pubic hair is lost.

Excess hair growth takes two forms:

- Hirsutism: in females with male-pattern growth of terminal hair, including facial and pubic hair extending towards the umbilicus (male escutcheon). It is a racial trait but may be idiopathic, and is rarely caused by an androgen-secreting tumour (Box 4.5). In these cases there are other features of virilisation, e.g. male-pattern hair loss, clitoromegaly or a deep voice.
- Hypertrichosis: in males or females with excess terminal hair growth in a non-androgenic distribution. It is uncommon and usually due to a systemic disorder, e.g. porphyria cutanea tarda, malignancy, anorexia nervosa, malnutrition or drugs, e.g. ciclosporin, minoxidil and phenytoin.

4.5 Causes of hirsutism

Type	Example
Pituitary	Acromegaly
Adrenal	Cushing's syndrome, virilising tumours, congenital adrenal hyperplasia
Ovarian	Polycystic ovary syndrome, virilising tumours
Drugs	Androgens, progestogens
Idiopathic	End-organ hypersensitivity to androgens

Nail abnormalities

Nail changes are useful in diagnosing internal conditions and skin diseases (Box 4.6). In chronic iron

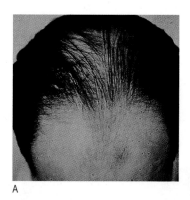
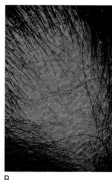
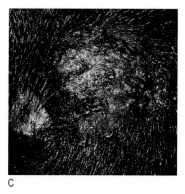

A   B   C

Fig. 4.14 Hair disorders. (A) Male-pattern baldness with hair loss from the temples and vertex of the scalp. **(B)** Alopecia areata with 'exclamation mark' hairs, which taper as they approach the skin. **(C)** Scalp ringworm with secondary bacterial infection and localised hair loss.

4.6 Nail changes in systemic disease and skin disorders

Change	Description of nail	Differential diagnosis
Beau's lines	Transverse grooves	Any severe systemic illness which affects growth of the nail matrix
Brittle nails	Nails break easily, usually at distal margin	Effect of water and detergent, iron deficiency, hypothyroidism, digital ischaemia
Clubbing	Loss of angle between nail fold and nail plate. Finger tip bulbous. Nail matrix feels spongy	Familial or may signify serious cardiac or respiratory disease
Colour changes	Blue Blue-green Brown Brown longitudinal streak	Cyanosis, antimalarials, haematoma *Pseudomonas* infection Fungal infection, staining from cigarettes, chlorpromazine, gold, Addison's disease Melanocytic naevus, malignant melanoma, Addison's disease, racial variant

4.6 Nail changes in systemic disease and skin disorders – _cont'd_

Change	Description of nail	Differential diagnosis
	Red streaks (splinter haemorrhages)	Infective endocarditis, trauma
	White spots	Trauma to nail matrix (not calcium deficiency)
	White/brown 'half and half' nails	Chronic kidney disease
	White (leukonychia)	Hypoalbuminaemia, e.g. associated with cirrhosis
	Yellow	Psoriasis, fungal infection, jaundice, tetracycline
	Yellow nail syndrome	Defective lymphatic drainage – pleural effusions may occur
Combination changes	Longitudinal ridges and triangular nicks at the distal nail	Darier's disease
Koilonychia	Spoon-shaped depression of nail plate	Iron deficiency anaemia, lichen planus, repeated exposure to detergents
Nail fold erythema and telangiectasia	Dilated capillaries and erythema at nail fold	Connective tissue disorders, including systemic sclerosis, SLE, dermatomyositis
Onycholysis	Nail separates from nail bed	Psoriasis, fungal infection, trauma, thyrotoxicosis, tetracyclines (photo-onycholysis)
Onychomycosis	Thickening of the nail plate with colour change, usually whitening or brown discoloration	Fungal infection
Pitting	Fine or coarse pits in the nail	Psoriasis, eczema, alopecia areata, lichen planus
Thimble pitting	A particular type of fine regular pitting, as seen on a thimble	Alopecia areata
Coarse pitting	Larger irregular pits in the nail plate	Eczema
Ridging	Transverse (across nail)	Beau's lines (see above), eczema, psoriasis, tic dystrophy, chronic paronychia
	Longitudinal (up/down)	Lichen planus, Darier's disease
Splinter haemorrhages	Small red streaks that lie longitudinally in the nail plate	Trauma, but can signify infective endocarditis

4

4.7 Causes of hypoalbuminaemia and leukonychia

Reduced albumin synthesis

- Chronic liver disease

Urinary protein loss

- Nephrotic syndrome

Protein-losing enteropathy

- Crohn's disease
- Ulcerative colitis
- Ménétrier's disease of the stomach
- Coeliac disease
- Intestinal lymphoma
- Bacterial overgrowth
- Radiation damage

Protein malnutrition

- Kwashiorkor

---

deficiency the nails become brittle, flat and eventually spoon-shaped (koilonychia) (Box 4.7). White nails (leukonychia) are a sign of hypoalbuminaemia. Beau's lines, due to arrest of nail growth, are transverse white grooves that appear on all nails shortly after a severe illness and which move out to the free margins as the nail grows. Although one or two splinter haemorrhages are commonly seen under the nails of manual workers, multiple lesions raise the possibility of bacterial endocarditis. Distal nail separation (onycholysis) is common

in psoriasis. Dilated capillaries in the proximal nail fold occur in vasculitic conditions, such as SLE (Fig. 4.15 and Box 4.6).

Mucous membranes and other sites

Changes in the mucous membranes of the mouth and genitalia accompany, and may be characteristic of, certain skin conditions, e.g. oral Wickham's striae in lichen planus, oral lesions in Kaposi's sarcoma (Fig. 4.16), vulval involvement with lichen sclerosus. Fully examine patients with skin lymphoma for lymphadenopathy and hepatosplenomegaly. In patients with leg ulcers, feel the leg and foot pulses to assess the arterial supply (Fig. 6.40).

THE HISTORY

Presenting complaint

Ask when, where and how the eruption or lesions began, about the initial appearance and what changes have occurred with time. Note associated features, such as itch and systemic upset, together with aggravating and relieving factors. Use SOCRATES to remember what to ask (Box 2.10).

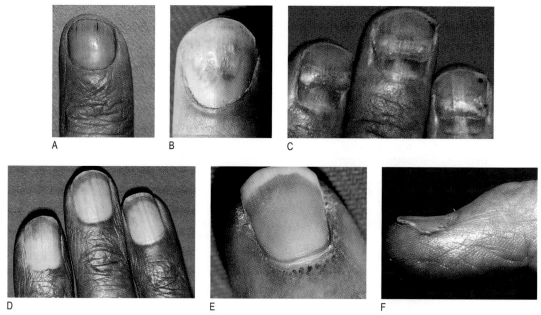

Fig. 4.15 The nail as a diagnostic aid. (A) Splinter haemorrhages. **(B)** Onycholysis with pitting in psoriasis. **(C)** Beau's lines. **(D)** Leukonychia. **(E)** Dilated proximal nail fold capillaries in systemic lupus erythematosus. **(F)** Koilonychia.

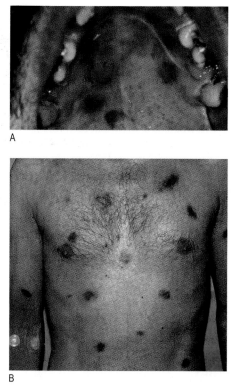

Fig. 4.16 Kaposi's sarcoma. (A) In the mouth and **(B)** on the skin.

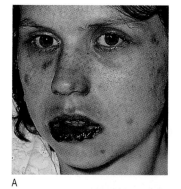

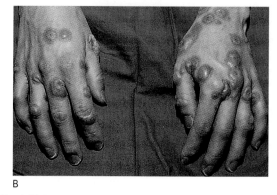

Fig. 4.17 Stevens–Johnson syndrome. (A) Facial and oral lesions. **(B)** 'Target lesions' on hands.

Past and drug histories

Ask about previous skin disease, atopic symptoms (hay-fever, asthma, childhood eczema), medical disorders that may involve the skin, e.g. Stevens–Johnson syndrome caused by drugs (Fig. 4.17) or have cutaneous features, and prescribed or self-medicated drugs, including creams and cosmetics.

Social, family and genetic histories

Foreign travel gives exposure to tropical infections or sunlight that could cause a photosensitive eruption. Does the patient have a fair skin type, i.e. does he burn easily and tan poorly or not at all? Skin cancers are commoner with a pale skin. Is there a family history of malignant melanoma or other skin cancer? A family history is found in 10% of patients with malignant melanoma. Psoriasis and atopic eczema also have strongly inherited traits.

Occupational and environmental histories

Chemicals encountered at work or leisure may cause contact dermatitis. Suspect industrial dermatitis if the eruption improves when the patient is away from work.

THE PHYSICAL EXAMINATION

General examination

Examining the skin is part of the general examination. When you examine the hands or face, note any abnormalities of the skin.

Ensure a warm, well-lit, private place is available. Offer a chaperone; record the chaperone's name or if the patient declines the offer. For widespread lesions ask the patient to undress to his underclothes. Use a hand lens to examine individual lesions. A dermoscope, using a ×10 magnification illuminated lens system, is helpful for pigmented lesions (Fig. 4.18).

The skin, hair and nails

Examination sequence

Stand back and look at the skin in its entirety: is it abnormal?
 Note the distribution of lesions.
 Pick a typical individual lesion and check:
- size (with a tape measure if need be)
- shape
- colour
- border changes
- spatial interrelationships: are lesions confluent or separate?
 Palpate with your finger tips to establish its consistency, putting on gloves if the skin is broken.

If any pigmented lesion (mole) has recently changed, note the distribution of pigment within it and whether it is inflamed or ulcerated. Malignant melanoma commonly shows variation in pigmentation and has an irregular or diffuse edge. Remember 'ABCDE' – **A**symmetry, **B**order irregular, **C**olour irregular and **D**iameter >6 mm, **E**nlargement (Fig. 4.19 and Box 4.8). Examine the entire skin as abnormal moles are more common in patients with a malignant melanoma.

Look at:
- nails on hands and feet
- different areas of the scalp (ask the patient to point to the problem to localise, then part the patient's hair to see)
- mucous membranes.

Examine local lymph nodes in any patient with a potential squamous cell cancer, malignant melanoma or cutaneous T-cell lymphoma (Fig. 3.21).

Take a skin scraping for microscopy and culture if you suspect fungal infection.

PUTTING IT ALL TOGETHER

In order to diagnose skin disease familiarise yourself with the patterns of skin conditions and then mentally test multiple hypotheses for the best fit against the facts of the history and examination. Not all historic or physical findings match the classic descriptions. Investigations, such as a skin biopsy, are sometimes required to establish a diagnosis.

INVESTIGATIONS

See Box 4.9.

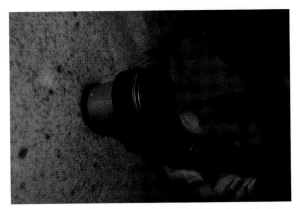

Fig. 4.18 A dermoscope. This is helpful when looking at suspicious pigmented lesions.

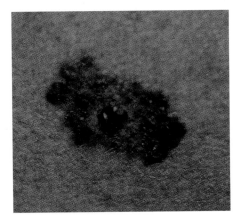

Fig. 4.19 Malignant melanoma. A darkly pigmented nodule, with irregular margins and variability of pigmentation.

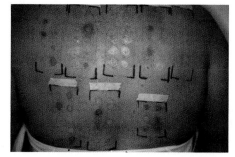

Fig. 4.20 Patch testing. Known allergens are applied to the patient's back and read at 2 and 4 days.

> **EBE** 4.8 **An enlarging mole**
>
> In a patient with an enlarging mole, use the ABCDE checklist. Any single positive finding justifies a biopsy or referral for specialist advice.
>
> Whited JD, Grichnik JM. Does this patient have a mole or a melanoma? JAMA 1998;279:696-701.

4.9 Investigations in skin disease

Investigation	Indication/comment
Wood's light	Vitiligo, fungal infection Hand-held ultraviolet lamp shows vitiligo not apparent in ordinary light, or fluorescence in fungal infection
Blood tests, including haematology and biochemistry	Systemic disease Anaemia, kidney, liver and thyroid function may confirm systemic disease. Monitor blood parameters in patients on systemic drugs
Serology	Autoimmune disease and eczema SLE and rheumatic disease. Serum IgE or allergen-specific IgE in some patients with atopic eczema
Microscopy and fungal culture	Rashes Use a disposable scalpel to scrape the active margin of the rash, dislodging scales on to a piece of black paper
Surgical biopsy	Rashes or nodules Histology or direct immunofluorescence (vasculitis)
Doppler studies	Leg ulcers An index of the dorsalis pedis blood pressure over brachial blood pressure of <0.8 helps suggests arterial disease
Photography	Pigmented lesions Compare the development of the lesion over time
Patch tests	Delayed-type contact allergy, e.g. to fragrances Prepared allergens on small aluminium discs are applied to the upper back and the skin reviewed 2 and 4 days later (Fig. 4.20)
Prick tests	Immediate allergy, e.g. to latex Prepared allergen solutions are pricked into the dermis and reviewed 15 minutes later. Histamine and saline solutions are used as positive and negative controls

John Bevan

The endocrine system

.5

ENDOCRINE EXAMINATION

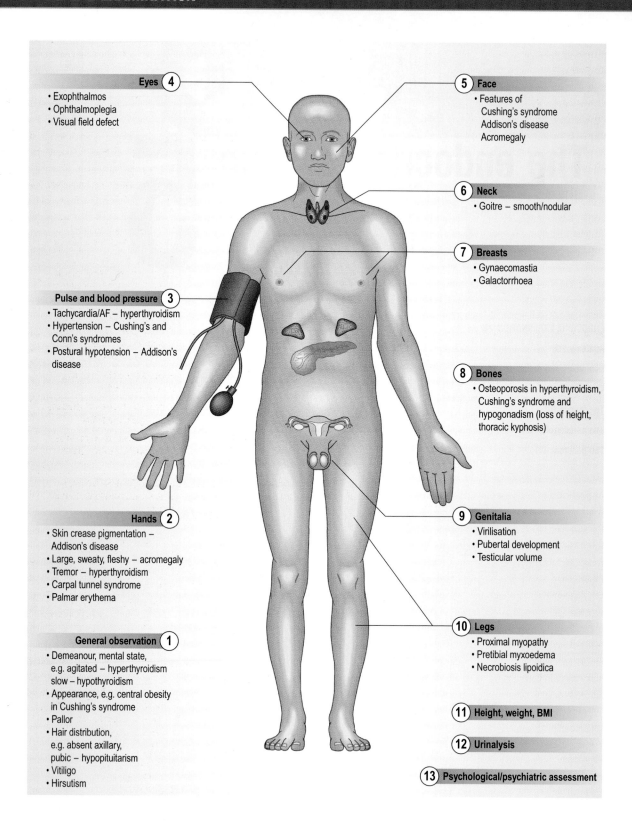

Eyes (4)
- Exophthalmos
- Ophthalmoplegia
- Visual field defect

(5) **Face**
- Features of
  Cushing's syndrome
  Addison's disease
  Acromegaly

(6) **Neck**
- Goitre – smooth/nodular

(7) **Breasts**
- Gynaecomastia
- Galactorrhoea

Pulse and blood pressure (3)
- Tachycardia/AF – hyperthyroidism
- Hypertension – Cushing's and
  Conn's syndromes
- Postural hypotension – Addison's
  disease

(8) **Bones**
- Osteoporosis in hyperthyroidism,
  Cushing's syndrome and
  hypogonadism (loss of height,
  thoracic kyphosis)

Hands (2)
- Skin crease pigmentation –
  Addison's disease
- Large, sweaty, fleshy – acromegaly
- Tremor – hyperthyroidism
- Carpal tunnel syndrome
- Palmar erythema

(9) **Genitalia**
- Virilisation
- Pubertal development
- Testicular volume

(10) **Legs**
- Proximal myopathy
- Pretibial myxoedema
- Necrobiosis lipoidica

General observation (1)
- Demeanour, mental state,
  e.g. agitated – hyperthyroidism
  slow – hypothyroidism
- Appearance, e.g. central obesity
  in Cushing's syndrome
- Pallor
- Hair distribution,
  e.g. absent axillary,
  pubic – hypopituitarism
- Vitiligo
- Hirsutism

(11) **Height, weight, BMI**

(12) **Urinalysis**

(13) **Psychological/psychiatric assessment**

ANATOMY

The main endocrine glands are the pituitary, thyroid, parathyroids, pancreas, adrenals and gonads: testes and ovaries (Fig. 5.1). These glands synthesise hormones which are released into the circulation and act at distant sites. Disease may result from excessive or inadequate production of hormones, or target organ hypersensitivity or resistance to the hormone. Although some endocrine glands, e.g. parathyroid glands and pancreas, respond directly to metabolic signals, most are controlled by hormones released from the pituitary gland. A wide variety of molecules act as hormones:

- peptides, e.g. insulin
- glycoproteins, e.g. thyroid-stimulating hormone
- amines, e.g. adrenaline (epinephrine)
- steroid hormones, e.g. cortisol, aldosterone, oestradiol, testosterone
- thyroid hormones, e.g. levothyroxine (T_4) and tri-iodothyronine (T_3).

SYMPTOMS AND DEFINITIONS

Symptoms of endocrine disturbance are frequently non-specific and affect many body systems (Box 5.1). Endocrine conditions may be detected by chance, e.g. glycosuria on screening, or if the clinician sees a patient after a significant time interval and notices diagnostic facial features, e.g. in acromegaly or hypothyroidism.

Nevertheless, diagnosis often depends upon careful observation of a patient with non-specific symptoms prompting the recognition of specific features.

Apart from diabetes mellitus, thyroid disease and some reproductive conditions, endocrine disorders are uncommon. Most patients with tiredness, excessive sweating or sexual dysfunction, for example, do not have an underlying endocrine cause (Box 5.2).

5.1 Common clinical features in endocrine disease

Symptom, sign or problem	Differential diagnoses
Weight gain	Hypothyroidism, polycystic ovary syndrome (PCOS), Cushing's syndrome
Weight loss	Hyperthyroidism, diabetes mellitus, adrenal insufficiency
Short stature	Constitutional, non-endocrine systemic disease (e.g. coeliac disease), growth hormone deficiency
Delayed puberty	Constitutional, non-endocrine systemic disease, hypothyroidism, hypopituitarism, primary gonadal failure
Menstrual disturbance	PCOS, hyperprolactinaemia, thyroid dysfunction
Diffuse neck swelling	Simple goitre, Graves' disease, Hashimoto's thyroiditis
Excessive thirst	Diabetes mellitus or insipidus, hyperparathyroidism, Conn's syndrome
Hirsutism	Idiopathic, PCOS, Cushing's syndrome, congenital adrenal hyperplasia
'Funny turns'	Hypoglycaemia, phaeochromocytoma, neuroendocrine tumour
Sweating	Hyperthyroidism, hypogonadism, acromegaly, phaeochromocytoma
Flushing	Hypogonadism (especially menopause), carcinoid syndrome
Resistant hypertension	Conn's syndrome, Cushing's syndrome, phaeochromocytoma, acromegaly, renal artery stenosis
Erectile dysfunction	Primary or secondary hypogonadism, diabetes mellitus, non-endocrine systemic disease, medication-induced (e.g. beta-blockers, opiates)
Muscle weakness	Cushing's syndrome, hyperthyroidism, hyperparathyroidism, osteomalacia
Bone fragility and fractures	Hypogonadism, hyperthyroidism, Cushing's syndrome
Altered facial appearance	Hypothyroidism, Cushing's syndrome, acromegaly, PCOS

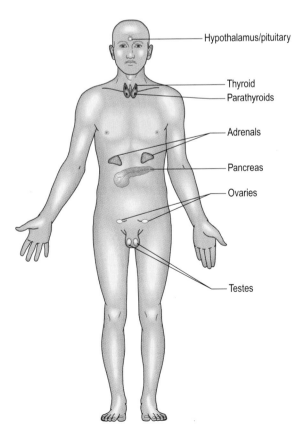

Fig. 5.1 The principal endocrine glands.

- Hypothalamus/pituitary
- Thyroid
- Parathyroids
- Adrenals
- Pancreas
- Ovaries
- Testes

5.2 Prevalence and incidence of endocrine conditions	
Condition	**Incidence/prevalence**
Common	
Type 2 diabetes mellitus	4–8% prevalence (increasing with obesity)
Primary hypothyroidism	2% prevalence (5% including subclinical disease); mostly women
Polycystic ovary syndrome	6–8% prevalence, depending on definition
Moderately common	
Hyperthyroidism	1% prevalence (80% Graves' disease, 80% in women)
Type 1 diabetes mellitus	0.5% prevalence (increasing in children)
Male hypogonadism	1–2% prevalence, depending on definition
Uncommon	
Hypopituitarism	Prevalence: 50–100 per million
Addison's disease	Prevalence: 50 per million (western countries, mostly autoimmune)
Differentiated thyroid cancer	Incidence: 5 new cases per 100 000 per year
Rare	
Carcinoid tumour	Incidence: 20 new cases per million per year
Pituitary-dependent Cushing's disease	Incidence: 5 new cases per million per year
Acromegaly	Incidence: 4 new cases per million per year

Common presenting symptoms are:
- appetite and/or weight change – in hyper/hypothyroidism, diabetes mellitus, Cushing's syndrome
- polydipsia (excessive thirst) and/or polyuria (passing >3 litres urine/day) – in diabetes mellitus, diabetes insipidus or hyperparathyroidism
- change in facial/body hair growth and distribution – in hypogonadism, hypopituitarism, adrenal insufficiency, androgen excess. Hirsutism is the excessive growth of thick terminal hair in an androgen-dependent distribution (upper lip, chin, chest, back, lower abdomen, thighs) in women
- change in skin and mucosal pigmentation and character: coarse dry skin in hypothyroidism; excessive pigmentation and/or vitiligo (areas of depigmented skin) in Addison's disease (Fig. 5.17D); soft-tissue overgrowth and skin tags in acromegaly; acanthosis nigricans (velvety thickening and pigmentation of the major flexures, especially the axillae and groins: Fig. 5.11A) in obesity, and type 2 diabetes
- increased sweating in acromegaly and phaeochromocytoma
- temperature intolerance – in hyperthyroidism (heat) and hypothyroidism (cold)

- change in sexual function:
  - erectile dysfunction or loss of libido in hypogonadism
  - gynaecomastia (breast tissue enlargement in men) in liver disease, Klinefelter's syndrome and drugs e.g. spironolactone, oestrogens
  - galactorrhoea (breast milk production in men, or in women outwith pregnancy or breastfeeding) in pituitary adenomas producing hyperprolactinaemia
  - primary or secondary amenorrhoea (p. 219) in pituitary or hypothalamic disease
- tiredness: can be a non-specific feature of diabetes mellitus, hypothyroidism or Addison's disease.

THE HISTORY

General points

Past history

Tuberculosis and HIV infection are associated with adrenal insufficiency.

Drug history

Excessive corticosteroid exposure causes cushingoid features and dopamine antagonist drugs such as haloperidol and domperidone cause hyperprolactinaemia.

Family history

Thyroid disease and diabetes mellitus may run in families. Multiple endocrine neoplasia syndromes are rare autosomal dominant conditions characterised by hyperplasia, adenoma formation and malignant change in multiple endocrine glands.

THE THYROID

Anatomy

The thyroid is butterfly-shaped with two symmetrical lobes joined by a central isthmus that normally covers the second and third tracheal rings (Fig. 5.2A). The gland may extend into the superior mediastinum, or may occasionally be entirely retrosternal. Rarely, it is located higher in the neck along the line of the thyroglossal duct. If situated at the back of the tongue (lingual goitre), it may be visible through the open mouth.

Symptoms and definitions

Goitre is enlargement of the thyroid gland. It is not necessarily associated with thyroid dysfunction and most patients with a goitre are euthyroid (Fig. 5.5).

Hyperthyroidism (thyrotoxicosis) is a clinical state caused by increased levels of circulating levels of the thyroid hormones, T_3 and T_4. Graves' disease is the commonest cause of hyperthyroidism. It is an autoimmune disease with a familial component, which is 5–10 times more common in women and usually presents between

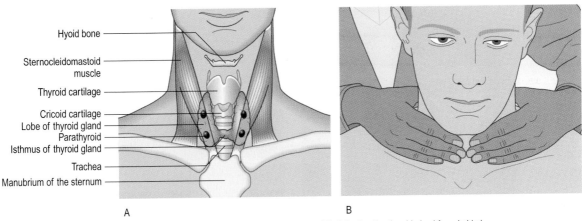

Fig. 5.2 **The thyroid gland. (A)** Anatomy of the gland and surrounding structures. **(B)** Palpating the thyroid gland from behind.

20 and 50 years of age. It has specific extrathyroid features (Fig. 5.3):

- Exophthalmos (proptosis) is increased protrusion of the eyeball from the orbit. It is caused by an inflammatory infiltration of the orbital contents (the soft tissues and extraocular muscles, not the globe). It is usually bilateral. Exophthalmos may lead to diplopia (Fig. 5.4A&B) and other features of Graves' ophthalmopathy: conjunctival oedema, conjunctivitis, corneal ulceration, ophthalmoplegia and optic atrophy (Ch. 12).
- Pretibial myxoedema is a raised, discoloured (usually pink or brown) indurated appearance over the lower legs (Fig. 5.4D). Note that, despite the name, it is associated with Graves' disease, not hypothyroidism.
- Thyroid acropachy is a periosteal hypertrophy of the distal phalanges which looks like finger clubbing (Fig. 5.4C).

Hypothyroidism (Fig. 5.3) is caused by reduced levels of thyroid hormones and is usually due to autoimmune Hashimoto's thyroiditis. Women are affected approximately six times more commonly than men. Many clinical features of hypothyroidism are produced by myxoedema (non-pitting oedema caused by tissue infiltration by mucopolysaccharides, chondroitin and hyaluronic acid) (Box 5.3 and Figs 5.3 and 5.7).

History

Presenting complaint

Ask about:

- recent weight loss/gain, appetite change, diarrhoea or constipation
- irritability, difficulty sleeping, hyperactivity or excessive fatigue
- heat or cold intolerance
- tremor, palpitation or excessive sweating
- skin or hair changes (excessive dryness or sweating, coarse dry hair or alopecia)
- eye symptoms: diplopia, pain, irritation or 'grittiness'.

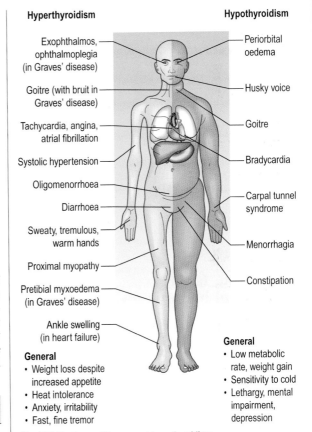

Fig. 5.3 Features of hyper- and hypothyroidism.

Hyperthyroidism

- Exophthalmos, ophthalmoplegia (in Graves' disease)
- Goitre (with bruit in Graves' disease)
- Tachycardia, angina, atrial fibrillation
- Systolic hypertension
- Oligomenorrhoea
- Diarrhoea
- Sweaty, tremulous, warm hands
- Proximal myopathy
- Pretibial myxoedema (in Graves' disease)
- Ankle swelling (in heart failure)

General
- Weight loss despite increased appetite
- Heat intolerance
- Anxiety, irritability
- Fast, fine tremor

Hypothyroidism

- Periorbital oedema
- Husky voice
- Goitre
- Bradycardia
- Carpal tunnel syndrome
- Menorrhagia
- Constipation

General
- Low metabolic rate, weight gain
- Sensitivity to cold
- Lethargy, mental impairment, depression

EBE 5.3 **Hypothyroidism**

The diagnosis of hypothyroidism is commonly delayed or missed because symptoms and signs develop insidiously over years.

Vaidya B, Pearce SHS. Management of hypothyroidism in adults. BMJ 2008;337:284–289.

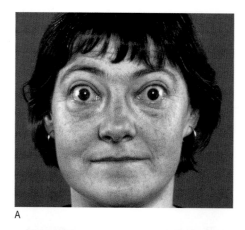

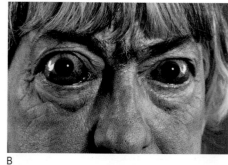

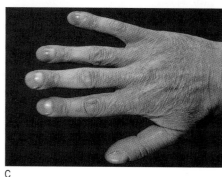

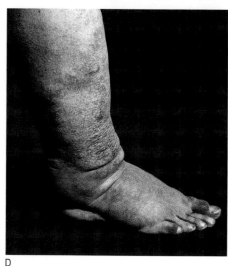

Fig. 5.4 Graves' hyperthyroidism. (A) Typical facies. **(B)** Severe inflammatory thyroid eye disease. **(C)** Thyroid acropachy. **(D)** Pretibial myxoedema.

Past drug, family and social history

Ask about:

- drug therapy (amiodarone and lithium are associated with hypothyroidism), antithyroid drugs
- family history of thyroid or autoimmune disease
- living in areas of iodine deficiency, e.g. the Andes, Himalayas, Central Africa, can cause goitre and, rarely, hypothyroidism.

Examination sequence

General
Look for:

- signs of weight loss or gain
- agitation, restlessness or apathy and lethargy
- the facial appearance and expression.

Examine:

- hands
- pulse and blood pressure (BP)
- arms and legs for: skin abnormalities, muscle power and the deep tendon reflexes (p. 261)

- the eyes for:
  - exophthalmos, diplopia, conjunctival oedema or conjunctivitis, corneal ulceration
  - lid retraction: this is present if the sclera is visible above the iris (Fig. 5.4A)
  - lid lag: ask the patient to follow your index finger as you move it from the upper to the lower part of his visual field (Fig. 12.13). Delay between the descent of the upper eyelid in relation to that of the eyeball is lid lag.

The thyroid gland

Examination sequence

- Inspect the neck from the front. Give the patient a glass of water and ask him to take a sip. Look for a swelling while he swallows.
- Ask the patient to sit with the neck muscles relaxed and stand behind him. Place your hands gently on the front of the neck, with your index fingers just touching (Fig. 5.2B). Ask him to swallow a sip of water and feel the gland as it moves upwards. Some patients find neck palpation uncomfortable, so be alert for any signs of distress.

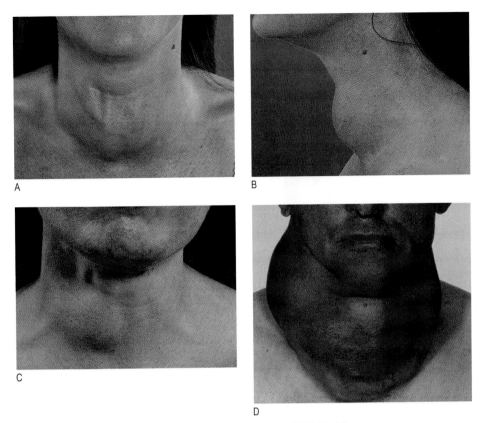

Fig. 5.5 Goitres. (A and B) Diffuse – Graves' disease. **(C)** Uninodular – toxic nodule. **(D)** Multinodular.

- Note the size, shape and consistency of any goitre and feel for any thrill.
- Measure any discrete nodules with callipers.
- Record the maximum neck circumference of a large goitre using a tape measure (objective measurements are useful for long-term follow-up).
- Auscultate with your stethoscope for a thyroid bruit. A thyroid bruit may be confused with other sounds: bruits from the carotid artery or transmitted from the aorta are louder along the line of the artery. Transient gentle pressure over the root of the neck will interrupt a venous hum from the internal jugular vein.

Normal findings

The normal thyroid gland is palpable in ~50% of women and 25% of men. Prominent skin folds may give a false impression of goitre. The thyroid (or a thyroglossal cyst) moves upwards on swallowing since it is enveloped in the pre-tracheal fascia, which is attached to the cricoid cartilage.

Abnormal findings

Shape, surface and consistency Simple goitres are relatively symmetrical in their earlier stages but often become nodular with time. In Graves' disease the surface of the thyroid gland is usually smooth and diffuse; it is irregular in uninodular or multinodular goitre (Fig. 5.5). Nodules in the substance of the gland may be large or small, and single or multiple, and are usually benign. A very hard consistency suggests malignancy. Large,

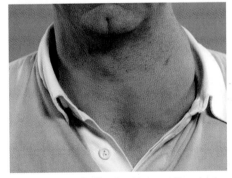

Fig. 5.6 Thyroid cancer. Papillary thyroid cancer with regional cervical lymphadenopathy.

firm lymph nodes near a goitre suggest thyroid cancer (Fig. 5.6). Diffuse tenderness is typical of viral thyroiditis. Localised tenderness may follow bleeding into a thyroid cyst.

Mobility Most goitres move upwards on swallowing. Very large goitres may be immobile, and invasive thyroid cancer may fix the gland to surrounding structures.

Thyroid bruit This may occur in hyperthyroidism and indicates abnormally high blood flow. There can be an associated palpable thrill.

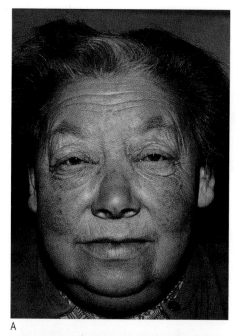

A

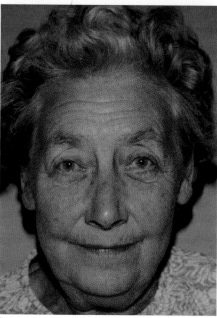

B

Fig. 5.7 Hypothyroidism. (A) Before treatment. **(B)** After levothyroxine replacement.

THE PARATHYROIDS

Anatomy

There are usually four parathyroid glands which lie posterior to the thyroid (Fig. 5.2A). Each is about the size of a pea and produces parathyroid hormone, a peptide which increases the level of calcium in the blood.

Symptoms and definitions

Parathyroid disease is commonly asymptomatic. In hyperparathyroidism, the commonest symptoms relate to hypercalcaemia: polyuria, polydipsia, renal stones, peptic ulceration, tender areas of bone fracture deformity ('Brown tumours': Fig. 5.8A), and confusion or psychiatric symptoms.

In hypoparathyroidism, hypocalcaemia may cause hyperreflexia or tetany (involuntary muscle contraction), most commonly in the hands or feet. Paraesthesiae of the hands and feet or around the mouth may occur. Hypoparathyroidism is most often caused by inadvertent damage to the glands during thyroid surgery.

Patients with the autosomal dominant condition pseudohypoparathyroidism have end-organ resistance to parathyroid hormone and typically have short stature, round face and shortening of some metacarpal bones.

History

Ask about:

- recent thyroid or neck surgery or irradiation
- polyuria, polydipsia or renal stones
- fractures
- abdominal pain or constipation
- muscle cramps
- confusion or psychiatric symptoms.

Examination sequence

- Look at the neck for scars of previous surgery.
- Assess mental state (p. 21).
- Take the BP and assess the state of hydration (p. 58).
- Look at the hands. Ask the patient to make a fist and assess the length of the metacarpals.
- Test for muscle weakness (p. 259) and hyperreflexia (p. 261).
- Test for latent tetany: place a BP cuff on the upper arm and inflate above systolic pressure for 3 minutes. In the hand, carpal muscle contraction produces a typical picture with the thumb adducted, the proximal interphalangeal and distal interphalangeal joints extended and the metacarpophalangeal joints flexed ('main d'accoucheur' (hand of the obstetrician) or Trousseau's sign: Fig 5.9).
- Look for evidence of recent fractures and bone tenderness.
- Use a slit lamp to look for corneal calcification.
- Perform urinalysis.

Abnormal findings

Parathyroid tumours are very rarely palpable.

Findings in hyperparathyroidism may include altered mental state, dehydration, proximal muscle weakness, fractures and bony tenderness. In long-standing hypercalcaemia, corneal calcification (band keratopathy) may be present (Fig. 5.8B). Renal stones may produce haematuria on stix testing.

In moderate/severe hypocalcaemia, hyperreflexia and a positive Trousseau's sign may be present. In pseudohypoparathyroidism the metacarpals of the ring and little fingers are shortened (Fig. 5.8C and D).

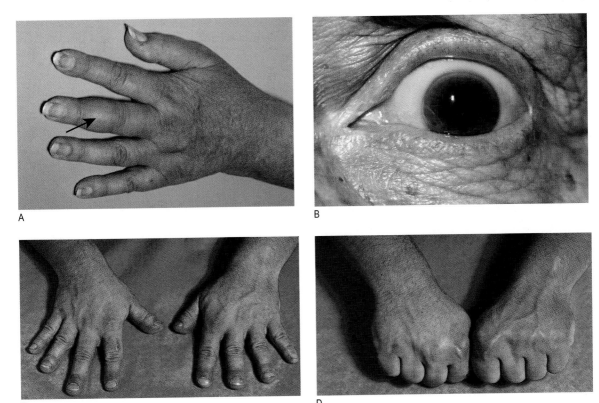

A

B

C

D

Fig. 5.8 Parathyroid disease. (A) 'Brown tumour' of the phalanx (middle finger) in hyperparathyroidism. **(B)** Corneal calcification in hyperparathyroidism. **(C)** Pseudohypoparathyroidism: short metacarpals. **(D)** These are best seen when the patient makes a fist.

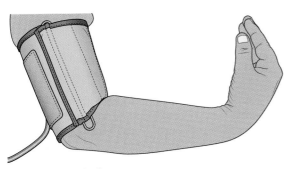

Fig. 5.9 Trousseau's sign.

THE PANCREAS

Anatomy

The pancreas lies behind the stomach on the posterior abdominal wall. Its endocrine functions include the production of insulin, glucagon, gastrin, somatostatin and vasoactive intestinal peptide. Its exocrine function is to produce alkaline secretions containing digestive enzymes.

Symptoms and definitions

Diabetes mellitus

This is characterised by hyperglycaemia due to absolute or relative insulin deficiency. Insulin-dependent patients are particularly susceptible to acute metabolic decompensation due to hypoglycaemia or ketoacidosis, both of which require prompt clinical and biochemical recognition and treatment.

There are two main subtypes:

- Type 1: severe insulin deficiency due to autoimmune destruction of the pancreatic islets.
- Type 2: commonly affects people who are obese and insulin-resistant, although impaired β-cell function is also important.

Diabetes mellitus may present with a classical triad of symptoms:

- Polyuria (and nocturia): due to osmotic diuresis caused by glycosuria.
- Thirst: due to the resulting loss of fluid and electrolytes.
- Weight loss: due to fluid depletion and breakdown of fat and muscle secondary to insulin deficiency.

Other common symptoms are tiredness, mood changes and blurred vision (due to glucose-induced changes in lens refraction). Bacterial and fungal skin infections are common because of the combination of hyperglycaemia, impaired immune resistance and tissue ischaemia. Itching of the genitalia (pruritus vulvae in women, balanitis in men) is due to *Candida* yeast infection (thrush).

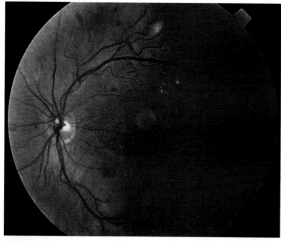

Fig. 5.10 Diabetic retinopathy. Note presence of yellow exudate due to leakage of plasma from abnormal retinal capillaries and multiple dot and blot haemorrhages indicating widespread capillary occlusion – a precursor of new vessel formation.

Examination sequence

- Look for evidence of weight loss and dehydration (p. 58).
- Smell the patient's breath for the sweet smell of ketones (diabetic ketoacidosis).
- Examine the skin: look for signs of infection and rashes. Look for xanthelasma and xanthomata (Fig. 6.8A and B). Examine insulin injection sites for evidence of lipohypertrophy (which may cause unpredictable insulin release), lipoatrophy (rare) or signs of infection (very rare).
- Measure pulse and BP and examine the cardiovascular and peripheral vascular systems.
- Examine the respiratory and gastrointestinal systems.
- Examine the central nervous system.
- Test visual acuity and examine the eyes and optic fundi (p. 285) (Fig. 5.10).
- Perform urinalysis.

Abnormal findings

Dehydration and Kussmaul respiration (hyperventilation with a deep, sighing respiratory pattern) are common in ketoacidosis.

Bacterial skin infections, e.g. cellulitis, boils, abscesses and fungal infections, may be seen. Acanthosis nigricans (Fig. 5.11A) occurs in hyperinsulinism and is seen frequently in patients with insulin-resistant type 2 diabetes.

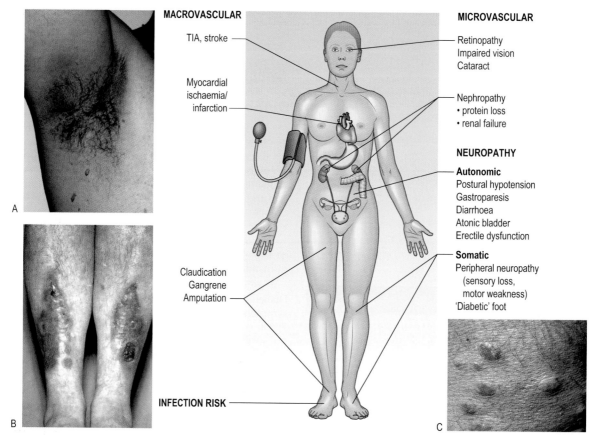

Fig. 5.11 Diabetes and the skin. (A) Acanthosis nigricans. **(B)** Necrobiosis lipoidica. **(C)** Eruptive xanthomata.

Necrobiosis lipoidica (a yellow indurated or ulcerated area surrounded by a red margin: Fig. 5.11B), due to collagen degeneration, may occur on the shins of some type 1 diabetic patients and often causes chronic ulceration. Xanthelasmata and xanthomata indicate significant hyperlipidaemia (Fig. 5.11C and Fig. 6.8).

Microvascular, neuropathic and macrovascular complications of hyperglycaemia (Fig. 5.11) can occur in patients with any type of diabetes mellitus, and may be present at diagnosis in patients with slow-onset type 2 disease. Careful examination of the eyes, cardiovascular, neurological and renal systems, and feet is essential.

Glycosuria suggests hyperglycaemia and, if accompanied by ketonuria (and Kussmaul respiration: Ch. 7) indicates ketoacidosis. Proteinuria occurs in diabetic nephropathy. Detection of nitrite ± haematuria suggests (often occult) urinary infection (Box 5.4).

The diabetic foot

Examination sequence

Diabetic patients have a 15% lifetime risk of foot ulcers, which are highly susceptible to infection. Early recognition of the 'at-risk' diabetic foot is essential. There are two main presentations:

- Neuropathic: where neuropathy predominates but the major arterial supply is intact.
- Neuro-ischaemic: where reduced arterial supply produces ischaemia and exacerbates neuropathy (Fig. 5.13).
  Infection complicates both presentations.
- Inspection:
  - Look for hair loss and nail dystrophy.
  - Examine the skin (including the interdigital clefts) for excessive callus, infections and ulcers.
  - Ask the patient to stand and assess the foot arch.
  - Look for deformation of the joints of the feet.
- Palpation:
  - Feel the temperature of the feet.
  - Examine the dorsalis pedis and posterior tibial pulses. If absent, arrange Doppler studies to evaluate ankle : brachial pressure index (Ch. 6).
- Test for peripheral neuropathy: use a nylon monofilament which buckles at a force of 10 g to apply a standard, reproducible stimulus. The technique and best sites to test are shown in Figure 5.12. Avoid areas of untreated callus.

Abnormal findings

Hair loss and nail dystrophy occur with ischaemia, causing nutritional changes. There may be skin fissures or tinea infection ('athlete's foot'). The foot arch may be

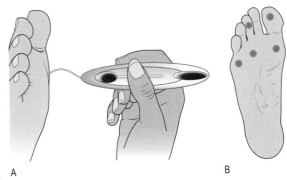

A   B

Fig. 5.12 Monofilament sensory testing of the diabetic foot.
(A) Technique. **(B)** Sites at highest risk (toes and metatarsal heads).

5

excessive in neuropathy or collapsed (rocker-bottom sole). Both conditions cause abnormal pressures and increase risk of plantar ulceration.

Warm feet occur in neuropathy and cold feet in ischaemia.

Sensory neuropathy is present if the patient cannot feel the monofilament in any of the sites. This means loss of protective pain sensation and is a good predictor of future ulceration.

Charcot's arthropathy is disorganised foot architecture, acute inflammation, fracture and bone thinning, usually in a patient with neuropathy but relatively good vascular supply to the lower limb. It presents acutely as a hot, red, swollen foot often impossible to distinguish clinically from infection.

Risk assessment

- Low – no risk factors (no sensation loss, peripheral vascular disease or other risk factors).
- Moderate – one risk factor present.
- High – previous ulceration or amputation, or more than one risk factor present.
- Active – ulceration, spreading infection, critical ischaemia, unexplained red, hot, swollen foot.

THE PITUITARY

Anatomy

The pituitary gland is enclosed in the sella turcica in the base of the skull beneath the hypothalamus. It is bridged over by a fold of dura mater (diaphragma sellae) with sphenoidal air spaces below and the optic chiasm above. The pituitary has two lobes:

- Anterior: which secretes several hormones (adrenocorticotrophic hormone (ACTH), prolactin, growth hormone (GH), thyroid-stimulating hormone and gonadotrophins (luteinising hormone (LH) and follicle-stimulating hormone (FSH)).
- Posterior: an extension of the hypothalamus, which secretes vasopressin (antidiuretic hormone) and oxytocin.

Acromegaly

Some pituitary tumours secrete excess GH. Before puberty, when long bone epiphyses close, this produces gigantism; after puberty, it causes acromegaly. GH

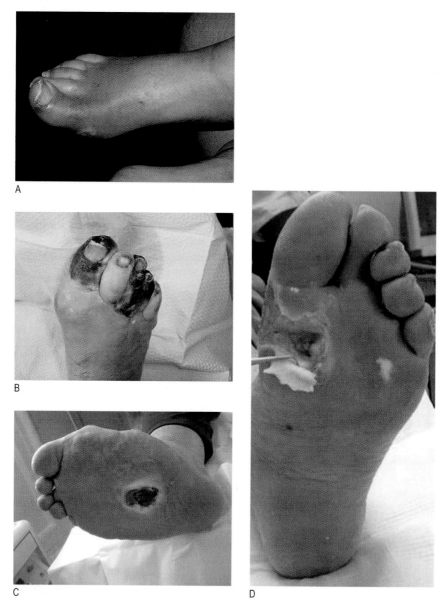

Fig. 5.13 Diabetic foot complications. (A) Infected foot ulcer with cellulitis and ascending lymphangitis. **(B)** Ischaemic foot – digital gangrene. **(C)** Charcot arthropathy with plantar ulcer. **(D)** Neuropathic ulcer (pressure ulcer below metatarsal head.

stimulates excessive insulin-like growth factor-1 production by the liver which is responsible for the clinical manifestations.

History

Ask about the most common symptoms – headache and excessive sweating.

Has the patient (or more often a relative or friend) noticed changes in his facial features? Photographs taken years earlier can be helpful to identify changes and the onset of the condition.

Has the patient noticed an increase in shoe, ring or glove size (Box 5.5)?

EBE 5.5 Acromegaly

Clinical presentations, such as carpal tunnel syndrome, sleep apnoea, with associated coarse facial features and symptoms, such as headache, sweating, an increase in ring or shoe size, should raise the possibility of acromegaly.

Reddy R, Hope S, Wass J. Acromegaly: easily missed? BMJ 2010;341:400–401.

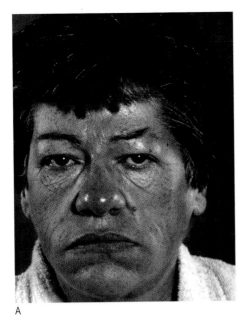

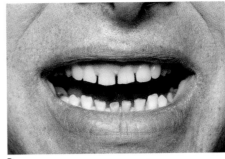

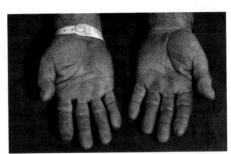

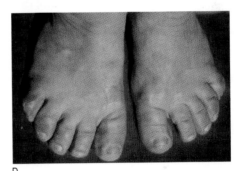

Fig. 5.14 Acromegaly. (A) Typical facies. **(B)** Separation of lower teeth. **(C)** Large fleshy hands. **(D)** Widening of the feet.

Examination sequence

- Look at the face for coarsening of features, thick greasy skin, enlargement of the nose, prognathism (protrusion of the mandible) and separation of the lower teeth (Fig. 5.14A, B).
- Examine the hands and feet. Look for soft-tissue enlargement and complications arising from this, e.g. tight-fitting rings or shoes, carpal tunnel syndrome (Fig. 5.14C, D).
- Assess the visual fields: expansion of the tumour can cause pressure on the optic chiasm, resulting in visual field defects, especially bitemporal hemianopia (Fig. 12.3).
- Check the BP and perform urinalysis. Hypertension and diabetes mellitus are common associations.

Hypopituitarism

Anterior hypopituitarism is due to compression of the pituitary by a macroadenoma, infarction after childbirth (Sheehan's syndrome), severe head trauma or cranial radiotherapy.

Apart from headache due to stretching of the diaphragma sellae and visual abnormalities, clinical presentation depends upon the deficiency of the specific anterior pituitary hormones involved. Individual or multiple hormones may be involved, so questioning in relation to the thyroid, adrenocortical and sexual function is needed.

Examination sequence

Look for:
- extreme skin pallor (a combination of mild anaemia and melanocyte-stimulating hormone deficiency)
- absent axillary hair
- reduced/absent secondary sexual hair (caused by gonadotrophin deficiency) (Fig. 5.15)
- testicular atrophy.
- Examine the eyes for: visual field defects (most often bitemporal hemianopia); optic atrophy or cranial nerve defects (III, IV and VI) caused by a tumour compressing the optic chiasm, optic nerve or cavernous sinus.

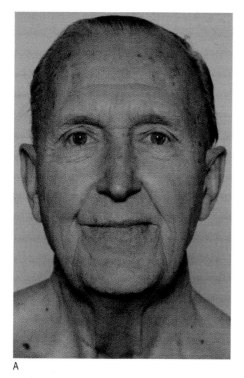
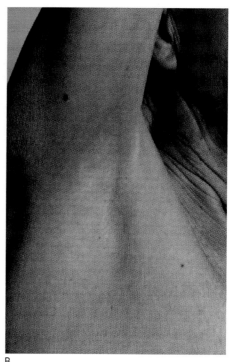

A   B

Fig. 5.15 Hypopituitarism. (A) Hypopituitarism due to a pituitary adenoma (note the fine pale skin). **(B)** Absent axillary hair.

THE ADRENALS

Anatomy

The adrenals are small pyramidal organs lying immediately above the kidneys on their posteromedial surface. The adrenal medulla is part of the sympathetic nervous system and secretes catecholamines. The adrenal cortex secretes cortisol, mineralocorticoids and androgens.

Symptoms and definitions

Cushing's syndrome

Cushing's syndrome is caused by excess exogenous or endogenous corticosteroid exposure. Most cases are iatrogenic due to side-effects of corticosteroid therapy. 'Endogenous' Cushing's usually results from an ACTH-secreting pituitary microadenoma. Other causes include a primary adrenal tumour or 'ectopic' ACTH secretion.

The catabolic effects of steroids cause widespread tissue breakdown (particularly in skin, muscle and bone) with central accumulation of body fat. Proximal myopathy, fragility fractures, spontaneous purpura, skin thinning and susceptibility to infection are common (Fig. 5.16). Patients may be hypertensive.

Examination sequence

- Look at the face and general appearance for central obesity and a round face (Fig. 5.16).

EBE 5.6 **Cushing's syndrome**

Easy bruising, facial plethora, proximal myopathy and broad purple striae best discriminate Cushing's syndrome but these findings do not have high sensitivity. Furthermore, many features of Cushing's syndrome are common in the general population and are less discriminatory, e.g. obesity, dorsocervical fat pad, oedema, acne and hirsutism.

Nieman LK, Biller BMK, Findling JW et al. The diagnosis of Cushing's syndrome: an Endocrine Society clinical practice guideline. J Clin Endocrinol Metab 2008;93:1526–1540.

- Examine the skin for thinning, hyperpigmentation, acne, hirsutism, bruising, striae (especially abdominal) and signs of infection or poor wound healing.
- Check the BP.
- Examine the legs for evidence of proximal muscle weakness and oedema.
- Examine the eyes for cataracts, and hypertensive changes (Fig. 6.16).
- Perform urinalysis (Box 5.6).

Addison's disease

Addison's disease is due to inadequate secretion of cortisol, usually secondary to autoimmune destruction of the adrenal cortex. Symptoms are usually non-specific, but weakness, muscle cramps, nausea, vomiting, diarrhoea or constipation may occur.

5

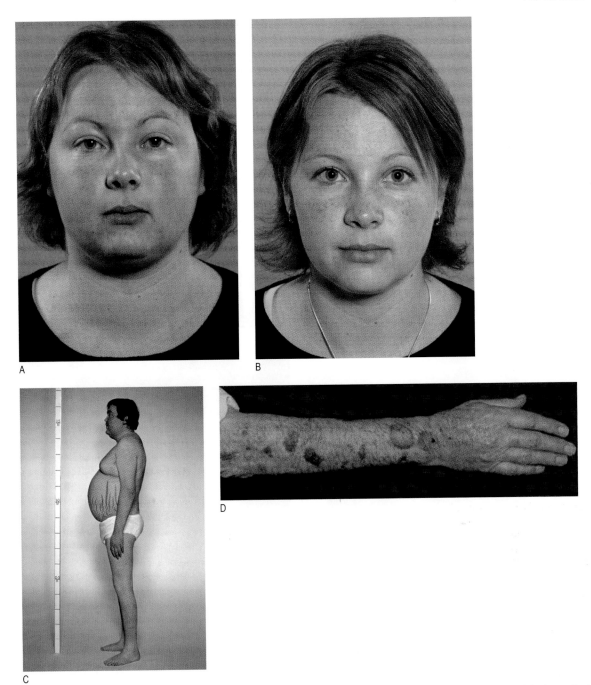

A

B

C

D

Fig. 5.16 Cushing's syndrome. (A) Cushingoid facies. **(B)** After curative pituitary surgery. **(C)** Typical features: facial rounding, central obesity, proximal muscle wasting and skin striae. **(D)** Skin thinning: purpura caused by wristwatch pressure.

Examination sequence

- Look for signs of weight loss.
- Examine the entire skin surface for abnormal or excessive pigmentation: this is most prominent in sun-exposed areas or epithelia subject to trauma or pressure – skin creases, buccal mucosa and recent scars (Fig. 5.17A–C). Excess pigmentation

is produced by melanocyte-stimulating hormone in primary adrenal insufficiency. It is most striking in white Europeans. Vitiligo (depigmentation of areas of skin) occurs in 10–20% of Addison's disease cases (Fig. 5.17D).

- Check the BP and test for postural hypotension (p. 114). Hypotension and postural hypotension result from reduced mineralocorticoid effects.

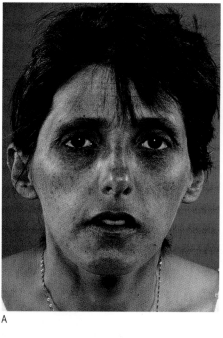

A

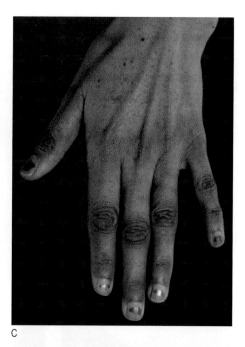

C

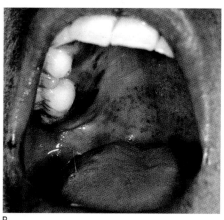

B

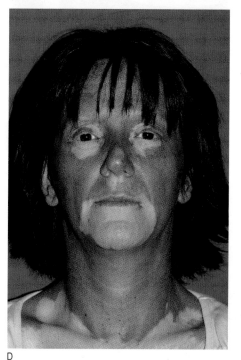

Fig. 5.17 Addison's disease. (A) Facial pigmentation.
(B) Buccal pigmentation. **(C)** Skin crease pigmentation.
(D) Vitiligo – particularly striking due to addisonian
pigmentation of the 'normal' skin.

D

THE GONADS

These glands secrete sex hormones (oestrogen and
testosterone) in response to gonadotrophin (FSH and
LH) release by the pituitary. They also contain the
germ cells.

Symptoms and definitions

Klinefelter's syndrome (47XXY) is the most common
cause of primary hypogonadism in men (1:600 live male
births). Diagnosis may be delayed until later life, by
which time features of prolonged testosterone deficiency
can be seen. Look for soft, finely wrinkled, hairless facial
skin and gynaecomastia and examine the genitalia
(pubic hair is often reduced/absent and the testes <3 ml
in volume; Fig. 5.18).

Hirsutism is common in women with polycystic ovary
syndrome (Fig. 5.19). Virilisation is temporal recession
of the scalp hair, deepening of the voice, breast atrophy,
increased muscle bulk and clitoromegaly (Fig. 5.20).
If present in women with a short history of severe
hirsutism, it suggests a possible testosterone-secreting
tumour.

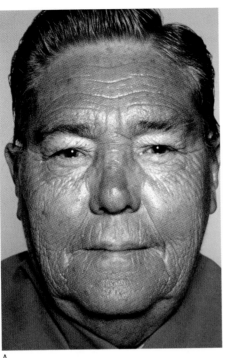

A

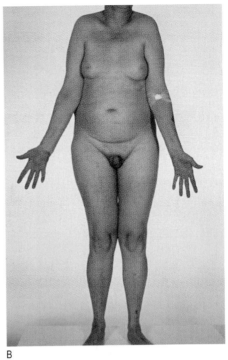

B

Fig. 5.18 Klinefelter's syndrome. (A) Hypogonadal facial skin. **(B)** Gynaecomastia, reduced pubic hair and small testes.

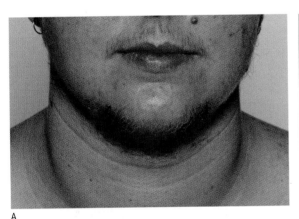

A

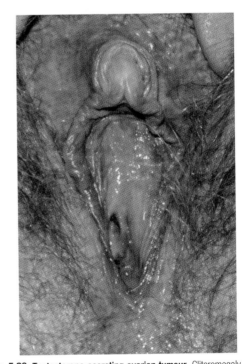

Fig. 5.20 Testosterone-secreting ovarian tumour. Clitoromegaly.

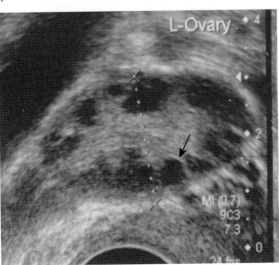

B

Fig. 5.19 Polycystic ovary syndrome. (A) Facial hirsutism.
(B) Ultrasound showing polycystic ovary (arrow).

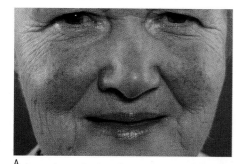

A

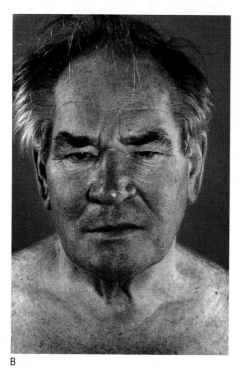

B

Fig. 5.21 Carcinoid syndrome. (A) Acute carcinoid flush. **(B)** Chronic telangiectasia.

OTHER ENDOCRINE DISORDERS

Carcinoid syndrome

Liver metastases from mid-gut carcinoid tumour release vasoactive chemicals into the systemic circulation which cause flushing, diarrhoea and bronchospasm. Bending, exercise or even palpation of the enlarged liver may induce typical skin flushing. Permanent facial telangiectasia occurs after many years of carcinoid flushing (Fig. 5.21).

PUTTING IT ALL TOGETHER

Because of their wide diversity of clinical features, keep alert to the possibility of endocrine disease in non-specific presentations. Perhaps more than in any other area of medicine, pattern recognition is important.

A structured approach to the general endocrine examination

Examination sequence

Carefully observe the patient's overall appearance, manner and habitus for diagnostic clues:

- Is he restless and agitated (hyperthyroidism) or slow and lethargic (hypothyroidism)?
- Measure the height and weight and calculate the body mass index (p. 55). Use a stadiometer in children and adolescents (Fig. 15.20). If the patient is obese, is the adiposity centrally distributed, e.g. Cushing's syndrome or GH deficiency.
- Look for a thoracic kyphosis, which may be a sign of osteoporotic vertebral collapse.
- Inspect the face and eyes for a 'spot' endocrine diagnosis (Figs 5.4A, 5.7A, 5.14A, 5.16A, 5.17A, 5.18A).
- Look at the mouth for overgrowth of the chin and tongue (acromegaly) and for buccal pigmentation (Addison's disease).
- Examine the hands: the initial handshake may suggest a diagnosis, e.g. tremor and palmar sweating in hyperthyroidism. Look for soft-tissue overgrowth (acromegaly) or dysmorphism (abnormal metacarpal length in pseudohypoparathyroidism); skin crease pigmentation (Addison's disease); wasting of the thenar muscles due to carpal tunnel syndrome (hypothyroidism, acromegaly) (Fig. 14.29B).
- Examine the entire skin surface: look for abnormal pallor (hypopituitarism), vitiligo, skin or scar pigmentation (Addison's disease), plethora (Cushing's or carcinoid syndrome). Patients with Cushing's syndrome often have thin, fragile skin with bruising after trivial trauma (Fig. 5.16D). Inspect the axillae and groins for acanthosis nigricans (obesity, diabetes mellitus) (Fig. 5.11A).
- Is the body hair normal in quality and amount? Look for hirsutism in females (polycystic ovary syndrome: Fig. 5.19) and for loss of hair in the axillae and groins (hypopituitarism) (Fig. 5.15B).
- Assess the pulse rate, rhythm and volume. Tachycardia and atrial fibrillation may suggest thyrotoxicosis.
- Record the BP. Hypertension is a feature of several endocrine conditions, e.g. Cushing's syndrome, phaeochromocytoma, Conn's syndrome (primary hyperaldosteronism) (Box 5.1). Postural hypotension (p. 114) occurs in adrenal insufficiency.
- Examine the eyes: look for features of thyroid disease. Assess visual acuity and perform fundoscopy in patients with diabetes mellitus. Assess visual acuities and fields (p. 286) in patients with suspected pituitary tumours (to detect bitemporal hemianopia due to compression of the optic chiasm). Look for optic atrophy in patients with longstanding optic pathway compression (Fig. 12.31A).
- Examine the neck for goitre. If present, record its size, surface and consistency.
- Look for gynaecomastia (common in Klinefelter's syndrome: Fig. 5.18) and galactorrhoea: Gently massage the breast tissue towards the nipple to see if milk is expressed. Explain beforehand why you are performing this examination and watch the patient carefully since this may be uncomfortable.

- Examine the abdomen: look for purple striae (Cushing's syndrome). Carcinoid syndrome is associated with a palpable, nodular liver, which is sometimes massively enlarged. Adrenal tumours may occasionally be palpable, but be cautious if you suspect phaeochromocytoma, as palpation may precipitate a hypertensive paroxysm.
- Inspect the legs for pretibial myxoedema (Graves' disease: Fig. 5.4D), proximal muscle wasting or weakness (Cushing's syndrome and hyperthyroidism) and delayed tendon reflexes (hypothyroidism).
- Examine the feet for signs of diabetic neuropathy, ischaemia and ulcers.
- Examine the external genitalia (p. 223). Inspect the amount of pubic hair and make a pubertal staging of all adolescents using Tanner gradings (Ch. 10). In men, record testicular size and consistency (p. 236). In women, look for virilising features.

- Test the urine for glucose, ketones, protein and nitrite.
- Formal psychological evaluation (p. 25) may be appropriate in selected patients (Cushing's syndrome, hyperparathyroidism).

INVESTIGATIONS

Measure serum hormone levels to assess over- or underactivity. Suppression tests can determine whether hormonal secretion is autonomous. Stimulation tests assess hormonal reserve (or lack of it in deficiency states). Modern imaging enables visualisation of small endocrine tumours, sometimes only millimetres in diameter (Box 5.7 and Fig. 5.22).

5.7 Investigations in endocrine disease

Investigation	Indication/comment
Bedside	
Urinalysis	Glycosuria in diabetes mellitus Proteinuria in hypertensive renal damage
Capillary blood glucose	High in diabetes mellitus
Blood	
Calcium	High in hyperparathyroidism
Free thyroxine	High in hyperthyroidism Low in hypothyroidism
Thyroxine-stimulating hormone	Undetectable in hyperthyroidism High in primary hypothyroidism
Serum cortisol	Low in hypoadrenalism, usually with reduced Synacthen response Loss of diurnal rhythm in Cushing's Reduced dexamethasone suppressibility in Cushing's
Gonadotrophins	High in primary hypogonadism in both sexes
Imaging	
Ultrasound	Thyroid, parathyroid, ovary, testis
Magnetic resonance imaging	Pituitary, pancreas
Computed tomography	Pancreas, adrenal
Radionuclide	Thyroid (^{123}I), parathyroid (^{99m}Tc-sesta-MIBI), adrenal (^{123}I-mIBG), neuroendocrine tumours (^{123}I-octreotide)
Positron emission tomography (PET)	Thyroid and neuroendocrine tumours
Invasive	
Fine-needle aspiration cytology	Thyroid nodule
Inferior petrosal sinus sampling for adrenocorticotrophic hormone (ACTH)	ACTH-dependent Cushing's

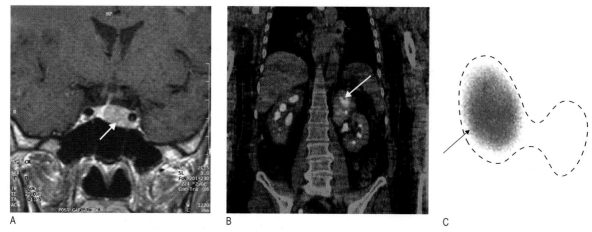

Fig. 5.22 Endocrine imaging. (A) Magnetic resonance imaging showing pituitary macroadenoma (arrow). **(B)** Positron emission tomography-computed tomography scan showing an adrenal cancer (arrow). **(C)** ^{99m}Technetium radionuclide scan confirming unilateral toxic thyroid adenoma (arrowed) – dotted line shows outline of thyroid.

Neil Grubb
James Spratt
Andrew Bradbury

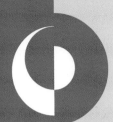

The cardiovascular system

6

CARDIOVASCULAR EXAMINATION

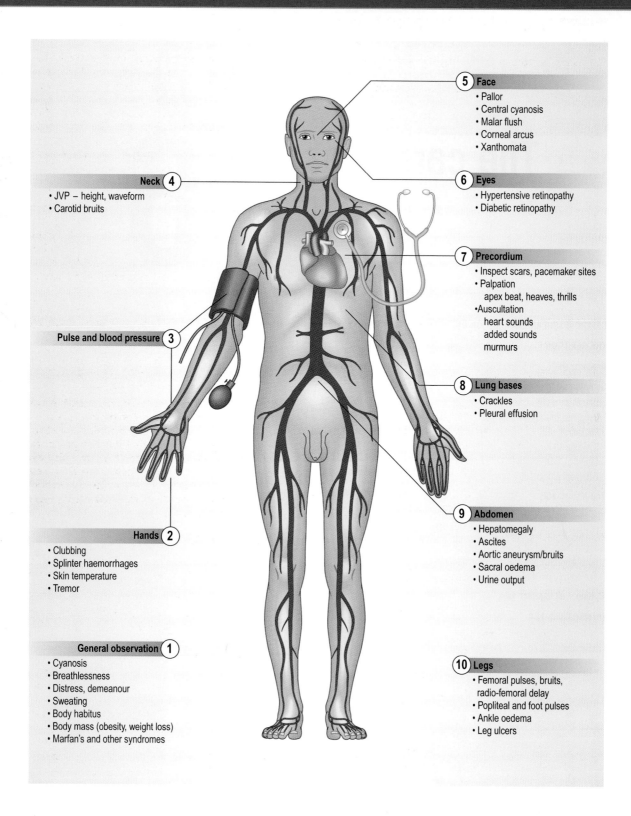

5 Face
- Pallor
- Central cyanosis
- Malar flush
- Corneal arcus
- Xanthomata

6 Eyes
- Hypertensive retinopathy
- Diabetic retinopathy

7 Precordium
- Inspect scars, pacemaker sites
- Palpation
  apex beat, heaves, thrills
- Auscultation
  heart sounds
  added sounds
  murmurs

8 Lung bases
- Crackles
- Pleural effusion

9 Abdomen
- Hepatomegaly
- Ascites
- Aortic aneurysm/bruits
- Sacral oedema
- Urine output

10 Legs
- Femoral pulses, bruits, radio-femoral delay
- Popliteal and foot pulses
- Ankle oedema
- Leg ulcers

Neck 4
- JVP – height, waveform
- Carotid bruits

Pulse and blood pressure 3

Hands 2
- Clubbing
- Splinter haemorrhages
- Skin temperature
- Tremor

General observation 1
- Cyanosis
- Breathlessness
- Distress, demeanour
- Sweating
- Body habitus
- Body mass (obesity, weight loss)
- Marfan's and other syndromes

THE HEART

ANATOMY

The heart comprises two muscular pumps working in series, covered in a serous sac (pericardium) which allows free movement with each heart beat and respiration. The heart delivers blood to both pulmonary and systemic circulations (Fig. 6.1). The right heart (right atrium and ventricle) pumps deoxygenated blood returning from the systemic veins into the pulmonary circulation at relatively low pressures. The left heart (left atrium and ventricle) receives blood from the lungs and pumps it round the body to the tissues at higher pressures (Fig. 6.2). The heart muscle (myocardium) is thicker in the ventricles than in the atria and in the left ventricle than the right ventricle, to generate higher pressures.

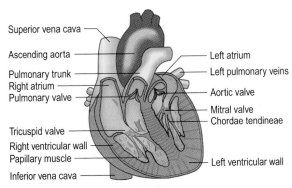

Fig. 6.1 The heart chambers and valves.

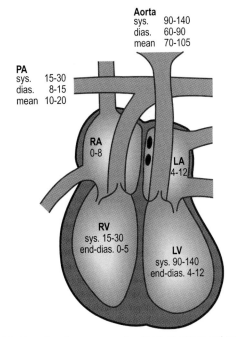

Fig. 6.2 Normal resting pressures (mmHg) in the heart and great vessels. PA, pulmonary artery; RA, right atrium; LA, left atrium; RV, right ventricle; LV, left ventricle; sys., systolic; dias., diastolic.

Heart valves

Atrioventricular valves (tricuspid on the right side, mitral on the left) separate the atria from the ventricles. They are attached to papillary muscles in the ventricular myocardium by chordae tendineae (Fig. 6.1) which prevent them from prolapsing into the atria when the ventricle contracts. The pulmonary valve on the right side of the heart and the aortic valve on the left separate the ventricles from the pulmonary and systemic arterial systems respectively. Each has three half-moon-shaped cusps called semilunar valves. Cardiac contraction is coordinated by specialised groups of cells (Fig. 6.3). The cells in the sinoatrial node normally act as the cardiac pacemaker. Subsequent spread of impulses through the heart ensures that atrial contraction is complete before ventricular contraction (systole) begins. At the end of systole the atrioventricular valves open, allowing blood to flow from the atria to refill the ventricles (diastole).

SYMPTOMS AND DEFINITIONS

See Box 6.1.

Chest pain and discomfort

Chest pain and discomfort are crucial symptoms because of their association with major pathology such as coronary artery disease and aortic dissection. Use a systematic history to distinguish serious from benign causes. Patients often describe discomfort rather than pain, and the severity of discomfort does not necessarily reflect the severity of the underlying problem. Coronary artery disease may produce no symptoms in its early phases and in elderly or diabetic patients.

Angina pectoris

Angina pectoris is the most common cardiac pain. It is usually due to myocardial ischaemia from obstructed

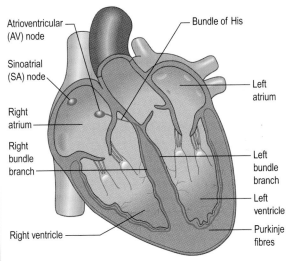

Fig. 6.3 Conducting system of the heart.

6.1 Common symptoms of heart disease

Symptom	Cardiovascular causes	Other causes
Chest discomfort	Myocardial infarction Angina Pericarditis Aortic dissection	Oesophageal spasm Pneumothorax Musculoskeletal pain
Breathlessness	Heart failure Angina Pulmonary embolism Pulmonary hypertension	Respiratory disease Anaemia Obesity Anxiety
Palpitation	Tachyarrhythmias Ectopic beats	Anxiety Hyperthyroidism Drugs
Syncope/ dizziness	Arrhythmias Postural hypotension Aortic stenosis Hypertrophic cardiomyopathy Atrial myxoma	Simple faints Epilepsy Anxiety
Oedema	Heart failure Constrictive pericarditis Venous stasis Lymphoedema	Nephrotic syndrome Liver disease Drugs Immobility

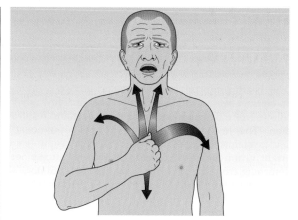

Fig. 6.4 Site and radiation of angina.

- Unstable angina is limiting angina of abrupt onset, or of increasing severity, duration or frequency. It may occur with minimal exertion or at rest. It is a medical emergency, as it may herald myocardial infarction.
- Crescendo angina occurs at increasing frequency at lower workloads, but not at rest.
- Nocturnal or decubitus angina occurs at night or on lying flat. It is caused either by increased venous return or reducing efficacy of antiangina drugs, which are often taken in the morning and may wear off overnight. It indicates severe coronary artery disease.

It may be difficult to distinguish between angina pectoris and non-cardiac causes of chest pain, such as oesophageal pain (Box 6.2).

Myocardial infarction causes symptoms that are similar to, but more severe and prolonged than, those of angina pectoris. Other features include restlessness, breathlessness and a feeling of impending death (angor animi). Autonomic stimulation produces sweating, pallor, nausea, vomiting and diarrhoea, particularly in inferior wall infarction. Pain is absent in up to 30% of patients with myocardial infarction, especially the elderly and those with diabetes mellitus.

Pericardial pain is a sharp anterior central chest pain exacerbated by inspiration and movement, particularly lying down and relieved by sitting forward. It may be confused with angina but both may coexist. It is caused by inflammation of the pericardium secondary to myocardial infarction, viral infection, or after surgery, catheter ablation, angioplasty or radiotherapy.

Aortic dissection is a tear in the intima of the aorta that allows blood to penetrate the media under high pressure, cleaving the aortic wall. It is usually associated with abrupt onset of very severe, tearing chest pain which can radiate to the back (typically interscapular) and may be associated with profound autonomic stimulation. If the tear involves the coronary, cranial or upper limb arteries, it may cause myocardial infarction, syncope, stroke and upper limb pulse asymmetry. If the tear extends into the thoracoabdominal aorta it can affect the intercostal, visceral, lumbar, renal and iliac arteries, leading to paraplegia, mesenteric infarction, renal failure and lower limb ischaemia (often with an absent femoral

flow in an epicardial coronary vessel, but can occur in conditions such as aortic stenosis or hypertrophic cardiomyopathy when there is increased myocardial oxygen demand due to increased left ventricular afterload (Box 6.2). Characteristically angina is an ache or dull discomfort, felt diffusely in the centre of the anterior chest, lasting <10 minutes. Patients describe a tight or pressing 'band-like' sensation, similar to a heavy weight, which can be confused with indigestion. It may radiate down one or both arms and into the throat, jaw and teeth (Fig. 6.4). It is not affected by inspiration, twisting or turning. The severity of the discomfort is a poor guide to prognosis. It may be precipitated by anything that increases the force of cardiac contraction, heart rate or blood pressure (BP) and increases myocardial oxygen demand. Triggers include:

- exercise
- cold or windy weather (causes peripheral vasoconstriction)
- walking uphill or carrying a heavy load (increases cardiac output and BP)
- exercise following a heavy meal (postprandial angina) causing redistribution of myocardial blood flow.

Angina is relieved by rest and glyceryl trinitrate (GTN), and is more likely to occur early during exercise. Some patients describe 'walk-through' angina, as peripheral vasodilatation during exercise decreases myocardial workload. Use an objective assessment of the impact of angina on the patient's activity (Box 6.3):

6.2 Cardiovascular causes of chest pain and their characteristics

	Angina	Myocardial infarction	Aortic dissection	Pericardial pain	Oesophageal pain
Site	Retrosternal	Retrosternal	Interscapular/ retrosternal	Retrosternal or left-sided	Retrosternal or epigastric
Onset	Over 1–2 minutes	Rapid over a few minutes	Very sudden	Gradual, postural change may suddenly aggravate	Over 1–2 minutes; can be sudden (spasm)
Character	Constricting, heavy	Constricting, heavy	Tearing or ripping	Sharp, 'stabbing', pleuritic	Gripping, tight or burning
Radiation	Sometimes arm(s), neck, epigastrium	Often to arm(s), neck, jaw, sometimes epigastrium	Back, between shoulders	Left shoulder or back	Often to back, sometimes to arms
Associated features	Breathlessness	Sweating, nausea, vomiting, breathlessness, feeling of impending death (angor animi)	Sweating, syncope, focal neurological signs, signs of limb ischaemia, mesenteric ischaemia	Flu-like prodrome, breathlessness, fever	Heartburn, acid reflux
Timing	2–10 minutes	Prolonged	Prolonged	Gradual onset, variable duration	Nighttime common, variable duration
Exacerbating/ relieving factors	Triggered by emotion, exertion, especially if cold, windy. Relieved by rest, nitrates	'Stress' and exercise rare triggers, usually spontaneous. Not relieved by rest or nitrates	Spontaneous No manoeuvres relieve pain	Pleuritic Sitting up/lying down may affect intensity Non-steroidal anti-inflammatory drugs (NSAIDs) help	Lying flat some foods may trigger Not relieved by rest; nitrates sometimes relieve
Severity	Mild to moderate	Usually severe	Very severe	Can be severe	Usually mild but oesophageal spasm can mimic myocardial infarction
Cause	Coronary artery disease, aortic stenosis, hypertrophic cardiomyopathy	Plaque rupture and coronary artery occlusion	Thoracic aortic dissection rupture	Pericarditis (usually viral, also post myocardial infarction)	Oesophageal spasm, reflux, hiatus hernia

6.3 Canadian Cardiovascular Society: functional classification of stable angina

Grade 1	Ordinary physical activity, such as walking and climbing stairs, does not cause angina. Angina with strenuous or rapid or prolonged exertion at work or recreation
Grade 2	Slight limitation of ordinary activity. Walking or climbing stairs rapidly, walking uphill, walking or stair climbing after meals, in cold, in wind, or when under emotional stress, or only during the few hours after awakening
Grade 3	Marked limitation of ordinary physical activity. Walking 1–2 blocks on the level and climbing less than one flight in normal conditions
Grade 4	Inability to carry on any physical activity without discomfort; angina may be present at rest

pulse on the affected side if the dissection extends into the iliac artery). Predisposing factors include smoking, hypertension and connective tissue disorders such as Marfan's syndrome (Fig. 3.28).

Dyspnoea (breathlessness)

This is an awareness of increased drive to breathe and is normal on exercise. It is pathological if it occurs at a significantly lower threshold than expected. Breathlessness is a non-specific symptom and may be caused by cardiac, respiratory, neuromuscular and metabolic conditions, or by toxins or anxiety (Ch. 7).

Dyspnoea may be caused by myocardial ischaemia and is known as 'angina equivalent'. It may occur instead of, or with, chest discomfort, especially in elderly and diabetic patients. It has identical precipitants to angina and may be relieved by GTN. Dyspnoea in heart

6.4 Some mechanisms and causes of heart failure

Mechanism	Cause
Reduced ventricular contractility (systolic dysfunction)	Myocardial ischaemia Myocardial infarction Cardiomyopathy Myocarditis Drugs with negative inotropic actions, e.g. beta-blockers
Impaired ventricular filling (diastolic dysfunction)	Left ventricular hypertrophy Constrictive pericarditis
Increased metabolic and cardiac demand	Pregnancy* Anaemia* Fever* Thyrotoxicosis Arteriovenous fistulae Paget's disease
Arrhythmia	Tachycardia, especially atrial fibrillation Bradycardia
Valvular or structural cardiac lesions	Mitral and/or aortic valve disease Tricuspid and/or pulmonary valve disease (rare) Ventricular septal defect Hypertrophic cardiomyopathy
Fluid overload	Excessive intravenous infusion Drugs, e.g. non-steroidal anti-inflammatory drugs, steroids
Other	Intercurrent non-cardiac illness in patients with cardiac disease

*Aggravating factors which rarely cause heart failure alone.

6.5 New York Heart Association classification of heart failure symptom severity

Class I	No limitations. Ordinary physical activity does not cause undue fatigue, dyspnoea or palpitation (asymptomatic left ventricular dysfunction)
Class II	Slight limitation of physical activity. Such patients are comfortable at rest. Ordinary physical activity results in fatigue, palpitation, dyspnoea or angina pectoris (symptomatically 'mild' heart failure)
Class III	Marked limitation of physical activity. Less than ordinary physical activity will lead to symptoms (symptomatically 'moderate' heart failure)
Class IV	Symptoms of congestive heart failure are present, even at rest. With any physical activity increased discomfort is experienced (symptomatically 'severe' heart failure)

but patients with heart failure may also produce frothy, blood-stained sputum.

Platypnoea is breathlessness on sitting upright. It is much rarer than orthopnoea and is usually associated with deoxygenation (platypnoea–orthodeoxia syndrome). It requires both anatomical and functional abnormalities. The anatomical component is usually an intracardiac communication, e.g. atrial septal defect. Platypnoea then develops when a right-to-left shunt occurs because of the functional component. This may be cardiac, e.g. pericardial effusion; pulmonary, e.g. pneumonectomy; abdominal, e.g. liver cirrhosis; or vascular, e.g. aortic aneurysm.

Palpitation

Palpitation is an unexpected awareness of the heart beating in the chest. It may be rapid, forceful or irregular, and described as thumping, pounding, fluttering, jumping, racing or skipping. The patient may be able to mimic the rhythm by tapping it out.

Palpitation may occur in sinus rhythm with anxiety, with intermittent irregularity of the heart beat, e.g. extrasystoles, or with an abnormal rhythm (arrhythmia). Not all patients with arrhythmia experience palpitation, e.g. atrial fibrillation often occurs in the elderly but rarely causes palpitation. The history helps distinguish different types of palpitation (Box 6.6).

Healthy people are occasionally aware of their heart beating with normal (sinus) rhythm, e.g. after exercise, or when waiting for an interview or examination. The sensation is more common in bed at night when external visual and auditory inputs are minimal and visceral sensations are more prominent. Slim people may notice it when lying on their left side.

Palpitation can be induced by excessive caffeine or nicotine intake. Prescription or 'over-the-counter' drugs can cause palpitation, e.g. decongestants, antihistamines, as can stimulant recreational drugs, e.g. amphetamines, ecstasy and cocaine. Carotid artery disease may cause an intermittent whooshing noise (bruit) heard in the affected side of the head during an arrhythmia.

Ectopic beats (extrasystoles) are a benign cause of palpitation at rest and are abolished by exercise. Patients

failure may be associated with fatigue. Pulmonary oedema (accumulation of fluid in the alveoli) occurs with left heart failure because increased left atrial end-diastolic pressure leads to elevated pressure in the pulmonary veins and capillaries (Box 6.4). Patients with acute pulmonary oedema usually prefer to be upright. Those with pulmonary embolism are often more comfortable lying flat and may faint (syncope) if made to sit upright. Use the New York Heart Association grading system to assess the degree of symptomatic limitation caused by the exertional breathlessness of heart failure (Box 6.5). Other cardiovascular causes of acute breathlessness include pulmonary embolism and arrhythmias.

Orthopnoea is dyspnoea on lying flat and is a sign of advanced heart failure. Lying flat increases venous return and in patients with left ventricular impairment may precipitate pulmonary oedema. The severity can be graded by the number of pillows used at night, e.g. 'three-pillow orthopnoea'.

Paroxysmal nocturnal dyspnoea is sudden breathlessness waking the patient from sleep (Fig. 6.5). It is caused by accumulation of alveolar fluid. Patients may choke or gasp for air, sit on the edge of the bed and open windows in an attempt to relieve their distress. It may be confused with asthma, which can also cause night-time dyspnoea, chest tightness, cough and wheeze,

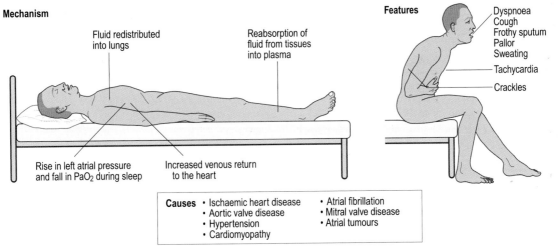

Fig. 6.5 Paroxysmal nocturnal dyspnoea.

6.6 Descriptions of arrhythmias

	Extrasystoles	Sinus tachycardia	Supraventricular tachycardia	Atrial fibrillation	Ventricular tachycardia
Site	–	–	–	–	–
Onset	Sudden	Gradual	Sudden, with 'jump'	Sudden	Sudden
Character	'Jump', missed beat or flutter	Regular, fast	Regular, fast	Irregular, usually fast; slower in elderly	Regular, fast
Radiation	–	–	–	–	–
Associated features	Nil	Anxiety	Polyuria, lightheadedness, chest tightness	Polyuria, breathlessness. Syncope uncommon	Presyncope, syncope, chest tightness
Timing	Brief	A few minutes	Minutes to hours	Variable	Variable
Exacerbating/ relieving factors	Fatigue, caffeine, alcohol may trigger. Often relieved by walking (increases sinus rate)	Exercise or anxiety may trigger	Usually at rest, trivial movements, e.g. bending, may trigger. Vagal manoeuvres may relieve	Exercise or alcohol may trigger; often spontaneous	Exercise may trigger; often spontaneous
Severity	Mild (usually)	Mild to moderate	Moderate to severe	Very variable, may be asymptomatic	Often severe

may describe 'missed beats', sometimes followed by a particularly strong heart beat. The ectopic beat produces a small stroke volume and an impalpable impulse due to incomplete left ventricular filling. The subsequent compensatory pause leads to ventricular overfilling and a forceful contraction with the next beat.

Supraventricular tachycardia produces sudden paroxysms of rapid, regular palpitation which can sometimes be terminated with breathing manoeuvres or carotid sinus pressure. Supraventricular tachycardia often affects young patients with no other underlying cardiac disease.

Ventricular tachycardia can produce similar symptoms but is more often associated with presyncope or syncope, and tends to affect patients with cardiomyopathy or previous myocardial infarction.

Urgently investigate palpitation with any high-risk features, including:

- Recent (<3 months) myocardial infarction, percutaneous coronary intervention or cardiac surgery
- Associated syncope or severe chest pain
- Family history of syncope or sudden death
- Wolff–Parkinson–White syndrome, or inherited channelopathy, e.g. long QT syndrome
- Significant structural heart disease, e.g. hypertrophic cardiomyopathy, aortic stenosis.

Syncope

Syncope is a loss of consciousness due to cerebral hypoperfusion. Dizziness may be due to vertigo or

6.7 Symptoms related to medication

Symptom	Medication
Dyspnoea	Beta-blockers in patients with asthma Exacerbation of heart failure by beta-blockers, some calcium channel antagonists (verapamil, diltiazem), NSAIDs
Dizziness	Vasodilators, e.g. nitrates, alpha-blockers, angiotensin-converting enzyme (ACE) inhibitors and angiotensin II receptor antagonists
Angina	Aggravated by thyroxine or drug-induced anaemia, e.g. aspirin or NSAIDs
Oedema	Steroids, NSAIDs, some calcium channel antagonists, e.g. nifedipine, amlodipine
Palpitation	Tachycardia and/or arrhythmia from thyroxine, β_2 stimulants, e.g. salbutamol, digoxin toxicity, hypokalaemia from diuretics, tricyclic antidepressants

NSAIDs, non-steroidal anti-inflammatory drugs.

6.8 Causes of unilateral and bilateral leg oedema

Unilateral

- Deep vein thrombosis
- Soft-tissue infection
- Trauma
- Immobility, e.g. hemiplegia
- Lymphoedema

Bilateral

- Heart failure
- Chronic venous insufficiency
- Hypoproteinaemia, e.g. nephrotic syndrome, kwashiorkor, cirrhosis
- Lymphatic obstruction, e.g. pelvic tumour, filariasis
- Drugs, e.g. NSAIDs, nifedipine, amlodipine, fludrocortisone
- Inferior vena caval obstruction
- Thiamine (vitamin B_1) deficiency (wet beriberi)
- Milroy's disease (unexplained lymphoedema which appears at puberty; more common in females)
- Immobility

lightheadedness (p. 243). Vertigo is rarely caused by heart disease. Lightheadedness, syncope or a feeling of impending loss of consciousness (presyncope) may be cardiovascular in origin. The main causes are:

- postural hypotension
- neurocardiogenic syncope
- arrhythmias
- mechanical obstruction to cardiac output.

Patients with vascular disease affecting the carotid and/or vertebral arteries may present with non-focal cerebral symptoms due to hypoperfusion. Common precipitating factors are head turning, getting up quickly from sitting or lying and starting or increasing antihypertensive drugs.

Postural hypotension is a fall of >20 mmHg in systolic BP on standing. It can be caused by hypovolaemia, antihypertensive drug therapy, especially diuretics and vasodilators (Box 6.7), and autonomic neuropathy. Postural hypotension is common in the elderly, affecting up to 30% of individuals aged >65 years.

Neurocardiogenic syncope is a group of conditions caused by abnormal autonomic reflexes. A simple **faint** occurs in healthy people forced to stand for a long time in a warm environment or subject to painful or emotional stimuli, e.g. the sight of blood. It results from sudden slow heart rate (bradycardia) and/or vasodilatation. There may be a prior history of fainting with a prodrome of lightheadedness, tinnitus, nausea, sweating and facial pallor and a darkening of vision from the periphery as the retinal blood supply (the most oxygen-sensitive part of the nervous system) is reduced,. The person then slides to the floor, losing consciousness. When laid flat to aid cerebral circulation, the individual wakes up, often flushing from vasodilatation and nauseated or even vomiting due to vagal overactivity. If held upright by misguided bystanders, continued cerebral hypoperfusion delays recovery and may lead to a seizure and a mistaken diagnosis of epilepsy.

Frequent fainting caused by minor stimuli may be due to malignant vasovagal syndrome or hypersensitive carotid sinus syndrome (HCSS). In patients with HCSS, gentle pressure over the carotid sinus may reproduce the symptoms by triggering bradycardia.

Arrhythmias can cause syncope or presyncope. The most common cause is bradyarrhythmia, due to sinoatrial disease or to atrioventricular block, i.e. Stokes–Adams attacks. Drugs, including digoxin, beta-blockers and rate-limiting calcium channel blockers, e.g. verapamil, diltiazem are a common cause of bradyarrhythmia. Supraventricular tachyarrhythmias, e.g. atrial fibrillation, rarely cause syncope. Ventricular tachycardia often causes syncope or presyncope, especially in patients with impaired left ventricular function.

Mechanical obstruction to cardiac output, including severe aortic stenosis and hypertrophic cardiomyopathy, can obstruct left ventricular outflow causing syncope or presyncope, especially on exertion when cardiac output cannot meet the increased metabolic demand.

Pulmonary embolism can obstruct outflow from the right ventricle, and is a frequently overlooked cause of recurrent syncope. Cardiac tumours, e.g. atrial myxoma, and thrombosis or failure of prosthetic heart valves are rare causes of syncope.

Oedema

Excess fluid in the interstitial space causes oedema (tissue swelling). It is usually gravity-dependent and so especially seen around the ankles, or over the sacrum in patients lying in bed. The most common causes of lower limb swelling are chronic venous disease and lymphoedema. Other causes include heart failure and vasodilator medications (Box 6.8 and Box 3.16). In general, if the jugular venous pressure (JVP) is not elevated, then oedema is not cardiogenic.

Infective endocarditis is microbial infection of the heart valves (natural or prosthetic), the lining of the cardiac chambers or blood vessels or a congenital abnormality, e.g. septal defect. The causative organism is usually bacterial, but may be fungal, rickettsial or

6

6.9 Cardiovascular disease presenting with 'non-cardiac' symptoms		
System	**Symptom**	**Cause**
Central nervous system	Stroke	Cerebral embolism Endocarditis Hypertension
Gastrointestinal	Jaundice Abdominal pain	Liver congestion secondary to heart failure Mesenteric embolism
Renal	Oliguria	Heart failure

Chlamydia. The presentation may be acute or subacute. Many features of infective endocarditis are thought to result from circulating immune complexes or emboli, e.g. petechial rash, haematuria, splinter haemorrhages, cerebral emboli. Features such as fever, splenomegaly and clubbing may occur.

Other symptoms

Non-cardiac symptoms occur in heart disease (Box 6.9). Infective endocarditis may present with non-specific symptoms, including weight loss, tiredness, fever and night sweats, and atrial fibrillation with symptoms and signs of cerebral or systemic embolisation (commonly legs, arms or viscera).

THE HISTORY

Heart disease commonly occurs without abnormal physical findings so the history is critical in making a diagnosis. Examination may confirm a cardiac diagnosis, e.g. murmur or signs of heart failure but, even in serious disease, physical signs may be completely absent.

- Patients with severe carotid artery stenosis may have no neck bruit due to low volume flow.
- Large abdominal aortic aneurysms (AAAs) can be impalpable in the obese.
- Patients with extensive deep vein thrombosis (DVT) often appear to have normal legs.

Presenting complaint

Establish the frequency, duration and severity of symptoms, exacerbating and relieving factors. Urgently attend to breathlessness, recent chest or lower limb pain. As many cardiovascular diseases are slowly progressive, the evolution of symptoms guides the timing of investigations and treatment, e.g. surgery for carotid artery disease is most effective soon after a cerebral event; and heart valve surgery is indicated for significantly limiting symptoms.

Functional impairment

How do symptoms affect your patient's functional capacity? Establish the intensity of exercise required to induce symptoms.

- Are symptoms provoked by gentle walking or strenuous exercise like climbing hills or stairs?
- Can patients keep up when walking with their peers?
- Do patients feel frustrated or restricted by their symptomatic limitation?
- How are domestic (cooking, cleaning, shopping), social (hobbies, sport) and occupational activities limited?

Lightheadedness and syncope may impair confidence, raise fear of physical injury and have safety implications when driving.

Calf leg pain on walking (intermittent claudication) from lower limb arterial disease is the most common symptom of peripheral vascular disease (p. 127):

- How far can the patient walk before the pain comes on? Is this on the flat or uphill?

Past history

Ask about rheumatic fever or heart murmurs during childhood and associated conditions, including:

- Hypertension
- Diabetes mellitus
- Kidney disease
- Thyrotoxicosis (atrial fibrillation)
- Marfan's syndrome (aortic regurgitation or aortic dissection).

In suspected infective endocarditis ask about potential causes of bacteraemia e.g. skin infection; recent dental work; intravenous drug use and penetrating trauma.

Consider possible links between other diseases and cardiovascular illness. Examples include patients with renal failure or cancer and pericardial effusion; cytotoxic drugs and heart failure; radiotherapy and radiation arteritis. Patients with chronic lung disease may develop right-sided heart failure (cor pulmonale; p. 115) or atrial fibrillation. Connective tissue diseases, e.g. rheumatoid arthritis, are associated with Raynaud's phenomenon (Fig. 6.38) and pericarditis.

Drug history

Drugs may cause or aggravate symptoms such as breathlessness, chest pain, oedema, palpitation or syncope (Box 6.7). Starting thyroxine for hypothyroidism may precipitate or exacerbate angina. 'Recreational' drugs such as cocaine and amphetamines can cause arrhythmias, chest pain, occlusive and aneurysmal peripheral arterial disease (PAD) and even myocardial infarction. Ask about 'over-the-counter' purchases such as NSAIDs, alternative and herbal medicines, as these may have cardiovascular actions. Beta-blockers and antihypertensives may impair the peripheral circulation and aggravate symptoms of intermittent claudication.

Family history

Many cardiac disorders have a genetic component (Box 6.10). Ask about premature coronary artery disease in first-degree relatives (<60 years in a female or <55 years in a male) or sudden unexplained death at a young age, raising the possibility of a cardiomyopathy or inherited arrhythmia disorder. Patients with venous thrombosis

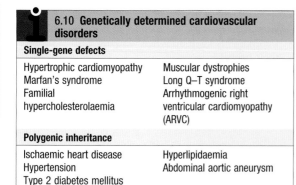

6.10 Genetically determined cardiovascular disorders

Single-gene defects	
Hypertrophic cardiomyopathy	Muscular dystrophies
Marfan's syndrome	Long Q–T syndrome
Familial hypercholesterolaemia	Arrhythmogenic right ventricular cardiomyopathy (ARVC)
Polygenic inheritance	
Ischaemic heart disease	Hyperlipidaemia
Hypertension	Abdominal aortic aneurysm
Type 2 diabetes mellitus	

6.11 Occupational aspects of cardiovascular disease

Occupational exposure associated with cardiovascular disease
- Organic solvents: arrhythmias, cardiomyopathy
- Vibrating machine tools: Raynaud's phenomenon
- Publicans: alcohol-related cardiomyopathy

Occupational exposure exacerbating pre-existing cardiac conditions
- Cold exposure: angina, Raynaud's disease
- Deep-sea diving: embolism through foramen ovale

Occupational requirements for high standards of cardiovascular fitness
- Pilots
- Public transport/heavy goods vehicle drivers
- Armed forces
- Police

may have inherited thrombophilia, e.g. factor V Leiden mutation. Familial hypercholesterolaemia is associated with premature arterial disease.

Social history

Smoking is the strongest risk factor for coronary artery and PAD. Take a detailed smoking history (p. 16).

Alcohol can induce atrial fibrillation and, in excess, is associated with obesity, hypertension and dilated cardiomyopathy. Excess alcohol intake with poor nutrition also predisposes to PAD. Intravenous drug use can damage peripheral arteries and veins, causing infected false aneurysms, e.g. of the common femoral artery in the groin, which can act as a source for infective endocarditis.

Occupational history

Heart disease may impair physical activity and affect employment. This may be a source of anxiety and an indication for treatment. The diagnosis of heart disease and/or PAD has significant consequences in certain occupations, e.g. commercial drivers and pilots (Box 6.11). Workers exposed to occupational vibration through the use of air-powered tools may develop hand–arm vibration syndrome, which presents with vasospastic symptoms, e.g. Raynaud's phenomenon, and neurosensory (numbness, tingling) symptoms.

THE PHYSICAL EXAMINATION

Tailor the sequence and extent of examination to the patient's condition:
- Patients with cardiac or respiratory arrest or requiring immediate emergency: manage first and leave more detailed examination for later (Fig. 19.9).
- Stable patients: examine thoroughly first.

General examination

- Look at the patient's general appearance. Does he look:
  - unwell?
  - breathless or cyanosed?
  - frightened or distressed?
- Check the temperature (p. 61).
- Perform urinalysis.

Hands and skin

Examination sequence

- Look for signs of tobacco staining (Fig. 7.8).
- Look for peripheral cyanosis.
- Feel the temperature.
- Check for clubbing (p. 49).
- Look at the nails for splinter haemorrhages (linear, reddish-brown marks along the axis of the finger and toenails, thought to be due to circulating immune complexes.
- Look at the palmar aspect of the hands for:
  - Janeway lesions – painless red spots, which blanch on pressure, on the thenar/hypothenar eminences of the palms, and soles of the feet.
  - Osler's nodes – painful raised erythematous lesions which are rare but found most often on the pads of the fingers and toes.
- Look at the palmar and extensor surfaces of the hands for xanthomata (yellow skin or tendon nodules from lipid deposits).
- Look at the entire skin surface for petechiae.

Normal findings

The hands usually feel dry at ambient temperature. Peripheral cyanosis (p. 45) is common in healthy patients when the hands are cold. One or two isolated splinter haemorrhages are common in healthy individuals from trauma.

Abnormal findings

Fever is a feature of infective endocarditis and pericarditis and may occur after myocardial infarction. With autonomic stimulation the hands may feel warm and sweaty; with hypotension and shock they may be cold and clammy.

Splinter haemorrhages are found in infective endocarditis and some vasculitic disorders.

A petechial rash (caused by vasculitis), most often present on the legs and conjunctivae (Fig. 6.6), is a transient finding in endocarditis and can be confused with the rash of meningococcal disease (Fig. 17.2A). Janeway lesions, Osler's nodes, nail fold infarcts and finger

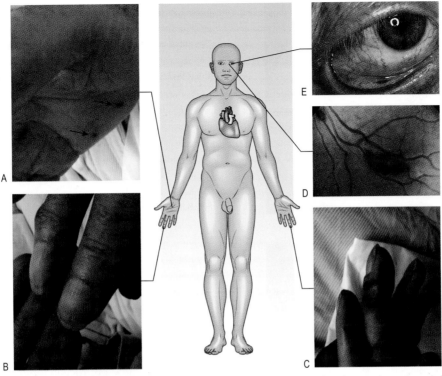

Fig. 6.6 **Clinical features which may be present in infective endocarditis: (A)** Janeway lesions on hypothenar eminence (arrows), **(B)** Splinter haemorrhages, **(C)** Osler's nodes, **(D)** Roth's spot on fundoscopy, **(E)** Petechial haemorrhages on conjunctiva.

clubbing are uncommon features of endocarditis (Ch. 3 and Fig. 6.6).

Urinalysis is necessary to check haematuria (endocarditis, vasculitis), glucose (diabetes) and protein (hypertension and renal disease).

The face and eyes

Examination sequence

Look:

- in the mouth for central cyanosis.
- at the eyelids for xanthelasmata (soft yellowish plaques periorbitally and on the medial aspect of the eyelids associated with hyperlipidaemia).
- at the iris for a corneal arcus.
- at the conjunctivae for petechiae.
- Examine the fundi (p. 291) for features of hypertension (Fig. 6.16), diabetes and Roth's spots (flame-shaped retinal haemorrhages with a 'cotton-wool' centre).

Abnormal findings

Central cyanosis may be due to heart failure or, rarely, congenital heart disease, where it is associated with right-to-left shunting and finger clubbing (p. 49).

Xanthelasmata are an important predictor of cardiovascular disease (Figs 6.7 and 6.8A). If present, also check the patellar and Achilles tendons for xanthomata (Fig. 6.8B).

Corneal arcus is a creamy yellow discoloration at the boundary of the iris and cornea caused by cholesterol deposition. It is more common in men and black

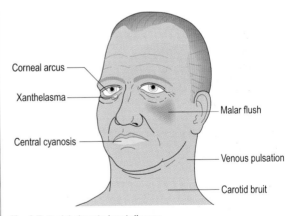

Fig. 6.7 Facial clues to heart disease.

patients (Fig. 6.8C). Both xanthelasmata and corneal arcus can, however, occur in normolipidaemic patients (Box 6.12).

Roth's spots (Fig. 6.6) are caused by a similar mechanism to splinter haemorrhages and can also occur in anaemia or leukaemia.

Arterial pulses

Anatomy

Ejection of blood from the left ventricle into the systemic arterial circulation (Fig. 6.9) creates a pressure wave that can be felt as a 'pulse' where the arteries are superficial

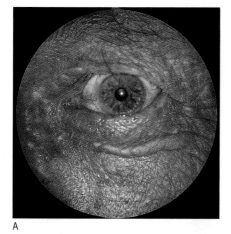

A

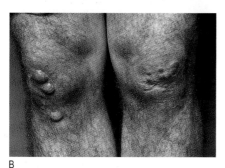

B

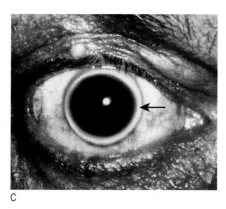

C

Fig. 6.8 Features of hyperlipidaemia. **(A)** Xanthelasma. **(B)** Skin xanthomata over knees. **(C)** Corneal arcus (arrow).

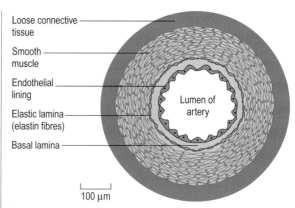

Loose connective tissue

Smooth muscle

Endothelial lining

Elastic lamina (elastin fibres)

Basal lamina

Lumen of artery

|⎯⎯⎯|
100 μm

Fig. 6.9 Cross-section of an artery.

---

or they pass over bone. This pressure wave is not the same as, and travels faster than, the blood flow itself. It can be possible, therefore, to feel a 'pulse' even if there is no flow in the artery being palpated. The pulse waveform depends upon heart rate, stroke volume, left ventricular outflow obstruction, arterial elasticity and peripheral resistance.

Use the larger (brachial, carotid or femoral) pulses to assess the pulse volume and character (Box 6.13). When taking a pulse, assess:

- Rate
- Rhythm
- Volume
- Character.

Record individual pulses as:

- Normal +
- Reduced ±
- Absent –
- Aneurysmal + +

If you are in any doubt about whose pulse you are feeling, palpate your own pulse at the same time. If it is not synchronous with yours, it is the patient's.

Radial pulse

Examination sequence

- Place the pads of your index and middle fingers over the right radial artery.
- Assess rate, and rhythm (Fig. 6.10A).
- Count the pulse rate over 30 seconds; multiply by 2 to obtain the beats per minute (bpm).
- To detect a collapsing pulse: first, check that the patient has no shoulder or arm pain or restriction on movement. Feel the pulse with the base of your fingers, then raise the patient's arm vertically above the patient's head (Fig. 6.10B).
- Palpate both radial pulses simultaneously, assessing any delay between the two, and any difference in pulse volume.
- Palpate the radial and femoral pulses simultaneously, again noting any timing and volume differences.

EBE **6.12 Risk predictors of cardiovascular disease**

The presence of xanthelasma predicts risk of myocardial infarction, coronary heart disease and death in the general population independently of well-known cardiovascular risk factors such as plasma cholesterol and triglyceride concentrations. Corneal arcus, however, is not an independent risk factor.

Christofferson M, Frikke-Schmidt R, Schnohr P et al. Xanthelasmata, arcus cornea and ischaemic vascular disease and death in the general population: prospective cohort study. BMJ 2011;343:731.

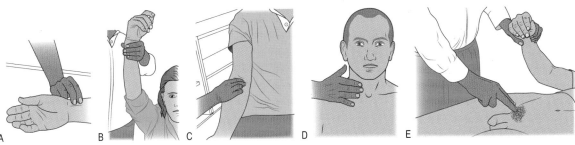

Fig. 6.10 The radial, brachial and carotid pulses. (A) Locating and palpating the radial pulse. **(B)** Feeling for a collapsing radial pulse. **(C)** Assessing the brachial pulse. **(D)** Locating the right carotid pulse with the fingers. **(E)** Examining the femoral artery, while simultaneously checking for radio-femoral delay.

6

6.13 Surface markings of the arterial pulses

Artery	Surface marking
Radial	At the wrist, lateral to the flexor carpi radialis tendon
Brachial	In the antecubital fossa, medial to the biceps tendon
Carotid	At the angle of the jaw, anterior to the sternocleidomastoid muscle
Femoral	Just below the inguinal ligament, midway between the anterior superior iliac spine and the pubic symphysis (the mid inguinal point). It is immediately lateral to the femoral vein and medial to the femoral nerve
Popliteal	Lies posteriorly in relation to the knee joint, at the level of the knee crease, deep in the popliteal fossa
Posterior tibial	Located 2 cm below and posterior to the medial malleolus, where it passes beneath the flexor retinaculum between flexor digitorum longus and flexor hallucis longus
Dorsalis pedis	Passes lateral to the tendon of extensor hallucis longus and is best felt at the proximal extent of the groove between the first and second metatarsals. It may be absent or abnormally sited in 10% of normal subjects, sometimes being 'replaced' by a palpable perforating peroneal artery

Brachial pulse

Examination sequence

- Use your index and middle fingers to palpate this over the lower end of the humerus just above the elbow joint. Assess the character and volume.

Carotid pulse

Some clinicians consider routine examination of the carotid pulse is inappropriate because it may cause distal vascular events, e.g. transient ischaemic attack, or induce reflex, vagally mediated bradycardia. In assessing a patient who may have had a cardiac arrest, however, it is the pulse of choice.

If you do examine the carotid pulse do this gently and never assess both carotids simultaneously.

Examination sequence

- Explain what you are going to do.
- Lie the patient semirecumbent in case you induce a reflex bradycardia.
- Gently place the tips of your fingers between the larynx and the anterior border of the sternocleidomastoid muscle and feel the pulse (Fig 6.10D).
- Listen for bruits over both carotid arteries, using the diaphragm of your stethoscope during held inspiration.

Femoral pulse

Examination sequence

- Lie the patient supine if possible and explain what you are going to do.
- Place your index and middle fingers over the femoral artery, which is just inferior to the midpoint between the anterior superior iliac spine and the pubis (Fig. 6.10E).
- Check for radiofemoral delay (coarctation of the aorta, Fig. 6.11) by simultaneously feeling the radial pulse.
- Listen for bruits over both femoral arteries, using the diaphragm of the stethoscope.

Normal findings

Rate Assess the pulse rate in the clinical context. A pulse rate of 40 bpm can be normal in a fit young adult, whereas a pulse rate of 65 bpm may be abnormally low in acute heart failure. Resting heart rate is normally 60–90 bpm.

Bradycardia is a pulse rate <60 bpm; tachycardia is a rate of >100 bpm.

Rhythm Sinus rhythm originates from the sinoatrial node and produces a regular rhythm (Fig. 6.12A). It varies slightly with the respiratory cycle, mediated by the vagus nerve, and is most pronounced in children, young adults or athletes (sinus arrhythmia). During inspiration, parasympathetic tone falls and the heart rate increases; on expiration, the heart rate decreases (Box 6.14).

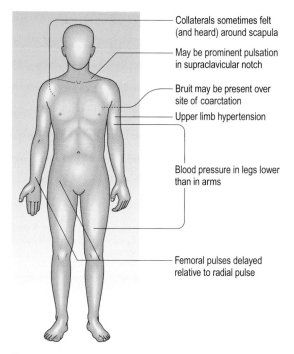

Collaterals sometimes felt (and heard) around scapula

May be prominent pulsation in supraclavicular notch

Bruit may be present over site of coarctation

Upper limb hypertension

Blood pressure in legs lower than in arms

Femoral pulses delayed relative to radial pulse

Fig. 6.11 Features of coarctation of the aorta.

6.14 Haemodynamic effects of respiration		
	Inspiration	**Expiration**
Pulse/heart rate	Accelerates	Slows
Systolic blood pressure	Falls (up to 10 mmHg)	Rises
Jugular venous pressure	Falls	Rises
Second heart sound	Splits	Fuses

Volume Volume refers to the perceived degree of pulsation and reflects the pulse pressure.

Character Character refers to the waveform or shape of the arterial pulse.

Abnormal findings

Rate The most common causes of bradycardia are medication, athletic conditioning, and sinoatrial or atrioventricular node dysfunction. The most common cause of tachycardia is sinus tachycardia (Box 6.15).

Rhythm The pulse may be regular or irregular (Box 6.16). If irregular, it may be regularly irregular, due to an ectopic beat occurring at a regular interval or to second-degree atrioventricular block (Fig. 6.12B). Atrial fibrillation is the most common cause of an irregularly irregular pulse (Box 6.17 and Fig. 6.12C). The rate in atrial fibrillation depends on the number of beats conducted by the atrioventricular node. Untreated, the ventricular rate may be very fast (up to 200 bpm). The variability of the pulse rate (and therefore ventricular filling) explains why the pulse volume varies and there may be a pulse deficit, with some cycles not felt at the

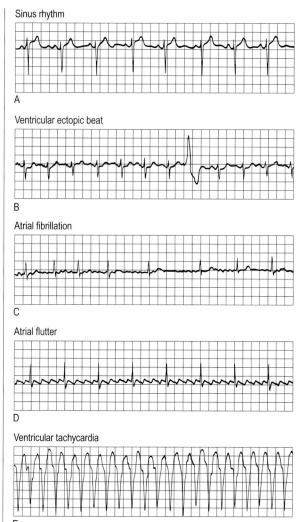

Sinus rhythm

A

Ventricular ectopic beat

B

Atrial fibrillation

C

Atrial flutter

D

Ventricular tachycardia

E

Fig. 6.12 Electrocardiogram rhythm strip. **(A)** Sinus rhythm. **(B)** Ventricular ectopic beat. **(C)** Atrial fibrillation with 'controlled' ventricular response. **(D)** Atrial flutter: note the regular 'saw-toothed' atrial flutter waves at about 300/min. **(E)** Ventricular tachycardia, with ventricular rate of about 200/min.

radial artery. Calculate the pulse deficit by counting the radial pulse rate and subtracting this from the apical heart rate assessed by auscultation (Fig. 6.12D and E).

Volume The ventricles fill during diastole. Longer diastolic intervals are associated with increased stroke volume, which is reflected by increased pulse volume on examination. This is why pulse volume and BP vary widely during atrial fibrillation, and why the 'compensatory pause' following a premature ectopic beat is sometimes felt by the patient.

A large pulse volume is a reflection of a large pulse pressure, which can be physiological or pathological (Box 6.18). The most common cause of a large pulse pressure is arteriosclerosis, which is seen in patients with widespread vascular disease, hypertension and advanced age.

A low pulse volume may be due to reduced stroke volume and occurs in left ventricular failure, hypovolaemia or peripheral arterial disease.

6.15 Causes of a fast or slow pulse

Heart rate	Sinus rhythm	Arrhythmia
Fast (tachycardia, >100 bpm)	Exercise Pain Excitement/anxiety Fever Hyperthyroidism Medication: Sympathomimetics, e.g salbutamol Vasodilators	Atrial fibrillation Atrial flutter Supraventricular tachycardia Ventricular tachycardia
Slow (bradycardia, <60 bpm)	Sleep Athletic training Hypothyroidism Medication: Beta-blockers Digoxin Verapamil, diltiazem	Carotid sinus hypersensitivity Sick sinus syndrome Second-degree heart block Complete heart block

6.16 Causes of an irregular pulse

- Sinus arrhythmia
- Atrial extrasystoles
- Ventricular extrasystoles
- Atrial fibrillation
- Atrial flutter with variable response
- Second-degree heart block with variable response

6.17 Common causes of atrial fibrillation

- Hypertension
- Heart failure
- Myocardial infarction
- Thyrotoxicosis
- Alcohol-related heart disease
- Mitral valve disease
- Infection, e.g. respiratory, urinary
- Following surgery, especially cardiothoracic surgery

6.18 Causes of increased pulse volume

Physiological

- Exercise
- Pregnancy
- Advanced age
- Increased environmental temperature

Pathological

- Hypertension
- Fever
- Thyrotoxicosis
- Anaemia
- Aortic regurgitation
- Paget's disease of bone
- Peripheral atrioventricular shunt

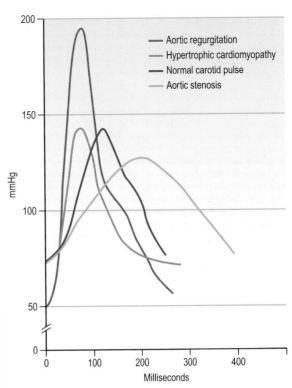

Fig. 6.13 Pulse waveforms.

Coarctation is a congenital narrowing of the aorta, usually distal to the left subclavian artery. The clinical signs depend on the location and severity of the narrowing and the patient's age. In children, the upper limb pulses are usually normal with reduced volume lower limb pulses, which are delayed relative to the upper limb pulses (radio-femoral delay) (Fig. 6.11). In adults, coarctation usually presents with hypertension and heart failure.

Character A collapsing pulse is when the peak of the pulse wave arrives early and is followed by a rapid descent. This rapid fall imparts the 'collapsing' sensation. This is exaggerated by raising the patient's arm above the level of the heart (Fig. 6.10B). It occurs in severe aortic regurgitation and is associated with wide pulse pressure (systolic BP – diastolic BP >80 mmHg).

A slow-rising pulse has a gradual upstroke with a reduced peak occurring late in systole, and is a feature of severe aortic stenosis.

Pulsus bisferiens is an increased pulse with a double systolic peak separated by a distinct mid-systolic dip. Causes include aortic regurgitation, and concomitant aortic stenosis and regurgitation (Fig. 6.13).

Pulsus alternans is a beat-to-beat variation in pulse volume with a normal rhythm. It is rare and occurs in advanced heart failure.

Pulsus paradoxus is an exaggeration of the normal variability of pulse volume with breathing. Pulse volume normally increases in expiration and decreases during inspiration due to intrathoracic pressure changes affecting venous return to the heart. This variability in exaggerated diastolic filling of both ventricles is impeded by increased intrapericardial pressure. This occurs in cardiac tamponade because of accumulation of pericardial fluid and in constrictive pericarditis.

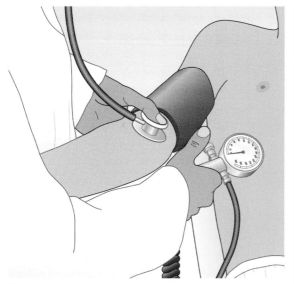

Fig. 6.14 Measuring the blood pressure.

Examination sequence

- Place a BP cuff and inflate until no sounds are heard.
- Decrease the cuff pressure until sounds are heard only on expiration. Note the reading.
- Decrease the cuff pressure again until sounds are heard throughout the respiratory cycle; again note the reading.
- A difference >10 mmHg on inspiration is pulsus paradoxus.

Blood pressure

BP is a measure of the pressure that the circulating blood exerts against the arterial walls. Systolic BP is the maximal pressure that occurs during ventricular contraction (systole). During ventricular filling (diastole), arterial pressure is maintained at a lower level by the elasticity and compliance of the vessel wall. The lowest value (diastolic BP) occurs immediately before the next cycle.

BP is usually measured using a sphygmomanometer (Fig. 6.14). In certain situations, such as the intensive care unit, it is measured invasively using an indwelling intra-arterial catheter connected to a pressure sensor.

BP is measured in mmHg and recorded as systolic pressure/diastolic pressure, together with where, and how, the reading was taken, e.g. BP: 146/92 mmHg, right arm, supine.

BP is an important guide to cardiovascular risk and provides vital information on the haemodynamic condition of acutely ill or injured patients. BP constantly varies and rises with stress, excitement and environment. 'White-coat hypertension' occurs in patients only when a patient is seeing a healthcare worker. Ambulatory BP measurement, using a portable device at intervals during normal daytime activity and at night, is better at determining cardiovascular risk.

Hypertension

Abnormal elevation of BP is defined by the British Hypertension Society (Box 6.19). Normal BP is defined

6.19 British Hypertension Society classification of blood pressure (BP) levels		
BP	**Systolic BP (mmHg)**	**Diastolic BP (mmHg)**
Optimal	<120	<80
Normal	<130	<85
High normal	130–139	85–89
Hypertension		
Grade 1 (mild)	140–159	90–99
Grade 2 (moderate)	160–179	100–109
Grade 3 (severe)	>180	>110
Isolated systolic hypertension		
Grade 1	140–159	<90
Grade 2	>160	<90

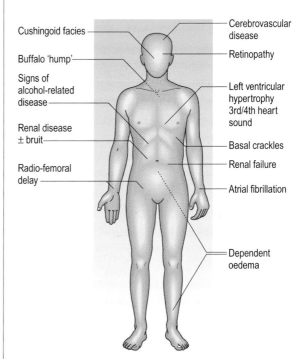

Fig. 6.15 Physical signs which may be associated with hypertension.

as <130/85 mmHg. Hypertension is extremely common, affecting 20–30% of the UK adult population, with higher rates in black Africans (Box 6.22).

Hypertension is asymptomatic although, rarely in severe hypertension, headaches and visual disturbances occur (Fig. 6.15). It is associated with significant morbidity and mortality from vascular disease (heart failure, coronary artery disease, cerebrovascular disease and renal failure). The risk rises progressively with increasing systolic and diastolic pressure; for example, isolated grade 1 systolic hypertension has a two- to threefold increased risk of cardiac mortality. Lowering BP lowers vascular risk regardless of the starting value. In most hypertensive patients there is no identifiable cause

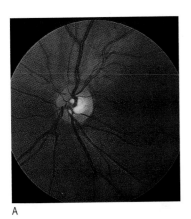

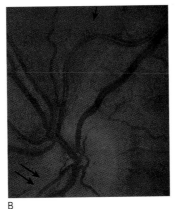

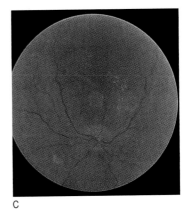

A

B

C

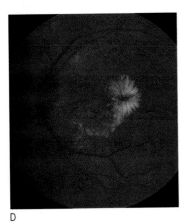

D

Fig. 6.16 Hypertensive retinopathy. (A) Grade 1: early changes: increased tortuosity of a retinal vessel and increased reflectiveness (silver wiring) of a retinal artery are seen at 1 o'clock. **(B)** Grade 2: increased tortuosity and silver wiring (double arrow) with 'nipping' of the venules at arteriovenous crossings (single arrow). **(C)** Grade 3: similar to grade 2 plus flame-shaped retinal haemorrhages and soft 'cotton-wool' exudates. **(D)** Grade 4: swelling of the optic disc (papilloedema), retinal oedema and hard exudates around the fovea, producing a 'macular star'.

6.20 Causes of secondary hypertension

Renal arterial disease, including renal artery stenosis	Suspect if there is other evidence of vascular disease
Phaeochromocytoma	Neuroendocrine tumour that secretes catecholamines, causing hypertension, headaches, sweating and palpitation
Conn's syndrome	Tumour of the adrenal cortex that secretes aldosterone
Cushing's syndrome	Microadenoma of the pituitary that secretes adrenocorticotrophic hormone (ACTH)
Coarctation of the aorta	
Adult polycystic kidney disease (p. 202)	

– so-called 'essential hypertension'. Secondary hypertension is rare, occurring in <1% of the hypertensive population (Box 6.20).

Assess the hypertensive patient for:
- Any underlying cause
- End-organ damage:
  - cardiac: heart failure
  - renal: chronic kidney disease
  - eye: hypertensive retinopathy – four grades (Fig. 6.16)
- Overall risk of vascular disease, i.e. of stroke, myocardial infarction, heart failure.

Korotkoff sounds

These sounds are produced between systole and diastole because the artery collapses completely and reopens with each heart beat, producing a snapping or knocking sound. The first appearance of sounds (phase 1) during cuff deflation indicates systole. As pressure is gradually reduced, the sounds muffle (phase 4) and then disappear (phase 5). Interobserver agreement is better for phase 5 and this is the diastolic BP. Occasionally, muffled sounds persist (phase 4) and do not disappear; in this case, record phase 4 as the diastolic pressure (Fig. 6.17).

Examination sequence

- Rest the patient for 5 minutes.
- Always measure BP in both arms (brachial arteries); the higher of the two is closest to central aortic pressure and should be used to determine treatment.
- With the patient seated or lying down, support the patient's arm comfortably at about heart level, with no tight clothing constricting the upper arm. You can measure over thin clothing, as it makes no difference to the result.
- The usual sphygmomanometer cuff has a bladder width of 12.5 cm and length of 30–35 cm. Apply the cuff to the upper arm, with the centre of the bladder over the brachial artery.

- Palpate the brachial pulse.
- Inflate the cuff until the pulse is impalpable. Note the pressure on the manometer; this is a rough estimate of systolic pressure.
- Inflate the cuff another 30 mmHg and listen through the diaphragm of the stethoscope placed over the brachial artery.
- Deflate the cuff slowly (2–3 mmHg/s) until you hear a regular tapping sound (phase 1 Korotkoff sounds). Record the reading to the nearest 2 mmHg. This is the systolic pressure.
- Continue to deflate the cuff slowly until the sounds disappear.
- Record the pressure at which the sounds completely disappear as the diastolic pressure (phase 5). If muffled sounds persist (phase 4) and do not disappear, use the point of muffling as the diastolic pressure.

Common problems in BP measurement

- BP is different in each arm: a difference >10 mmHg suggests the presence of aortic or subclavian artery disease. Unequal brachial BP is a marker of increased cardiovascular morbidity and mortality (Box 6.21). Record the highest pressure and use this to guide management
- Wrong cuff size: the bladder should be approximately 80% of the length and 40% of the width of the upper arm circumference. A standard adult cuff has a bladder approximately 13 × 30 cm and suits an arm circumference 22–26 cm. In obese patients a standard adult cuff will overestimate BP,

so use a large adult (bladder 16 × 38 cm) or thigh cuff (20 × 42 cm)

- Auscultatory gap: up to 20% of elderly hypertensive patients have Korotkoff sounds which appear at systolic pressure and disappear for an interval between systolic and diastolic pressure. If the first appearance of the sound is missed, the systolic pressure will be recorded at a falsely low level. Avoid this by palpating the systolic pressure first
- Patient's arm at the wrong level: the patient's elbow should be level with the heart. Hydrostatic pressure causes ~5 mmHg change in recorded systolic and diastolic BP for a 7 cm change in arm elevation
- Terminal digit preference: record the true reading rather than rounding values to the nearest 0 or 5
- Postural change: the pulse increases by about 11 bpm, systolic BP falls by 3–4 mmHg and diastolic BP rises by 5–6 mmHg when a healthy person stands. The BP stabilises after 1–2 minutes. Check the BP after a patient has been standing for 2 minutes; a drop of >20 mmHg on standing is postural hypotension
- Atrial fibrillation: makes BP assessment more difficult because of beat-to-beat variability. Deflate the cuff at 2 mmHg per beat and repeat measurement if necessary.

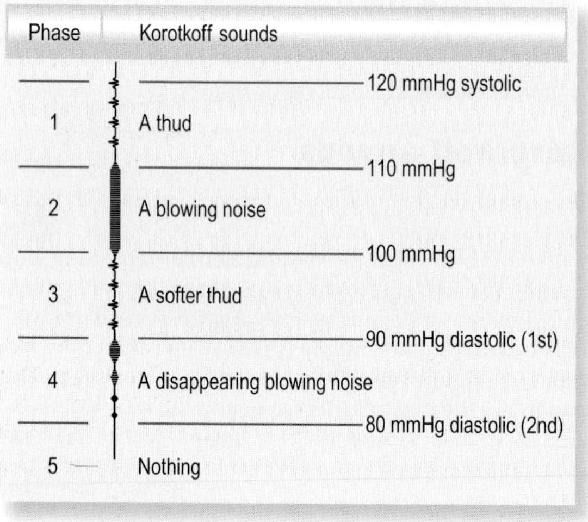

Jugular venous pressure and waveform

Anatomy

The internal jugular vein enters the neck behind the mastoid process. It runs deep to the sternocleidomastoid muscle before entering the thorax between the sternal and clavicular heads and should be examined with the neck muscles relaxed. A pulsation is visible when the pressure in the internal jugular vein is elevated.

The external jugular vein is more superficial, prominent and easier to see. It can be kinked or obstructed as it traverses the deep fascia of the neck but, when visible, pulsatile and not obstructed, it can be used to estimate the JVP in difficult cases.

Estimate the JVP by observing the level of pulsation in the internal jugular vein. The normal waveform has two main peaks per cycle, which helps to distinguish it from the carotid arterial pulse (Box 6.23).

The JVP level reflects right atrial pressure (normally <7 mmHg/9 cmH$_2$O). The sternal angle is approximately 5 cm above the right atrium, so the JVP in health should be ≤4 cm above this angle when the patient lies at 45°. If right atrial pressure is low, the patient may have to lie flat for the JVP to be seen; if high, the patient may need to sit upright (Fig. 6.18).

Phase	Korotkoff sounds	
1	A thud	120 mmHg systolic
		110 mmHg
2	A blowing noise	
		100 mmHg
3	A softer thud	
		90 mmHg diastolic (1st)
4	A disappearing blowing noise	
		80 mmHg diastolic (2nd)
5	Nothing	

Fig. 6.17 Korotkoff sounds.

EBE 6.21 Aortic dissection

The presence of: (1) chest pain that is tearing or ripping; (2) a difference in blood pressure of >20mmHg between arms; and (3) mediastinal or aortic widening on chest X-ray is pathognomonic of aortic dissection.

Von Kodolitsch Y, Schwartz AG, Nienaber CA. Clinical prediction of acute aortic dissection. Arch Intern Med 2000;160:2977–2982.

EBE 6.22 Hypertension

If the clinic blood pressure is 140/90 mmHg or higher, offer ambulatory blood pressure monitoring to confirm the diagnosis of hypertension.

NICE. Hypertension. Clinical management of primary hypertension in adults. 2011. Available online at: www.nice.org.uk/guidance/CG127.

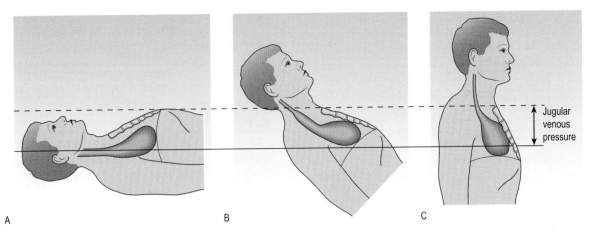

Fig. 6.18 Jugular venous pressure in a healthy subject. (A) Supine: jugular vein distended, pulsation not visible. **(B)** Reclining at 45°: point of transition between distended and collapsed vein can usually be seen to pulsate just above the clavicle. **(C)** Upright: upper part of vein collapsed and transition point obscured.

6.23 Differences between carotid artery and jugular venous pulsation

Carotid	Jugular
Rapid outward movement	Rapid inward movement
One peak per heart beat	Two peaks per heart beat (in sinus rhythm)
Palpable	Impalpable
Pulsation unaffected by pressure at the root of the neck	Pulsation diminished by pressure at the root of the neck
Independent of respiration	Height of pulsation varies with respiration
Independent of position of patient	Varies with position of patient
Independent of abdominal pressure	Rises with abdominal pressure

Examination sequence

The JVP is best seen on the patient's right side.

- Position the patient supine, reclined at 45°, with the head on a pillow to relax the sternocleidomastoid muscles.
- Look across the patient's neck from the right side (Fig. 6.19A). Use oblique lighting if the JVP is difficult to see.
- Identify the jugular vein pulsation in the suprasternal notch or behind the sternocleidomastoid muscle.
- Use the abdomino-jugular test or occlusion to confirm it is the JVP.
- The JVP is the vertical height in centimetres between the upper limit of the venous pulsation and the sternal angle (junction of the manubrium and sternum at the level of the second costal cartilages) (Fig. 6.19B).
- Identify the timing and waveform of the pulsation and note any abnormality.

Normal findings

Aids to differentiate the jugular venous waveform from arterial pulsation:

- Abdomino-jugular test: firmly press over the abdomen. This increases venous return to the right side of the heart temporarily and the JVP normally rises.
- Changes with respiration: the JVP normally falls with inspiration due to decreased intrathoracic pressure.
- Waveform (Fig. 6.19C): the normal JVP waveform has two distinct peaks per cardiac cycle:
  - 'a' wave corresponds to right atrial contraction and occurs just before the first heart sound. In atrial fibrillation the 'a' wave is absent.
  - 'v' wave is caused by atrial filling during ventricular systole when the tricuspid valve is closed.
  - Rarely, a third peak ('c' wave) may be seen due to closure of the tricuspid valve.
- Occlusion: the JVP waveform is obliterated by gently occluding the vein at the base of the neck with your finger.

Abnormal findings

The JVP is primarily a sign of right ventricular function. It is elevated in states of fluid overload, notably in heart failure and in conditions with right heart dilatation, e.g. acute pulmonary embolism and chronic obstructive pulmonary disease (when it is called cor pulmonale). Mechanical obstruction of the superior vena cava (most often caused by lung cancer) may cause extreme, non-pulsatile elevation of the JVP. Here the JVP no longer reflects right atrial pressure and the abdominojugular test will be negative (Box 6.24).

Kussmaul's sign: a paradoxical rise of JVP on inspiration seen in pericardial constriction or tamponade, severe right ventricular failure and restrictive cardiomyopathy.

Prominent 'a' wave: caused by delayed or restricted right ventricular filling, e.g. pulmonary hypertension or tricuspid stenosis.

Cannon waves: giant 'a' waves occur when the right atrium contracts against a closed tricuspid valve. Irregular cannon waves are seen in complete heart block and are due to atrio-ventricular dissociation. Regular cannon

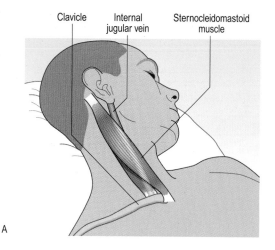

A

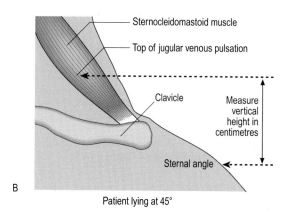

B

Patient lying at 45°

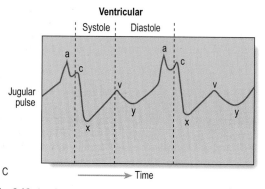

C

Time

Fig. 6.19 Jugular venous pressure. (A) Inspecting the jugular venous pressure from the side (the internal jugular vein lies deep to the sternocleidomastoid muscle). **(B)** Measuring the height of the jugular venous pressure. **(C)** Form of the venous pulse wave tracing from the internal jugular vein: a, atrial systole; c, closure of the tricuspid valve; v, peak pressure in right atrium immediately prior to opening of tricuspid valve; a–x, descent, due to downward displacement of the tricuspid ring during systole; v–y, descent at commencement of ventricular filling.

waves occur during junctional rhythm and with some ventricular and supraventricular tachycardias.

'cv' wave: a fusion of the 'c' and 'v' waves resulting in a large systolic wave and associated with a pulsatile liver is seen in tricuspid regurgitation.

6.24 Abnormalities of the jugular venous pulse	
Condition	**Abnormalities**
Heart failure	Elevation, sustained abdominojugular reflux >10 seconds
Pulmonary embolism	Elevation
Pericardial effusion	Elevation, prominent 'y' descent
Pericardial constriction	Elevation, Kussmaul's sign
Superior vena caval obstruction	Elevation, loss of pulsation
Atrial fibrillation	Absent 'a' waves
Tricuspid stenosis	Giant 'a' waves
Tricuspid regurgitation	Giant 'v' waves
Complete heart block	'Cannon' waves

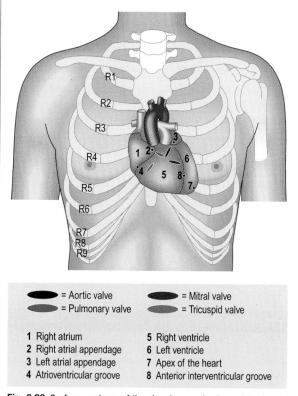

= Aortic valve   = Mitral valve
= Pulmonary valve   = Tricuspid valve

1 Right atrium
2 Right atrial appendage
3 Left atrial appendage
4 Atrioventricular groove
5 Right ventricle
6 Left ventricle
7 Apex of the heart
8 Anterior interventricular groove

Fig. 6.20 Surface anatomy of the chambers and valves of the heart.

The precordium

The precordium is the anterior chest surface overlying the heart and great vessels (Fig. 6.20).

Learn the surface anatomy of the heart to understand how and where the sounds and murmurs radiate and basic cardiac physiology to appreciate their timing (Figs 6.20 and 6.21). The auscultatory areas (aortic, pulmonary, apex and left sternal border) do not correspond with the location of cardiac structures, but are where transmitted sounds and murmurs are best heard (Box 6.25).

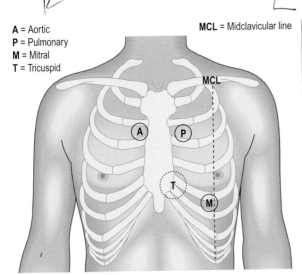

A = Aortic
P = Pulmonary
M = Mitral
T = Tricuspid

MCL = Midclavicular line

MCL

Fig. 6.21 Sites for auscultation. Sites at which murmurs from the relevant valves are usually, but not preferentially, heard.

6.25 Cardiac auscultation: the best sites for hearing abnormality

Site	Sound
Cardiac apex	First heart sound Third and fourth heart sounds Mid-diastolic murmur of mitral stenosis
Lower left sternal border	Early diastolic murmurs of aortic and tricuspid regurgitation Opening snap of mitral stenosis Pansystolic murmur of ventricular septal defect
Upper left sternal border	Second heart sound Pulmonary valve murmurs
Upper right sternal border	Systolic ejection (outflow) murmurs, e.g. aortic stenosis, hypertrophic cardiomyopathy
Left axilla	Radiation of the pansystolic murmur of mitral regurgitation
Below left clavicle	Continuous 'machinery' murmur of a persistent patent ductus arteriosus

Chest wall abnormalities

Pectus excavatum (funnel chest), a posterior displacement of the lower sternum, and pectus carinatum (pigeon chest) may displace the heart and affect palpation and auscultation (Fig. 7.14).

A midline sternotomy scar usually indicates previous coronary artery bypass surgery or aortic valve replacement. A left submammary scar is usually the result of mitral valvotomy. Infraclavicular scars are seen after pacemaker or defibrillator implantation, and the bulge of the device may be obvious.

Apex beat

The apex beat is the most lateral and inferior position where the cardiac impulse can be felt. The cardiac impulse results from the left ventricle moving forward and striking the chest wall during systole. The apex beat is normally in the fifth left intercostal space at, or medial to, the mid-clavicular line (halfway between the suprasternal notch and the acromioclavicular joint).

A thrill is the tactile equivalent of a murmur and is a palpable vibration.

A heave is a palpable impulse that noticeably lifts your hand.

Examination sequence

- Explain that you wish to examine the chest and ask the patient to remove all clothing above the waist. Keep a female patient's chest covered with a sheet as far as possible.
- Inspect the precordium with the patient sitting at a 45° angle with shoulders horizontal. Look for surgical scars, visible pulsations and chest deformity.
- Place your right hand flat over the precordium to obtain a general impression of the cardiac impulse (Fig. 6.22A).
- Locate the apex beat by lying your fingers on the chest parallel to the rib spaces; if you cannot feel it, ask the patient to roll on to his left side (Fig. 6.22B).
- Assess the character of the apex beat and note its position.
- Apply the heel of your right hand firmly to the left parasternal area and feel for a right ventricle heave. Ask the patient to hold his breath in expiration (Fig. 6.22C).
- Palpate for thrills at the apex and both sides of the sternum using the flat of your fingers.

Normal findings

A normal apical impulse briefly lifts your fingers and is localised. There should be no parasternal heave or thrill.

Abnormal findings

The apex beat may be impalpable in overweight or muscular people or in patients with asthma or emphysema because the lungs are hyperinflated. It may be diffusely displaced inferiorly and laterally in left ventricular dilatation, e.g. after myocardial infarction, with aortic stenosis, severe hypertension and dilated cardiomyopathy or in chest deformity. In dextrocardia, with a prevalence of 1:10 000, the cardiac apex is on the right side.

Left ventricular hypertrophy, e.g. with hypertension, aortic stenosis, produces a forceful, undisplaced apical impulse. This thrusting apical 'heave' is quite different from the diffuse impulse of left ventricular dilatation. Pulsation over the left parasternal area (right ventricular heave) indicates right ventricular hypertrophy or dilatation, most often accompanying pulmonary hypertension. The 'tapping' apex beat in mitral stenosis represents a palpable first heart sound, and is not usually displaced. A double apical impulse is characteristic of hypertrophic cardiomyopathy.

The most common thrill is that of aortic stenosis which may be palpable at the apex, at the lower sternum or in the neck. The thrill caused by a ventricular septal defect is best felt at the left and right sternal edges. Diastolic thrills are very rare.

Heart sounds

Normal heart valves make a sound only when they close. The 'lub-dub' sounds are caused by closure of the

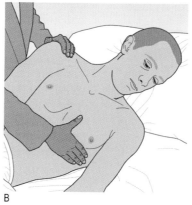
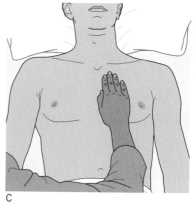

A   B   C

Fig. 6.22 Palpating the heart. (A) Use your hand to palpate the cardiac impulse. **(B)** Localise the apex beat with your finger (roll the patient, if necessary, into the left lateral position). **(C)** Palpate from apex to sternum for parasternal pulsations.

atrioventricular (mitral and tricuspid) valves followed by the outlet (aortic and pulmonary) valves.

The bell of the stethoscope transmits all sounds well but in some patients with high-frequency murmurs any additional low-frequency sound masks the high-frequency murmur. The bell is particularly useful at the apex and left sternal edge to listen for the diastolic murmur of mitral stenosis and third and fourth heart sounds.

The diaphragm attenuates all frequencies equally, therefore making some low-frequency sounds less audible. Use the diaphragm to identify high-pitched sounds, e.g. early diastolic murmur of aortic regurgitation. Listen with it over the whole precordium for a pericardial friction rub.

Examination sequence

Make sure the room is quiet when you auscultate. Your stethoscope should fit comfortably with the earpieces angled slightly forward. The tubing should be ~25 cm long and thick enough to reduce external sound.

- Listen with your stethoscope diaphragm at the:
  - apex
  - lower left sternal border
  - upper right and left sternal borders.
- Listen with your stethoscope bell at the:
  - apex
  - lower left sternal border.
- Listen over the carotid arteries (ejection systolic murmur of aortic stenosis) and in the left axilla (pansystolic murmur of mitral regurgitation).
- At each site identify the S_1 and S_2 sounds. Assess their character and intensity; note any splitting of the S_2. Palpate the carotid pulse to time any murmur. The S_1 barely precedes the upstroke of the carotid pulsation, while the S_2 is clearly out of phase with it.
- Concentrate in turn on systole (the interval between S_1 and S_2) and diastole (the interval between S_2 and S_1). Listen for added sounds and then for murmurs. Soft diastolic murmurs are sometimes described as the 'absence of silence'.

- Roll the patient on to his left side. Listen at the apex using light pressure with the bell, to detect the mid-diastolic and presystolic murmur of mitral stenosis (Fig. 6.23A).
- Ask the patient to sit up and lean forwards, then to breathe out fully and hold his breath (Fig. 6.23B). Listen over the right second intercostal space and over the left sternal edge with the diaphragm for the murmur of aortic regurgitation.
- Note the character and intensity of any murmur heard.
- Develop a routine for auscultation so that you do not overlook subtle abnormalities. Identify and describe the following:
  - the first and second heart sounds (S_1 and S_2)
  - extra heart sounds (S_3 and S_4)
  - additional sounds, e.g. clicks and snaps
  - pericardial rubs
  - murmurs in systole and/or diastole.

Normal findings

- First heart sound (S_1), 'lub', is caused by closure of the mitral and tricuspid valves at the onset of ventricular systole. It is best heard at the apex.
- Second heart sound (S_2), 'dub', is caused by closure of the pulmonary and aortic valves at the end of ventricular systole and is best heard at the left sternal edge. It is louder and higher-pitched than the S_1 'lub', and the aortic component is normally louder than the pulmonary one. Physiological splitting of S_2 occurs because left ventricular contraction slightly precedes that of the right ventricle so that the aortic valve closes before the pulmonary valve. This splitting increases at end-inspiration because increased venous filling of the right ventricle further delays pulmonary valve closure. This separation disappears on expiration (Fig. 6.24). Splitting of S_2 is best heard at the left sternal edge. On auscultation, you hear 'lub d/dub' (inspiration) 'lub-dub' (expiration)
- Third heart sound (S_3) is a low-pitched early diastolic sound best heard with the bell at the apex. It coincides with rapid ventricular filling immediately after opening of the atrioventricular valves and is therefore heard after the second as 'lub-dub-dum'. It is a normal finding in children, young adults and during pregnancy.

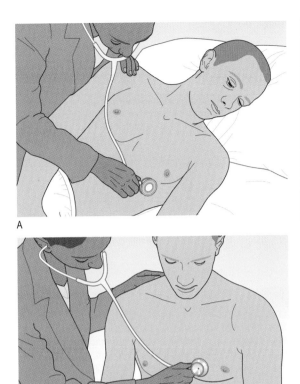

A

B

Fig. 6.23 Auscultating the heart. (A) Listen for the murmur of mitral stenosis with the lightly applied bell with the patient in the left lateral position. **(B)** Listen for the murmur of aortic regurgitation with the diaphragm with the patient leaning forward.

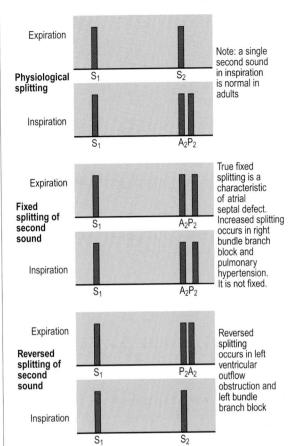

Note: a single second sound in inspiration is normal in adults

True fixed splitting is a characteristic of atrial septal defect. Increased splitting occurs in right bundle branch block and pulmonary hypertension. It is not fixed.

Reversed splitting occurs in left ventricular outflow obstruction and left bundle branch block

Fig. 6.24 Normal and pathological splitting of the second heart sound.

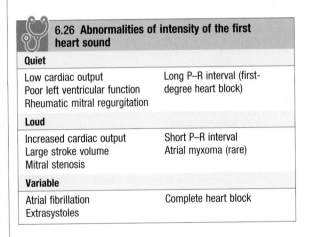

6.26 Abnormalities of intensity of the first heart sound

Quiet	
Low cardiac output Poor left ventricular function Rheumatic mitral regurgitation	Long P–R interval (first-degree heart block)

Loud	
Increased cardiac output Large stroke volume Mitral stenosis	Short P–R interval Atrial myxoma (rare)

Variable	
Atrial fibrillation Extrasystoles	Complete heart block

6

Abnormal findings

First heart sound: In mitral stenosis the intensity of S_1 is increased due to elevated left atrial pressure (Box 6.26).

Second heart sound: The aortic component of S_2 is sometimes quiet or absent in calcific aortic stenosis and reduced in aortic regurgitation (Box 6.27). The aortic component is loud in systemic hypertension, and the pulmonary component increased in pulmonary hypertension.

Wide splitting of S_2, but with normal respiratory variation, occurs in conditions which delay right ventricular emptying, e.g. right bundle branch block. Fixed splitting, i.e. no variation with respiration of S_2, is a feature of atrial septal defect (Fig. 6.25). In this condition the right ventricular stroke volume is larger than the left, and the splitting is fixed because the defect equalises the pressure between the two atria throughout the respiratory cycle.

In reversed splitting the two components of S_2 occur together on inspiration and separate on expiration. This occurs when left ventricular emptying is delayed so that the aortic valve closes after the pulmonary valve. Examples include left bundle branch block and right ventricular pacing.

Third heart sound: This is usually pathological after the age of 40 years (Box 6.28). The most common causes are left ventricular failure, when it is an early sign, and mitral regurgitation, due to volume loading of the ventricle. In heart failure S_3 occurs with a tachycardia, referred to as a 'gallop' rhythm, and S_1 and S_2 are quiet (lub-da-dub; Box 6.29).

Fourth heart sound: This is less common. It is soft and low-pitched, best heard with the stethoscope bell at the apex. It occurs just before S_1 (da-lub-dub). It is always pathological and is caused by forceful atrial contraction against a non-compliant or stiff ventricle. An S_4 is most often heard with left ventricular hypertrophy (due to

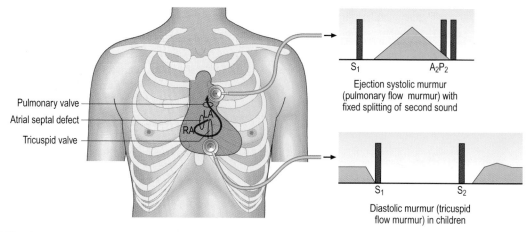

Ejection systolic murmur
(pulmonary flow murmur) with
fixed splitting of second sound

Diastolic murmur (tricuspid
flow murmur) in children

Fig. 6.25 Atrial septal defect. RA, right atrium; LA, left atrium.

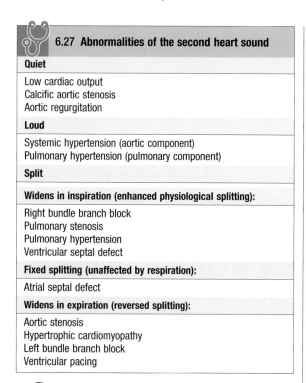

6.27 Abnormalities of the second heart sound

Quiet

Low cardiac output
Calcific aortic stenosis
Aortic regurgitation

Loud

Systemic hypertension (aortic component)
Pulmonary hypertension (pulmonary component)

Split

Widens in inspiration (enhanced physiological splitting):

Right bundle branch block
Pulmonary stenosis
Pulmonary hypertension
Ventricular septal defect

Fixed splitting (unaffected by respiration):

Atrial septal defect

Widens in expiration (reversed splitting):

Aortic stenosis
Hypertrophic cardiomyopathy
Left bundle branch block
Ventricular pacing

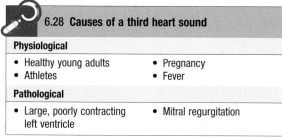

6.28 Causes of a third heart sound

Physiological

• Healthy young adults   • Pregnancy
• Athletes   • Fever

Pathological

• Large, poorly contracting   • Mitral regurgitation
  left ventricle

hypertension, aortic stenosis or hypertrophic cardiomyopathy). It cannot occur when there is atrial fibrillation.

Both an S_3 and an S_4 cause a 'triple' or 'gallop' rhythm.

Added sounds

An opening snap is commonly heard in mitral (rarely tricuspid) stenosis. It results from sudden opening of a

EBE 6.29 Heart failure

In an adult with acute breathlessness a third heart sound is highly suggestive of heart failure with depressed left ventricular ejection fraction. Other useful signs, if present, are raised jugular venous pressure, peripheral oedema and basal lung crackles.

McGee S. Evidence based physical diagnosis. St Louis, MO: Saunders/ Elsevier, 2007, pp. 436–440.

stenosed valve and occurs early in diastole, just after the S_2 (Fig. 6.26A). It is best heard by the diaphragm at the apex.

Ejection clicks are high-pitched sounds best heard by the diaphragm. They occur early in systole just after the S_1, in patients with congenital pulmonary or aortic stenosis (Fig. 6.26B). The mechanism is similar to that of an opening snap. Ejection clicks do not occur in calcific aortic stenosis because the cusps are rigid.

Mid-systolic clicks are high-pitched and best heard at the apex by the diaphragm. They occur in mitral valve prolapse (Fig. 6.26C) and may be associated with a late systolic murmur.

Mechanical heart valves can make a sound when they close or open. The closure sound is normally louder, especially with modern valves. The sounds are high-pitched, 'metallic' and often palpable, and may be heard even without a stethoscope. A mechanical mitral valve replacement makes a metallic S_1 and a sound like a loud opening snap (Fig. 6.26D). Mechanical aortic valves have a loud, metallic S_2 and an opening sound like an ejection click (Fig. 6.26E). They are normally associated with a flow murmur.

Pericardial rub (friction rub) is a coarse scratching sound, often with systolic and diastolic components. It is best heard using the diaphragm with the patient holding his breath in expiration. It may be audible over any part of the precordium but is often localised. It is most often heard in acute viral pericarditis and sometimes 24–72 hours after myocardial infarction. Pericardial rubs vary in intensity over time, and with the position of the patient.

A pleuro-pericardial rub is a similar sound that occurs in time with the cardiac cycle but is also influenced by

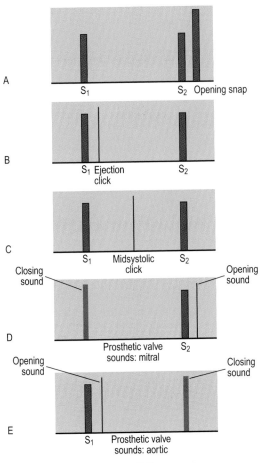

Fig. 6.26 'Added sounds' on auscultation.

Figure labels (A–E):

A — S_1 ... S_2 Opening snap

B — S_1 Ejection click ... S_2

C — S_1 Midsystolic click ... S_2

D — Closing sound / Opening sound — Prosthetic valve sounds: mitral S_2

E — Opening sound / Closing sound — S_1 Prosthetic valve sounds: aortic

6.30	Grades of intensity of murmur
Grade 1	Heard by an expert in optimum conditions
Grade 2	Heard by a non-expert in optimum conditions
Grade 3	Easily heard; no thrill
Grade 4	A loud murmur, with a thrill
Grade 5	Very loud, often heard over wide area, with thrill
Grade 6	Extremely loud, heard without stethoscope

respiration and is pleural in origin. Occasionally a 'crunching' noise can be heard caused by gas in the pericardium (pneumo-pericardium).

Murmurs

Heart murmurs are produced by turbulent flow across an abnormal valve, septal defect or outflow obstruction. 'Innocent' murmurs caused by increased volume or velocity of flow through a normal valve occur when stroke volume is increased, e.g. during pregnancy, in athletes with resting bradycardia or children with fever.

Examination sequence

Timing
Identify the S_1 and S_2 sounds. It may help to palpate the patient's carotid pulse while listening to the precordium.

Determine whether the murmur is systolic or diastolic:

- **Systole** begins with the S_1 (mitral and tricuspid valve closure). This occurs when left and right ventricular pressures exceed the corresponding atrial pressures. For a short period all four heart valves are closed (pre-ejection period). Ventricular pressures continue to rise until they exceed those of the aorta and pulmonary artery, causing the aortic and pulmonary valves to open. Systole ends with the closure of these valves, producing the S_2.
- **Diastole** is the interval between S_2 and S_1. Physiologically it is divided into three phases:
  - early diastole (isovolumic relaxation): the time from the closure of the aortic and pulmonary valves until the opening of the mitral and tricuspid valves
  - mid-diastole: the early period of ventricular filling when atrial pressures exceed ventricular pressures
  - pre-systole: coinciding with atrial systole.

Murmurs of aortic (and pulmonary) regurgitation start in early diastole and extend into mid-diastole. The murmurs of mitral or tricuspid stenosis cannot start before mid-diastole. Likewise, S_3 occurs in mid-diastole and S_4 in pre-systole.

Duration
The murmurs of mitral and tricuspid regurgitation start with S_1, sometimes muffling or obscuring it, and continue throughout systole (pansystolic) (Fig. 6.27). The murmur produced by mitral valve prolapse does not begin until the mitral valve leaflet has prolapsed during systole, producing a late systolic murmur. The ejection systolic murmur of aortic or pulmonary stenosis begins after S_1 reaches maximal intensity in mid-systole, then fades, stopping before S_2 (Fig. 6.27).

Character and pitch
The quality of a murmur is subjective, but terms such as harsh, blowing, musical, rumbling, high- or low-pitched can help. High-pitched murmurs often correspond with high-pressure gradients, so the diastolic murmur of aortic regurgitation is higher-pitched than that of mitral stenosis.

Intensity
Describe any murmur according to its grade of intensity (Box 6.30). Diastolic murmurs are rarely louder than grade 3. The intensity of a murmur does not correlate with severity of valve dysfunction; for instance, the murmur of critical aortic stenosis can be quiet and occasionally inaudible. Changes in intensity with time are important, as they can denote progression of a valve lesion. Rapidly changing murmurs can occur with infective endocarditis because of valve destruction.

Location
Record the site(s) where you hear the murmur best. This helps to differentiate diastolic murmurs (mitral stenosis at the apex, aortic regurgitation at the left sternal edge), but is less helpful with systolic murmurs, which are often loud over all the precordium (Fig. 6.21).

Radiation
Murmurs radiate in the direction of the blood flow to specific sites outside the precordium. Differentiate this from location. The pansystolic murmur of mitral regurgitation radiates towards the left axilla, the murmur of ventricular septal defect towards the right sternal edge, and that of aortic stenosis to the aortic area and the carotid arteries.

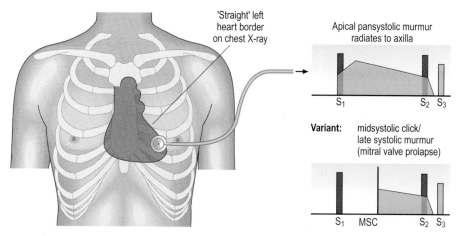

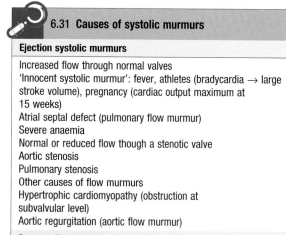

Fig. 6.27 Mitral regurgitation. The murmur begins at the moment of valve closure and may obscure the first heart sound. It varies little in intensity throughout systole. In mitral valve prolapse, the murmur begins in mid or late systole and there is often a mid-systolic click (MSC).

6.31 Causes of systolic murmurs

Ejection systolic murmurs

Increased flow through normal valves
'Innocent systolic murmur': fever, athletes (bradycardia → large stroke volume), pregnancy (cardiac output maximum at 15 weeks)
Atrial septal defect (pulmonary flow murmur)
Severe anaemia
Normal or reduced flow though a stenotic valve
Aortic stenosis
Pulmonary stenosis
Other causes of flow murmurs
Hypertrophic cardiomyopathy (obstruction at subvalvular level)
Aortic regurgitation (aortic flow murmur)

Pansystolic murmurs

All caused by a systolic leak from a high- to a lower-pressure chamber:
• Mitral regurgitation
• Tricuspid regurgitation
• Ventricular septal defect
• Leaking mitral or tricuspid prosthesis

Abnormal findings

Systolic murmurs Ejection systolic murmurs are caused by increased stroke volume (flow murmur), or stenosis of the aortic or pulmonary valve (Box 6.31). An ejection murmur is also a feature of hypertrophic cardiomyopathy and is accentuated by exercise. An atrial septal defect is characterised by a pulmonary flow murmur during systole.

The murmur of aortic stenosis is often audible all over the precordium (Fig. 6.28). It is harsh, high-pitched and musical, and radiates to the upper right sternal edge and carotid arteries. It is usually loud and there may be a thrill.

Pansystolic murmurs are usually caused by mitral regurgitation. The murmur is often loud and blowing in character, best heard at the apex and radiating to the axilla. With mitral valve prolapse, regurgitation begins in mid-systole, producing a late systolic murmur (Fig. 6.27). The murmur of tricuspid regurgitation is heard at the lower left sternal edge; if significant, it is associated with a 'v' wave in the JVP and a pulsatile liver.

Ventricular septal defect also causes a pansystolic murmur. Small congenital defects produce a loud murmur audible at the left sternal border, radiating to the right sternal border and often associated with a thrill. Rupture of the interventricular septum can complicate myocardial infarction, producing a harsh pansystolic murmur. Other murmurs heard after myocardial infarction include acute mitral regurgitation due to papillary muscle rupture, functional mitral regurgitation caused by left ventricular dilatation and a pericardial rub.

Diastolic murmurs

Early diastolic murmurs The term 'early diastolic murmur' is misleading; usually the murmur lasts throughout diastole, but is loudest in early diastole. It is typically caused by aortic regurgitation (Fig. 6.29), and is best heard at the left sternal edge with the patient leaning forward holding the breath in expiration. In general the duration of the aortic regurgitation murmur is inversely proportional to lesion severity. Since the regurgitant blood volume must be ejected during the subsequent systole, significant aortic regurgitation leads to increased stroke volume and is almost always associated with a systolic flow murmur.

Pulmonary regurgitation is uncommon. It may be caused by pulmonary artery dilatation in pulmonary hypertension (Graham Steell murmur) or a congenital defect of the pulmonary valve.

Mid-diastolic murmurs A mid-diastolic murmur is usually caused by mitral stenosis. This is a low-pitched, rumbling sound which may follow an opening snap (Fig. 6.30). It is best heard with the stethoscope bell at the apex with the patient rolled to the left side. The murmur is accentuated by exercise. The cadence sounds like 'lup-ta-ta-rru'; 'lup' is the loud S_1, 'ta-ta' the S_2, and opening snap and 'rru' the mid-diastolic murmur. If the patient is in sinus rhythm, left atrial contraction increases

6

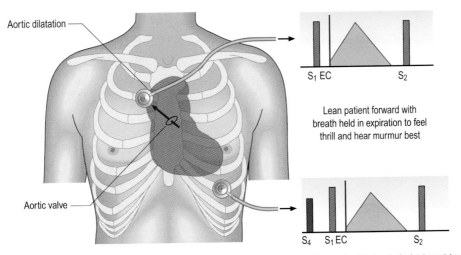

Fig. 6.28 Aortic stenosis. There is a systolic pressure gradient across the stenosed aortic valve. The resultant high-velocity jet (arrow) impinges on the wall of the aorta, and is best heard with the diaphragm in the aortic area. Alternatively, the bell may be placed in the suprasternal notch. The ejection systolic murmur precedes an ejection click (EC). A fourth heart sound may be heard at the apex.

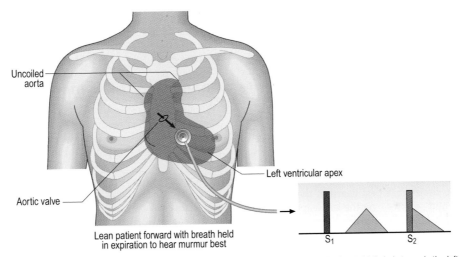

Fig. 6.29 Aortic regurgitation. The pulse pressure is usually increased; the jet from the aortic valve is directed inferiorly towards the left ventricular outflow tract (arrow) during diastole, producing a high-pitched early diastolic murmur, best heard with the diaphragm. An associated systolic murmur is common because of the increased flow through the aortic valve in systole.

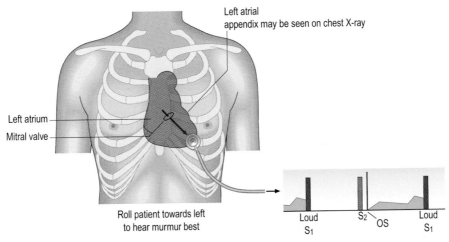

Fig. 6.30 Mitral stenosis. There is a pressure gradient across the mitral valve; in this example it continues throughout diastole. This causes a sharp movement of the tethered anterior cusp of the mitral valve at the time when the flow commences, and an opening snap (OS) results. The jet through the stenosed valve (arrow) strikes the endocardium at the cardiac apex.

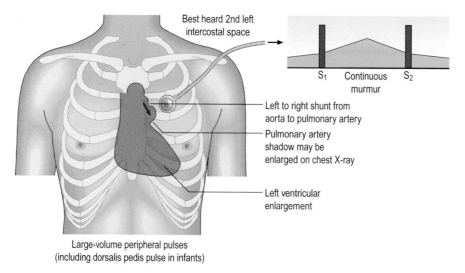

Fig. 6.31 Persistent patent ductus arteriosus. A continuous 'machinery' murmur is heard because aortic pressure always exceeds pulmonary arterial pressure, resulting in continuous ductal flow. The pressure difference is greatest in systole, producing a louder systolic component to the murmur.

the blood flow across the stenosed valve, leading to presystolic accentuation of the murmur. The murmur of tricuspid stenosis is similar but rare.

An Austin Flint murmur is a mid-diastolic murmur that accompanies aortic regurgitation. It is caused by the regurgitant jet striking the anterior leaflet of the mitral valve, restricting inflow to the left ventricle.

Continuous murmurs Continuous murmurs are rare in adults. The most common cause is a patent ductus arteriosus. In the fetus this connects the upper descending aorta and pulmonary artery and normally closes just after birth. The murmur is best heard at the upper left sternal border and radiates over the left scapula. Its continuous character is 'machinery-like' (Fig. 6.31).

PUTTING IT ALL TOGETHER

Auscultation remains an important clinical skill despite the ready availability of echocardiography. You must be able to detect abnormal signs to prompt appropriate investigation. Auscultatory signs, e.g. S_3 or S_4 and pericardial friction rubs, have no direct equivalent on echocardiography but are diagnostically important. Some patients, especially those with rheumatic heart disease, have multiple heart valve defects, and the interpretation of more subtle physical signs is important. For example, a patient with mixed mitral stenosis and regurgitation will probably have dominant stenosis if the S_1 is loud, but dominant regurgitation if there is an S_3.

INVESTIGATIONS

See Box 6.32.

Electrocardiography (ECG)

The standard 12-lead ECG (Fig. 6.32) uses recordings made from six precordial electrodes (V_1–V_6) and six

different recordings from the limb electrodes (left arm, right arm and left leg). The right leg electrode is used as a reference.

Ambulatory ECG monitoring

This is a continuous ECG recording that lasts 24–48 hours and is read by computer. Patient-activated recorders capture occasional arrhythmias and are activated only when symptoms occur (Fig. 6.33).

Exercise ECG

An exercise ECG may unmask evidence of coronary artery disease. Severe ECG abnormalities, or changes that occur during minor exertion, are of prognostic significance and may require invasive investigation with coronary angiography.

Ambulatory BP monitoring

A portable device is worn by the patient at home: this device takes at least two BP measurements per hour during the person's usual waking hours. The average value of at least 14 measurements is used to confirm a diagnosis of hypertension.

Chest X-ray

An enlarged heart, as judged by the cardiothoracic ratio (Fig. 7.22), is common in valvular heart disease and heart failure. In heart failure this is often accompanied by distension of the upper lobe pulmonary veins, diffuse shadowing within the lungs due to pulmonary oedema and Kerley B lines (horizontal engorged lymphatics at the periphery of the lower lobes) (Fig. 6.34A). A widened mediastinum may indicate a thoracic aneurysm.

Echocardiography

Echocardiography uses high-frequency sound waves to evaluate valve abnormalities, left ventricular function

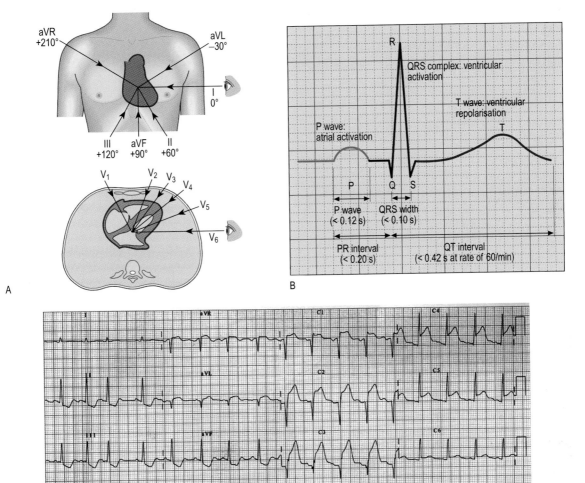

Fig. 6.32 Electrocardiography. (A) Diagram to show the directions from which the 12 standard leads 'look at the heart'. The transverse section is viewed from below like a computed tomography scan. **(B)** Normal PQRST complex. **(C)** Acute anterior myocardial infarction. Note ST elevation in leads V_1–V_6 and aVL, and 'reciprocal' ST depression in leads II, III and aVF.

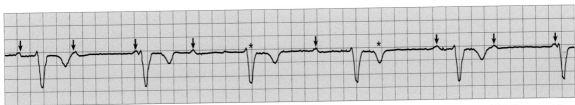

Fig. 6.33 Printout from 24-hour ambulatory electrocardiogram recording, showing complete heart block. Arrows indicate visible P waves; at times these are masked by the QRS complex or T wave (*).

6

6.32 Investigations in cardiac disease

Investigation	Indication/comment
Blood tests	
Full blood count and erythrocyte sedimentation rate	Anaemia unmasking angina and connective tissue disease
Urine and electrolytes	Renal function
Blood glucose	Hypertension more common in diabetes
Lipids	Hyperlipidaemia
Cardiac enzymes	Troponins rise after myocardial infarction
Serology	Connective tissue disease, streptococcal infection
Blood culture	Infective endocarditis
Electrophysiology	
Electrocardiogram (ECG)	Cardiac rhythm, conduction, e.g. left bundle branch block Myocardial infarction and ischaemia (usually normal in angina) Assess left ventricular hypertrophy
Exercise ECG	Ischaemia, prognosis post myocardial infarction
Ambulatory ECG monitoring	Confirms if palpitation coincides with arrhythmia
Radiology	
Chest X-ray	Cardiothoracic ratio (maximum width of the cardiac silhouette/widest part of lung fields) increased in heart failure and valve disease
Echocardiography (transoesophageal echocardiogram more sensitive)	Quantifies valvular defects; assesses left ventricular function (heart failure); valve vegetations in infective endocarditis
Radionuclide studies	Left ventricular function; myocardial ischaemia; pulmonary embolism
Invasive tests	
Cardiac catheterisation	Coronary angiography (angina) determines therapy, prior to surgery in valve disease to assess coronary anatomy, and severe heart failure for cardiac transplantation

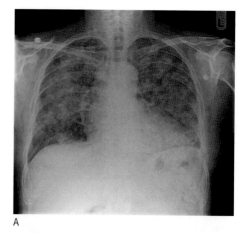

A

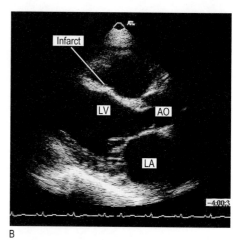

B

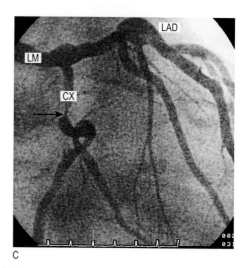

C

and blood flow (Doppler echocardiography). Most scans are performed through the anterior chest wall (transthoracic) (Fig. 6.34B). Transoesophageal echocardiography requires sedation, but gives high resolution of posterior structures, e.g. left atrium, tricuspid valve and descending aorta.

Radionuclide studies

Technetium-99 is injected intravenously and detected using a gamma camera to assess left ventricular function. Thallium and sesta-MIBI are taken up by

Fig. 6.34 Cardiovascular imaging. (A) Chest X-ray in heart failure. This shows cardiomegaly with patchy alveolar shadowing of pulmonary oedema and Kerley B lines (engorged lymphatics) at the periphery of both lungs. **(B)** Transthoracic echocardiogram in parasternal long-axis view. This shows thinning of the interventricular septum, which has an irregular shape and bright echoes indicating fibrous scarring. This is the site of an old infarct. LA, left atrium; LV, left ventricle; AO, aortic root. **(C)** Coronary angiography. The arrow indicates a severe discrete stenosis in the circumflex coronary artery. LM, left main; LAD, left anterior descending; CX, circumflex.

myocardial cells and indicate myocardial perfusion at rest and exercise.

Cardiac catheterisation

A fine catheter is introduced under local anaesthetic via a peripheral artery (usually the brachial or femoral) and advanced to the heart under X-ray guidance. Although measurements of intracardiac pressures and therefore estimates of valvular and cardiac function are possible, the primary application of this technique is coronary arterial imaging, using contrast medium. This is performed to inform revascularisation, either by coronary angioplasty or bypass grafting (Fig. 6.34C).

Computed tomography (CT) and magnetic resonance imaging (MRI)

CT, with its superior temporal resolution of the coronary arteries, is particularly useful to investigate symptomatic patients at low-intermediate risk of coronary artery disease. It can also reduce the need for invasive investigation in patients, with a low probability of occlusive coronary disease, awaiting valve surgery. MRI provides superior tissue resolution and is the imaging modality of choice for investigating heart muscle disease (cardiomyopathy).

PERIPHERAL VASCULAR SYSTEM

PERIPHERAL ARTERIAL SYSTEM

See Figures 6.9 and 6.35.

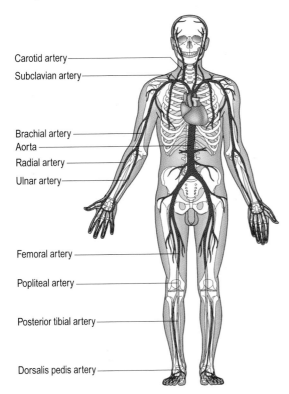

Carotid artery
Subclavian artery

Brachial artery
Aorta
Radial artery
Ulnar artery

Femoral artery

Popliteal artery

Posterior tibial artery

Dorsalis pedis artery

Fig. 6.35 The arterial system.

CLINICAL PRESENTATION

Lower limb

Approximately 20% of people aged >60 years in developed countries have PAD but only a quarter of these are symptomatic. The underlying pathology is usually atherosclerosis (hardening of the arteries) affecting large and medium-sized vessels.

Identifying patients with PAD is important for the following reasons:

- PAD, even if asymptomatic, is a powerful marker for premature vascular death
- The first manifestation of PAD may be a life- or limb-threatening complication, e.g. stroke, acute limb ischaemia or ruptured AAA
- Modifying vascular risk factors dramatically improves outcomes
- PAD may affect medical and surgical treatment for other conditions, e.g. prescription of a beta-blocker may precipitate intermittent claudication.

PAD affects the legs eight times more commonly than the arms for the following reasons:

- The arterial supply to the legs is less well developed in relation to the muscle mass
- The lower limb is more frequently affected by atherosclerosis.

There are four stages of lower limb lack of blood supply (ischaemia) (Box 6.33).

Asymptomatic ischaemia

Haemodynamically significant lower limb ischaemia is defined as an ankle to brachial pressure index (ABPI) <0.9 at rest. Most of these patients are asymptomatic, either because they choose not to walk very far, or because their exercise tolerance is limited by other comorbidity. Although asymptomatic, these patients are at high risk of 'vascular' complications and should be assessed and treated medically as if they have intermittent claudication.

6.33 Classification of lower limb ischaemia	
I	Asymptomatic
II	Intermittent claudication
III	Night/rest pain
IV	Tissue loss (ulceration/gangrene)

6

6.34 The clinical features of arterial, neurogenic and venous claudication

	Arterial	Neurogenic	Venous
Pathology	Stenosis or occlusion of major lower limb arteries	Lumbar nerve root or cauda equina compression (spinal stenosis)	Obstruction to the venous outflow of the leg due to iliofemoral venous occlusion
Site of pain	Muscles, usually the calf but may involve thigh and buttocks	Ill defined. Whole leg. May be associated with numbness and tingling	Whole leg. 'Bursting' in nature
Laterality	Unilateral if femoropopliteal, and bilateral if aortoiliac disease	Often bilateral	Nearly always unilateral
Onset	Gradual after walking the 'claudication distance'	Often immediate on walking or standing up	Gradual, from the moment walking starts
Relieving features	On stopping walking, the pain disappears completely in 1–2 minutes	Bending forwards and stopping walking. May sit down for full relief	Leg elevation
Colour	Normal or pale	Normal	Cyanosed. Often visible varicose veins
Temperature	Normal or cool	Normal	Normal or increased
Oedema	Absent	Absent	Always present
Pulses	Reduced or absent	Normal	Present but may be difficult to feel owing to oedema
Straight-leg raising	Normal	May be limited	Normal

Intermittent claudication

Intermittent claudication is pain felt in the legs on walking due to arterial insufficiency and is the most common symptom of PAD. The pain typically occurs in the calf secondary to femoropopliteal disease but may be felt in the thigh and/or buttock in proximal (aorto-iliac) obstruction. Patients describe tightness or 'cramp-like' pain which develops after a relatively constant distance; the distance is often shorter if walking uphill, in the cold and after meals. The pain disappears completely within a few minutes of rest but recurs on walking. The 'claudication distance' is how far patients say they can walk before the pain stops them from walking.

There are two other types of claudication

- Neurogenic claudication is due to neurological and musculoskeletal disorders of the lumbar spine
- Venous claudication is due to venous outflow obstruction from the leg, following extensive DVT.

Neurogenic and venous claudication are much less common than arterial claudication, and can be distinguished on history and examination (Box 6.34).

Night/rest pain

The patient goes to bed, falls asleep, but is then woken 1–2 hours later with severe pain in the foot, usually in the instep. The pain is due to poor perfusion resulting from the loss of the beneficial effects of gravity on lying down and the reduction in heart rate, BP and cardiac output that occurs when sleeping. Patients often obtain relief by hanging the leg out of bed or by getting up and walking around. However, on return to bed, the pain recurs and patients often choose to sleep in a chair. This leads to dependent oedema, increased interstitial tissue pressure, a further reduction in tissue perfusion and ultimately a worsening of the pain.

Rest (night) pain indicates severe, multilevel lower limb PAD and is a 'red flag' symptom that mandates urgent referral to a vascular surgeon as failure to revascularise the leg usually leads to the development of critical limb ischaemia with tissue loss (gangrene, ulceration) and amputation.

In diabetic patients it may be difficult to differentiate between rest pain and diabetic neuropathy as both may be worse at night. Neuropathic pain is not usually confined to the foot, is associated with burning and tingling, is not relieved by dependency and is associated with dysaesthesia (pain or uncomfortable sensations sometimes described as burning, tingling or numbness). Many patients cannot even bear the pressure of bedclothes on their feet.

Tissue loss (ulceration and/or gangrene)

In patients with severe lower limb PAD, even trivial injuries to the feet fail to heal. This allows bacteria to enter, leading to gangrene and/or ulceration. This usually progresses rapidly and, without revascularisation, often leads quickly to amputation and/or death.

Signs of lower limb PAD

Ischaemic signs include absence of hair, thin skin and brittle nails (Box 6.34). The presence of foot pulses does not completely exclude significant lower limb PAD but they are almost always diminished or absent. If the history is convincing but pulses are felt, ask the patient to walk until the claudication pain stops him and then recheck the pulses; if they have disappeared then PAD is very likely.

6.35 Signs of acute limb ischaemia

Soft signs

- **P**ulseless
- **P**allor
- **P**erishing cold

Hard signs (indicating a threatened limb)

- **P**araesthesia
- **P**aralysis
- **P**ain on squeezing muscle

6.36 Acute limb ischaemia: embolus versus thrombosis in situ

	Embolus	Thrombosis
Onset and severity	Acute (seconds or minutes), ischaemia profound (no pre-existing collaterals)	Insidious (hours or days), ischaemia less severe (pre-existing collaterals)
Embolic source	Present (usually atrial fibrillation)	Absent
Previous claudication	Absent	Present
Pulses in contralateral leg	Present	Often absent
Diagnosis	Clinical	Angiography
Treatment	Embolectomy and anticoagulation	Medical, bypass surgery, thrombolysis

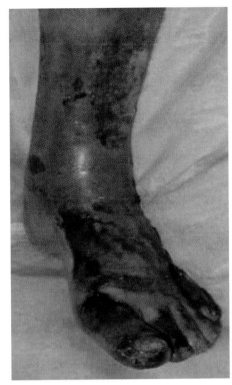

Fig. 6.36 Gangrene of the foot.

Patients with critical limb ischaemia (rest pain, tissue loss) typically have an ankle BP <50 mmHg and a positive Buerger's test.

Acute limb ischaemia

The classical features of acute limb ischaemia are the 'six Ps' (Box 6.35). Paralysis (inability to wiggle the toes/fingers) and paraesthesia (loss of light touch sensation over the forefoot/dorsum of the hand) are the most important and indicate severe ischaemia affecting nerve function. Muscle tenderness is a grave sign indicating impending muscle infarction. A limb with these features will usually become irreversibly damaged unless the circulation is restored within a few hours.

The commonest causes of acute limb ischaemia are:

- Thromboembolism: usually from the left atrium in association with atrial fibrillation
- Thrombosis in situ: thrombotic occlusion of an already narrowed atherosclerotic arterial segment (Box 6.36).

Acute arterial occlusion produces intense spasm in the arterial tree distal to the blockage. The limb appears 'marble white'. Over a few hours, the spasm relaxes and the skin microcirculation fills with deoxygenated blood, leading to light blue or purple mottling, which has a fine reticular pattern and blanches on pressure. As ischaemia progresses, blood coalesces in the skin, producing a coarser pattern of mottling which is dark purple, almost black, and does not blanch. Finally, large patches of fixed staining lead to blistering and liquefaction. Fixed mottling of an anaesthetic, paralysed limb, with muscle rigidity and turgor, indicates irreversible ischaemia; amputation or end-of-life care is the only option (Fig. 6.36).

Compartment syndrome occurs where there is increased pressure within the fascial compartments of the limb, most commonly the calf, which compromises perfusion and viability of muscle and nerves. The two commonest causes are lower trauma, e.g. fractured tibia, and reperfusion following treatment of acute lower limb ischaemia. Failure to recognise and treat compartment syndrome may require limb amputation. The key symptom is severe pain often unrelieved by opioids and exacerbated by active or passive movement. Peripheral pulses are usually present.

Stroke

Stroke is a focal central neurological deficit of vascular cause. Approximately 80% of strokes are ischaemic rather than haemorrhagic. Transient ischaemic attack (TIA) describes a stroke in which symptoms resolve within 24 hours. The term 'stroke' is reserved for those events in which symptoms last for more than 24 hours.

Carotid artery territory (anterior circulation)

Up to half of all strokes and TIAs are due to embolism from an atheromatous plaque at the origin of the internal

| EBE | **6.37 Imaging in suspected carotid territory transient ischaemic attack (TIA) or stroke** |

All patients with suspected carotid territory TIA or stroke should undergo urgent duplex Doppler ultrasound imaging as the finding of a carotid bruit is unreliable in detecting or excluding significant carotid disease that may be an indication for endarterectomy.

Sauve J-S, Laupacis A, Ostbye T et al. Does this patient have a clinically important carotid bruit? In: Simel D, Rinne D (eds) The rational clinical examination. New York: JAMA and Archives Journals/McGraw-Hill Professional, 2008, pp. 103–110.

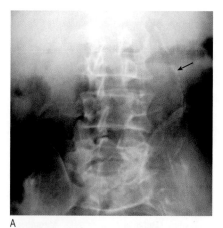

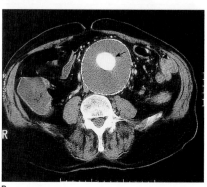

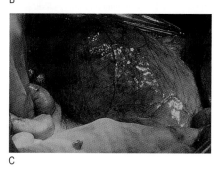

Fig. 6.37 Abdominal aortic aneurysm. (A) Abdominal X-ray showing calcification (arrow). **(B)** Computed tomography of the abdomen showing an abdominal aortic aneurysm (arrow). **(C)** At laparotomy the aorta is seen to be grossly and irregularly dilated.

carotid artery. Clinical features vary according to the cerebral area involved but can include motor deficit, visual field defect, e.g. homonymous hemianopia (Fig. 12.3), or difficulty with speech (dysphasia, p. 248) (Box 6.37).

Vertebrobasilar artery territory (posterior circulation)

TIAs and strokes in this territory cause giddiness, collapse with or without loss of consciousness, transient occipital blindness or complete loss of vision in both eyes (Ch. 11). Subclavian artery stenosis or occlusion proximal to the origin of the vertebral artery may cause vertebrobasilar symptoms as part of the 'subclavian steal' syndrome. This happens when the arm is exercised. The increased blood supply requirement in the arm is met by blood travelling up the carotid arteries and then, via the circle of Willis (Fig. 11.29), down the vertebral artery into the arm, so 'stealing' blood from the posterior cerebral circulation. Signs of this include asymmetry of the pulses and BP in the arms, sometimes with a bruit over the subclavian artery in the supraclavicular fossa.

Abdominal symptoms

Mesenteric angina

Because of the rich collateral circulation, usually two of the three major visceral arteries (coeliac axis, superior and inferior mesenteric arteries) must be critically stenosed or occluded before symptoms and signs of chronic mesenteric arterial insufficiency occur. Severe central abdominal pain typically develops 10–15 minutes after eating. The patient becomes scared of eating and significant weight loss is a universal finding. Diarrhoea may occur and visceral ischaemia may mimic a whole range of gastrointestinal pathologies. The patient may have had numerous investigations, even laparotomy, before the diagnosis is made and confirmed by angiography. Any patient suspected of visceral ischaemia should undergo urgent angiography.

Acute mesenteric ischaemia is a surgical emergency. The patient presents with severe abdominal pain, shock, bloody diarrhoea and profound metabolic acidosis. Rarely, renal angle pain occurs from renal infarction or ischaemia, and is associated with microscopic or macroscopic haematuria.

Abdominal aortic aneurysm

AAA is an abnormal dilatation of the aorta (Fig. 6.37) and is present in 5% of men aged >65 years. The main risk factors are smoking and hypertension; there is also a familial/genetic element to the disease. AAA is three times more common in men than women. Most patients are asymptomatic until the aneurysm ruptures, although they may present with abdominal and/or back pain or an awareness of abdominal pulsation.

Clinical examination is unreliable in establishing the presence or size of an AAA; if in any doubt, obtain an ultrasound scan of the aorta. In the UK there is now an ultrasound-based AAA screening programme for men as they reach their 65th birthday.

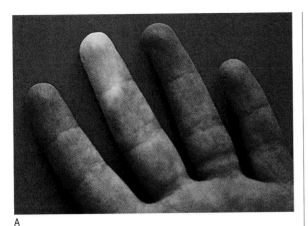

A

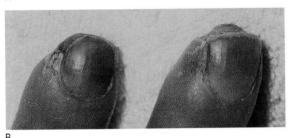

B

Fig. 6.38 Raynaud's syndrome. (A) The acute phase, showing severe blanching of the tip of one finger. **(B)** Primary Raynaud's syndrome occasionally progresses to fingertip ulceration or even gangrene.

> **6.38 Diseases associated with secondary Raynaud's syndrome**
>
> - Connective tissue syndromes, e.g. systemic sclerosis, CREST (calcinosis, Raynaud's phenomenon, oesophageal dysfunction, sclerodactyly, telangiectasia) and systemic lupus erythematosus
> - Atherosclerosis/embolism from proximal source, e.g. subclavian artery aneurysm
> - Drug-related, e.g. nicotine, beta-blockers, ergot
> - Thoracic outlet syndrome
> - Malignancy
> - Hyperviscosity syndromes, e.g. Waldenström's macroglobulinaemia, polycythaemia
> - Vibration-induced disorders (power tools)
> - Cold agglutinin disorders

A ruptured AAA can be difficult to diagnose because many patients do not have the classical features of abdominal and/or back pain, pulsatile abdominal mass and shock (hypotension). The most common misdiagnosis is renal colic (a man, >60 years, presenting with 'renal colic' has a ruptured AAA until proved otherwise). If there is any suspicion of a ruptured AAA speak to a vascular surgeon straight away who will probably request an immediate contrast-enhanced CT of the abdomen (if the patient is cardiovascularly stable).

Athero-embolism from an AAA can cause 'blue toe syndrome', characterised by purple discoloration of the toes and forefoot of both feet. There is usually a full set of pedal pulses.

Vasospastic symptoms

Raynaud's phenomenon is digital ischaemia induced by cold and emotion and has three phases (Fig. 6.38):
- Pallor: due to digital artery spasm and/or obstruction
- Cyanosis: due to deoxygenation of static venous blood (this phase may be absent)
- Redness: due to reactive hyperaemia.

Raynaud's phenomenon may be primary (Raynaud's disease) and due to idiopathic digital artery vasospasm, or secondary (Raynaud's syndrome) (Box 6.38).

Patients >40 years old presenting with unilateral Raynaud's phenomenon have underlying PAD unless proven otherwise, especially if they have risk factors (smoking, diabetes).

THE HISTORY

Ask about risk factors for atheroma (smoking, hypercholesterolaemia, hypertension, diabetes mellitus) and any family history of premature arterial disease. Specifically ask about diabetes because it is associated with the early development and rapid progression of widespread atheroma.

The impact of intermittent claudication relates to the patient's age and lifestyle. A postman/postwoman who can walk only 400 metres has a serious problem, but an elderly person who simply wants to cross the road to the shops may cope well. Rather than focusing upon absolute distances, ask specific questions like:
- Can you walk to the clinic from the bus stop or car park without stopping?
- Can you do your own shopping?
- What can't you do because of the pain?

Ask about the patient's other medical conditions. There is little point in subjecting patients with intermittent claudication to the risks of vascular surgery, only to find that they are then equally limited by osteoarthritis of the hip, angina or severe breathlessness.

Male patients with buttock (gluteal) intermittent claudication due to internal iliac disease have erectile dysfunction. Ask about sexual function as many men and their partners are extremely concerned by erectile dysfunction yet too embarrassed to mention it.

THE PHYSICAL EXAMINATION

Follow the routine described for the heart, looking for evidence of anaemia or cyanosis, signs of heart failure, and direct or indirect evidence of PAD (Box 6.39). Then perform a detailed examination of the arterial pulses. Abnormally prominent pulsation in the neck of an elderly person is rarely of clinical significance and is normally caused by tortuous arteries rather than a carotid aneurysm or carotid body tumour. However, if in any doubt, arrange for a duplex ultrasound scan.

6.39 Signs suggesting vascular disease

Sign	Implication
Hands and arms	
Tobacco stains	Smoking
Purple discoloration of the fingertips	Atheroembolism from a proximal subclavian aneurysm
Pits and healed scars in the finger pulps	Secondary Raynaud's syndrome
Calcinosis and visible nailfold capillary loops	Systemic sclerosis and CREST (calcinosis, Raynaud's phenomenon, oesophageal dysfunction, sclerodactyly, telangiectasia)
Wasting of the small muscles of the hand	Thoracic outlet syndrome
Face and neck	
Corneal arcus and xanthelasma	Hypercholesterolaemia
Horner's syndrome	Carotid artery dissection or aneurysm
Hoarseness of the voice and 'bovine' cough	Recurrent laryngeal nerve palsy from a thoracic aortic aneurysm
Prominent veins in the neck, shoulder and anterior chest	Axillary/subclavian vein occlusion
Abdomen	
Epigastric/umbilical pulsation	Aortoiliac aneurysm
Mottling of the abdomen	Ruptured abdominal aortic aneurysm or saddle embolism occluding aortic bifurcation
Evidence of weight loss	Visceral ischaemia

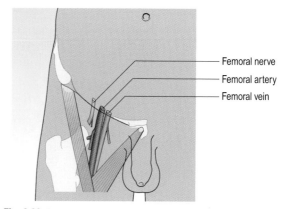

Femoral nerve
Femoral artery
Femoral vein

Fig. 6.39 Femoral triangle: vessels and nerves.

■ Look specifically between the toes for ulcers and at the heels for ischaemic changes (commonest site of 'pressure sores').

Femoral pulse
■ Ask the patient to lie down and explain what you are going to do.
■ Place the pads of your index and middle fingers over the femoral artery. It can be difficult to feel in the obese.
■ Listen for bruits over both femoral arteries, using the stethoscope diaphragm (Figs 6.39 and 6.40A).

Popliteal pulse
■ Ask the patient to lie on a firm comfortable surface and relax.
■ Flex the patient's knee to 30°.
■ With your thumbs in front of the knee and your fingers behind, press firmly in the midline over the popliteal artery.
■ Then slide your fingers 2–3 cm below the knee crease and try to compress the artery against the back of the tibia as it passes under the soleal arch (Fig. 6.40B).

Posterior tibial pulse
■ Feel 2 cm below and 2 cm behind the medial malleolus, using the pads of your middle three fingers (Fig. 6.40C).

Dorsalis pedis pulse
■ Using the pads of your middle three fingers, feel in the middle of the dorsum of the foot just lateral to the tendon of extensor hallucis longus (Fig. 6.40D).

Buerger's test

 Examination sequence

■ With the patient lying supine, stand at the foot of the bed. Raise the patient's feet and support the legs at 45° to the horizontal for 2–3 minutes.
■ Watch for pallor with emptying or 'guttering' of the superficial veins.
■ Ask the patient to sit up and hang the legs over the edge of the bed.
■ Watch for reactive hyperaemia on dependency; the loss of pallor and spreading redness is a positive test.

Ankle to brachial pressure index

Assessing pulse status can be unreliable in patients with obesity or oedema. Routinely measure ABPI in all patients with difficulty palpating lower limb pulses or where PAD is suspected on the basis of history.

 Examination sequence

Start at the patient's head and work down the body, using the sequence and principles of inspection, palpation and auscultation for each area.

The arms
■ Examine the radial and brachial pulses (p. 108 and Fig. 6.10).
■ Measure the BP in both arms.

The abdomen
■ Look for obvious pulsation.
■ Palpate and listen over the abdominal aorta. The aortic bifurcation is at the level of the umbilicus, so feel in the epigastrium for a palpable AAA. If the aorta is easily palpable, consider the possibility of an AAA. In thin patients a tortuous but normal-diameter aorta can feel aneurysmal. If in any doubt, arrange a duplex ultrasound scan. A pulsatile mass below the umbilicus suggests an iliac aneurysm.

The legs
■ Inspect and feel the legs and feet for changes of ischaemia, including temperature and colour changes.
■ Note scars from previous vascular or non-vascular surgery and the position, margin, depth and colour of any ulceration.

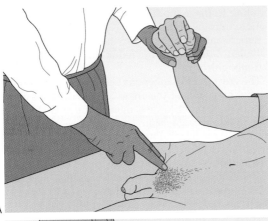

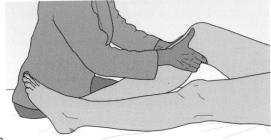

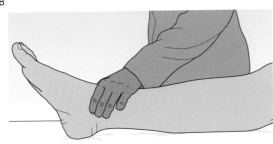

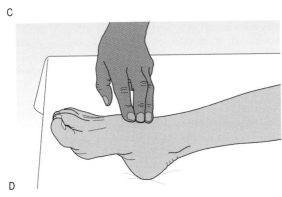

Fig. 6.40 Examination of the femoral, popliteal, posterior tibial and dorsalis pedis arteries. (A) Examine the femoral artery, while simultaneously checking for radiofemoral delay. **(B)** Feel the popliteal artery with the fingertips, having curled the fingers into the popliteal fossa. **(C)** Examination of the posterior tibial artery. **(D)** Examination of the dorsalis pedis artery.

- Use a hand-held Doppler and a sphygmomanometer
- Hold the probe over the posterior tibial artery
- Inflate a BP cuff round the ankle
- Note the pressure when Doppler signal disappears. This is the systolic pressure in that artery as it passes under the cuff

6.40 Investigations in peripheral arterial disease

Investigation	Indication/comment
Blood tests	
Full blood count and erythrocyte sedimentation rate	Anaemia unmasking symptoms and connective tissue disease
Urine and electrolytes	Renal function
Blood glucose	Hypertension more common in diabetes
Serology	Connective tissue disease
Microbiology	
Bacteriology	Swab base of ulcer
Radiology	
Doppler ultrasound	Ankle pressure, ankle to brachial pressure index, pulse waveform analysis
B-mode ultrasound	Abdominal aortic aneurysm, popliteal artery aneurysm
Duplex ultrasound	Carotid artery stenosis, vein bypass graft surveillance
Computed tomography	Abdominal aortic aneurysm, detection of cerebral infarct/haemorrhage
Magnetic resonance imaging	Arteriovenous malformations, carotid artery stenosis
Angiography	Acute and chronic limb ischaemia, carotid artery stenosis

- Repeat holding the probe over dorsalis pedis, and then the perforating peroneal (Box 6.13)
- Measure the brachial BP in both arms, holding the Doppler probe over the brachial artery at the elbow or the radial artery at the wrist.

Normal findings The ratio of the highest pedal artery pressure to the highest brachial artery pressure is the ABPI. In health, the ABPI is >1.0 when the patient is supine. The popliteal artery is always hard to feel – if you feel it easily, consider an aneurysm.

Abnormal findings

Typical values in intermittent claudication and critical limb ischaemia are <0.9 and <0.4 respectively. Absolute values may be less informative than the trend over time.

Patients with lower limb PAD, particularly those with diabetes mellitus, often have incompressible, calcified crural arteries with falsely elevated pedal pressures and ABPI. Use a Doppler ultrasound probe to detect the foot arteries while elevating the foot. The Doppler signal disappears at a height (in cm) above the bed that approximates to the perfusion pressure (in mmHg).

Choose further tests to provide the most information at the least risk to the patient and at least expense. In most situations duplex Doppler ultrasound has replaced angiography as the first-line investigation of choice (Box 6.40).

6

PERIPHERAL VENOUS SYSTEM

Whereas venous return from the head and neck is passive, that from the legs must be actively pumped back up to the heart against gravity. Pressure on the sole of the foot on walking, together with contraction of muscles in the calf (the 'calf muscle pump'), and, to a lesser extent in the thighs and buttocks, forces venous blood back up deep (90%) and superficial (10%) veins. Backward flow (reflux) is prevented by valves which divide the long column of blood from the foot to the right atrium into a series of short low-pressure segments. As a result, the 'ambulatory venous pressure' in the feet in health is usually <20 mmHg. The great majority of lower limb venous symptoms and signs are due to failure of the muscle pump and/or valves and the resulting 'ambulatory venous hypertension'.

Deep veins follow the course of the main arteries; are often paired; and may be affected by primary or postthrombotic (following DVT) valvular insufficiency. DVT often leads to deep venous obstruction as well as reflux (leading to the symptoms and signs of the postthrombotic syndrome).

Superficial veins may also be affected by primary valvular failure and by reflux following superficial thrombophlebitis.

The great (long) saphenous vein passes anterior to the medial malleolus at the ankle, up the medial aspect of the calf to behind the knee, then up the medial aspect of the thigh to join the common femoral vein in the groin at the saphenofemoral junction (Fig. 6.41).

The lesser (short) saphenous vein passes behind the lateral malleolus at the ankle and up the posterior aspect of the calf. It commonly joins the popliteal vein at the saphenopopliteal junction, which usually lies 2 cm above the posterior knee crease.

There are numerous intercommunications between the long and short saphenous, and between the deep and superficial venous (via perforating or communicating veins) systems; and the venous anatomy of the leg is highly variable.

CLINICAL PRESENTATION

Lower limb venous disease presents in four ways:

- Varicose veins
- Superficial thrombophlebitis
- DVT
- Chronic venous insufficiency and ulceration.

The severity of symptoms and signs may bear little relationship to the severity of the underlying pathology and the physical signs. Life-threatening DVT may be asymptomatic, while apparently trivial varicose veins may be associated with significant complaints.

Pain

Patients with uncomplicated varicose (dilated, tortuous, superficial) veins often complain of aching leg discomfort, itching and a feeling of swelling. Symptoms are aggravated by prolonged standing and are often worse towards the end of the day. Once established, DVT causes pain and tenderness in the affected part (usually the calf). Superficial thrombophlebitis produces a red, painful area overlying the vein involved. Varicose ulceration may be surprisingly painless; if it is painful, this may be relieved by limb elevation (but exclude coexisting arterial disease) (Box 6.41). Bandaging for a leg ulcer is contraindicated unless there is documented evidence of adequate arterial circulation. Do this by feeling the pulses or by measuring the ABPI.

Swelling

Swelling (or oedema), or a 'feeling of swelling', may be associated with lower limb venous disease.

Discoloration

Chronic venous insufficiency is associated with lipodermatosclerosis, which results from the deposition of haemosiderin (from the breakdown of extravasated blood) in the skin. Lipodermatosclerosis varies in colour

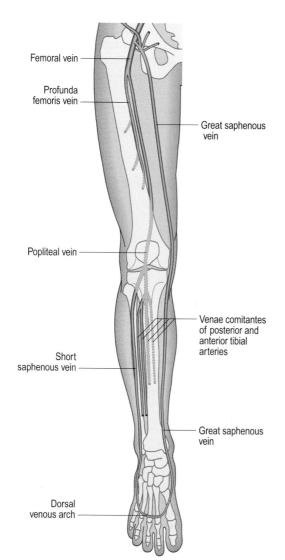

Femoral vein

Profunda femoris vein

Great saphenous vein

Popliteal vein

Venae comitantes of posterior and anterior tibial arteries

Short saphenous vein

Great saphenous vein

Dorsal venous arch

Fig. 6.41 Veins of the lower limb.

6.41 Clinical features of venous and arterial ulceration

Clinical feature	Venous ulceration	Arterial ulceration
Age	Develops at age 40–45 but may not present for years; multiple recurrences common	First presents in over-60s
Sex	More common in women	More common in men
Past medical history	Deep vein thrombosis (DVT) or suggestive of occult DVT, i.e. leg swelling after childbirth, hip/knee replacement or long bone fracture	Peripheral arterial disease, cardio- and cerebrovascular disease
Risk factors	Thrombophilia, family history, previous DVT	Smoking, diabetes, hypercholesterolaemia and hypertension
Pain	One-third have pain (not usually severe) that improves with elevating the leg	Severe pain, except in diabetics with neuropathy; improves on dependency
Site	Gaiter areas; usually medial to long saphenous vein; 20% are lateral to short saphenous vein	Pressure areas (malleoli, heel, fifth metatarsal base, metatarsal heads and toes)
Margin	Irregular, often with neoepithelium (appears whiter than mature skin)	Regular, indolent, 'punched out'
Base	Often pink and granulating under green slough	Sloughy (green) or necrotic (black), with no granulation
Surrounding skin	Lipodermatosclerosis always present	No venous skin changes
Veins	Full and usually varicose	Empty with 'guttering' on elevation
Swelling (oedema)	Usually present	Absent
Temperature	Warm	Cold
Pulses	Present, but may be difficult to feel	Absent

from deep blue/black to purple or bright red and usually affects the medial aspect of the lower third of the leg, although it may be lateral if superficial reflux predominates in the lesser saphenous vein.

Chronic venous ulceration

In developed countries about 70–80% of leg ulcers are due primarily to venous disease. Other causes include pyoderma gangrenosum, syphilis, tuberculosis, leprosy, sickle cell disease and tropical conditions. Chronic venous ulceration usually affects the medial aspect, is shallow; is pink (granulation tissue) or yellow/green (slough); has an irregular margin; and is always associated with other skin changes of chronic venous insufficiency (varicose eczema, lipodermatosclerosis) (Fig. 6.42).

Deep vein thrombosis

The leg

The clinical features of DVT depend upon its site, extent and whether it is occlusive or not (Box 6.42). The so-called 'classical' features of DVT relate to well-established occlusive thrombus. Most patients who die from pulmonary embolism have non-occlusive thrombosis and the leg is normal on clinical examination. Non-occlusive DVT poses the greatest threat of pulmonary embolism as the clot lies within a flowing stream of venous blood, is more likely to propagate and has not yet induced an inflammatory response in the vein wall to anchor it in place. Risk factors for DVT are listed in Box 6.43. Perform an urgent duplex Doppler ultrasound scan of the leg in any patient with a suspected DVT.

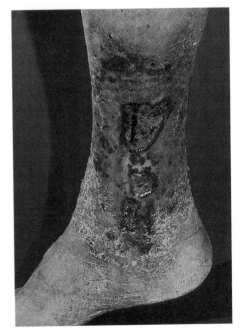

Fig. 6.42 Venous ulceration.

The arm

Axillary subclavian vein thrombosis can occur as a result of repetitive trauma at the thoracic outlet due to vigorous, repetitive exercise. Upper limb DVT may also complicate indwelling subclavian/jugular venous catheters. Symptoms include arm swelling and discomfort, often exacerbated by activity, especially when holding the arm overhead.

6.42 Features of deep vein thrombosis of the lower limb

Clinical feature	Non-occlusive thrombus	Occlusive thrombus
Pain	Often absent	Usually present
Calf tenderness	Often absent	Usually present
Swelling	Absent	Present
Temperature	Normal or slightly increased	Increased
Superficial veins	Normal	Distended
Pulmonary embolism	High risk	Low risk

6.43 Risk factors for deep vein thrombosis

- Recent bed rest or operations (especially to the leg, pelvis or abdomen)
- Recent travel, especially long flights
- Previous trauma to the leg, especially long-bone fractures, plaster of Paris splintage and immobilisation
- Pregnancy or features to suggest pelvic disease
- Malignant disease
- Previous deep vein thrombosis
- Family history of thrombosis
- Recent central venous catheterisation, injection of drugs, etc.

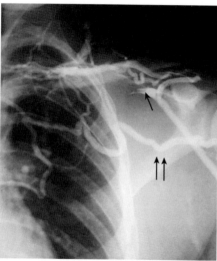

A

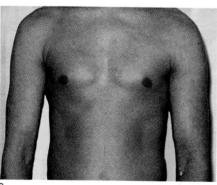

B

Fig. 6.43 Axillary vein thrombosis. (A) Angiogram. Single arrow shows site of thrombosis. Double arrows show dilated collateral vessels. **(B)** Clinical appearance with swollen left arm and dilated superficial veins.

The arm is swollen and the skin is cyanosed and mottled, especially when dependent. Look for superficial distended veins (acting as collaterals) in the upper arm, over the shoulder region and on the anterior chest wall (Fig. 6.43).

Superficial venous thrombophlebitis

This condition affects up to 10% of patients with severe varicose veins and is more common during pregnancy. Recurrent superficial venous thrombophlebitis, especially affecting different areas sequentially and non-varicose veins, may be associated with underlying malignancy. It may propagate into the deep system, leading to DVT and pulmonary embolism.

The physical examination

Examination sequence

Expose the patient's legs and examine them with the patient standing and then lying supine.

- Inspect the skin for colour changes, swelling and superficial venous dilatation and tortuosity.
- Feel for any temperature difference.
- Press with your fingertip above the ankle medially for a few seconds (gently, as this can be painful; do not do this near an ulcer) and then see if your finger has left a pit (pitting oedema).
- If the leg is grossly swollen, press at a higher level to establish how far oedema extends.
- If you find oedema, check the JVP (p. 114). If the JVP is raised, this suggests cardiac disease or pulmonary hypertension as a cause.
- Elevate the limb to about 15° above the horizontal and note the rate of venous emptying.
- If appropriate, perform the Trendelenburg test to detect saphenofemoral junction reflux.

The Trendelenburg test

Examination sequence

- Ask the patient to sit on the edge of the examination couch.
- Elevate the limb as far as is comfortable for the patient and empty the superficial veins by 'milking' the leg towards the groin.
- With the patient's leg still elevated, press with your thumb over the sapheno-femoral junction (2–3 cm below and 2–3 cm lateral to the pubic tubercle). A high thigh tourniquet can be used instead.
- Ask the patient to stand while you maintain pressure over the saphenofemoral junction.
- If saphenofemoral junction reflux is present, the patient's varicose veins will not fill until your digital pressure, or the tourniquet, is removed.

Clinical examination is unreliable, and all patients being considered for treatment should undergo a colour flow duplex, Doppler ultrasound scan before intervention.

Graham Devereux
Graham Douglas

The respiratory system

7

RESPIRATORY EXAMINATION

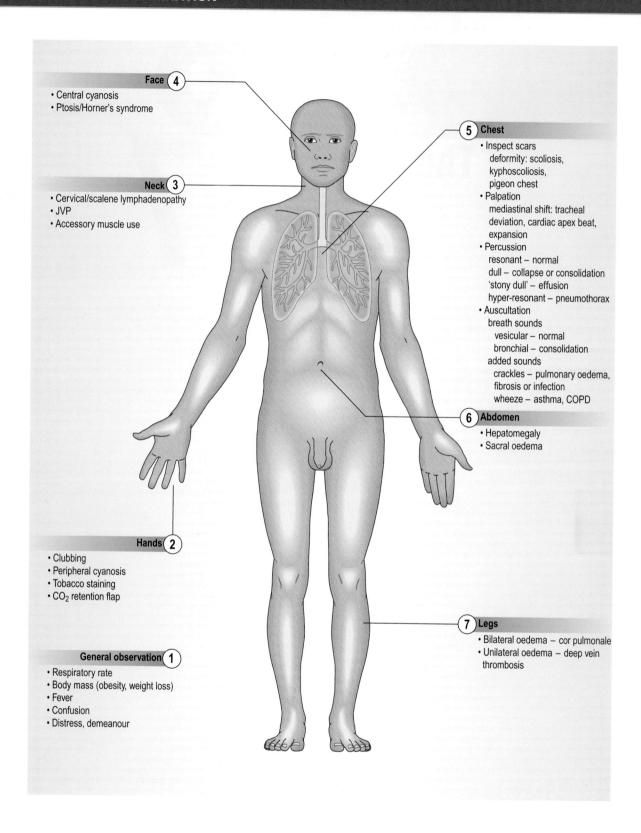

Face 4
- Central cyanosis
- Ptosis/Horner's syndrome

Neck 3
- Cervical/scalene lymphadenopathy
- JVP
- Accessory muscle use

Hands 2
- Clubbing
- Peripheral cyanosis
- Tobacco staining
- CO_2 retention flap

General observation 1
- Respiratory rate
- Body mass (obesity, weight loss)
- Fever
- Confusion
- Distress, demeanour

5 **Chest**
- Inspect scars
  deformity: scoliosis,
  kyphoscoliosis,
  pigeon chest
- Palpation
  mediastinal shift: tracheal
  deviation, cardiac apex beat,
  expansion
- Percussion
  resonant – normal
  dull – collapse or consolidation
  'stony dull' – effusion
  hyper-resonant – pneumothorax
- Auscultation
  breath sounds
    vesicular – normal
    bronchial – consolidation
  added sounds
    crackles – pulmonary oedema,
    fibrosis or infection
    wheeze – asthma, COPD

6 **Abdomen**
- Hepatomegaly
- Sacral oedema

7 **Legs**
- Bilateral oedema – cor pulmonale
- Unilateral oedema – deep vein
  thrombosis

ANATOMY

The respiratory system comprises the upper airway; the nose, mouth, oropharynx and larynx, and the lower airway; the trachea and lungs. The left lung only contains 45% of the total surface area available for gas exchange, because the heart lies principally within the left side of the chest. The right lung has three lobes (upper, middle and lower) and the left, two (upper and lower) (Fig. 7.1).

The airways (bronchi) transport air to the alveoli on inspiration and carry waste gases, e.g. carbon dioxide, away on expiration. The gas exchange unit of the lung is the acinus, with branching bronchioles leading to clusters of alveoli (Fig. 7.2). Alveoli are tiny air sacs lined by flattened epithelial cells (type I pneumocytes) and covered in capillaries where gas exchange occurs. The alveoli and capillaries have extremely thin walls and come into very close contact (the alveolar–capillary membrane); carbon dioxide and oxygen readily diffuse between them. There are approximately 300 million alveoli in each lung, with a total surface area for gas exchange of 40–80 m^2.

The lung has two blood supplies: the bronchial arteries arise from the aorta and supply oxygenated blood to the bronchial walls. The pulmonary arteries circulate deoxygenated blood to the capillaries surrounding the alveoli.

SYMPTOMS AND DEFINITIONS

Cough

Cough is a characteristic sound caused by a forced expulsion against an initially closed glottis. Acute cough is one lasting less than 3 weeks; chronic cough lasts more than 8 weeks. The most common cause of acute cough is acute upper respiratory tract viral infection. Acute cough is usually self-limiting and benign, but may occur in more serious conditions (Box 7.1). Chronic cough in a non-smoker with a normal chest X-ray is usually caused by gastro-oesophageal reflux disease, chronic sinus disease with postnasal drip or angiotensin-converting enzyme inhibitors (Box 7.2).

Severe asthma or chronic obstructive pulmonary disease (COPD) causes prolonged wheezy cough and often a paroxysmal dry cough after a viral infection that lasts several months (bronchial hyperreactivity).

A feeble non-explosive 'bovine' cough with hoarseness suggests lung cancer invading the left recurrent laryngeal nerve causing left vocal cord paralysis, but may also occur with respiratory muscle weakness due to neuromuscular disorders.

Laryngeal inflammation, infection or tumour causes harsh, barking or painful coughs and associated hoarseness and the rasping or croaking inspiratory sound of stridor (p. 140). A moist cough suggests secretions in the upper and larger airways from bronchial infection and bronchiectasis. A persistent moist 'smoker's cough' first thing in the morning is typical of chronic bronchitis. Smokers often consider this normal but any change in this cough may indicate lung cancer. Tracheitis and

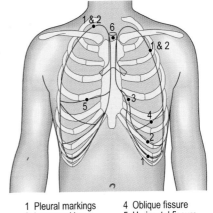

A
1 Pleural markings   4 Oblique fissure
2 Lung markings   5 Horizontal fissure
3 Cardiac notch   6 Trachea

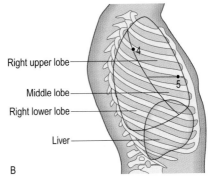

B
Right upper lobe
Middle lobe
Right lower lobe
Liver

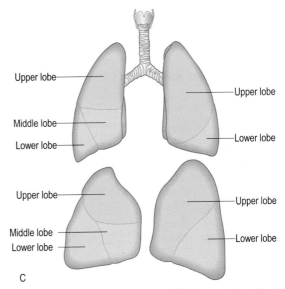

C
Upper lobe
Middle lobe
Lower lobe
Upper lobe
Lower lobe
Upper lobe
Middle lobe
Lower lobe
Upper lobe
Lower lobe

Fig. 7.1 Surface anatomy of the thorax. (A) Surface markings of the lungs and pleura, trachea and bronchi. The trachea is normally central. The bifurcation of the trachea corresponds on the anterior chest wall with the sternal angle, the transverse bony ridge at the junction of the sternum and manubrium sternum. Count the ribs downwards from the second costal cartilage at the level of the sternal angle. **(B)** Surface markings of the right lung and underlying viscera. **(C)** Lobes of the lungs: anterior view (upper) and lateral view (lower).

7

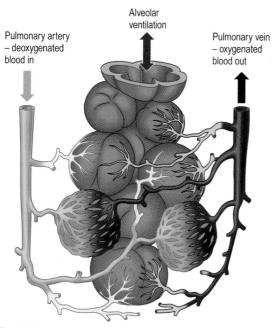

Pulmonary artery – deoxygenated blood in

Alveolar ventilation

Pulmonary vein – oxygenated blood out

Fig. 7.2 The acinus: the basic gas exchange unit of the lung.

7.1 'Red flag' symptoms associated with cough

- Haemoptysis
- Breathlessness
- Fever
- Chest pain
- Weight loss

7.2 Causes of cough

	Normal chest X-ray	Abnormal chest X-ray
Acute cough (<3 weeks)	Viral respiratory tract infection Bacterial infection (acute bronchitis) Inhaled foreign body Inhalation of irritant dusts/fumes	Pneumonia Inhaled foreign body Acute hypersensitivity pneumonitis
Chronic cough (>8 weeks)	Gastro-oesophageal reflux disease Asthma Postviral bronchial hyperreactivity Rhinitis/sinusitis Cigarette smoking Drugs, especially angiotensin-converting enzyme inhibitors Irritant dusts/fumes	Lung tumour Tuberculosis Interstitial lung disease Bronchiectasis

pneumonia cause dry, centrally painful and non-productive cough.

Chronic dry cough occurs in interstitial lung disease, e.g. idiopathic pulmonary fibrosis (formerly fibrosing alveolitis).

Timing and associated features

Nocturnal cough disrupting sleep is a feature of asthma. Occupational asthma and exposure to dusts and fumes cause a chronic cough which improves during weekends and holidays. Coughing during and after swallowing liquids suggests neuromuscular disease of the oropharynx.

Cough syncope may result from raised intrathoracic pressure impairing venous return to the heart, reducing cardiac output.

Dysphonia (hoarseness)

Dysphonia (hoarseness) is most commonly caused by laryngitis. Damage to the left recurrent laryngeal nerve by lung cancer at the left hilum causes hoarseness with a prolonged, low-pitched, 'bovine' cough as the left vocal cord cannot adduct to the midline (Ch. 13).

Wheeze

Wheeze is a high-pitched whistling sound produced by air passing through narrowed small airways. It occurs with expiration, but patients may call rattling sounds from secretions in the upper airways or larynx or the inspiratory sound of stridor wheeze. Wheeze on exercise is common in asthma and COPD. Night wakening with wheeze suggests asthma or paroxysmal nocturnal dyspnoea, but wheeze after wakening in the morning suggests COPD.

Stridor

Stridor is a high-pitched, often harsh noise produced by airflow turbulence through a partial obstruction of the upper airway. It occurs most commonly on inspiration but also on expiration or biphasically. Inspiratory stridor indicates narrowing at the vocal cords; biphasic stridor suggests tracheal obstruction, while stridor on expiration suggests tracheobronchial obstruction. Narrowing of smaller, peripheral airways produces wheeze (Fig. 13.22). Stridor always needs investigation. Common causes include infection/inflammation, e.g. acute epiglottitis in children and young adults, and tumours of the trachea and main bronchi or extrinsic compression by lymph nodes in older adults. Rarer causes include anaphylaxis and foreign body.

Stertor

Stertor, or muffled 'hot potato' speech, occurs with naso- or oropharyngeal blockage, e.g. quinsy.

Sputum

Sputum is mucus produced from the respiratory tract. The normal lung produces about 100 ml of clear sputum each day, which is transported to the oropharynx and swallowed. There are four main types of sputum (Box 7.3).

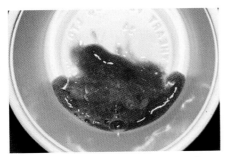

Fig. 7.3 Rusty red sputum of pneumococcal pneumonia.

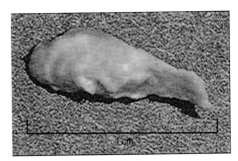

Fig. 7.4 Mucus plug from a patient with asthma.

7.3 Types of sputum

Type	Appearance	Cause
Serous	Frothy, pink	Acute pulmonary oedema
	Clear, watery/rarely copious (bronchorrhea)	Bronchioloalveolar cancer
Mucoid	Clear, grey	Chronic bronchitis/chronic obstructive pulmonary disease
	White, viscid	Asthma
Purulent	Yellow	Acute bronchopulmonary infection Asthma (eosinophils)
	Green	Longer-standing infection Pneumonia Bronchiectasis Cystic fibrosis Lung abscess
Rusty	Rusty red	Pneumococcal pneumonia

7.4 Causes of haemoptysis

Tumour

Malignant	Benign
• Lung cancer	• Bronchial carcinoid
• Endobronchial metastases	

Infection

• Bronchiectasis	• Mycetoma
• Tuberculosis	• Cystic fibrosis
• Lung abscess	

Vascular

• Pulmonary infarction	• Arteriovenous malformation
• Vasculitis	• Goodpasture's syndrome
• Polyangiitis	• Iatrogenic
• Trauma	• Bronchoscopic biopsy
• Inhaled foreign body	• Transthoracic lung biopsy
• Chest trauma	• Bronchoscopic diathermy
• Cardiac	• Acute left ventricular failure
• Mitral valve disease	• Anticoagulation
• Haematological	
• Blood dyscrasias	

Colour

- Clear or 'mucoid' sputum is produced in chronic bronchitis and COPD with no active infection.
- Yellow sputum occurs in acute lower respiratory tract infection (live neutrophils) and in asthma (eosinophils).
- Green purulent sputum (dead neutrophils) indicates chronic infection, e.g.in COPD or bronchiectasis. Purulent sputum is green because lysed neutrophils release the green-pigmented enzyme, verdoperoxidase. The first sputum produced in the morning by a patient with COPD may be green because of nocturnal stagnation of neutrophils.
- Rusty red sputum can occur in early pneumococcal pneumonia, as pneumonic inflammation causes lysis of red cells (Fig. 7.3).

Amount

Bronchiectasis causes large volumes of purulent sputum, which varies with posture. Suddenly coughing up large amounts of purulent sputum on a single occasion suggests rupture of a lung abscess or empyema into the bronchial tree. Large volumes of watery sputum with a pink tinge in an acutely breathless patient suggest pulmonary oedema but, if occurring over weeks (bronchorrhoea), suggests alveolar cell cancer.

Taste or smell

Foul-tasting or smelling sputum suggests anaerobic bacterial infection, and occurs in bronchiectasis, lung abscess and empyema. In bronchiectasis a change of sputum taste may indicate an infective exacerbation.

Solid material

In asthma and allergic bronchopulmonary aspergillosis thick secretions can accumulate in airways and be coughed up as 'worm-like' structures that are casts of the bronchi (Fig. 7.4). Other solid matter sometimes coughed up includes necrotic tumour and inhaled foreign bodies, e.g. food, teeth and tablets.

Haemoptysis

Haemoptysis is coughing up blood from the respiratory tract and always requires investigation (Box 7.4).

Amount and appearance

Blood-streaked clear sputum or clots in sputum for more than a week suggest lung cancer. Haemoptysis with purulent sputum suggests infection. Coughing up large

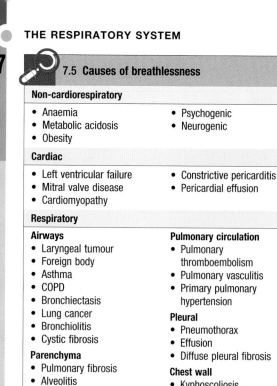

7.5 Causes of breathlessness

Non-cardiorespiratory

- Anaemia
- Metabolic acidosis
- Obesity
- Psychogenic
- Neurogenic

Cardiac

- Left ventricular failure
- Mitral valve disease
- Cardiomyopathy
- Constrictive pericarditis
- Pericardial effusion

Respiratory

Airways
- Laryngeal tumour
- Foreign body
- Asthma
- COPD
- Bronchiectasis
- Lung cancer
- Bronchiolitis
- Cystic fibrosis

Parenchyma
- Pulmonary fibrosis
- Alveolitis
- Sarcoidosis
- Tuberculosis
- Pneumonia
- Diffuse infections, e.g. *Pneumocystis jiroveci* pneumonia
- Tumour (metastatic, lymphangitis)

Pulmonary circulation
- Pulmonary thromboembolism
- Pulmonary vasculitis
- Primary pulmonary hypertension

Pleural
- Pneumothorax
- Effusion
- Diffuse pleural fibrosis

Chest wall
- Kyphoscoliosis
- Ankylosing spondylitis

Neuromuscular
- Myasthenia gravis
- Neuropathies
- Muscular dystrophies
- Guillain–Barré syndrome

7.6 Breathlessness: modes of onset, duration and progression

Minutes
- Pulmonary thromboembolism
- Pneumothorax
- Asthma
- Inhaled foreign body
- Acute left ventricular failure

Hours to days
- Pneumonia
- Asthma
- Exacerbation of COPD

Weeks to months
- Anaemia
- Pleural effusion
- Respiratory neuromuscular disorders

Months to years
- COPD
- Pulmonary fibrosis
- Pulmonary tuberculosis

---

amounts of pure blood is rare but potentially life-threatening; causes include lung cancer, bronchiectasis and tuberculosis and, less commonly, lung abscess, mycetoma, cystic fibrosis, aortobronchial fistula and granulomatosis with polyangiitis (formerly Wegener's granulomatosis).

Duration and frequency

Bronchiectasis causes intermittent haemoptysis associated with copious purulent sputum over years. Daily haemoptysis for a week or more is a symptom of lung cancer; other causes include tuberculosis and lung abscess.

Single episodes of haemoptysis, if associated with symptoms, e.g. pleuritic chest pain and breathlessness, suggest pulmonary thromboembolism and infarction and need immediate investigation.

Dyspnoea

Dyspnoea (breathlessness) is undue awareness of breathing and is normal with strenuous physical exercise. Patients use terms such as 'shortness of breath', 'difficulty getting enough air in', or 'tiredness' (Box 7.5).

Mode of onset, duration and progression

Psychogenic breathlessness may occur suddenly at rest or while talking. Patients often say they cannot get enough air into their chest and need to take deep breaths. The resultant hypocapnia causes lightheadedness, dizziness, tingling in the fingers and round the mouth and chest tightness. These symptoms, in turn, aggravate anxiety and exacerbate the situation (Box 7.6 and Ch. 2).

Variability and aggravating/relieving factors

Breathlessness when lying flat (orthopnoea) is usually associated with left ventricular failure. It can also be a feature of respiratory muscle weakness, large pleural effusion, massive ascites, morbid obesity or any severe lung disease.

Breathlessness on sitting up (platypnoea) with relief on lying down is rare and due to right-to-left shunting through a patent foramen ovale, atrial septal defect or a large intrapulmonary shunt.

Breathlessness when lying on one side (trepopnoea) is due to unilateral lung disease (patient prefers the healthy lung down), dilated cardiomyopathy (patient prefers right side down) or tumours compressing central airways and major blood vessels.

Breathlessness that wakes the patient from sleep is typical of asthma and left ventricular failure (paroxysmal nocturnal dyspnoea). Patients with asthma typically wake between 3 and 5 a.m. and have associated wheezing. Breathlessness worse on waking is more typical of COPD and may improve after coughing up sputum.

Patients with exercise-induced asthma may notice that the breathlessness continues to worsen for 5–10 minutes after stopping activity. If you suspect asthma, ask about exposure to allergens, smoke, perfumes, fumes, cold air or drugs, e.g. aspirin, non-steroidal anti-inflammatory drugs. Common allergens are house dust mite (shaking bedding, hoovering), animals (cats, dogs, horses) and grass pollens (mowing the lawn, the 'hayfever season') and tree pollens. Breathlessness improving at weekends or holidays suggests occupational asthma. Ask about symptoms that accompany the breathlessness, e.g. chest pain, cough, wheeze (Box 7.9).

7.7	Medical Research Council (MRC) breathlessness scale
Grade 1	Breathless when hurrying on the level or walking up a slight hill
Grade 2	Breathlessness when walking with people of own age or on level ground
Grade 3	Walks slower than peers, or stops when walking on the flat at own pace
Grade 4	Stops after walking 100 metres, or a few minutes, on the level
Grade 5	Too breathless to leave the house
(Grade 5b)	Too breathless to wash or dress

7.8 Causes of chest pain

Non-central

Pleural
- Infection: pneumonia, bronchiectasis, tuberculosis
- Malignancy: lung cancer, mesothelioma, metastatic
- Pneumothorax
- Pulmonary infarction
- Connective tissue disease: rheumatoid arthritis, SLE

Chest wall
- Malignancy: lung cancer, mesothelioma, bony metastases
- Persistent cough/ breathlessness
- Muscle sprains/tears
- Bornholm's disease (Coxsackie B infection)
- Tietze's syndrome (costochondritis)
- Rib fracture
- Intercostal nerve compression
- Thoracic shingles (herpes zoster)

Central

Tracheal
- Infection
- Irritant dusts

Cardiac
- Massive pulmonary thromboembolism
- Acute myocardial infarction/ ischaemia

Oesophageal
- Oesophagitis
- Rupture

Great vessels
- Aortic dissection

Mediastinal
- Lung cancer
- Thymoma
- Lymphadenopathy
- Metastases
- Mediastinitis

Severity

Breathlessness while walking on the flat, up gentle inclines or stairs indicates a significant condition. Severely breathless patients are dyspnoeic at rest, walking around the house, washing, dressing and even eating (Box 7.7).

COPD is characterised by airflow obstruction that is usually progressive and not fully reversible. It is defined as a reduced post-bronchodilator forced expiratory volume in 1 second (FEV_1)/forced vital capacity (FVC) ratio of <70%.

Asthma is reversible airways obstruction.

Chest pain

Chest pain can originate from the parietal pleura, the chest wall and mediastinal structures (Box 7.8). The lungs do not cause pain because their innervation is exclusively autonomic.

Pleural pain is sharp, stabbing and intensified by inspiration or coughing. Irritation of the parietal pleura of the upper six ribs causes localised pain. Irritation of the parietal pleura overlying the central diaphragm innervated by the phrenic nerve is referred to the neck or shoulder tip. The lower six intercostal nerves innervate the parietal pleura of the lower ribs and the outer diaphragm, and pain from these sites may be referred to the upper abdomen. Common causes of pleuritic chest pain are pulmonary embolism, pneumonia, pneumothorax and fractured ribs.

Chest wall pain which is sudden and localised after vigorous coughing or direct trauma is characteristic of rib fractures or intercostal muscle injury. Prevesicular herpes zoster and intercostal nerve root compression can cause chest pain in a thoracic dermatomal distribution. Chest wall pain due to direct invasion by lung cancer, mesothelioma or rib metastasis is typically dull, aching or gnawing, unrelated to respiration, progressively worsens and disrupts sleep. Pancoast's tumour of the lung apex may involve the first rib and the brachial plexus, causing referred pain down the medial side of the ipsilateral arm.

Mediastinal pain is central, retrosternal and unrelated to respiration or cough. Irritant dusts or infection of the tracheobronchial tree produce a raw, burning retrosternal pain worse on coughing. A dull, aching retrosternal pain that disturbs sleep is a feature of cancer invading mediastinal lymph nodes or an enlarging thymoma. Massive pulmonary thromboembolism acutely increasing right ventricular pressure may produce central chest pain similar to myocardial ischaemia (Ch. 6).

Respiratory pattern

Respiratory rate

Tachypnoea is a respiratory rate >25 breaths/min. It is caused by increased ventilatory drive in fever, acute asthma and exacerbation of COPD, or reduced ventilatory capacity in pneumonia, pulmonary oedema and interstitial lung disease (Boxes 7.17 and Box 7.18). A slow respiratory rate of <10 breaths/min (bradypnoea) occurs in opioid toxicity, hypercapnia, hypothyroidism, raised intracranial pressure and hypothalamic lesions.

Breathing patterns

Periodic breathing (Cheyne–Stokes respiration) is cyclical with increasing rate and depth of breathing, followed by diminishing respiratory effort and rate, ending in a period of apnoea or hypopnoea. This relates to altered sensitivity of the respiratory centre to CO_2 and delay in circulation time between the lung and chemoreceptors.

Hyperventilation is a common response to acute anxiety or emotional distress, and is often associated with respiratory alkalosis with hypocapnia. Breathing is deep, irregular and sighing, and patients feel unable to fill their lungs completely. When acute hyperventilation

7

7

7.9 Acute breathlessness: commonly associated symptoms

No chest pain

- Pulmonary embolism
- Pneumothorax
- Metabolic acidosis
- Hypovolaemia/shock
- Acute left ventricular failure/pulmonary oedema

Pleuritic chest pain

- Pneumonia
- Pneumothorax
- Pulmonary embolism
- Rib fracture

Central chest pain

- Myocardial infarction with left ventricular failure
- Massive pulmonary embolism/infarction

Wheeze and cough

- Asthma
- COPD

7.10 Symptoms of obstructive sleep apnoea/hypopnoea syndrome (OSAHS)

- Snoring
- Excessive daytime sleepiness
- Witnessed apnoeas
- Impaired concentration
- Unrefreshing sleep
- Choking episodes during sleep
- Restless sleep
- Irritability/personality change
- Nocturia
- Decreased libido

is sustained, tetany and occasionally grand mal seizure can occur. Hyperventilation with deep, sighing respirations (Kussmaul respiration) occurs in metabolic acidosis caused by diabetic ketoacidosis, acute renal failure, lactic acidosis, and salicylate and methanol poisoning. Although patients may not be aware of breathlessness, their respiratory rate increases and they appear to have 'air hunger'.

Apnoea is the absence of breathing; hypopnoea is a reduction in airflow or respiratory movements by >50% for 10 seconds or more. Obstructive sleep apnoea/hypopnoea syndrome (OSAHS) is the combination of excessive daytime sleepiness and recurrent upper airway obstruction with sleep fragmentation caused by upper airway obstruction from collapse of the retropharynx. A total of 2–4% of middle-aged men and 1–2% of middle-aged women (Box 7.10) have OSAHS with multiple apnoeas during sleep. They usually describe loud snoring, then a pause in breathing followed by a grunting noise and restoration of snoring. Simple (benign) snoring is more common than OSAHS, affecting 40% of middle-aged men and 20% of middle-aged women. Urgently investigate patients with daytime sleepiness and drowsiness while driving, especially if they have a heavy goods or public service vehicle licence.

THE HISTORY

Presenting complaint

Cough

Ask about the duration of the cough and when, during the day, it is most severe. Cough on lying down in the evening may be due to gastro-oesophageal reflux; cough disrupting sleep is typical of asthma; cough on rising in the morning can be caused by rhinosinusitis and post-nasal drip.

Wheeze

Ask about precipitating factors such as exercise and exposure to allergens (pets, pollens) and relationship to occupation.

Sputum

Ask patients specifically about sputum as they may find it difficult to discuss or may swallow it. Ask about the colour of any sputum produced and how many teaspoonfuls are coughed up daily.

Haemoptysis

Establish the volume and nature of the blood. Clarify whether the blood was coughed up from the respiratory tract, vomited (upper gastrointestinal tract) or suddenly appeared in the mouth without coughing (nasopharyngeal).

Breathlessness

Use the Medical Research Council grading scale to characterise breathlessness (Box 7.7). How far can the patient walk before stopping to rest? Get an estimate of the time taken to walk a given distance and the number of stops involved: say, from home to a local shop. Ask about the effect on work and hobbies such as golf, gardening, dancing, swimming or hill walking, Can the patient walk up hills or keep up with contemporaries? Box 7.9 outlines some combinations of symptoms in acutely breathless patients.

Chest pain

Characterise chest pain using SOCRATES (Box 2.10).

Respiratory pattern

Ask about any change in the rate or pattern of breathing. If the patient has daytime sleepiness, ask the patient's bed partner about apnoea, loud snoring, nocturnal restlessness, irritability and personality change (Box 7.11).

Past history

Enquire about previous respiratory and non-respiratory illnesses (Box 7.12).

Drug history

Detail the type of inhaler, dose in micrograms (not puffs) and frequency. Ask patients to demonstrate how they use the inhaler to check that they are doing this correctly. Note the effectiveness of previously prescribed medications, e.g. oral corticosteroids and β-agonist inhalers and current and previous medications, if you suspect drug-induced respiratory disease (Box 7.13).

7.11 The Epworth sleepiness scale

For each of the situations outlined in recent everyday life, ask the patient to grade the likelihood of dozing off or falling asleep:
0 = Would never doze
1 = Slight chance of dozing
2 = Moderate chance of dozing
3 = High chance of dozing

Situation	Chance of dozing
• Sitting and reading	
• Watching television	
• Sitting inactive in a public place, e.g. a theatre or meeting	
• As passenger in a car for 1 hour without a break	
• Lying down for a rest in the afternoon when circumstances permit	
• Sitting and talking to someone	
• Sitting quietly after a lunch without alcohol	
• In a car, whilst stopped for a few minutes in traffic	

Total: A score of > 10 is abnormal

ESS © MW Johns 1990–1997. Used under license

Family history

Cystic fibrosis is the most common severe autosomal recessive disease in Europeans, with a carrier rate of 1:25 and an incidence of ~1:2500 live births. α_1-antitrypsin deficiency (associated with emphysema and COPD) also has recessive inheritance.

A family history of asthma, eczema and hayfever increases the chance of a predisposition to form excess IgE in response to allergen (atopy). 'Asthma' in parents or grandparents who were smokers may have been misdiagnosed COPD. A family history of tuberculosis can represent significant past exposure that may reactivate later in life. Patients with asbestos-related disease and no obvious occupational exposure may have had significant exposure through asbestos-contaminated work clothes brought home for cleaning by a relative in a relevant occupation.

Social history

Smoking

Although cigarette smoking has declined in the UK, the current prevalence of COPD and incidence of lung cancer reflect historical smoking patterns. Establish when patients started and stopped smoking and their average tobacco consumption as cigarettes/day or ounces/grams of 'roll-up' tobacco/week. Calculate the 'pack year' consumption: smoking 1 pack of 20 cigarettes per day for 1 year equates to 1 pack year (Box 2.20). Patients with COPD usually have smoked >20 pack years. Stopping smoking at any age is crucial to improving health; beyond 40 years people lose, on average, 3 months of life expectancy for every further year they continue smoking.

7.12 Previous history of illness

History	Current implications
Eczema, hayfever	Allergic tendency relevant to asthma
Childhood asthma	In the past asthma was commonly termed 'wheezy bronchitis'
Recurrent childhood viral-associated wheeze	Relevant to adult-onset (recurrence of) asthma
Whooping cough, measles	Recognised causes of bronchiectasis, especially if complicated by pneumonia
Pneumonia, pleurisy	Recognised cause of bronchiectasis Recurrent episodes may be a manifestation of bronchiectasis
Tuberculosis	Reactivation if not previously treated effectively Respiratory failure may complicate thoracoplasty Mycetoma in lung cavity may present with haemoptysis
Connective tissue disorders, e.g. rheumatoid arthritis	Lung diseases are recognised complications, e.g. pulmonary fibrosis, effusions, bronchiectasis
Previous malignancy	Recurrence, metastatic/pleural disease Chemotherapeutic agents recognised causes of pulmonary fibrosis Radiotherapy-induced pulmonary fibrosis
Recent travel, immobility, cancer	Pulmonary thromboembolism
Recent surgery, loss of consciousness	Aspiration of foreign body, gastric contents Pneumonia, lung abscess
Neuromuscular disorders	Respiratory failure Aspiration

Pets

Ask about exposure to pets. Hair and fur from dogs, cats, rodents and horses may aggravate asthma. Hypersensitivity pneumonitis and psittacosis are associated with birds.

Occupational history

Occupation is important in many respiratory disorders. Record all the occupations, full- and parttime, since the patient left school and the number of years spent in each job (Box 7.14). Find out exactly what the job entailed and the length of any exposure. Exposure to a recognised hazard helps diagnosis, has implications for current employment and may be the basis for compensation.

7.13 Examples of drug-induced respiratory conditions

Respiratory condition	Drug
Bronchoconstriction	Beta-blockers Opioids NSAIDs
Cough	Angiotensin-converting enzyme inhibitors
Bronchiolitis obliterans	Penicillamine
Diffuse parenchymal lung disease	Cytotoxic agents: bleomycin, methotrexate Anti-inflammatory agents: sulfasalazine, penicillamine, gold salts, aspirin Cardiovascular drugs: amiodarone, hydralazine Antibiotics: nitrofurantoin Intravenous drug misuse Radiation
Pulmonary thromboembolism	Oestrogens
Pulmonary hypertension	Oestrogens Dexfenfluramine, fenfluramine
Pleural effusion	Amiodarone Nitrofurantoin Phenytoin Methotrexate Pergolide
Respiratory depression	Opioids Benzodiazepines

Asbestos was widely used in shipyards, building construction and plumbing until the 1970s, and asbestos-related lung disease, e.g. mesothelioma and asbestosis, is the greatest single cause of work-related death in the UK. Occupation is particularly important in adult-onset asthma, e.g. baker's asthma due to flour dust, and interstitial lung disease, e.g. farmer's lung. Some occupational diseases are worse at the beginning of the working week, e.g. byssinosis due to cotton dust and humidifier fever due to organism-contaminated water in air-conditioning systems. Occupational asthma gets better on holidays away from work.

THE PHYSICAL EXAMINATION

General examination

Observe patients as you first meet them. Look for breathlessness, weight loss, cyanosis and their mental state.

Examination sequence

- Measure the respiratory rate in all patients with breathlessness (Box 7.16).
- Note if the patient is breathless at rest and count the respiratory rate (breaths/min) for 30–60 seconds while you feel the pulse and assess chest movements.
- Notice if the patient is using the accessory muscles of respiration.

7.14 Examples of occupational lung disease

Lung disease	Exposure	Occupation
Pulmonary fibrosis	Asbestos	Shipyard/construction workers, plumbers, boilermakers
	Quartz (silica)	Miners, quarry workers, stone masons
	Coal	Coal miners
	Beryllium	Nuclear, aerospace industries
COPD	Coal	Coal miners
Malignancy	Asbestos	Shipyard/construction workers, plumbers, boilermakers
	Radon	Metal miners
Byssinosis	Cotton, flax, hemp	Cotton, flax, hemp manufacturing
Hypersensitivity pneumonitis Farmer's lung	Fungal spores of thermophilic actinomycetes or *Micropolyspora faeni*	Farm workers exposed to mouldy hay
Malt worker's lung	*Aspergillus clavatus*	Exposure to whisky maltings
Bird fancier's lung	Bloom on birds' feathers/excreta	Pigeon fanciers, bird owners
Asthma	Animals	Vets, laboratory workers
	Grains, flour	Farmers, bakers, millers
	Hardwood dusts	Joiners, carpenters
	Colophony	Soldering, welders
	Enzymes	Detergent manufacturing, pharmaceuticals
	Isocyanates	Spray painting, varnishing
	Epoxy resins	Adhesives, varnishing
	Drugs	Pharmaceutical industry
	Formaldehyde, paraldehyde, latex	Hospital workers

EBE **7.15 Mortality predictor in community-acquired pneumonia**

CURB-65 (1 point each for: **c**onfusion; blood **u**rea >7 mmol/l; **r**espiratory rate >30 breaths/min; diastolic **b**lood pressure <60 mmHg; and age **65** years or older) predicts mortality in patients with community-acquired pneumonia.

Guidelines for the management of community-acquired pneumonia in adults: update 2009. Thorax 2009;64(Suppl. III):26–27.

EBE **7.16 Respiratory rate and community-acquired pneumonia**

Respiratory rate >30 breaths/min is an important adverse prognostic sign in community-acquired pneumonia (Box 7.17).

Garcia-Ordonez MA, Garcia-Jiminez JM, Paez F et al. Clinical aspects and prognostic factors in elderly patients hospitalised for community-acquired pneumonia. Eur J Clin Microbiol Infect Dis 2001;20:14–19.
Neill AM, Martin IR, Weir R et al. Community acquired pneumonia: aetiology and usefulness of severity criteria on admission. Thorax 1996;51:1010–1016.

Normal findings

Muscles of respiration During normal (resting) respiration women use the intercostal muscles more than the diaphragm, and their respiratory movements are predominantly thoracic. Men rely more on the diaphragm and their respiratory movements are predominantly abdominal.

Abnormal findings

The sternocleidomastoid, platysma and trapezius muscles are accessory muscles of respiration and their use is an early sign of airways obstruction. If the patient sits forward with the hands/arms on the thighs or knees to 'fix' the shoulder girdle, he raises the clavicles and upper chest, increasing lung volume and negative intrathoracic pressure. Use of accessory muscles is characteristic in severe COPD and acute severe asthma.

In severe respiratory failure or, rarely, bilateral phrenic nerve lesions causing diaphragmatic palsy, the abdomen and chest move paradoxically; during inspiration the abdomen moves inwards as the chest wall moves out.

Some patients with severe COPD appear to breathe with 'pursed lips'. This manoeuvre increases positive end-expiratory pressure, reducing small-airway collapse and improving ventilation.

Stridor

Examination sequence

- Ask the patient to cough and then breathe deeply in and out with the mouth wide open. Listen closely to the patient's mouth, for stridor.

Cyanosis

Examination sequence

Lips and tongue
- Ask the patient to open his mouth and look at the lips and the underside of the tongue for a purplish blue discoloration in natural light (Fig. 7.5).

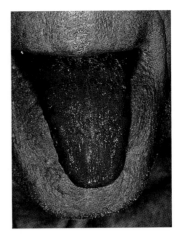

Fig. 7.5 Central cyanosis of the tongue.

 7.17 Features of severe community-acquired pneumonia (CRB-65)

- **C**onfusion
- **R**espiratory rate >30 breaths/min
- **B**lood pressure – diastolic <60 mmHg
- Age >**65** years

Abnormal findings

Cyanosis is the blue colour caused by an absolute concentration of deoxygenated haemoglobin of >50 g/l.

Central cyanosis reflects arterial hypoxaemia. With a normal haemoglobin concentration, central cyanosis occurs when the arterial oxygen saturation falls below 90%, corresponding to a PaO_2 of approximately 8 kPa (60 mmHg). In anaemic or hypovolaemic patients, you may not see cyanosis because severe hypoxia is required to produce the necessary concentration of deoxygenated haemoglobin. Patients with polycythaemia become cyanosed at higher arterial oxygen tensions. Rarely, central cyanosis is caused by methaemoglobinaemia due to intravascular haemolysis or drugs.

Peripheral cyanosis is only seen in the fingers and toes and is usually due to circulatory disorders or cold, but can also occur in patients with severe central cyanosis.

Blood pressure

Examination sequence

- Measure blood pressure and check the pulse (Ch. 6).

Abnormal findings

Diastolic pressure of <60 mmHg is associated with increased mortality in community-acquired pneumonia (Boxes 7.15 and 7.17). In pneumothorax, hypotension may indicate the development of 'tension' with reduction in venous return to the heart and risk of cardiac arrest. Pulsus paradoxus is an exaggeration of the normal variability of pulse volume with the respiratory cycle (Box 7.18). A fall in pulse volume and consequent fall in systolic blood pressure of >10 mmHg during inspiration is abnormal and can occur in cardiac tamponade (Ch. 6).

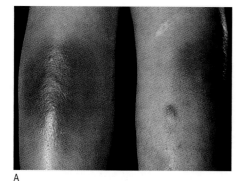

A

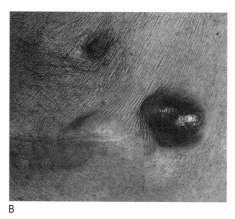

B

Fig. 7.6 Skin lesions associated with respiratory conditions.
(A) Erythema nodosum on the shins. **(B)** Metastatic skin nodes of lung cancer.

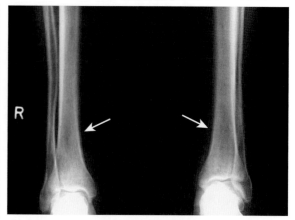

Fig. 7.7 X-ray of the lower legs in hypertrophic pulmonary osteoarthropathy. Arrows show periosteal reaction.

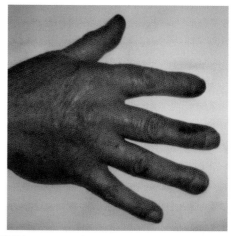

Fig. 7.8 Tobacco 'tar'-stained fingers.

EBE 7.18 Pulsus paradoxus and acute asthma
Pulsus paradoxus is a poor indicator of the severity of acute asthma.
Pearson MG, Spence DP, Ryland I et al. Value of pulsus paradoxus in assessing acute severe asthma. BMJ 1993;307:659.

Skin appearances

Erythema nodosum over the shins is a feature of acute sarcoidosis and tuberculosis (Fig. 7.6A). Raised, firm, non-tender subcutaneous nodules may occur in patients with disseminated cancer (Fig. 7.6B).

Hands

Clubbing

The majority of patients with finger clubbing have thoracic disease (lung cancer, bronchiectasis, interstitial lung disease) but it is also associated with gastrointestinal disorders and can be familial (Box 3.10). Rarely, clubbing develops relatively quickly over several weeks, in empyema.

Hypertrophic pulmonary osteoarthropathy is rare and almost always associated with lung cancer, usually squamous cancer. Pronounced clubbing of fingers and toes occurs, with pain and swelling affecting the wrists and ankles. X-rays of the distal forearm and lower legs show subperiosteal new bone formation separate from the cortex of the long bones (Fig. 7.7).

Discoloration of the fingers and nails

A brownish stain on the fingers and nails in cigarette smokers is caused by tar, not nicotine (Fig. 7.8). The rare 'yellow nail syndrome' is associated with lymphoedema and an exudative pleural effusion (Fig. 7.9).

A fine finger tremor is often caused by excessive use of β-agonist or theophylline bronchodilator drugs.

A coarse flapping tremor (asterixis) is seen with severe ventilatory failure and carbon dioxide retention. This is the result of intermittent failure of parietal mechanisms required to maintain posture. Unilateral asterixis is due to structural abnormality in the contralateral cerebral hemisphere.

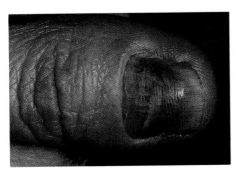

Fig. 7.9 Yellow nail syndrome.

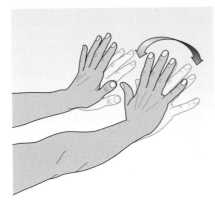

Fig. 7.10 **Asterixis.** Hand and arm position for observing the 'flapping tremor' of CO_2 retention.

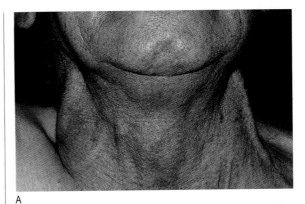

A

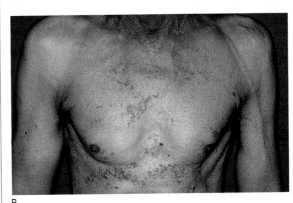

B

Fig. 7.11 **Superior vena caval obstruction. (A)** Distended neck veins. **(B)** Dilated superficial veins over chest.

Examination sequence

- Ask the patient to hold out his arms with the hands extended at the wrists (Fig. 7.10). Look for a jerky, flapping tremor (asterixis).
- Alternatively, ask the patient to squeeze your index and middle fingers and maintain this for 30–60 seconds. Patients with a flapping tremor cannot maintain their grip.

Neck

Jugular venous pressure (JVP)

Abnormal findings

The JVP is raised in right-sided heart failure. Chronic hypoxia in COPD leads to pulmonary arterial vasoconstriction, pulmonary hypertension, right heart dilatation and peripheral oedema with elevation of the JVP. This is cor pulmonale. The JVP is high if the intrathoracic pressure is raised in tension pneumothorax or severe acute asthma. Massive pulmonary embolism may cause the JVP to be so high that the patient has to be sitting upright to see it.

In superior vena caval obstruction (SVCO) (Fig. 7.11A) the JVP is raised and non-pulsatile, and the abdominojugular reflex is absent. Most cases are due to lung cancer compressing the superior vena cava. Other causes include lymphoma, thymoma and mediastinal fibrosis. Facial flushing, distension of neck veins and

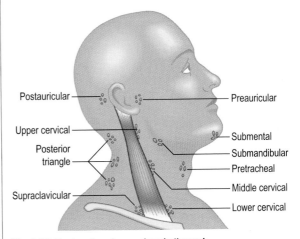

Fig. 7.12 **The lymph node groupings in the neck.**

stridor can occur in SVCO when the arms are raised above the head.

Neck nodes

Examination sequence

- Look for enlargement of the cervical, supraclavicular and scalene lymph nodes (Figs 7.12 and 7.13).
- Palpate the neck (p. 53). Note the size and consistency of any palpable node and whether it is fixed to surrounding structures.

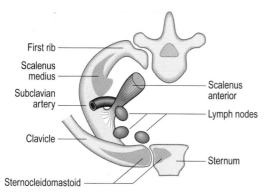

First rib
Scalenus medius
Subclavian artery
Clavicle
Sternocleidomastoid
Scalenus anterior
Lymph nodes
Sternum

Fig. 7.13 Relation of lymph nodes to scalenus anterior.

EBE 7.19 Lymphadenopathy and lung cancer

In a patient with lung cancer, a palpable supraclavicular node strongly suggests metastatic spread.

van Overhagen H, Brakel K, Heijenbrok MW et al. Metastases in supraclavicular lymph nodes in lung cancer: assessment with palpation, US and CT. Radiology 2004;232:75–80.

Abnormal findings

Scalene lymph node enlargement may be the first evidence of metastatic lung cancer and localised cervical lymphadenopathy is a common presenting feature of lymphoma. In Hodgkin's disease, the lymph nodes are typically 'rubbery'; in dental sepsis and tonsillitis they are usually tender; in tuberculosis and metastatic cancer they are often 'matted' together to form a mass; and calcified lymph nodes feel stony hard. Palpable lymph nodes, fixed to deep structures or skin, are usually malignant (Box 7.19).

Thorax

Ask the patient to sit over the edge of a bed or on a chair if possible with the chest and upper abdomen fully exposed. Fully examine the back of the chest first and then the front.

Examination sequence

- Look at the chest and the relationship of anteroposterior diameter to lateral diameter.
- Look for scars of previous heart or lung surgery, and for swellings, marks and spots on the skin.

Chest shape

Normal findings

The chest should be symmetrical and elliptical in cross-section. The anteroposterior diameter should be less than the lateral diameter.

Abnormal findings

When the anteroposterior diameter is greater than the lateral diameter, the chest is 'barrel-shaped'. This is

associated with lung hyperinflation in patients with severe COPD (Fig. 7.14A), although the degree of deformity does not correlate with the severity of airways obstruction or lung function.

Kyphosis is an exaggerated anterior curvature of the spine and scoliosis is lateral curvature. Kyphoscoliosis, involving both deformities (Fig. 7.14B), may be idiopathic or secondary to childhood poliomyelitis or spinal tuberculosis, and may be grossly disfiguring and disabling. It may reduce ventilatory capacity and increase the work of breathing. These patients develop progressive ventilatory failure with carbon dioxide retention and cor pulmonale at an early age.

Pectus carinatum (pigeon chest) is a localised prominence of the sternum and adjacent costal cartilages, often accompanied by indrawing of the ribs to form symmetrical horizontal grooves (Harrison's sulci) above the costal margin (Fig. 7.14C). These result from lung hyperinflation with repeated vigorous contractions of the diaphragm while the bony thorax is in a pliable prepubertal state. It is most often caused by severe and poorly controlled childhood asthma but can occur in osteomalacia and rickets.

Pectus excavatum (funnel chest) is a developmental deformity with a localised depression of the lower end of the sternum (Fig. 7.14D) or, less commonly, of the whole length of the sternum. Patients are usually asymptomatic but concerned about their appearance. In severe cases the heart is displaced to the left and the ventilatory capacity is reduced.

Skin

Subcutaneous lesions may be visible, including metastatic tumour nodules, neurofibromas and lipomas, as may vascular anomalies, e.g. the dilated venous vascular channels of SVCO (Fig. 7.11B).

Palpation

Determine the position of the mediastinum by examining the trachea and cardiac apex beat (Box 7.20).

Examination sequence

- With the patient looking directly forwards, look for any deviation of the trachea.
- Gently place the tip of your right index finger into the suprasternal notch and palpate the trachea (Fig. 7.15). This can be uncomfortable; be gentle and explain what you are doing. Slight displacement to the right is common in healthy people.
- Measure the distance between the suprasternal notch and cricoid cartilage, normally 3–4 finger breadths; any less suggests lung hyperinflation.

Abnormal findings

Shift of the upper mediastinum causes tracheal deviation. Displacement of the cardiac apex beat may indicate shift of the lower mediastinum (Ch. 6). Displacement of the cardiac impulse without tracheal deviation is usually due to left ventricular enlargement but can occur in scoliosis, kyphoscoliosis or severe pectus excavatum. The cardiac apex beat may be difficult to localise in obesity,

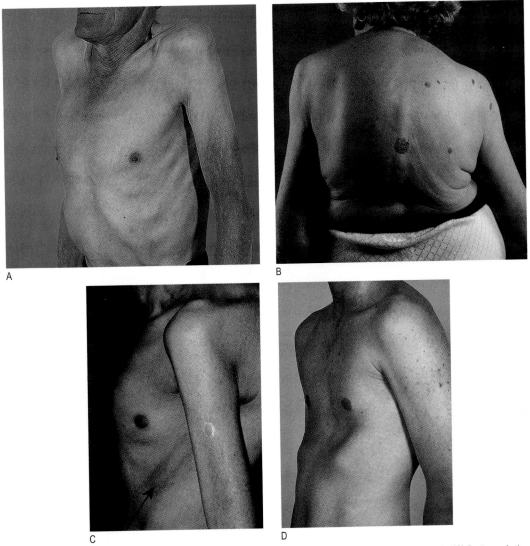

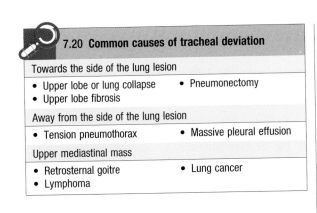

Fig. 7.14 Abnormalities in the shape of the chest. (A) Hyperinflated chest with intercostal indrawing. **(B)** Kyphoscoliosis. **(C)** Pectus carinatum with prominent Harrison's sulcus (arrow). **(D)** Pectus excavatum.

7.20 Common causes of tracheal deviation

Towards the side of the lung lesion	
• Upper lobe or lung collapse	• Pneumonectomy
• Upper lobe fibrosis	

Away from the side of the lung lesion	
• Tension pneumothorax	• Massive pleural effusion

Upper mediastinal mass	
• Retrosternal goitre	• Lung cancer
• Lymphoma	

pericardial effusion, poor left ventricular function or lung hyperinflation, as in COPD. The heave of right ventricular hypertrophy, found in severe pulmonary hypertension, is best felt at the left sternal edge (Fig. 6.22C).

A 'tracheal tug' is found in severe hyperinflation; resting on the patient's trachea, your fingers move inferiorly with each inspiration.

Chest expansion

Examination sequence

- Stand behind the patient and assess expansion of the upper lobes by watching the clavicles during tidal breathing.
- Assess expansion of the lower lobes by placing your hands firmly on the chest wall. Extend your fingers around the sides of the patient's chest (Fig. 7.16). Your thumbs should almost meet in the midline and hover just off the chest so they can move freely with respiration.
- Ask the patient to take a deep breath. Your thumbs should move symmetrically apart by at least 5 cm.
- With the patient supine, look for paradoxical inward movement of the abdomen during inspiration.

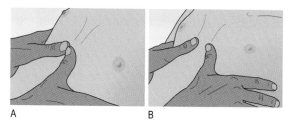

Fig. 7.15 Examining for tracheal shift.

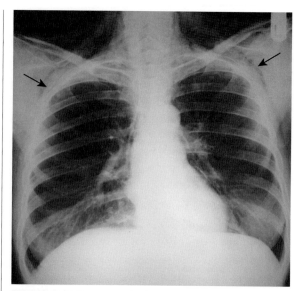

Fig. 7.17 Subcutaneous emphysema seen over the neck and chest wall on chest X-ray (arrowed).

A   B

Fig. 7.16 Assessing chest expansion from the front. (A) Expiration. **(B)** Inspiration.

Normal findings

Both sides of the thorax should expand equally during normal (tidal) breathing and maximal inspiration.

Abnormal findings

Reduced expansion on one side indicates abnormality on that side: for example, pleural effusion, lung or lobar collapse, pneumothorax and unilateral fibrosis. Bilateral reduction in chest wall movement is common in severe COPD and diffuse pulmonary fibrosis.

Paradoxical inward movement may indicate diaphragmatic paralysis or, more commonly, severe COPD. Double fracture of a series of ribs or of the sternum allows the chest wall between the fractures to become mobile or 'flail' (Fig. 19.6).

Subcutaneous emphysema produces a characteristic crackling sensation over gas-containing tissue (Fig. 7.17) and there may be diffuse swelling of the chest wall, neck and face. It may complicate severe acute asthma, spontaneous or traumatic pneumothorax, or rupture of the oesophagus, and is a complication of intercostal drainage. Mediastinal emphysema occurs if air tracks into the mediastinum and is associated with a characteristic systolic 'crunching' sound on auscultating the precordium (Hamman's sign).

Tenderness over the costal cartilages is found in the costochondritis of Tietze's syndrome. Localised rib tenderness can be found over areas of pulmonary infarction or fracture.

Percussion

Percussion allows you to hear the pitch and loudness of the percussed note and to feel for postpercussive vibrations. Percuss in sequence over corresponding areas on both sides of the chest (Fig. 7.18).

Examination sequence

- Place the palm of your left hand on the chest, with your fingers slightly separated (Fig. 7.18C).
- Press the middle finger of your left hand firmly against the chest, aligned with the underlying ribs over the area to be percussed.
- Strike the centre of the middle phalanx of your left middle finger with the tip of your right middle finger, using a loose swinging movement of the wrist and not the forearm.
- Remove the percussing finger quickly so the note generated is not dampened.
- Percuss the lung apices by placing the palmar surface of your left middle finger across the anterior border of the trapezius muscle, overlapping the supraclavicular fossa and percussing downwards.
- Percuss the clavicle directly over the medial third, as percussing laterally is dull over the shoulder muscles.
- Ask the patient to fold the arms across the front of the chest, moving the scapulae laterally and percuss the upper posterior chest. Do not percuss near the midline, as solid structures of the thoracic spine and paravertebral musculature produce a dull note.
- Map out abnormal areas by percussing from resonant to dull. Percuss each side alternately and compare the note.

Normal findings

Normal lung produces a resonant note (Box 7.21).

Abnormal findings

A pneumothorax produces a hyperresonant note, whereas percussion over solid structures, e.g. liver, heart or a consolidated area of lung (pneumonia) produces a dull note. Percussion over fluid, e.g. pleural

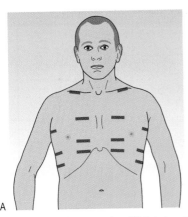
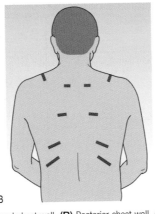
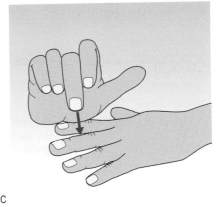

A   B   C

Fig. 7.18 Sites for percussion. (A) Anterior and lateral chest wall. **(B)** Posterior chest wall. **(C)** Technique of percussion.

7.21 Percussion note

Type	Detected over
Resonant	Normal lung
Hyperresonant	Pneumothorax
Dull	Pulmonary consolidation
	Pulmonary collapse
	Severe pulmonary fibrosis
Stony dull	Pleural effusion
	Haemothorax

effusion (Box 7.21), produces an extremely dull ('stony dull') note. Find the upper level of liver dullness by percussing down the anterior wall of the right chest; in adults the upper level of liver dullness is the fifth rib in the mid-clavicular line. Resonance below this is a sign of hyperinflation (COPD or severe asthma). The area of cardiac dullness over the left anterior chest may be decreased when the lungs are hyperinflated. Basal dullness due to elevation of the diaphragm is easily confused with pleural fluid.

Auscultation

Most sounds reaching the chest wall are low-frequency and best heard with the stethoscope bell. The diaphragm locates higher-pitched sounds, such as pleural friction rubs. Stretching the skin and hairs under the diaphragm during deep breathing can produce anomalous noises like crackles, and in thin patients it may be difficult to apply the diaphragm fully to the chest wall skin.

Examination sequence

■ Listen with the patient relaxed and breathing deeply through his open mouth. Avoid asking him to breathe deeply for prolonged periods, as this causes giddiness and even tetany. Auscultate each side alternately, comparing findings over a large number of equivalent positions to ensure that you do not miss localised abnormalities.

■ Listen:
  ■ anteriorly from above the clavicle down to the sixth rib
  ■ laterally from the axilla to the eighth rib
  ■ posteriorly down to the level of the 11th rib.
■ Assess the quality and amplitude of the breath sounds. Identify any gap between inspiration and expiration, and listen for added sounds. Avoid auscultation within 3 cm of the midline anteriorly or posteriorly, as these areas may transmit sounds directly from the trachea or main bronchi.

Normal findings

Turbulent flow in large airways causes normal breath sounds heard at the chest wall. Through a stethoscope they have a rustling (vesicular) quality. The larynx makes little contribution in quiet breathing but may accentuate the noise in deep respiration. The intensity of breath sounds relates to airflow and the tissue through which the sound travels.

The pattern and intensity of breath sounds reflect regional ventilation. Sounds are decreased through normal lungs since the parenchyma transmits sounds poorly. In an upright patient breath sounds are normally loudest at the apex in early inspiration and at the bases in mid-inspiration. During expiration, normal breath sounds rapidly fade as airflow decreases.

Abnormal findings

Diminished vesicular breathing occurs in obesity, pleural effusion, marked pleural thickening, pneumothorax, hyperinflation due to COPD and over an area of collapse where the underlying major bronchus is occluded (Box 7.22). If breath sounds appear reduced, ask the patient to cough. If the reduced breath sounds are due to bronchial obstruction by secretions, they are likely to become more audible after coughing.

Bronchial breathing is a high-pitched breath sound with a hollow or blowing quality similar to that heard over the trachea and larynx during tidal breathing. The breath sounds are of similar length and intensity in inspiration and expiration, with a characteristic pause between the two phases (Fig. 7.19). Bronchial breath sounds are found when normal lung tissue is replaced by uniformly conducting tissue and the underlying major bronchus is patent (Box 7.27), so it tends to exclude the possibility of an obstructing lung cancer. Bronchial

7.22 Causes of diminished vesicular breathing

Reduced conduction

- Obesity/thick chest wall
- Pleural effusion or thickening
- Pneumothorax

Reduced airflow

- Generalised, e.g. COPD
- Localised, e.g. collapsed lung due to occluding lung cancer

7.23 Simplified Well's score for pulmonary embolism

Risk factors	Points
• Previous pulmonary embolism or deep vein thrombosis	1.5
• Immobilisation or major surgery in previous 4 weeks	1.5
• Cancer	1
Clinical findings	
• Haemoptysis	1
• Heart rate >100 bpm	1.5
• Signs of deep vein thrombosis	3
Alternative diagnosis is less likely than pulmonary embolism	3

Interpretation of total score; 0 or 1 point = low probability; 2–6 points = moderate probability; 7 or more points = high probability.

7.24 Major risk factors for pulmonary thromboembolism

- Fracture of the hip, pelvis or leg
- Hip or knee replacement
- Major abdominal or pelvic surgery
- Major trauma
- Spinal cord injury
- Malignancy

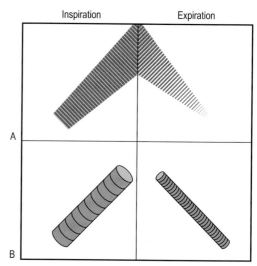

Fig. 7.19 Diagrammatic representation of breath sounds.
(A) Vesicular. (B) Bronchial. Note the gap between inspiration and expiration and change in pitch and the blowing, tubular quality of bronchial breath sounds.

7.25 Causes of crackles

Phase of inspiration	Cause
Early	Small airways disease, as in bronchiolitis
Middle	Pulmonary oedema
Late	Pulmonary fibrosis (fine) Pulmonary oedema (medium) Bronchial secretions in COPD, pneumonia, lung abscess, tubercular lung cavities (coarse)
Biphasic	Bronchiectasis (coarse)

breathing and whispering pectoriloquy are heard over pulmonary consolidation (pneumonia), at the top of a pleural effusion and over areas of dense fibrosis.

Aegophony is a bleating or nasal sound heard over consolidated lung (pneumonia) or at the upper level of a pleural effusion. It is due to enhanced transmission of high-frequency noise across abnormal lung, with lower frequencies filtered out (Box 7.28).

Added sounds

Crackles are interrupted non-musical sounds and result from collapse of peripheral airways on expiration. On inspiration, air rapidly enters these distal airways, and the alveoli and small bronchi open abruptly, producing the crackling noise.

Note when crackles occur within the respiratory cycle (Box 7.25). Early inspiratory crackles suggest small airways disease and can occur in bronchiolitis. In pulmonary oedema crackles occur in mid-inspiration. Fine late inspiratory crackles, which sound similar to rubbing hair between your fingers, are characteristic of pulmonary fibrosis. Bronchiectasis can cause crackles throughout inspiration and expiration.

Crackles may be heard when air bubbles through secretions in major bronchi, dilated bronchi in bronchiectasis or in pulmonary cavities. These crackles sound coarse, have a gurgling quality and change if the secretions are dislodged by coughing.

Wheeze is caused by continuous oscillation of opposing airway walls and has a musical quality. Wheezes imply airway narrowing and are timed in relation to the respiratory cycle. They are louder on expiration because airways normally dilate during inspiration and narrow on expiration. Inspiratory wheeze implies severe airway narrowing. High-pitched wheeze arises from smaller airways and has a whistling quality. Low-pitched wheeze originates from larger bronchi. Distinguish wheeze from the harsh rasping sound of stridor (p. 140).

Wheeze is characteristic of asthma and COPD, but is a poor guide to severity of airflow obstruction. In severe airways obstruction wheeze may be absent because of

EBE 7.26 **Predictors of pulmonary thromboembolism**

No single symptom or sign is predictive of pulmonary thromboembolism. Use a validated multivariate test such as the Modified Wells Score (Box 7.23).

Wells PS, Ginsberg JS, Anderson DR et al. Use of a clinical model for safe management of patients with suspected pulmonary embolism. Ann Intern Med 1998;129:997–1005.
Wells PS, Anderson DR, Rodger M et al. Excluding pulmonary embolism at the bedside without diagnostic imaging: management of patients with suspected pulmonary embolism presenting to the emergency department by using a simple clinical model and D-dimer. Ann Intern Med 2001;135:98–107.

 7.27 **Causes of bronchial breath sounds**

Common
- Lung consolidation (pneumonia)

Uncommon
- Localised pulmonary fibrosis
- At the top of a pleural effusion
- Collapsed lung (where the underlying major bronchus is patent)

EBE 7.28 **Clinical diagnosis of pneumonia**

Bronchial breath sounds and aegophony in a febrile patient with a cough strongly suggest pneumonia.

Heckerling PS, Tape TG, Wigton RS et al. Clinical prediction rule for pulmonary infiltrates. Ann Intern Med 1990;113:664–670.

reduced airflow, producing a 'silent chest'. A fixed bronchial obstruction, most commonly due to lung cancer, may cause localised wheeze with a single musical note that does not clear on coughing.

A pleural friction rub is a creaking sound similar to that produced by bending stiff leather or treading in fresh snow. It is produced when inflamed parietal and visceral pleurae move over one another and is best heard with the stethoscope diaphragm. It may be heard only on deep breathing at the end of inspiration and beginning of expiration. A pleural rub is usually associated with pleuritic pain and may be heard over areas of inflamed pleura in pulmonary infarction due to pulmonary embolism. Pulmonary embolism is obstruction of part of the pulmonary vascular tree by thrombus that has travelled from a distant site, e.g. deep veins in the legs or pelvis (Figs 7.18 and 7.19; Boxes 7.23 and 7.24). Pulmonary embolism is frequently unrecognised and fewer than one-third of patients have symptoms or signs of deep vein thrombosis (Box 7.26). A pleural friction rub may be heard in pneumonia or pulmonary vasculitis. If the pleura adjacent to the pericardium is involved, a pleuropericardial friction rub may also be heard. Pleural friction rubs disappear if an effusion separates the pleural surfaces.

A pneumothorax click is a rhythmical sound, synchronous with cardiac systole, and produced when there is air between the two layers of pleura overlying the heart.

A mid-expiratory 'squeak' is characteristic of obliterative bronchiolitis – a rare complication of rheumatoid arthritis – where small airways are narrowed or obliterated by chronic inflammation and fibrosis.

Vocal resonance

Examination sequence

- Ask the patient to say 'one, one, one' while you auscultate to assess the quality and amplitude of vocal resonance.
- Ask the patient to whisper 'one, one, one' while you continue to listen.

Normal findings

Over normal lung the low-pitched components of speech are heard and high-pitched components attenuated so that whispering is not heard.

Abnormal findings

Over consolidated lung (pneumonia) the spoken numbers are clearly audible. Over an effusion or area of collapse they are muffled.

Whispering is not heard over the normal lung, but in consolidation (pneumonia) the sound is transmitted, producing 'whispering pectoriloquy'.

PUTTING IT ALL TOGETHER

Examination sequence

- Note the patient's general appearance and demeanour.
- Look for central cyanosis of the lips and tongue.
- Examine the skin for rashes and nodules.
- Listen for hoarseness and stridor.
- Examine the hands for finger clubbing, peripheral cyanosis and tremor.
- Measure the blood pressure.
- Examine the neck for raised JVP and cervical lymphadenopathy.
- Record the respiratory rate.
- Observe the breathing pattern, and look for use of accessory muscles.
- Inspect the chest front and back for abnormalities of shape and scars.
- Feel the trachea and cardiac apex beat for evidence of mediastinal shift.
- Percuss the chest front and back for areas of dullness or hyperresonance.
- Listen to the chest front and back for altered breath sounds and added sounds.

Certain groups of physical signs are typically associated with particular pathological changes in the lungs (Figs 7.20 and 7.21).

INVESTIGATIONS

See Box 7.29.

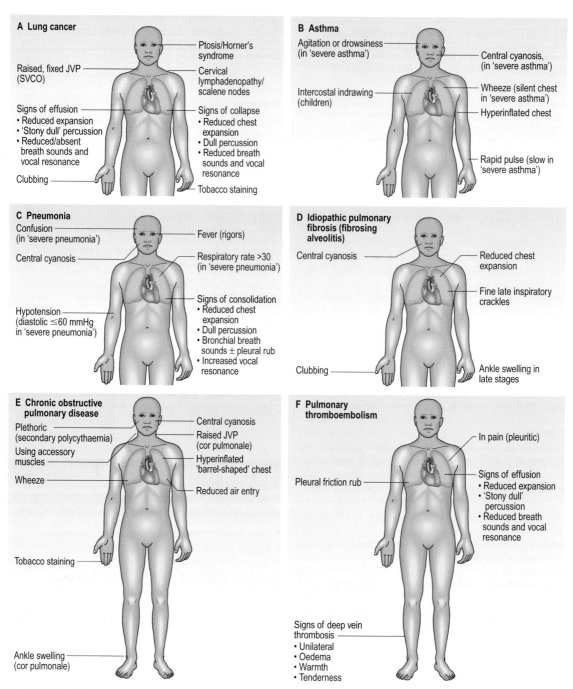

A Lung cancer

Ptosis/Horner's syndrome

Raised, fixed JVP (SVCO)

Cervical lymphadenopathy/ scalene nodes

Signs of effusion
• Reduced expansion
• 'Stony dull' percussion
• Reduced/absent breath sounds and vocal resonance

Signs of collapse
• Reduced chest expansion
• Dull percussion
• Reduced breath sounds and vocal resonance

Clubbing

Tobacco staining

B Asthma

Agitation or drowsiness (in 'severe asthma')

Central cyanosis, (in 'severe asthma')

Intercostal indrawing (children)

Wheeze (silent chest in 'severe asthma')

Hyperinflated chest

Rapid pulse (slow in 'severe asthma')

C Pneumonia

Confusion (in 'severe pneumonia')

Central cyanosis

Fever (rigors)

Respiratory rate >30 (in 'severe pneumonia')

Hypotension (diastolic ≤60 mmHg in 'severe pneumonia')

Signs of consolidation
• Reduced chest expansion
• Dull percussion
• Bronchial breath sounds ± pleural rub
• Increased vocal resonance

D Idiopathic pulmonary fibrosis (fibrosing alveolitis)

Central cyanosis

Reduced chest expansion

Fine late inspiratory crackles

Clubbing

Ankle swelling in late stages

E Chronic obstructive pulmonary disease

Plethoric (secondary polycythaemia)

Using accessory muscles

Wheeze

Central cyanosis

Raised JVP (cor pulmonale)

Hyperinflated 'barrel-shaped' chest

Reduced air entry

Tobacco staining

Ankle swelling (cor pulmonale)

F Pulmonary thromboembolism

In pain (pleuritic)

Signs of effusion
• Reduced expansion
• 'Stony dull' percussion
• Reduced breath sounds and vocal resonance

Pleural friction rub

Signs of deep vein thrombosis
• Unilateral
• Oedema
• Warmth
• Tenderness

Fig. 7.20 Clinical signs of common respiratory conditions. JVP, jugular venous pressure; SVCO, superior vena caval obstruction.

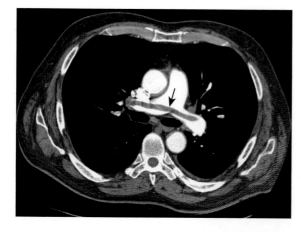

Fig. 7.21 (CT) pulmonary angiogram showing large embolus within the main pulmonary artery (arrowed).

7.29 Investigations in respiratory disease

Investigation	Indication/comment
Bedside	
Peak flow rate Oximetry	Monitoring of asthma/acute asthma Respiratory failure Assessment of oxygen requirements
Blood tests	
White cell count	High in lower respiratory tract infection
Haematocrit	Elevated in polycythaemia

Eosinophil count	High in:
	  Allergic asthma
	  Pulmonary eosinophilia
	  Allergic bronchopulmonary aspergillosis
	  Churg–Strauss syndrome

C-reactive protein	High in:
	  Pneumonia
	  Empyema

Serum sodium	Reduced in:
	  Small cell lung cancer (inappropriate antidiuretic hormone (ADH) secretion)
	  Legionnaire's disease and any severe pneumonia

Blood and urine osmolality	Inappropriate ADH secretion
Serum calcium	Elevated in bony metastases, sarcoidosis and squamous cell lung cancer
Liver function tests	Metastatic liver disease
Immunoglobulins	Deficiencies in bronchiectasis
Angiotensin-converting enzyme activity	Elevated in sarcoidosis
Alpha-1-antitrypsin	Deficiency in hereditary panacinar emphysema
Total and specific (radioallergosorbent test) IgE	Atopic status (asthma)
Antinuclear factor	Idiopathic pulmonary fibrosis (fibrosing alveolitis)

Antineutrophil cytoplasmic antibody (ANCA)
  Proteinase 3 (cANCA)
  Myeloperoxidase (pANCA)
	Granulomatosis with polyangiitis (Wegener's granulomatosis)
	Microscopic polyangiitis
	Churg–Strauss syndrome

Farmer's lung and avian precipitins	Hypersensitivity pneumonitis (extrinsic allergic alveolitis)
Cold agglutinins (IgM)	*Mycoplasma* infection
Serology (IgG antibodies)	Viral respiratory tract infection, e.g. influenza, respiratory syncytial virus Small bacterial infection, e.g. *Mycoplasma, Legionella, Chlamydia*
D-dimer	Venous thromboembolism
Immunoreactive trypsin	Screening for cystic fibrosis
Complement fixation transmembrane regulator (CFTR) genotyping	Cystic fibrosis
Gamma-interferon release assay	Latent infection with *Mycobacterium tuberculosis*
Urine tests	
Pneumococcal capsular antigen	Pneumococcal bacteraemia
Legionella urinary antigen	Legionnaire's disease
Skin tests	
Mantoux test	Exposure to *Mycobacterium tuberculosis*
Allergen skin prick tests	Atopic status (asthma)
Sweat test	Cystic fibrosis in children

Continued

7

7.29 Investigations in respiratory disease – *cont'd*

Investigation	Indication/comment
Respiratory function	
Arterial blood gas tensions	Respiratory failure, acid–base balance
Spirometry	Diagnosis/monitoring of COPD and asthma

Carbon monoxide gas transfer	Reduced in:
	    Interstitial lung disease
	    Emphysema/COPD

Flow–volume curves	Detection of extra- and intrathoracic large airway obstruction
Maximal mouth pressures	Respiratory neuromuscular disorders
Erect and supine forced vital capacity	Respiratory neuromuscular disorders
Exercise test	
6-minute run	Diagnosis of asthma in children and young adults
6-minute walk test	Assessment of disability, e.g. in COPD
Cardiopulmonary exercise test	Peak oxygen consumption (VO_2) Differentiates breathlessness due to lung disease from that due to heart disease
Bronchial challenge test	Exclusion of asthma
Bronchial provocation studies	Asthma, especially occupational asthma
Exhaled nitric oxide	Inhaled steroid dosage in asthma
Overnight sleep study	Sleep apnoea/hypopnoea syndrome
Radiology	
CT thorax	Pulmonary or mediastinal mass Staging of lung cancer Pleural disease
High-resolution CT	Interstitial lung disease Bronchiectasis
Isotope VQ lung scan	Pulmonary thromboembolism
CT pulmonary angiogram	Pulmonary thromboembolism Pulmonary hypertension
Echocardiogram	Right heart dilatation (cor pulmonale)
Ultrasound of chest wall	Localisation of pleural effusion
Positron emission tomography/CT	Staging of lung cancer
Invasive	
Lymph node aspiration	Cervical lymphadenopathy
Bronchoscopy	Suspected lung cancer Suspected foreign-body inhalation Obtaining specimens for microbiology
Transbronchial lung biopsy	Suspected pulmonary sarcoidosis Suspected diffuse malignancy
Pleural aspiration and biopsy	Undiagnosed pleural effusion
Percutaneous fine-needle lung aspiration	Peripheral lesion/suspected lung cancer
Mediastinoscopy	Staging of lung cancer Mediastinal mass
Thoracoscopy	Undiagnosed pleural disease
Lung biopsy (open or video-assisted thoracoscopic surgery)	Interstitial lung disease

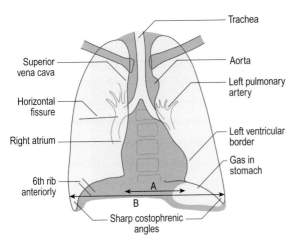

Superior vena cava

Horizontal fissure

Right atrium

6th rib anteriorly

Trachea

Aorta

Left pulmonary artery

Left ventricular border

Gas in stomach

Sharp costophrenic angles

Fig. 7.22 Normal posteroanterior chest X-ray. Note vertebral outlines just seen through the heart shadow. A/B: the cardiothoracic ratio should be <50%.

Chest X-ray

The standard chest X-ray is a posteroanterior (PA) view taken with the film in front of the anterior chest and the X-ray source 2 metres behind the patient (Fig. 7.22). In an anteroposterior (AP) film the X-ray source is in front of the patient, which tends to enlarge anterior structures such as the heart. Always compare an abnormal chest X-ray with previous films to see if abnormalities are resolving or longstanding.

Examination sequence

Systematically check:

■ Name, date and orientation of the film: AP films are usually marked as such. Otherwise assume PA.

■ Lung fields: should be equally translucent. Identify the horizontal fissure running from the right hilum to the sixth rib in the axillary line.

■ Lung apices: look specifically for masses, cavitation and consolidation above and behind the clavicles.

■ Trachea: confirm this is central, midway between the ends of the clavicles. Look for paratracheal masses, retrosternal goitre.

■ Heart: check that the heart shape is normal and the maximum diameter is less than half the internal transthoracic diameter (cardiothoracic ratio). Look specifically for any retrocardiac masses.

■ Hila: the left hilum should be higher than the right. Compare the shape and density of the two hila; both should appear concave laterally. A convex appearance suggests a mass or lymphadenopathy.

■ Diaphragms: the right hemidiaphragm should be higher than the left. The anterior end of the right sixth rib should cross the mid-diaphragm. If not, the lungs are hyperinflated.

■ Costophrenic angles: these should be well-defined, acute angles. Loss of one or both suggests pleural fluid or pleural thickening.

■ Soft tissues: note the presence of both breast shadows in female patients. Look around the chest wall for any soft-tissue masses or subcutaneous emphysema.

■ Bones: look closely at the ribs, scapulae and vertebrae for fractures and metastatic deposits in each bone (Figs 7.23 and 7.24).

Sputum examination

Inpatients with respiratory symptoms should have a sputum pot for inspection.

Gram stain helps rapid identification of the causative organism: for example, Gram-positive – pneumococcus or staphylococcus; Gram-negative – *Haemophilus influenzae*. If the patient's symptoms and chest X-ray suggest tuberculosis send several sputum samples urgently for auramine staining (screening); if these are positive, obtain a Ziehl–Neelsen stain. Positive samples indicate a high degree of infectivity; the patient should be urgently isolated and treated, and the condition notified.

Pulse oximetry

An oximeter is a spectrophotometric device that measures arterial oxygen saturation (SpO_2) by determining the differential absorption of light by oxyhaemoglobin and deoxyhaemoglobin. Modern oximeters use a probe incorporating a light source and sensor attached to a patient's ear or finger (Fig. 7.25).

Oximeters are easy to use, portable, non-invasive and inexpensive. They are widely used for the continuous measurement of SpO_2 and to adjust oxygen therapy. In acutely ill patients with no risk of CO_2 retention, SpO_2 should be maintained at 94–98%. Movement artifact, poor tissue perfusion, hypothermia and nail varnish can lead to spuriously low SpO_2 values. Dark skin pigmentation and raised levels of bilirubin or carboxyhaemoglobin can result in falsely high SpO_2. Oximetry is less accurate with saturations <75%.

Arterial blood gas analysis

Arterial blood gas (PaO_2, $PaCO_2$) and acid–base (pH and HCO_3^-) status are obtained from heparinised samples of arterial blood from the radial, brachial or femoral artery (Box 7.30 and Fig. 7.26).

Respiratory acidosis

An acute rise in $PaCO_2$ caused by alveolar hypoventilation associated with a decrease in pH occurs in severe acute asthma, severe pneumonia, exacerbations of COPD and neuromuscular disorders. Elevation of $PaCO_2$ for more than 2–3 days may occur in COPD, respiratory muscle weakness due to neuromuscular disorders and thoracic skeletal deformities, and leads to renal retention of HCO_3^- and normalisation of pH, i.e. compensated respiratory acidosis. In some patients with COPD low PaO_2 levels drive respiratory effort. Removal of this stimulus by excessive oxygen therapy may result in alveolar hypoventilation with further increase in $PaCO_2$, which can lead to deterioration and death.

7

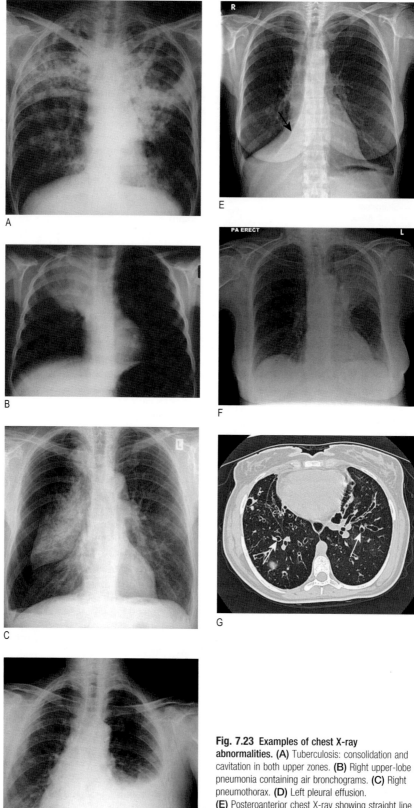

Fig. 7.23 Examples of chest X-ray abnormalities. **(A)** Tuberculosis: consolidation and cavitation in both upper zones. **(B)** Right upper-lobe pneumonia containing air bronchograms. **(C)** Right pneumothorax. **(D)** Left pleural effusion. **(E)** Posteroanterior chest X-ray showing straight line of collapsed right middle lobe (arrowed). **(F)** Left upper-lobe collapse. **(G)** CT thorax showing bronchiectasis: typical dilated bronchi which are larger than adjacent pulmonary artery (signet ring sign) (arrows).

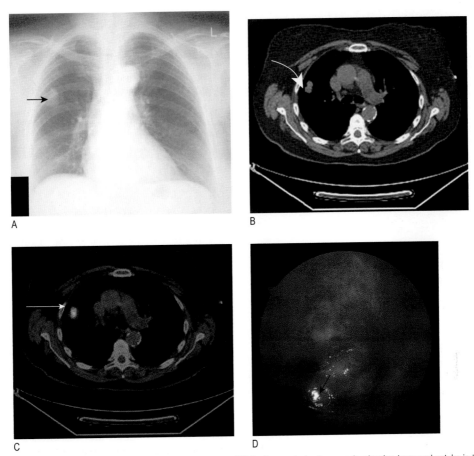

Fig. 7.24 Lung cancer in right lung. (A) Chest X-ray. **(B)** CT of thorax. **(C)** Positron emission tomography showing increased uptake in tumour. **(D)** Lung cancer seen through a bronchoscope (arrow).

7.30 Common causes of acid–base disturbance

Disturbance	pH	CO$_2$	HCO$_3^-$	Cause

Respiratory acidosis	↓	↑	↑	Acute ventilatory failure with:
				  Severe acute asthma
				  Severe pneumonia
				  Exacerbation of COPD
				  Thoracic skeletal abnormality, e.g. kyphoscoliosis
				  Neuromuscular disorders, e.g. muscular dystrophy

Respiratory alkalosis	↑	↓	↓	Hyperventilation due to anxiety/panic Central nervous system causes, e.g. stroke, subarachnoid haemorrhage Salicylate poisoning, early phase

Metabolic acidosis	↓	↓	↓	Increased production of organic acids:
				  Diabetic ketoacidosis
				  Poisoning: alcohol, methanol, ethylene glycol, iron, salicylate
				  Acute renal failure
				  Lactic acidosis, e.g. shock, post cardiac arrest
				Loss of bicarbonate:
				  Renal tubular acidosis, severe diarrhoea, Addison's disease

Metabolic alkalosis	↑	↑	↑	Loss of acid:
				  Severe vomiting, nasogastric suction
				Loss of potassium:
				  Excess diuretic therapy, hyperaldosteronism, Cushing's syndrome, liquorice
				  ingestion, excess alkali ingestion: milk–alkali syndrome

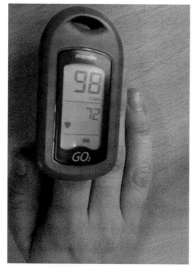

Fig. 7.25 Pulse oximeter with probe on finger.

and decrease in pH. The decrease in pH stimulates arterial chemoreceptors, resulting in alveolar hyperventilation with a consequent decrease in $PaCO_2$.

Metabolic alkalosis

The primary abnormality of metabolic alkalosis is retention of HCO_3^-, often related to renal tubular K^+ depletion or loss of H^+, resulting in an increase in pH. The increase in pH induces alveolar hypoventilation via arterial chemoreceptors, with consequent increase in $PaCO_2$.

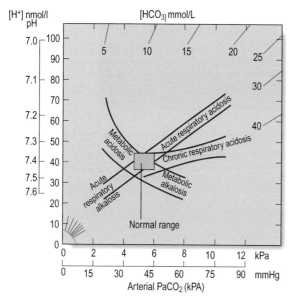

Fig. 7.26 Acid–base diagram. Acid–base nomogram showing the relationships between pH (H^+), $PaCO_2$ and bicarbonate. The bands represent 95% confidence limits of acid–base disturbance.

Respiratory alkalosis

Hyperventilation occurs with respiratory conditions (asthma, pulmonary thromboembolism, pleurisy), high altitude and acute anxiety. Alveolar hyperventilation leads to decrease in $PaCO_2$ and a consequent increase in pH. If hyperventilation persists, as occurs with stays at high altitude, increased renal excretion of HCO_3^- results in normalisation of pH, i.e. compensated respiratory alkalosis.

Metabolic acidosis

In acute renal failure, diabetic ketoacidosis and lactic acidosis, metabolic acidosis results from loss of HCO_3^-

Spirometry

Dynamic lung volumes are measured by inhaling to total lung capacity and then exhaling into a spirometer with maximal effort to residual volume. The volume exhaled in the first second is the FEV₁ and the total volume exhaled is the FVC. Normal predictive values for FEV₁ and FVC are influenced by age, gender, height and race. In healthy young and middle-aged adults the FEV₁/FVC ratio is usually >75%. In the elderly the ratio is usually 70–75%. Reduction in the FEV₁/FVC ratio indicates airway obstruction. The severity of obstruction is represented by the absolute FEV₁ expressed as a percentage of predicted. Airway obstruction that reverses with inhaled β₂-agonist or oral steroid over 5 days or more (an absolute increase in FEV₁ >200 ml that is >15% of baseline) favours a diagnosis of asthma over COPD (Box 7.31).

In interstitial lung disorders, e.g. idiopathic pulmonary fibrosis, pulmonary sarcoidosis or hypersensitivity pneumonitis, there is a decrease in FVC with preservation of FEV₁/FVC ratio, a restrictive defect (Fig. 7.27).

Peak expiratory flow

Peak expiratory flow (PEF) is measured by inhaling to total lung capacity and exhaling into a peak flow meter with maximal effort. Measuring PEF is essential in the assessment of acute asthma and for the diagnosis of occupational asthma where falls in PEF occur during the working week but improve during weekends and holidays. Early-morning falls in PEF of >60 L/min (>20% maximal PEF) are very suggestive of asthma. A >60 L/min fall in PEF (>15% baseline) after exercise is diagnostic of asthma (Box 7.29).

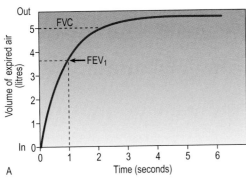

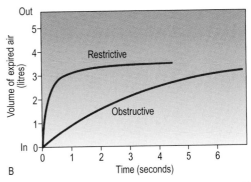

Fig. 7.27 Volume–time curves obtained using a wedge-bellows spirometer. (A) The patient takes a full inspiration and exhales forcibly and fully. Maximal flow decelerates as forced expansion proceeds. **(B)** Obstructive and restrictive patterns. In obstruction, FEV_1/FVC is low; in restriction, it is normal or high. FEV_1, forced expiratory volume in 1 second; FVC, forced vital capacity.

Alastair MacGilchrist
John Iredale
Rowan Parks

The gastrointestinal system

8

GASTROINTESTINAL EXAMINATION

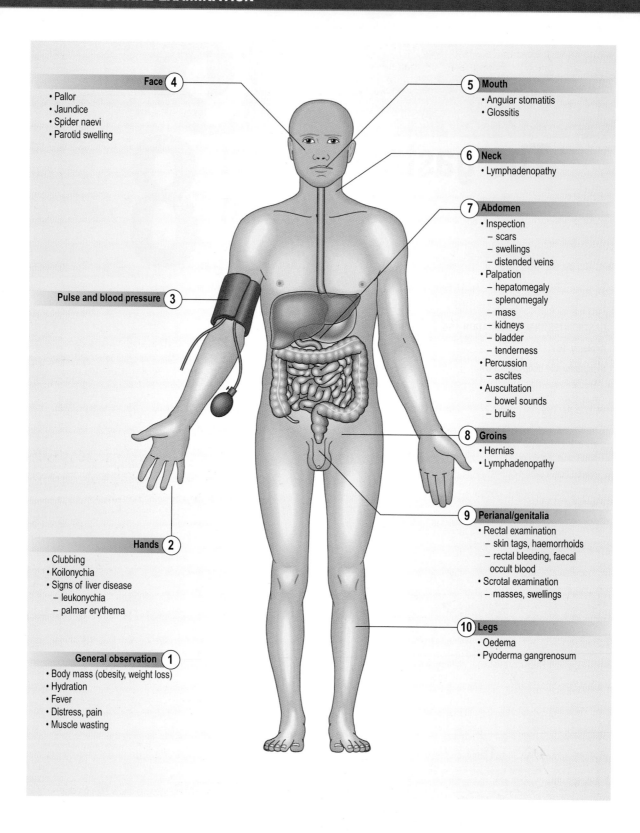

Face 4
- Pallor
- Jaundice
- Spider naevi
- Parotid swelling

5 **Mouth**
- Angular stomatitis
- Glossitis

6 **Neck**
- Lymphadenopathy

7 **Abdomen**
- Inspection
  - scars
  - swellings
  - distended veins
- Palpation
  - hepatomegaly
  - splenomegaly
  - mass
  - kidneys
  - bladder
  - tenderness
- Percussion
  - ascites
- Auscultation
  - bowel sounds
  - bruits

Pulse and blood pressure 3

8 **Groins**
- Hernias
- Lymphadenopathy

9 **Perianal/genitalia**
- Rectal examination
  - skin tags, haemorrhoids
  - rectal bleeding, faecal occult blood
- Scrotal examination
  - masses, swellings

Hands 2
- Clubbing
- Koilonychia
- Signs of liver disease
  - leukonychia
  - palmar erythema

10 **Legs**
- Oedema
- Pyoderma gangrenosum

General observation 1
- Body mass (obesity, weight loss)
- Hydration
- Fever
- Distress, pain
- Muscle wasting

ANATOMY

The gastrointestinal system comprises the alimentary tract plus the liver and biliary system (including the gallbladder), the pancreas and the spleen. The alimentary tract extends from the mouth to the anus and includes the oesophagus, stomach, small intestine (which is also called the small bowel, and comprises duodenum, jejunum and ileum), colon (also called the large intestine, or large bowel) and rectum (Figs 8.1–8.2 and Box 8.1).

The abdomen

The abdomen can be divided into nine regions by the intersection of imaginary planes: two horizontal and two vertical (Fig. 8.3).

SYMPTOMS AND DEFINITIONS

See Box 8.2.

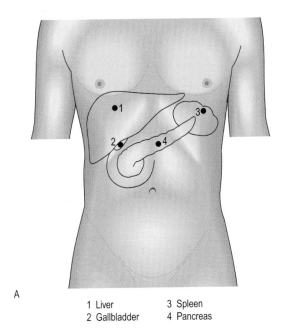

A

1 Liver	3 Spleen
2 Gallbladder	4 Pancreas

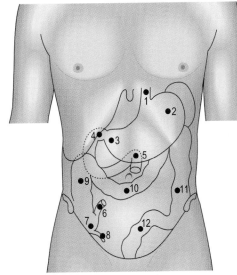

B

1 Oesophagus	7 Caecum
2 Stomach	8 Appendix (in pelvic position)
3 Pyloric antrum	9 Ascending colon
4 Duodenum	10 Transverse colon
5 Duodenojejunal flexure	11 Descending colon
6 Terminal ileum	12 Sigmoid colon

Fig. 8.1 Surface anatomy. (A) Surface markings of non-alimentary tract abdominal viscera. **(B)** Surface markings of the alimentary tract.

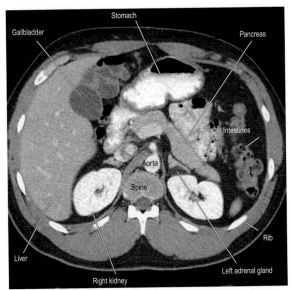

Fig. 8.2 Normal computed tomography (CT) scan of the abdomen at L1 level.

8.1 Surface markings of the gastrointestinal system

Structure	Position
Liver	Upper border: fifth right intercostal space on full expiration Lower border: at the costal margin in the mid-clavicular line on full inspiration
Spleen	Underlies left ribs 9–11, posterior to the mid-axillary line
Gallbladder	At the intersection of the right lateral vertical plane and the costal margin, i.e. tip of the ninth costal cartilage
Pancreas	Neck of the pancreas lies at the level of L1; head lies below and right; tail lies above and left
Kidneys	Upper pole lies deep to the 12th rib posteriorly, 7 cm from the midline; the right is 2–3 cm lower than the left

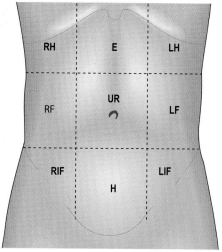

Fig. 8.3 Regions of the abdomen. RH, right hypochondrium; RF, right flank or lumbar region; RIF, right iliac fossa; E, epigastrium; UR, umbilical region; H, hypogastrium or suprapubic region; LH, left hypochondrium; LF, left flank or lumbar region; LIF, left iliac fossa.

8.3 Energy requirements

Males	2500 cal/day
Females	2000 cal/day
Calorie deficit of 500 cal/day = weight loss of 0.5 kg/week	
No calorie intake at all = weight loss of approximately 2 kg/week	

8.4 Causes of a painful mouth

Idiopathic

- Recurrent aphthous mouth ulcers

Infections

- Candidiasis
- Dental sepsis
- Herpes simplex virus (HSV1 and 2)
- Coxsackie A virus: herpangina; hand, foot and mouth; Vincent's angina (ulcerative gingivitis)

Miscellaneous

- Trauma from teeth/dentures
- Leukoplakia

Associated with systemic disorder

- Drug allergies, e.g. sulphonamides, gold, cytotoxics
- Iron, folate, vitamin B_{12} deficiency
- Leucopenia, acute leukaemia
- Reactive arthritis, Behçet's disease
- Crohn's disease, ulcerative colitis
- Coeliac disease

Associated with skin disorder

- Lichen planus, erythema multiforme
- Pemphigoid, pemphigus vulgaris

8.2 Other gastrointestinal terms

Symptom	Definition
Upper gastrointestinal	
Xerostomia	Dry mouth
Halitosis	Bad breath due to gingival, dental or pharyngeal infection
Dysgeusia	Altered taste sensation
Cacageusia	Foul taste sensation, e.g. rotting food
Hiccups	Persistent hiccups suggest diaphragmatic disorder
Lower gastrointestinal	
Steatorrhoea	Fatty stools, pale, greasy, difficult to flush
Haematochezia	Rectal bleeding
Anismus/dyschezia	Difficulty emptying the rectum despite prolonged straining

Anorexia and weight loss

Anorexia is loss of appetite and/or a lack of interest in food. Weight loss is usually the result of reduced energy intake, not increased energy expenditure (Box 8.3). Reduced energy intake arises from dieting, loss of appetite or malabsorption and malnutrition. Energy loss occurs in uncontrolled diabetes mellitus due to marked glycosuria. Increased energy expenditure occurs in hyperthyroidism, fever or the adoption of a more energetic lifestyle. A net calorie deficit of 1000 kcal/day produces a weight loss of approximately 1 kg/week (7000 kcal ≈ 1 kg of fat). Greater weight loss during the initial stages of energy restriction arises from salt and water loss and depletion of hepatic glycogen stores, and not from fat loss. Rapid weight loss over days suggests loss of body fluid as a result of vomiting, diarrhoea or diuretic therapy (1 litre of water = 1 kg).

Weight loss, in isolation, is rarely associated with serious organic disease and loss of <3 kg in the previous 6 months is rarely significant. It does not specifically indicate gastrointestinal disease but is common in many upper gastrointestinal disorders, including malignancy and liver disease. Weight loss with amenorrhoea in an adolescent female may suggest anorexia nervosa but menstrual irregularity is common in women who lose weight from any cause.

Pain

Painful mouth

There are many causes of sore lips, tongue or buccal mucosa, including iron, folate, vitamin B_{12} or vitamin C deficiencies, dermatological disorders, e.g. lichen planus, chemotherapy, isolated aphthous ulcers and infective stomatitis (Box 8.4 and Fig. 8.4). Inflammatory bowel disease and gluten enteropathy are associated with mouth ulcers.

Heartburn and reflux

Heartburn is a hot, burning retrosternal discomfort which radiates upwards. When heartburn is the principal symptom, gastro-oesophageal reflux disease (GORD)

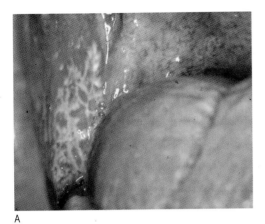

A

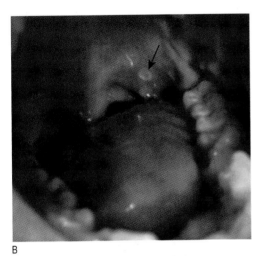

B

Fig. 8.4 Some causes of a painful mouth. (A) Lichen planus.
(B) Small, 'punched-out' aphthous ulcer (arrow).

is the likeliest diagnosis. A sour taste in the mouth from regurgitating gastric acid is called reflux. Differentiate heartburn from cardiac chest pain by its burning quality, upward radiation, association with acid reflux and its occurrence on lying flat or bending forward. Waterbrash is the sudden appearance of fluid in the mouth due to reflex salivation as a result of GORD or, rarely, peptic ulcer disease.

Dyspepsia

Dyspepsia is pain or discomfort centred in the upper abdomen. In contrast, 'indigestion' is a term commonly used for ill-defined symptoms from the upper gastro-intestinal tract. Dyspepsia affects up to 80% of the population at some time. In the majority, no identifiable cause is found (functional dyspepsia). Clusters of symptoms are used to classify dyspepsia:

- reflux-like dyspepsia (heartburn-predominant dyspepsia)
- ulcer-like dyspepsia (epigastric pain relieved by food or antacids)
- dysmotility-like dyspepsia (nausea, belching, bloating and premature satiety).

There is considerable overlap and it is impossible to diagnose functional dyspepsia on history alone, without investigation. Dyspepsia that is worse with an empty

stomach and eased by eating is the classical symptom of peptic ulceration. The patient may indicate a single localised point in the epigastrium (pointing sign), and complain of nausea and abdominal fullness which is worse after meals with a high spice or fat content. 'Fat intolerance' is common in all causes of dyspepsia, including gallbladder disease.

Odynophagia

Odynophagia is pain on swallowing, often precipitated by drinking hot liquids. It can be present with or without dysphagia and may indicate active oesopha-geal ulceration from peptic oesophagitis or oesophageal candidiasis. It implies intact mucosal sensation, making oesophageal cancer unlikely.

8

Abdominal pain

Site

Visceral abdominal pain from distension of hollow organs, mesenteric traction or excessive smooth-muscle contraction is deep and poorly localised in the midline. It is conducted via sympathetic splanchnic nerves. Somatic pain from the parietal peritoneum and abdomi-nal wall is lateralised and localised to the area of inflam-mation. It is conducted via intercostal (spinal) nerves.

Pain arising from foregut structures (stomach, pan-creas, liver and biliary system) is localised above the umbilicus (Fig. 8.5). Central abdominal pain arises from midgut structures, e.g. small bowel and appendix. Lower abdominal pain arises from hindgut structures, e.g. colon. Inflammation may cause localised pain, e.g. left iliac fossa pain due to diverticular disease of the sigmoid colon.

Pain from an unpaired structure, such as the pancreas, is midline and radiates through to the back. Pain from paired structures is felt on and radiates to the affected side, e.g. renal colic. Boys with abdominal pain may have torsion of the testis (Fig. 10.51). In women, consider gynaecological causes, e.g. ruptured ovarian cyst, pelvic inflammatory disease, endometriosis or an ectopic pregnancy.

Onset

The sudden onset of severe abdominal pain, rapidly pro-gressing to become generalised and constant, suggests a hollow viscus perforation, a ruptured abdominal aortic aneurysm or mesenteric infarction. Preceding constipa-tion suggests colorectal cancer or diverticular disease as the cause of perforation and prior dyspepsia suggests peptic ulceration. Coexisting peripheral vascular disease, hypertension, heart failure or atrial fibrillation may suggest aortic aneurysm or mesenteric ischaemia.

Development of circulatory failure following the onset of pain suggests intra-abdominal sepsis or bleeding, e.g. ruptured aortic aneurysm or ectopic pregnancy. Torsion of the testis or ovary produces severe acute abdominal pain and nausea. Torsion of the caecum or sigmoid colon (volvulus) presents with sudden abdominal pain associ-ated with acute intestinal obstruction.

Character

Inflammation and obstruction are the principal pathological processes producing acute abdominal pain. Inflammation usually produces constant pain

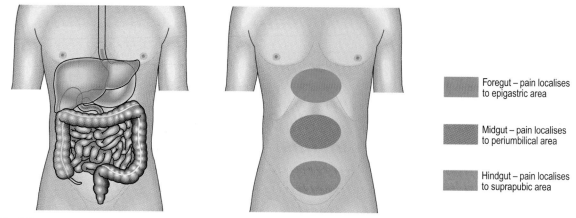

Fig. 8.5 **Abdominal pain.** Perception of visceral pain is localised to the epigastric, umbilical or suprapubic region, according to the embryological origin of the affected organ.

Foregut – pain localises to epigastric area

Midgut – pain localises to periumbilical area

Hindgut – pain localises to suprapubic area

8.5 Diagnosing abdominal pain

	Disorder			
	Peptic ulcer	**Biliary colic**	**Acute pancreatitis**	**Renal colic**
Site	Epigastrium	Epigastrium/right hypochondrium	Epigastrium/left hypochondrium	Loin
Onset	Gradual	Rapidly increasing	Sudden	Rapidly increasing
Character	Gnawing	Constant	Constant	Constant
Radiation	Into back	Below right scapula	Into back	Into genitalia and inner thigh
Timing				
Frequency/periodicity	Remission for weeks/ months	Able to enumerate attacks	Able to enumerate attacks	Usually a discrete episode
Special times	Nocturnal and especially when hungry	Unpredictable	After heavy drinking	Following periods of dehydration
Duration	½–2 hours	4–24 hours	>24 hours	4–24 hours
Exacerbating factors	Stress, spicy foods, alcohol, non-steroidal anti-inflammatory drugs (NSAIDs)	Unable to eat during bouts	Alcohol Unable to eat during bouts	
Relieving factors	Food, antacids, vomiting		Eased by sitting upright	
Severity	Mild to moderate	Severe	Severe	Severe

exacerbated by movement or coughing. Colicky pain arises from hollow structures, e.g. small or large bowel obstruction, or the uterus during labour. It lasts for a short period of time (seconds or minutes), eases off and then returns.

Biliary and renal 'colic' are misnamed, as the pain is rarely colicky; pain rapidly increases to a peak intensity and persists over several hours before gradually resolving (Box 8.5).

Biliary or renal colic is usually promptly relieved by parenteral analgesia. Dull, vague and poorly localised pain is more typical of an inflammatory process or low-grade infection, e.g. salpingitis, appendicitis or diverticulitis.

Radiation

Pain radiating from the right hypochondrium to the shoulder or interscapular region may reflect diaphragmatic irritation, e.g. in acute cholecystitis (Fig. 8.6). Pain radiating from the loin to the groin and genitalia is typical of renal colic. Central upper abdominal pain radiating through to the back, partially relieved by sitting forward, is common in pancreatitis. Central abdominal pain, which later shifts into the right iliac fossa, occurs in acute appendicitis (Fig. 8.27). The combination of severe back and abdominal pain may indicate a ruptured or dissecting abdominal aortic aneurysm.

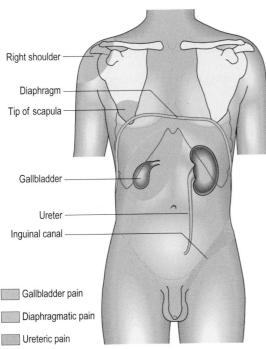

Right shoulder

Diaphragm

Tip of scapula

Gallbladder

Ureter

Inguinal canal

◼ Gallbladder pain

◼ Diaphragmatic pain

◼ Ureteric pain

Fig. 8.6 Characteristic radiation of pain from the gallbladder, diaphragm and ureters.

8.6 Non-alimentary causes of abdominal pain	
Disorder	**Clinical features**
Myocardial infarction	Epigastric pain without tenderness Angor animi (feeling of impending death), hypotension, cardiac arrhythmias
Dissecting aortic aneurysm	Tearing interscapular pain Angor animi, hypotension Asymmetry of femoral pulses
Acute vertebral collapse	Lateralised pain restricting movement Tenderness overlying the involved vertebra
Cord compression	Pain on percussion of thoracic spine Hyperaesthesia in dermatomal distribution Spinal cord signs
Pleurisy	Lateralised pain on coughing Chest signs, e.g. pleural rub
Herpes zoster	Hyperaesthesia in dermatomal distribution Vesicular eruption
Diabetic ketoacidosis	Cramp-like pain, vomiting, air hunger Tachycardia, ketotic breath
Salpingitis or tubal pregnancy	Suprapubic and iliac fossa pain, localised tenderness, nausea, vomiting, fever
Torsion of the testis/ovary	Lower abdominal pain Nausea, vomiting, localised tenderness

Associated symptoms

Anorexia, nausea and vomiting are common but non-specific symptoms reflecting the nature and severity of pain; they may be absent, even in advanced intra-abdominal disease. Severe vomiting without significant pain suggests gastric outlet or proximal small-bowel obstruction. Faeculent vomiting, of small-bowel contents (not faeces), is a late feature of distal small-bowel or colonic obstruction. In peritonitis, the vomitus is usually small in volume but persistent. Severe vomiting with retching may result in laceration at the gastro-oesophageal junction (Mallory–Weiss tear) or oesophageal rupture (Boerhaave's syndrome).

Timing

During the first hour or two after perforation, a 'silent interval' may occur when abdominal pain resolves transiently. The initial chemical peritonitis may subside before bacterial peritonitis becomes established. In acute appendicitis, pain is initially periumbilical (visceral pain) and moves to the right iliac fossa when localised inflammation of the parietal peritoneum becomes established (somatic pain). If the appendix ruptures, generalised peritonitis may develop. Occasionally, a localised appendix abscess develops, with a palpable mass and localised pain in the right iliac fossa.

Change in the pattern of symptoms suggests either that the initial diagnosis was wrong, or that complications have developed. In acute small-bowel obstruction, a change from typical intestinal colic to persistent pain with abdominal tenderness suggests intestinal ischaemia, e.g. strangulated hernia, an indication for urgent surgical intervention.

Exacerbating and relieving factors

Pain exacerbated by movement or coughing suggests inflammation. Patients tend to lie still in order not to exacerbate the pain. Patients with colic typically move around or draw their knees up towards the chest during painful spasms. Abdominal pain persisting for hours or days suggests an inflammatory disorder, such as acute appendicitis, cholecystitis or diverticulitis.

Accompanying features

Nausea and vomiting may accompany any very severe pain. Abdominal pain due to irritable bowel syndrome, diverticular disease or colorectal cancer is invariably accompanied by an alteration in bowel habit. Other features such as breathlessness or palpitation suggest non-alimentary causes (Box 8.6).

Severity

Excruciating pain, poorly relieved by opioid analgesia, suggests an ischaemic vascular event, e.g. bowel infarction or ruptured abdominal aortic aneurysm. Severe pain rapidly eased by potent analgesia is more typical of acute pancreatitis or peritonitis secondary to a ruptured viscus.

8

Dysphagia

Dysphagia (Boxes 8.7 and 8.8) is difficulty swallowing. Always investigate it. Do not confuse dysphagia with early satiety, the inability to complete a full meal because of premature fullness, or globus, the feeling of a lump in the throat. Globus does not interfere with swallowing and is not related to eating.

Neurological dysphagia resulting from bulbar or pseudobulbar palsy is worse for liquids than for solids, and may be accompanied by choking, spluttering and fluid regurgitating from the nose.

Neuromuscular dysphagia, or oesophageal dysmotility, presents in middle age, is worse for solids and may be helped by liquids and sitting upright. Achalasia, when the lower oesophageal sphincter fails to relax normally, leads to progressive oesophageal dilatation above the sphincter. Overflow of secretions and food into the respiratory tract may then occur, especially at night when the patient lies down, and cause aspiration pneumonia. Oesophageal dysmotility can cause oesophageal spasm and central chest pain which may be confused with cardiac pain.

'Mechanical' dysphagia is often due to oesophageal stricture. With weight loss, a short history and no reflux symptoms, suspect oesophageal cancer. Longstanding dysphagia without weight loss but accompanied by heartburn is more likely to be due to benign peptic stricture. Record the site at which the patient feels the food sticking but this is not a reliable guide to the site of oesophageal obstruction.

8.7 Causes of dysphagia

Oral

- Tonsillitis, glandular fever, pharyngitis, peritonsillar abscess
- Painful mouth ulcers

Neurological

- Bulbar or pseudobulbar palsy
- Cerebrovascular accident

Neuromuscular

- Achalasia
- Pharyngeal pouch
- Myasthenia gravis
- Oesophageal dysmotility

Mechanical

- Oesophageal cancer
- Peptic oesophagitis
- Other benign strictures, e.g. after prolonged nasogastric intubation
- Extrinsic compression, e.g. lung cancer
- Systemic sclerosis

8.8 Symptom checklist in dysphagia

- Is dysphagia painful or painless?
- Is dysphagia intermittent or progressive?
- How long is the history of dysphagia?
- Is there a previous history of dysphagia or heartburn?
- Is the dysphagia for solids or liquids or both?
- At what level does food stick?
- Is there complete obstruction with regurgitation?

Nausea and vomiting

Nausea is the sensation of feeling sick. Vomiting is the expulsion of gastric contents via the mouth. Both are associated with pallor, sweating and hyperventilation. Nausea and vomiting, particularly with abdominal pain or discomfort, suggest upper gastrointestinal disorders. Remember to consider non-gastrointestinal causes of nausea and vomiting, especially adverse drug effects, pregnancy and vestibular disorders (Boxes 8.9 and 8.10).

Dyspepsia causes nausea without vomiting. Peptic ulcers seldom cause painless vomiting unless complicated by pyloric stenosis. Gastric outlet obstruction causes projectile vomiting of large volumes of gastric content that is not bile-stained (green). Obstruction distal to the pylorus produces bile-stained vomit. The more distal the level of intestinal obstruction, the more marked the accompanying symptoms of abdominal distension and intestinal colic.

Vomiting is common in gastroenteritis, cholecystitis, pancreatitis and hepatitis. Vomiting is typically preceded by nausea, but in raised intracranial pressure may occur without warning. Severe pain may cause it, e.g. renal or biliary colic, myocardial infarction, as well as systemic disease, metabolic disorders and drug therapy.

Anorexia nervosa and bulimia are eating disorders characterised by undisclosed, self-induced vomiting. In bulimia, weight is maintained or increased, unlike in anorexia nervosa, where weight loss is obvious.

8.9 Non-alimentary causes of vomiting

Neurological

- Raised intracranial pressure, e.g. meningitis, brain tumour
- Labyrinthitis and Ménière's disease
- Migraine
- Vasovagal syncope, shock, fear and severe pain, e.g. renal colic, myocardial infarction

Drugs

- Alcohol, opioids, theophyllines, digoxin, cytotoxic agents, antidepressants
- Consider any drug

Metabolic/endocrine

- Pregnancy
- Diabetic ketoacidosis
- Renal failure
- Liver failure
- Hypercalcaemia
- Addison's disease

Psychological

- Anorexia nervosa
- Bulimia

8.10 Symptom checklist in vomiting

- What medications has the patient been taking?
- Is vomiting:
  - heralded by nausea or occurring without warning?
  - associated with dyspepsia or abdominal pain?
  - relieving dyspepsia or abdominal pain?
  - related to mealtimes, early morning or late evening?
  - bile-stained, blood-stained or faeculent?

Wind and flatulence

Belching, excessive or offensive flatus, abdominal distension and borborygmi (audible bowel sounds) are often called 'wind' or flatulence. Clarify exactly what patients mean. Belching is due to air swallowing (aerophagy) and has no medical significance. It may indicate anxiety, but sometimes occurs in an attempt to relieve abdominal pain or discomfort, and accompanies GORD.

Normally 200–2000 ml of flatus is passed each day. Flatus is a mixture of gases derived from swallowed air and from colonic bacterial fermentation of poorly absorbed carbohydrates. Excessive flatus occurs particularly in lactase deficiency and intestinal malabsorption. No flatus is passed with intestinal obstruction.

Borborygmi result from movement of fluid and gas along the bowel. Loud borborygmi, particularly if associated with colicky discomfort, suggest small-bowel obstruction or dysmotility.

Abdominal distension

Abdominal girth slowly increasing over months or years is usually due to obesity, but in a patient with weight loss it suggests intra-abdominal disease (Box 8.11).

Ascites is an accumulation of fluid in the peritoneal cavity. Exudates from the peritoneal membrane have a higher protein content than transudates and indicate inflammatory or malignant disease (Fig. 8.7 and Box 8.12).

Functional bloating is fluctuating abdominal distension that develops during the day and resolves overnight. It is rarely due to organic disease and usually occurs in irritable bowel syndrome.

Chronic simple constipation rarely produces painful distension, unless associated with the irritable bowel syndrome. Painless abdominal distension in women may be the presenting symptom of ovarian pathology or a concealed pregnancy.

Altered bowel habit

Diarrhoea

Diarrhoea is the frequent passage of loose stools. Normal bowel movement frequency ranges from three times daily to once every 3 days.

High-volume diarrhoea (>1 litre per day) occurs when stool water content is increased (the principal site of water absorption being the colon) and may be:

- secretory, due to intestinal inflammation, e.g. infection, or inflammatory bowel disease
- osmotic, due to malabsorption, adverse drug effects or motility disorders (Box 8.13).

If the patient fasts, osmotic diarrhoea stops but secretory diarrhoea persists. Steatorrhoea is diarrhoea associated with fat malabsorption. The stools are greasy, pale and bulky, and float, making them difficult to flush away.

Low-volume diarrhoea is associated with the irritable bowel syndrome (Box 8.14). The diagnosis of irritable bowel syndrome is based on a pattern of gastrointestinal symptoms (Box 8.15). Abdominal bloating, dyspepsia and often non-alimentary symptoms commonly accompany irritable bowel symptoms.

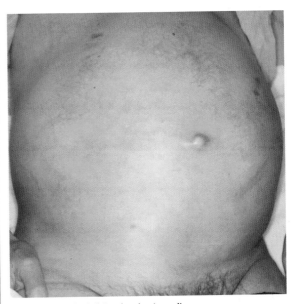

Fig. 8.7 Abdominal distension due to ascites.

8.11 Causes of abdominal distension

Factor	Consider
Fat	Obesity
Flatus	Pseudo-obstruction, obstruction
Faeces	Subacute obstruction, constipation
Fluid	Ascites, tumours (especially ovarian), distended bladder
Fetus	Check date of the last menstrual period
Functional	Bloating, often associated with irritable bowel syndrome

8.12 Causes of ascites

Diagnosis	Comment
Common	
Hepatic cirrhosis with portal hypertension	Transudate
Intra-abdominal malignancy with peritoneal spread	Exudate, cytology may be positive
Uncommon	
Hepatic vein occlusion (Budd–Chiari syndrome)	Transudate in acute phase
Constrictive pericarditis and other right heart failure	Check jugular venous pressure and listen for pericarditic rub
Hypoproteinaemia (nephrotic syndrome, protein-losing enteropathy)	Transudate
Tuberculosis peritonitis	Low glucose content
Pancreatitis	Very high amylase content

8.13 Causes of diarrhoea

Acute

- Infective gastroenteritis, e.g. *Clostridium difficile*
- Drugs (especially antibiotics)

Chronic (>4 weeks)

- Irritable bowel syndrome
- Inflammatory bowel disease
- Parasitic infestations, e.g. *Giardia lamblia*, amoebiasis, *Cryptosporidium* spp.
- Colorectal cancer
- Autonomic neuropathy (especially diabetic)
- Laxative abuse and other drug therapies
- Hyperthyroidism
- Constipation and faecal impaction (overflow)
- Small-bowel or right colonic resection
- Malabsorption, e.g. lactose deficiency, coeliac disease

8.14 Symptom checklist in patients with diarrhoeal disorders

- Is diarrhoea acute, chronic or intermittent?
- Is there tenesmus, urgency or incontinence?
- Is the stool:
  - watery, unformed or semisolid?
  - large-volume and not excessively frequent, suggesting small-bowel disease?
  - small-volume and excessively frequent, suggesting large-bowel disease?
  - associated with blood, mucus or pus?
- Is sleep disturbed by diarrhoea, suggesting organic disease?
- Is there a history of:
  - contact with diarrhoea or of travel abroad?
  - relevant sexual contact ('gay bowel syndrome', human immunodeficiency virus (HIV))?
  - alcohol abuse or relevant drug therapy?
  - gastrointestinal surgery, gastrointestinal disease or inflammatory bowel disease?
  - family history of gastrointestinal disorder, e.g. gluten enteropathy, Crohn's?
  - any other gastrointestinal symptom, e.g. abdominal pain and vomiting?
  - systemic disease suggested by other symptoms, e.g. rigors or arthralgia?

8.15 Rome III criteria: diagnosis of irritable bowel syndrome

Recurrent abdominal pain, for at least the last 6 months, on at least 3 days per month in the last 3 months, associated with two or more of the following:
- Improvement with defecation
- Onset associated with a change in stool frequency
- Onset associated with a change in form of stool

Bloody diarrhoea may be due to inflammatory bowel disease, colonic ischaemia or infective gastroenteritis.

Constipation

Constipation is the infrequent passage of hard stools (Box 8.16) and may be due to impaired colonic motility, physical obstruction, impaired rectal sensation or

8.16 Symptom checklist in patients with constipation

- Has constipation been lifelong or is it of recent onset?
- How often do the bowels empty each week?
- How much time is spent straining at stool?
- Is there associated abdominal pain, anal pain on defecation or rectal bleeding?
- Has the shape of the stool changed, e.g. become pellet-like?
- Has there been any change in drug therapy?

8.17 Causes of constipation

- Lack of fibre in diet
- Irritable bowel syndrome
- Intestinal obstruction (cancer)
- Drugs (opioids, iron)
- Metabolic/endocrine (hypothyroidism, hypercalcaemia)
- Immobility (stroke, Parkinson's disease)

8.18 Symptom checklist in haematemesis and melaena

- Is there a previous history of dyspepsia, peptic ulceration, gastrointestinal bleeding or liver disease?
- Is there a history of alcohol, NSAIDs or corticosteroid ingestion?
- Did the vomitus comprise fresh blood or coffee ground-stained fluid?
- Was the haematemesis preceded by intense retching?
- Was blood staining of the vomitus apparent in the first vomit?

anorectal dysfunction causing anismus (impaired process of evacuation) (Box 8.17). Absolute constipation (no gas or bowel movements) suggests intestinal obstruction and is likely to be associated with pain, vomiting and distension. Tenesmus, the sensation of needing to defecate although the rectum is empty, suggests rectal inflammation or tumour.

Bleeding

Haematemesis

Haematemesis is vomiting blood, which can be fresh and red, or degraded by gastric pepsin, when it is dark brown in colour and resembles coffee grounds (Box 8.18). If the source of bleeding is above the gastro-oesophageal sphincter, e.g. from oesophageal varices, fresh blood may well up in the mouth, as well as being actively vomited. With a lower oesophageal mucosal tear due to the trauma of forceful retching (Mallory–Weiss syndrome), the patient vomits forcefully several times and fresh blood only appears after the patient has vomited several times.

Melaena

Melaena is the passage of tarry, shiny black stools with a characteristic odour and results from upper gastrointestinal bleeding. Distinguish this from the matt black stools associated with oral iron or bismuth therapy. Excessive alcohol ingestion may cause haematemesis from erosive gastritis, Mallory–Weiss tear or bleeding oesophageal varices. Peptic ulceration is a common cause of upper gastrointestinal bleeding (Box 8.19). The Rockall and Blatchford scores are used to assess the severity (Box 8.20). A profound upper gastrointestinal bleed may lead to the passage of purple stool, or, rarely, fresh blood (see below).

8.19 Causes of upper gastrointestinal bleeding

- Gastric or duodenal ulcer
- Mallory–Weiss oesophageal tear
- Oesophagitis, gastritis, duodenitis
- Oesophagogastric varices
- Oesophageal or gastric cancer
- Vascular malformation

8.20 Prediction of the risk of mortality in patients with upper gastrointestinal bleeding: Rockall score

Criterion	Score
Age	
<60 years	0
60–79 years	1
>80 years	2
Shock	
None	0
Pulse >100 bpm and systolic blood pressure (BP) >100 mmHg	1
Systolic BP <100 mmHg	2
Comorbidity	
None	0
Heart failure, ischaemic heart disease or other major illness	2
Renal failure or disseminated malignancy	3
Endoscopic findings	
Mallory–Weiss tear and no visible bleeding	0
All other diagnoses	1
Upper gastrointestinal malignancy	2
Major stigmata of recent haemorrhage	
None	0
Visible bleeding vessel/adherent clot	2
Total score	
Pre-endoscopy (maximum score = 7)	Score 4 = 25% mortality pre-endoscopy
Postendoscopy (maximum score = 11)	Score 8+ = 40% mortality postendoscopy

Rectal bleeding

Fresh rectal bleeding indicates a disorder in the anal canal, rectum or colon (Box 8.21). Blood may be mixed with stool, coat the surface of otherwise normal stool, or be seen on the toilet paper or in the pan. Melaena signifies blood loss from the upper gastrointestinal tract. During severe upper gastrointestinal bleeding, blood may pass through the intestine unaltered, causing fresh rectal bleeding.

Jaundice

Jaundice is a yellowish discoloration of the skin, sclerae (Fig. 8.8) and mucous membranes due to hyperbilirubinaemia (Box 8.22). There is no absolute level at which jaundice is clinically detected but, in good light, most clinicians will recognise jaundice when bilirubin levels exceed 50 μmol/l.

8.21 Causes of rectal bleeding

- Haemorrhoids
- Anal fissure
- Colorectal polyps
- Colorectal cancer
- Inflammatory bowel disease
- Ischaemic colitis
- Complicated diverticular disease
- Vascular malformation

8.22 Common causes of jaundice

Increased bilirubin production

- Haemolysis (unconjugated hyperbilirubinaemia)

Impaired bilirubin excretion

- Congenital
  - Gilbert's syndrome (unconjugated)
- Hepatocellular
  - Viral hepatitis
  - Cirrhosis
  - Drugs
  - Autoimmune hepatitis
- Intrahepatic cholestasis
  - Drugs
  - Primary biliary cirrhosis
- Extrahepatic cholestasis
  - Gallstones
  - Cancer: pancreas, cholangiocarcinoma

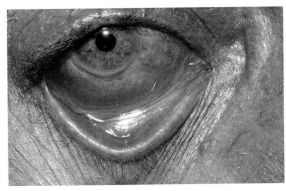

Fig. 8.8 Yellow sclera of jaundice.

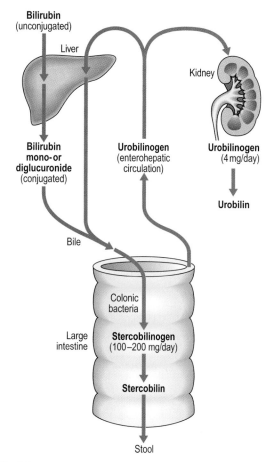

Fig. 8.9 Pathway of bilirubin excretion.

8.24 Checklist for the history of jaundice

- Appetite and weight change
- Abdominal pain, altered bowel habit
- Gastrointestinal bleeding
- Pruritus, dark urine, rigors
- Drug and alcohol history
- Past medical history (pancreatitis, biliary surgery)
- Previous jaundice or hepatitis
- Blood transfusions (hepatitis B or C)
- Family history, e.g. congenital spherocytosis, haemochromatosis
- Sexual and contact history (hepatitis B or C)
- Travel history and immunisations (hepatitis A)
- Skin tattooing (hepatitis B or C)

Prehepatic jaundice

In haemolytic disorders the accompanying anaemic pallor combined with jaundice may produce a pale lemon complexion. The stools and urine are normal in colour. Gilbert's syndrome is common and causes unconjugated hyperbilirubinaemia. Serum liver enzyme concentrations are normal and jaundice is mild (plasma bilirubin <100 μmol/l) but increases during prolonged fasting or intercurrent febrile illness.

Hepatic jaundice

Hepatocellular disease causes hyperbilirubinaemia that is both unconjugated and conjugated. Conjugated bilirubin is soluble and filtered by the kidney, so the urine is dark brown. The stools are normal in colour.

Posthepatic/cholestatic jaundice

In biliary obstruction, conjugated bilirubin in the bile does not reach the intestine, so the stools are pale. Obstructive jaundice may be accompanied by pruritus (generalised itch) due to skin deposition of bile salts. Obstructive jaundice with abdominal pain is usually due to gallstones; if fever or rigors also occur (Charcot's triad), ascending cholangitis is likely. Painless obstructive jaundice suggests malignant biliary obstruction, e.g. cholangiocarcinoma or cancer of the head of the pancreas. Obstructive jaundice can be due to intrahepatic as well as extrahepatic cholestasis, e.g. primary biliary cirrhosis, certain hepatotoxic drug reactions and profound hepatocellular injury (Boxes 8.24 and 8.25).

THE HISTORY

Presenting complaint

Gastrointestinal symptoms are common and are often caused by functional dyspepsia and irritable bowel syndrome. Explore the patient's ICE (p. 8) to understand the context in which symptoms have arisen. Alarm features raise the probability of a serious alternative or coexistent diagnosis (Box 8.26). The risk of serious disease increases with age, and patients >50 years should be investigated before a functional bowel disorder is diagnosed. Clarify exactly what patients mean by terms they use, especially constipation and diarrhoea.

8.23 Urine and stool analysis in jaundice

	Urine			Stools
	Colour	Bilirubin	Urobilinogen	Colour
Unconjugated	Normal	−	++++	Normal
Hepatocellular	Dark	++	++	Normal
Obstructive	Dark	++++	−	Pale

Unconjugated bilirubin is insoluble and transported in plasma bound to albumin; it is therefore not filtered by the renal glomeruli. In jaundice from unconjugated hyperbilirubinaemia, the urine is a normal colour (acholuric jaundice; Box 8.23).

Bilirubin is conjugated to form bilirubin diglucuronide in the liver, and excreted in bile, producing its characteristic green colour (Fig. 8.9). In conjugated hyperbilirubinaemia, the urine is dark brown in colour due to the presence of bilirubin diglucuronide. In the colon, conjugated bilirubin is metabolised by bacterial flora to stercobilinogen and stercobilin which are excreted in the stool, contributing to the brown colour of stool. Stercobilinogen is absorbed from the bowel and excreted in the urine as urobilinogen, a colourless, water-soluble compound.

8.25 Examples of drug-induced gastrointestinal conditions

Symptom	Drug
Weight gain	Oral corticosteroids
Dyspepsia and gastrointestinal bleeding	Aspirin NSAIDs
Nausea	Many drugs, including selective serotonin reuptake inhibitor antidepressants
Diarrhoea (pseudomembranous colitis)	Antibiotics Proton pump inhibitors
Constipation	Opioids
Jaundice: hepatitis	Paracetamol (overdose) Pyrazinamide Rifampicin Isoniazid
Jaundice: cholestatic	Flucloxacillin Chlorpromazine Co-amoxiclav
Liver fibrosis	Methotrexate

THE BRISTOL STOOL FORM SCALE

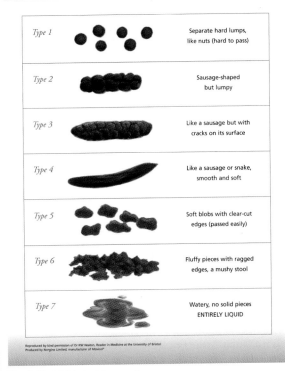

Fig. 8.10 Bristol stool form scale.

8.26 Gastrointestinal (GI) 'alarm features'

- Persistent vomiting
- Dysphagia
- Fever
- Weight loss
- GI bleeding
- Anaemia
- Painless, watery, high-volume diarrhoea
- Nocturnal symptoms disturbing sleep

8.27 Risk factors for viral hepatitis

- Intravenous drug use
- Tattoos
- Foreign travel
- Blood transfusion
- Sex between men or with prostitutes
- Multiple sexual partners

Anorexia and weight loss

In addition to asking about appetite, ask: 'Do you still enjoy your food?' Confirm subjective assessment of weight loss from ill-fitting clothes and by reviewing documented weights from the case records.

Dysphagia and odynophagia

Ask: 'Does food (or drink) stick when you swallow and is this painful?' Enquire if there is difficulty swallowing liquids (neuromuscular disorder) or solids (oesophageal obstruction due to cancer, peptic stricture, achalasia).

Vomiting

Ask about relation to meals and about associated symptoms such as abdominal pain, weight loss and haematemesis (Box 8.10).

Reflux symptoms and dyspepsia

Ask about reflux-like dyspepsia (heartburn-predominant dyspepsia), ulcer-like dyspepsia (epigastric pain relieved by food or antacids) and dysmotility-like dyspepsia (nausea, belching, bloating and premature satiety).

Haematemesis

Note recent ingestion of aspirin, NSAIDs and alcohol.

Abdominal pain

Characterise pain using SOCRATES (Box 2.10) and use the questions listed in Box 8.8.

Altered bowel habit

Clarify what the patient means by diarrhoea or constipation. Use the Bristol stool chart to ensure agreement (Fig. 8.10). Use questions listed in Box 8.14 for those with diarrhoea and Box 8.16 for those with constipation. For those with either diarrhoea or constipation, always ask: 'Have you noticed any red blood in the stools?'

Jaundice

Ask about alcohol intake, recent travel abroad, use of illicit or intravenous drugs and take a sexual history (Box 8.27). Always review recently prescribed drugs.

Ask about itching or dark urine or pale stools (obstructive jaundice) and whether there is associated weight loss, abdominal pain or fever.

Past history

History of a similar problem may suggest the diagnosis: for example, bleeding peptic ulcer or inflammatory bowel disease. Primary biliary cirrhosis and auto-immune hepatitis are associated with thyroid disease and non-alcoholic fatty liver disease (NAFLD) is associated with diabetes and obesity. Ask about previous abdominal surgery and radiological and other investigations.

Drug history

Ask about all prescribed medications, over-the-counter medicines and herbal preparations. Many drugs affect the gastrointestinal tract (Box 8.25) and are hepatotoxic.

Family history

Inflammatory bowel disease is more common in patients with a family history of either Crohn's disease or ulcerative colitis. Colorectal cancer in a first-degree relative increases the risk of colorectal cancer and polyps. Peptic ulcer disease is familial but this may be due to environmental factors, e.g. transmission of *Helicobacter pylori* infection. Gilbert's syndrome is an autosomal dominant condition; haemochromatosis and Wilson's disease are autosomal recessive disorders. Autoimmune diseases, particularly thyroid disease, are common in relatives of those with primary biliary cirrhosis and autoimmune hepatitis. A family history of diabetes is frequently seen in the context of NAFLD.

Social history

Take a dietary history and approximately assess the intake of calories and sources of essential nutrients (Box 8.28). Painless diarrhoea may indicate high alcohol intake, lactose intolerance or gluten enteropathy. Patients with irritable bowel syndrome often report specific food intolerances, including wheat, dairy products and others.

Calculate the patient's alcohol consumption in units (p. 17).

Smokers are at increased risk of oesophageal cancer, colorectal cancer, Crohn's disease and peptic ulcer, while patients with ulcerative colitis are less likely to smoke. Many disorders, particularly irritable bowel syndrome and dyspepsia, are exacerbated by stress and emotional ill health. Ask about potential sources of stress, as well as about the symptoms of anxiety and depression (Box 2.49).

In patients with liver disease, ask about specific risk factors (Box 8.27). Hepatitis B and C may present with chronic liver disease or cancer decades after the primary infection, so enquire about drug use and other risk factors in the distant as well as the recent past. Foreign travel is important in relation to diarrhoeal illnesses.

THE PHYSICAL EXAMINATION

Examination sequence

- Note the patient's demeanour and general appearance. Is he in pain or cachectic or obese? Look at his hands for clubbing, koilonychia (spoon-shaped nails) and signs of liver disease, including leukonychia and palmar erythema. Is the patient well nourished, obese or thin?
- Look for stigmata of iron deficiency, including angular cheilitis (painful hacks at the corners of the mouth) and atrophic glossitis (pale, smooth tongue). The tongue has a beefy, raw appearance in folate and vitamin B_{12} deficiency. Look at the mouth and throat for aphthous ulcers, which are common in gluten enteropathy and inflammatory bowel disease (Fig. 8.4B).
- Examine the cervical, axillary and inguinal lymph nodes; gastric and pancreatic cancer may spread to cause enlargement of the left supraclavicular lymph nodes (Troisier's sign). More widespread lymphadenopathy with hepatosplenomegaly suggests lymphoma.

Nutritional state

- Record the height, weight, waist circumference and the patient's body mass index (p. 55).
- Note whether obesity is truncal or generalised. Look for abdominal striae, which indicate rapid weight gain, previous pregnancy or, rarely, Cushing's syndrome. Loose skin folds signify recent weight loss.

Liver disease

If jaundice is not obvious, ask the patient to look down and retract the upper eyelid to expose the sclera; look to see if it is yellow in natural light (Fig. 8.8). Do not confuse the diffuse yellow sclerae of jaundice with small yellowish fat pads (pingueculae) sometimes seen at the periphery of the sclerae.

8.28 Calorie value of some food groups	
Food group	**Calorific value of food**
Dairy products (milk, butter, cheese, yoghurt)	Milk = 500 kcal/l Fat = 9 kcal/g
Wheat (bread, pasta)	Carbohydrates = 4 kcal/g
Meat, fish	Protein = 4 kcal/g
Alcohol	Wine = 500 kcal/70 cl Beer = 400 kcal/l

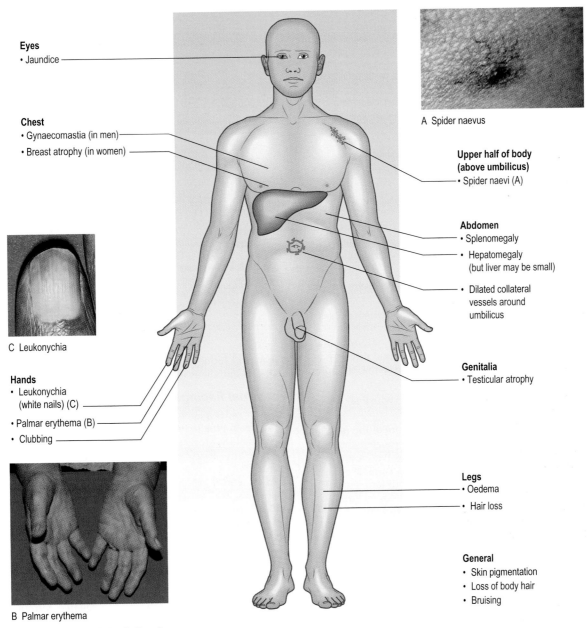

Eyes
• Jaundice

Chest
• Gynaecomastia (in men)
• Breast atrophy (in women)

A Spider naevus

Upper half of body (above umbilicus)
• Spider naevi (A)

Abdomen
• Splenomegaly
• Hepatomegaly (but liver may be small)
• Dilated collateral vessels around umbilicus

C Leukonychia

Genitalia
• Testicular atrophy

Hands
• Leukonychia (white nails) (C)
• Palmar erythema (B)
• Clubbing

Legs
• Oedema
• Hair loss

General
• Skin pigmentation
• Loss of body hair
• Bruising

B Palmar erythema

Fig. 8.11 Features of chronic liver disease.

Certain signs which suggest chronic liver disease (Fig. 8.11):

• Palmar erythema and spider naevi are due to excess oestrogen associated with reduced hepatic breakdown of sex steroids. Spider naevi are isolated telangiectases that characteristically fill from a central feeding vessel found in the distribution of the superior vena cava on the upper trunk, arms and face (Fig. 8.11). Women may have up to five spider naevi in health; palmar erythema and numerous spider naevi are normal during pregnancy. In men these signs suggest chronic liver disease (Box 8.29).

• Gynaecomastia (breast enlargement in males), with loss of body hair and testicular atrophy, may occur due to reduced breakdown of oestrogens.

EBE **8.29 Chronic liver disease**

In a jaundiced patient, finding spider naevi, palmar erythema and ascites all strongly suggests chronic liver disease rather than obstructive jaundice.

O'Connor KW, Snodgrass PJ, Swonder JE et al. A blinded prospective study comparing four current non-invasive approaches in the differential diagnosis of medical versus surgical jaundice. Gastroenterology 1983;84:1498–1504.

• Leukonychia (white nails), caused by hypoalbuminaemia, may also occur in protein calorie malnutrition (kwashiorkor), malabsorption due to protein-losing enteropathy, e.g. coeliac disease, or heavy and prolonged proteinuria (nephrotic syndrome).

8.30 Signs of liver failure

- Fetor hepaticus: stale 'mousy' smell of the volatile amine, dimethyl sulphide, on the breath
- Flapping tremor of outstretched arms with hands dorsiflexed ('asterixis')

Mental state varies from drowsiness with day/night pattern reversed, through confusion and disorientation, to unresponsive coma

- Late neurological features
  - Spasticity and extension of the arms and legs
  - Extensor plantar responses

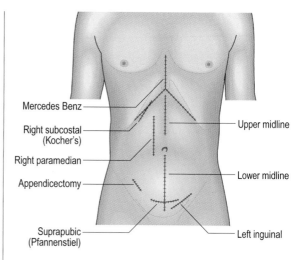

Fig. 8.12 **Some abdominal incisions.** The midline and oblique incisions avoid damage to innervation of the abdominal musculature and later development of incisional herniae. These incisions however have been widely superseded by laparascopic surgery.

- Finger clubbing is associated with liver cirrhosis, inflammatory bowel disease and malabsorption syndromes.

Signs which suggest liver failure include the following (Box 8.30):

- Asterixis is a coarse flapping tremor which occurs with hepatic encephalopathy (p. 148).
- Fetor hepaticus, a distinctive 'mousy' odour on the breath, is due to the volatile compound dimethyl sulphide and is evidence of portosystemic shunting (with or without encephalopathy).

Other signs which may be associated with liver disease include:

- Dupuytren's contracture (contracture of the palmar fascia; p. 49) is linked with alcohol-related chronic liver disease. More commonly, however, it is familial (autosomal dominant with variable penetrance) or associated with conditions causing microvascular pathology, e.g. diabetes mellitus, smoking, hyperlipidaemia, HIV infection.
- Bilateral parotid swelling due to sialoadenosis of the salivary glands may be a feature of chronic alcohol abuse or bulimia associated with recurrent vomiting.

The abdomen

Examination sequence

Inspection

- Examine the patient in good light and warm surroundings.
- Position the patient comfortably supine with the head resting on only one or two pillows to relax the abdominal wall muscles.
- Use extra pillows to support a patient with kyphosis or breathlessness.
- Look at the teeth, tongue and buccal mucosa and ask about mouth ulcers.
- Note any smell, e.g. alcohol, fetor hepaticus, uraemia, melaena or ketones.
- Expose the abdomen from the xiphisternum to the symphysis pubis, leaving the chest and legs covered.

Normal findings

The abdomen is normally flat or slightly scaphoid and symmetrical. At rest, respiration is principally diaphragmatic; the abdominal wall moves out and the liver, spleen and kidneys move downwards during inspiration. The umbilicus is usually inverted.

Abnormal findings

Skin In older patients, seborrhoeic warts, ranging in colour from pink to brown or black, and haemangiomas (Campbell de Morgan spots) are common and normal, but note any striae, bruising or scratch marks.

Visible veins Abnormally prominent veins on the abdominal wall suggest portal hypertension or vena caval obstruction. In portal hypertension, recanalisation of the umbilical vein along the falciform ligament produces distended veins which drain away from the umbilicus: the 'caput medusae'. The umbilicus may appear bluish and distended due to an umbilical varix. In contrast, an umbilical hernia is a distended and everted umbilicus which does not appear vascular and may have a palpable cough impulse. Dilated tortuous veins with blood flow superiorly are collateral veins due to obstruction of the inferior vena cava. Rarely, superior vena cava obstruction gives rise to similarly distended abdominal veins, but which all flow inferiorly.

Abdominal distension If the abdomen is distended, is this generalised or localised? In obesity, the umbilicus is usually sunken; in ascites, it is flat or everted. Look tangentially across the abdomen and from the foot of the bed for any asymmetry associated with a localised mass, such as an enlarged liver or bladder.

Abdominal scars and stomas Note any surgical scars or stomas and clarify what operations have been undertaken (Figs 8.12 and 8.13). A small infraumbilical incision is usually the result of previous laparoscopy. Puncture scars from the ports used for laparoscopic surgery may be visible. An incisional hernia at the site of a scar is palpable as a defect in the abdominal wall musculature and becomes more obvious as the patient raises the head off the bed or coughs.

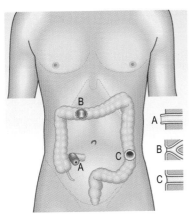

Fig. 8.13 Surgical stomas. A, An ileostomy is usually in the right iliac fossa and is formed as a spout. **B,** A loop colostomy is created to defunction the distal bowel temporarily. It is usually in the transverse colon and has afferent and efferent limbs. **C,** A colostomy may be terminal, i.e. resected distal bowel. It is usually flush and in the left iliac fossa.

Palpation

Examination sequence

- Ensure that your hands are warm.
- If the bed is low, kneel beside it.
- Ask the patient to show you where any pain is and to report any tenderness elicited during palpation.
- Ask the patient to place the arms by the sides to help relax the abdominal wall.
- Use your right hand, keeping it flat and in contact with the abdominal wall.
- Observe the patient's face for any sign of discomfort throughout the examination.
- Begin with light superficial palpation away from any site of pain.
- Palpate each region in turn, and then repeat with deeper palpation.
- Test abdominal muscle tone by light, dipping movements with your fingers.
- Describe any mass using the basic principles outlined in Chapter 3 (Box 3.11). Describe its site, size, surface, shape and consistency, and note whether it moves on respiration. Is the mass fixed or mobile?
- To determine if a mass is superficial and in the abdominal wall rather than within the abdominal cavity, ask the patient to tense the abdominal muscles by lifting his head.
- An abdominal wall mass will still be palpable, whereas an intra-abdominal mass will not.
- Decide whether the mass is an enlarged abdominal organ or separate from the solid organs.

Normal findings

A pulsatile mass palpable in the upper abdomen may be normal aortic pulsation in a thin person, a gastric or pancreatic tumour transmitting underlying aortic pulsation or an aortic aneurysm.

The normal liver is identified as an area of dullness to percussion over the right anterior chest between the fifth rib and the costal margin. The normal spleen is identified as an area of dullness to percussion posterior to the left mid-axillary line beneath the ninth, 10th and 11th ribs.

Abnormal findings

Tenderness Discomfort during palpation may vary and be accompanied by resistance to palpation. Consider the patient's level of anxiety when assessing the severity of pain and tenderness elicited. Tenderness in several areas on minimal pressure may be due to generalised peritonitis but is more often due to anxiety. Severe superficial pain with no tenderness on deep palpation or pain that disappears if the patient is distracted also suggests anxiety. With these exceptions, tenderness usefully indicates underlying pathology.

Voluntary guarding is the voluntary contraction of the abdominal muscles when palpation provokes pain. Involuntary guarding is the reflex contraction of the abdominal muscles when there is inflammation of the parietal peritoneum. If the whole peritoneum is inflamed (generalised peritonitis) due to a perforated viscus, the abdominal wall no longer moves with respiration; breathing becomes increasingly thoracic and the anterior abdominal wall muscles are held rigid (board-like rigidity).

The site of tenderness is important. Tenderness in the epigastrium suggests peptic ulcer; in the right hypochondrium, cholecystitis; in the left iliac fossa, diverticulitis; in the right iliac fossa, appendicitis or Crohn's ileitis. 'Rebound tenderness' is a sign of intra-abdominal disease but not necessarily of parietal peritoneal inflammation (peritonism). Ask the patient to cough or gently percuss the abdomen to elicit any pain or tenderness, rapidly removing your hand after deep palpation increases the pain (Fig. 8.14).

Palpable mass A pathological mass can usually be distinguished from palpable faeces as the latter are indentable and may disappear following defecation (Fig. 8.15). A hard subcutaneous nodule palpable at the umbilicus may indicate metastatic cancer ('Sister Mary Joseph's nodule').

Palpation for enlarged organs

Examine the liver, gallbladder, spleen and kidneys in turn during deep inspiration. Keep your examining hand still and wait for the organ to descend. Do not start palpation too close to the costal margin, missing the edge of the liver or spleen.

Hepatomegaly

Examination sequence

- Place your hand flat on the skin of the right iliac fossa.
- Point your fingers upwards and your index and middle fingers lateral to the rectus muscle, so that your fingertips lie parallel to the rectus sheath (Fig. 8.16). Keep your hand stationary.
- Ask the patient to breathe in deeply through the mouth.
- Feel for the liver edge as it descends on inspiration.
- Move your hand progressively up the abdomen, 1 cm at a time, between each breath the patient takes, until you reach the costal margin or detect the liver edge. The liver may be enlarged or displaced downwards by hyperinflated lungs (Fig. 8.17A).

8

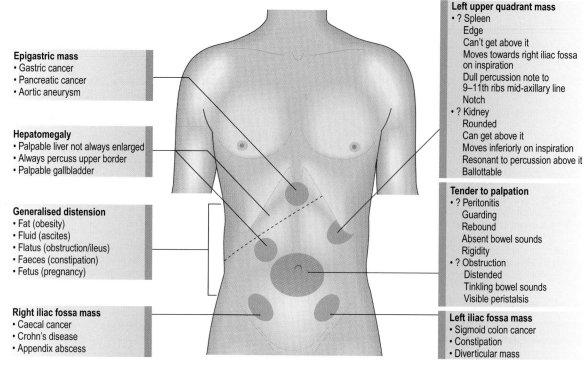

Epigastric mass
• Gastric cancer
• Pancreatic cancer
• Aortic aneurysm

Hepatomegaly
• Palpable liver not always enlarged
• Always percuss upper border
• Palpable gallbladder

Generalised distension
• Fat (obesity)
• Fluid (ascites)
• Flatus (obstruction/ileus)
• Faeces (constipation)
• Fetus (pregnancy)

Right iliac fossa mass
• Caecal cancer
• Crohn's disease
• Appendix abscess

Left upper quadrant mass
• ? Spleen
  Edge
  Can't get above it
  Moves towards right iliac fossa on inspiration
  Dull percussion note to 9–11th ribs mid-axillary line
  Notch
• ? Kidney
  Rounded
  Can get above it
  Moves inferiorly on inspiration
  Resonant to percussion above it
  Ballottable

Tender to palpation
• ? Peritonitis
  Guarding
  Rebound
  Absent bowel sounds
  Rigidity
• ? Obstruction
  Distended
  Tinkling bowel sounds
  Visible peristalsis

Left iliac fossa mass
• Sigmoid colon cancer
• Constipation
• Diverticular mass

Fig. 8.14 Palpable abnormalities in the abdomen.

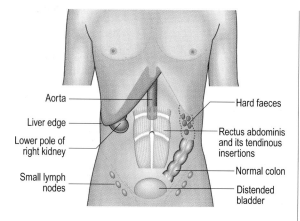

Aorta

Liver edge

Lower pole of right kidney

Small lymph nodes

Hard faeces

Rectus abdominis and its tendinous insertions

Normal colon

Distended bladder

Fig. 8.15 Palpable masses which may be physiological rather than pathological.

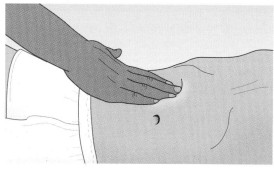

Fig. 8.16 Palpation of the liver.

■ If you feel a liver edge, describe:
  ■ size
  ■ surface: smooth or irregular
  ■ edge: smooth or irregular
  ■ consistency: soft or hard
  ■ tenderness
  ■ whether it is pulsatile.

Percussion

Examination sequence

■ Ask the patient to hold his breath in full expiration.
■ Percuss downwards from the right fifth intercostal space in the mid-clavicular line, listening for the dullness that indicates the upper border of the liver.
■ Measure the distance in centimetres below the costal margin in the mid-clavicular line or from the upper border of dullness to the palpable liver edge.

To feel for gallbladder tenderness (in cholecystitis):

■ Ask the patient to breathe in deeply and gently palpate the right upper quadrant of the abdomen in the mid-clavicular line. As the liver descends, the inflamed gallbladder contacts the fingertips, causing pain and the sudden arrest of inspiration (Murphy's sign) (Boxes 8.31 and 8.32).

Normal findings

You may feel the liver edge below the right costal margin. Other normal findings may include:

• The aorta may be palpable as a pulsatile swelling above the umbilicus
• The lower pole of the right kidney may be palpable in the right flank

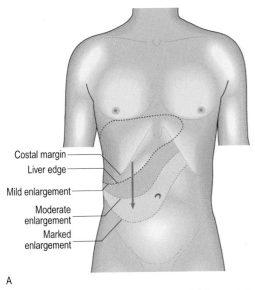
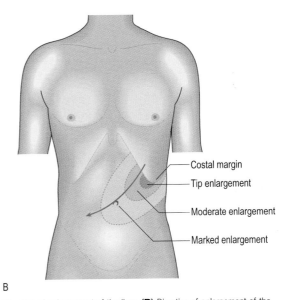

Fig. 8.17 Patterns of progressive enlargement of liver and of spleen. (A) Direction of enlargement of the liver. **(B)** Direction of enlargement of the spleen. The spleen moves downwards and medially during inspiration.

EBE 8.31 **Acute cholecystitis**

In a patient with right upper quadrant pain, a positive Murphy's sign modestly increases the probability of acute cholecystitis.

McGee S. Evidence based physical diagnosis. St Louis, MO: Saunders/Elsevier, 2007, p. 575–587.

EBE 8.32 **Jaundice and a palpable gallbladder**

In a jaundiced patient, a palpable gallbladder is likely to be due to extrahepatic obstruction, e.g. from pancreatic cancer or, more rarely, gallstones (Courvoisier's sign).

McGee S. Evidence based physical diagnosis. St Louis, MO: Saunders/Elsevier, 2007, p. 560–563.

8.33 **Causes of hepatomegaly**

Chronic parenchymal liver disease

- Alcoholic liver disease
- Hepatic steatosis
- Autoimmune hepatitis
- Viral hepatitis
- Primary biliary cirrhosis

Malignancy

- Primary hepatocellular cancer
- Secondary metastatic cancer

Right heart failure

Haematological disorders

- Lymphoma
- Leukaemia
- Myelofibrosis
- Polycythaemia

Rarities

- Amyloidosis
- Budd–Chiari syndrome
- Sarcoidosis
- Glycogen storage disorders

- Faecal scybala may be palpable in the sigmoid colon in the left iliac fossa
- A full bladder arising out of the pelvis may be palpable in the suprapubic region.

Abnormal findings

Hepatic enlargement can result from chronic parenchymal liver disease from any cause (Box 8.33). The liver is enlarged in early cirrhosis but often shrunken in advanced cirrhosis. Fatty liver (hepatic steatosis) can cause marked hepatomegaly. Hepatic enlargement due to metastatic tumour is hard and irregular. An enlarged left lobe may be felt in the epigastrium or even in the left hypochondrium. An audible bruit may be heard over the liver in hepatocellular cancer and sometimes in alcoholic hepatitis. In right heart failure, the congested liver is usually soft and tender; a pulsatile liver indicates tricuspid regurgitation. A bruit over the liver may be heard in acute alcoholic hepatitis, hepatocellular cancer and arteriovenous malformation. Liver failure produces associated symptoms and its severity can be graded (Box 8.34).

Resonance below the fifth intercostal space suggests emphysema or occasionally the interposition of the transverse colon between the liver and the diaphragm (Chilaiditi's sign).

Palpable distension of the gallbladder has a characteristic globular shape. It is rare and results from either obstruction of the cystic duct, as in a mucocoele or empyema of the gallbladder, or obstruction of the common bile duct (providing the cystic duct is patent), as in pancreatic cancer. In gallstone disease the gallbladder may be tender but impalpable because of fibrosis of the gallbladder wall.

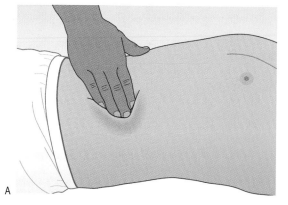
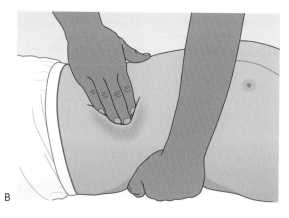

A   B

Fig. 8.18 Palpation of the spleen.

8.34 Grading of hepatic encephalopathy (West Haven)	
Stage	**State of consciousness**
0	No change in personality or behaviour No asterixis (flapping tremor)
1	Impaired concentration and attention span Sleep disturbance, slurred speech Euphoria or depression Asterixis present
2	Lethargy, drowsiness, apathy or aggression Disorientation, inappropriate behaviour, slurred speech
3	Confusion and disorientation, bizarre behaviour Drowsiness or stupor Asterixis usually absent
4	Comatose with no response to voice commands Minimal or absent response to painful stimuli

8.35 Causes of splenomegaly

Haematological disorders
- Lymphoma and lymphatic leukaemias
- Myeloproliferative diseases, polycythaemia rubra vera and myelofibrosis
- Haemolytic anaemia, congenital spherocytosis

Portal hypertension

Infections
- Glandular fever
- Malaria, kala azar (leishmaniasis)
- Brucellosis, tuberculosis, salmonellosis
- Bacterial endocarditis

Rheumatological conditions
- Rheumatoid arthritis (Felty's syndrome)
- Systemic lupus erythematosus

Rarities
- Sarcoidosis
- Amyloidosis
- Glycogen storage disorders

Splenomegaly

Examination sequence

- Place your hand over the umbilicus. Keep your hand stationary and ask the patient to breathe in deeply through the mouth.
- Feel for the splenic edge as it descends on inspiration (Fig. 8.18A).
- Move your hand diagonally upwards towards the left hypochondrium 1 cm at a time between each breath the patient takes.
- Feel the costal margin along its length, as the position of the spleen tip is variable.
- If you cannot feel the splenic edge, ask the patient to roll towards you and on to his right side and repeat the above. Palpate with your right hand, placing your left hand behind the patient's left lower ribs, pulling the ribcage forward (Fig. 8.18B).
- Feel along the left costal margin and percuss over the lateral chest wall to confirm or exclude the presence of splenic dullness.

Abnormal findings

The spleen has to increase in size threefold before it becomes palpable, so a palpable spleen always indicates splenomegaly. The normal spleen lies beneath the ninth and 11th ribs in the left mid-axillary line. It enlarges from under the left costal margin down and medially towards the umbilicus (Fig. 8.17B). A characteristic notch may be palpable midway along its leading edge, differentiating it from an enlarged left kidney.

Although there are many causes of splenomegaly (Boxes 8.35–8.37), massive enlargement in the developed world is usually due to myeloproliferative disease or haematological malignancy; worldwide, malaria is a common cause.

Ascites

Ascites is the accumulation of intraperitoneal fluid. Causes include intra-abdominal malignancy, chronic liver disease, severe heart failure, nephrotic syndrome and hypoproteinaemia.

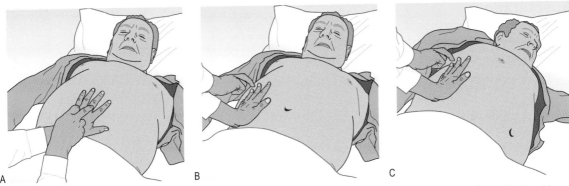

Fig. 8.19 Percussing for ascites. **(A and B)** Percuss towards the flank from resonant to dull. **(C)** Then ask the patient to roll on to his other side. In ascites, the note then becomes resonant.

8.36 Differentiating a palpable spleen from the left kidney

Distinguishing feature	Spleen	Kidney
Mass is smooth and regular in shape	More likely	Polycystic kidneys are bilateral irregular masses
Mass descends in inspiration	Yes, travels superficially and diagonally	Yes, moves deeply and vertically
Able to feel deep to the mass	Yes	No
Palpable notch on the medial surface	Yes	No
Bilateral masses palpable	No	Sometimes, e.g. polycystic kidneys
Percussion resonant over the mass	No	Sometimes
Mass extends beyond the midline	Sometimes	No (except with horseshoe kidney)

8.37 Causes of hepatosplenomegaly

- Lymphoma
- Myeloproliferative diseases
- Cirrhosis with portal hypertension
- Amyloidosis, sarcoidosis, glycogen storage disease

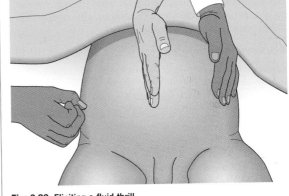

Fig. 8.20 Eliciting a fluid thrill.

EBE 8.38 Ascites

Weight gain, increased abdominal girth and shifting dullness together strongly suggest ascites.

Simel D, Rinne D (eds) The rational clinical examination. New York: JAMA and Archives Journals/McGraw-Hill Professional, 2008, pp. 65–72.

- Pause for 10 seconds to allow any ascites to gravitate, then percuss again. If the area of dullness is now resonant, shifting dullness is present, indicating ascites (Box 8.38).

Fluid thrill

- If the abdomen is tensely distended and you are not certain whether ascites is present, feel for a fluid thrill.
- Place the palm of your left hand flat against the left side of the patient's abdomen and flick a finger of your right hand against the right side of the abdomen.
- If you feel a ripple against your left hand, ask an assistant or the patient to place the edge of his hand on the midline of the abdomen (Fig. 8.20). This prevents transmission of the impulse via the skin rather than through the ascites. If you still feel a ripple against your left hand, a fluid thrill is present (only detected in gross ascites).

Examination sequence

Shifting dullness

- With the patient supine, percuss from the midline out to the flanks (Fig. 8.19). Note any change from resonant to dull, along with areas of dullness and resonance.
- Keep your finger on the site of dullness in the flank and ask the patient to turn on to his opposite side.

Auscultation

- With the patient supine, place your stethoscope diaphragm to the right of the umbilicus and do not move it.
- Listen for up to 2 minutes before concluding that bowel sounds are absent.
- Listen above the umbilicus over the aorta for arterial bruits.
- Now listen 2–3 cm above and lateral to the umbilicus for bruits from renal artery stenosis.
- Listen over the liver for bruits.
- A succussion splash sounds like a half-filled water bottle being shaken. Explain the procedure to the patient, then shake the patient's abdomen by lifting him with both hands under his pelvis.

Normal findings

Bowel sounds are gurgling noises from the normal peristaltic activity of the gut. They normally occur every 5–10 seconds, but the frequency varies.

Abnormal findings

Absence of bowel sounds implies paralytic ileus or peritonitis. In intestinal obstruction, bowel sounds occur with increased frequency and volume and have a high-pitched, tinkling quality. Bruits suggest an atheromatous or aneurysmal aorta or superior mesenteric artery stenosis. A friction rub, which sounds like rubbing your dry fingers together, may be heard over the liver (perihepatitis) or spleen (perisplenitis). An audible splash more than 4 hours after the patient has eaten or drunk anything indicates delayed gastric emptying, e.g. pyloric stenosis.

Hernias

Hernias are common and typically occur at openings of the abdominal wall, e.g. the inguinal, femoral and obturator canals, the umbilicus and the oesophageal hiatus. They may occur at sites of weakness of the abdominal wall or be related to previous surgical incisions.

An external abdominal hernia is an abnormal protrusion of bowel and/or omentum from the abdominal cavity. External hernias are more obvious when the pressure within the abdomen rises, e.g. when the patient is standing, coughing or straining at stool. Internal hernias occur through defects of the mesentery or into the retroperitoneal space and are not visible.

An impulse can often be felt in a hernia during coughing (cough impulse). Identify a hernia from its anatomical site and characteristics, and attempt to differentiate between direct and indirect inguinal types (Box 8.39).

Anatomy

The inguinal canal extends from the pubic tubercle to the anterior superior iliac spine (Fig. 8.21). It has an internal ring at the mid-inguinal point and an external ring at the pubic tubercle. The mid-inguinal point is midway between the pubic symphysis and the anterior superior iliac spine, not at the midpoint of the inguinal ligament. The femoral canal lies below the inguinal ligament and lateral to the pubic tubercle.

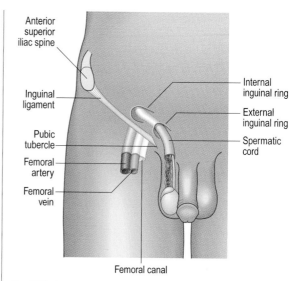

Fig. 8.21 Anatomy of the inguinal canal and femoral sheath.

 8.39 Causes of palpable swellings in the groin

- Inguinal hernia: indirect and direct
- Femoral hernia
- Lymph node(s)
- Saphena varix (a varicosity of the long saphenous vein)
- Skin and subcutaneous lumps, e.g. lipoma, sebaceous cyst
- Hydrocoele of spermatic cord
- Undescended testis
- Femoral aneurysm
- Psoas abscess

History

Groin hernias frequently present with a dull dragging discomfort, rather than acute pain, which is often exacerbated by straining. A swelling or lump in the groin may be the only presenting feature. Ask the patient about precipitating/exacerbating factors such as straining, e.g. due to chronic constipation, chronic cough, heavy manual labour, straining at micturition. Typically symptoms are worse at the end of a day when the patient has been standing or active for a prolonged period. Often patients can manually reduce the hernia by gentle pressure over the swelling or by lying flat.

Examination sequence

- Examine the groin with the patient standing upright.
- Inspect the inguinal and femoral canals and the scrotum for any lumps or bulges.
- Ask the patient to cough; look for an impulse over the femoral or inguinal canals and scrotum.
- Identify the anatomical relationships between the bulge, the pubic tubercle and the inguinal ligament to distinguish a femoral from an inguinal hernia.
- Palpate the external inguinal ring and along the inguinal canal for possible muscle defects. Ask the patient to cough and feel for a cough impulse.
- Now ask the patient to lie down and establish whether the hernia reduces spontaneously.

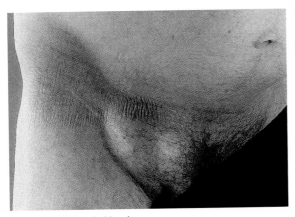

Fig. 8.22 Right inguinal hernia.

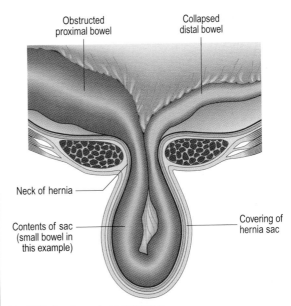

Fig. 8.23 Hernia: anatomical structure.

Labels on Fig. 8.23: Obstructed proximal bowel · Collapsed distal bowel · Neck of hernia · Contents of sac (small bowel in this example) · Covering of hernia sac

- If so, press two fingers over the internal inguinal ring at the mid-inguinal point and ask the patient to cough or stand up while you maintain pressure over the internal inguinal ring. If the hernia reappears, it is a direct hernia. If it can be prevented from reappearing, it is an indirect inguinal hernia.
- Examine the opposite side to exclude the possibility of asymptomatic hernias.

Abnormal findings

An indirect inguinal hernia bulges through the internal ring and follows the course of the inguinal canal. It may extend beyond the external ring and enter the scrotum. Indirect hernias comprise 85% of all hernias and are more common in younger men.

A direct inguinal hernia forms at a site of muscle weakness in the posterior wall of the inguinal canal and rarely extends into the scrotum. It is more common in older men and women (Fig. 8.22).

A femoral hernia projects through the femoral ring and into the femoral canal.

Inguinal hernias are palpable above and medial to the pubic tubercle. Femoral hernias are palpable below the inguinal ligament and lateral to the pubic tubercle.

In a reducible hernia the contents can be returned to the abdominal cavity, spontaneously or by manipulation; if they cannot, the hernia is irreducible. An abdominal hernia has a covering sac of peritoneum and the neck of the hernia is a common site of compression of the contents (Fig. 8.23). If bowel is contained within the hernia, obstruction may occur. If the blood supply to the contents of the hernia (bowel or omentum) is restricted, the hernia is strangulated. It is tense and tender and has no cough impulse; there may be bowel obstruction and, later, signs of sepsis and shock. A strangulated hernia is a surgical emergency and, untreated, will lead to bowel infarction and peritonitis.

Rectal examination

Digital examination of the rectum is important (Box 8.40). Do not avoid it because you or the patient finds it disagreeable.

8.40 Indications for rectal examination

Alimentary

- Suspected appendicitis, pelvic abscess, peritonitis, lower abdominal pain
- Diarrhoea, constipation, tenesmus or anorectal pain
- Rectal bleeding or iron deficiency anaemia
- Unexplained weight loss
- Bimanual examination of lower abdominal mass for diagnosis or staging
- Malignancies of unknown origin

Genitourinary

- Assessment of the prostate in prostatism or suspected prostatic cancer
- Dysuria, frequency, haematuria, epididymo-orchitis
- Instead of vaginal examination in patients where this would be inappropriate

Miscellaneous

- Unexplained bone pain, backache or lumbosacral nerve root pain
- Pyrexia of unknown origin
- Abdominal, pelvic or spinal trauma

Anatomy

The normal rectum is usually empty and smooth-walled, with the coccyx and sacrum lying posteriorly. In the male, anterior to the rectum from below upwards, lie the membranous urethra, the prostate and the base of the bladder. The normal prostate is smooth and has a firm consistency, with lateral lobes and a median groove between them. In the female, the vagina and cervix lie anteriorly. The upper end of the anal canal is marked by the puborectalis muscle, which is readily palpable and contracts as a reflex action on coughing or on conscious contraction by the patient. Beyond the anal canal, the rectum passes upwards and backwards along the curve of the sacrum.

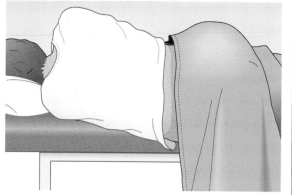

Fig. 8.24 The correct position of the patient before a rectal examination.

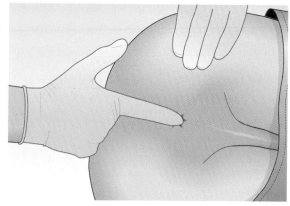

Fig. 8.25 Rectal examination. The correct method to insert your index finger in rectal examination.

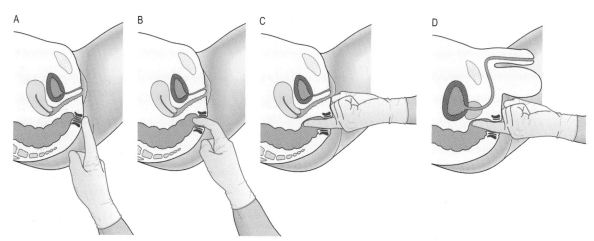

Fig. 8.26 Examination of the rectum. (A and B) Insert your finger, then rotate your hand. (C) The most prominent feature in the female is the cervix. (D) The most prominent feature in the male is the prostate.

Spasm of the external anal sphincter is common in anxious patients. When associated with local pain, it is probably due to an anal fissure (a mucosal tear). If you suspect an anal fissure, give the patient a local anaesthetic suppository 10 minutes before the examination to reduce the pain and spasm and to aid examination.

Examination sequence

- Explain what you are going to do, why it is necessary and ask for permission to proceed. Tell the patient that the examination may be uncomfortable but should not be painful.
- Offer a chaperone; record if this is refused. Record the name of the chaperone.
- Position the patient in the left lateral position with his buttocks at the edge of the couch, his knees drawn up to his chest and his heels clear of his perineum (Fig. 8.24).
- Put on gloves and examine the perianal skin, using an effective light source.
- Look for skin lesions, external haemorrhoids and fistulae.
- Lubricate your index finger with water-based gel.

- Place the pulp of your forefinger on the anal margin and apply steady pressure on the sphincter to push your finger gently through the anal canal into the rectum (Fig. 8.25).
- If anal spasm occurs, ask the patient to breathe in deeply and relax. If necessary insert a local anaesthetic suppository before trying again. If pain persists, examination under general anaesthesia may be necessary.
- Ask the patient to squeeze your finger with his anal muscles and note any weakness of sphincter contraction.
- Palpate systematically around the entire rectum; note any abnormality and examine any mass. Record the percentage of the rectal circumference involved by disease and its distance from the anus (Fig. 8.26).
- Identify the uterine cervix in women and the prostate in men; assess the size, shape and consistency of the prostate and note any tenderness.
- If the rectum contains faeces and you are in doubt about palpable masses, repeat the examination after the patient has defecated.
- Slowly withdraw your finger. Examine it for stool colour and the presence of blood or mucus (Box 8.41).

8.41 Causes of abnormal stool appearance

Stool appearance	Cause
Abnormally pale	Biliary obstruction
Pale and greasy	Steatorrhoea
Black and tarry (melaena)	Bleeding from the upper gastrointestinal tract
Grey/black	Oral iron or bismuth therapy
Silvery	Steatorrhoea plus upper gastrointestinal bleeding, e.g. pancreatic cancer
Fresh blood in or on stool	Large-bowel, rectal or anal bleeding
Stool mixed with pus	Infective colitis or inflammatory bowel disease
Ricewater stool (watery with mucus and cell debris)	Cholera

Abnormal findings

Haemorrhoids ('piles', congested venous plexuses around the anal canal) are only palpable if thrombosed. In patients with chronic constipation the rectum is often loaded with faeces. Faecal masses are often palpable, should be movable and can be indented. In women, a retroverted uterus and the normal cervix are often palpable through the anterior rectal wall and a vaginal tampon may be confusing. Cancer of the lower rectum is palpable as a mucosal irregularity. Obstructing cancer of the upper rectum may produce ballooning of the empty rectal cavity below. Metastases or colonic tumours within the pelvis may be mistaken for faeces and vice versa. Lateralised tenderness suggests pelvic peritonitis. Gynaecological malignancy may cause a 'frozen pelvis' with a hard, rigid feel to the pelvic organs due to extensive peritoneal disease, e.g. post-radiotherapy or metastatic cervical or ovarian cancer.

Benign prostatic hyperplasia often produces palpable symmetrical enlargement, but not if the hyperplasia is confined to the median lobe. A hard, irregular or asymmetrical gland with no palpable median groove suggests prostate cancer. Tenderness accompanied by a change in the consistency of the gland may be due to prostatitis or prostatic abscess. The prostate is abnormally small in hypogonadism.

Proctoscopy

Always undertake a digital rectal examination before visual examination of the anal canal by proctoscopy. If an examination of the rectal mucosa is required, flexible sigmoidoscopy is indicated rather than proctoscopy.

Examination sequence

- Place the patient in the left lateral position, as for digital rectal examination.
- With gloved hands, separate the buttocks with the forefinger and thumb of one hand: with your other hand, gently insert a lubricated proctoscope with its obturator in place into the anal canal and rectum in the direction of the umbilicus.
- Remove the obturator and examine the rectal mucosa carefully under good illumination, noting any abnormality.
- Carefully examine the anal canal for fissures, particularly if the patient has experienced pain during the procedure.
- Ask the patient to strain down as you slowly withdraw the instrument to detect any degree of rectal prolapse and the presence and severity of any haemorrhoids.

Abnormal findings

Proctoscopic examination of the anus and lower rectum can confirm or exclude the presence of haemorrhoids, anal fissures and rectal prolapse. Rectal mucosa looks like buccal mucosa, apart from the presence of prominent submucosal veins. During straining, haemorrhoids distend with blood and may prolapse. If the degree of protrusion is more than 3–4 cm, a rectal prolapse may be present.

THE ACUTE ABDOMEN

The majority of general surgical emergencies are patients with an 'acute abdomen'. Causes range from self-limiting conditions to severe life-threatening diseases (Box 8.42). Evaluate patients rapidly, then immediately resuscitate critically ill patients before undertaking further assessment and surgical intervention. Give parenteral opioid analgesia early to alleviate severe abdominal pain, as it will help, not hinder, clinical assessment. In a patient with undiagnosed acute abdominal pain, regularly reassess his clinical state, undertake urgent investigations and consider surgical intervention before administering repeat analgesia.

8.42 Common non-traumatic causes of the acute abdomen

Pathology	Organ	Disease
Inflammation	Appendix	Acute appendicitis
	Gallbladder	Acute cholecystitis
	Colon	Diverticulitis
	Fallopian tube	Salpingitis
	Pancreas	Acute pancreatitis
Obstruction	Intestine	Intestinal obstruction
	Gallbladder/bile duct	Biliary obstruction
	Ureter	Ureteric obstruction
	Urethra/bladder	Urinary retention
Ischaemia	Intestine	Strangulated hernia Volvulus Thromboembolism
	Ovary	Torsion of ovarian cyst
Perforation	Duodenum	Perforated peptic ulcer
	Stomach	Perforated ulcer/cancer
	Colon	Perforated diverticulum Perforated cancer
	Gallbladder	Biliary peritonitis
Rupture	Fallopian tube	Ruptured ectopic pregnancy
	Abdominal aorta	Ruptured aneurysm

8

Patients may be so occupied by recent and severe symptoms that they forget important details of the history unless you ask them directly (Box 8.43). Ask family or friends for additional information if severe pain, shock or altered consciousness makes it difficult to obtain an accurate history from the patient. Note any past history which may be relevant, e.g. acute perforation in a patient with known diverticular disease. Remember that disease outside the abdomen, e.g. myocardial infarction, pneumonia, diabetic ketoacidosis or herpes zoster, may present with acute abdominal pain (Box 8.5). Abdominal signs may be masked in patients taking steroids, immunosuppressants or anti-inflammatory drugs, in alcohol intoxication or in altered states of consciousness (Boxes 8.44 and 8.45).

INVESTIGATIONS

See Box 8.46 and Figures 8.29-33.

Stool

The stool can be tested for faecal occult blood (FOB). A positive FOB is produced by any gastrointestinal haemorrhage, e.g. bleeding peptic ulcer, colorectal cancer and inflammatory bowel disease. FOB tests are sensitive but not specific; false-positive tests occur after vigorous tooth brushing or after eating rare steak or other red meat. False-negative tests occur in patients with proven colorectal or gastric cancers, chronic upper

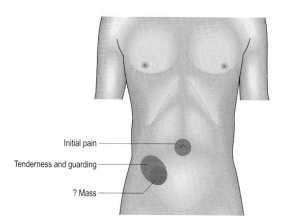

Initial pain ——

Tenderness and guarding ——

? Mass ——

Fig. 8.27 Acute appendicitis.

8.43 Typical clinical features in patients with an 'acute abdomen'

Condition	History	Examination
Acute appendicitis	Nausea, vomiting, central abdominal pain which later shifts to the right iliac fossa	Fever, tenderness, guarding or palpable mass in the right iliac fossa, pelvic peritonitis on rectal examination
Perforated peptic ulcer with acute peritonitis	Vomiting at onset associated with severe acute onset abdominal pain, previous history of dyspepsia, ulcer disease, NSAIDs or corticosteroid therapy	Shallow breathing with minimal abdominal wall movement, abdominal tenderness and guarding, board-like rigidity, abdominal distension and absent bowel sounds
Acute pancreatitis	Anorexia, nausea, vomiting, constant severe epigastric pain, previous alcohol abuse/cholelithiasis	Fever, periumbilical or loin bruising, epigastric tenderness, variable guarding, reduced or absent bowel sounds
Ruptured aortic aneurysm	Sudden onset of severe, tearing back/loin/abdominal pain, hypotension and past history of vascular disease and/or high blood pressure	Shock and hypotension, pulsatile, tender, abdominal mass, asymmetrical femoral pulses
Acute mesenteric ischaemia	Anorexia, nausea, vomiting, bloody diarrhoea, constant, abdominal pain, previous history of vascular disease and/or high blood pressure	Atrial fibrillation, heart failure, asymmetrical peripheral pulses, absent bowel sounds, variable tenderness and guarding
Intestinal obstruction	Colicky central abdominal pain, nausea, vomiting and constipation	Surgical scars, hernias, mass, distension, visible peristalsis, increased bowel sounds
Ruptured ectopic pregnancy	Premenopausal; delayed or missed menstrual period, hypotension, unilateral iliac fossa pain, pleuritic shoulder tip pain, 'prune juice'-like vaginal discharge	Suprapubic tenderness, periumbilical bruising, pain and tenderness on vaginal examination (cervical excitation), swelling/fullness in the fornix on vaginal examination
Pelvic inflammatory disease	Sexually active young female, previous history of sexually transmitted infection, recent gynaecological procedure, pregnancy or use of intrauterine contraceptive device, irregular menstruation, dyspareunia, lower or central abdominal pain, backache, pleuritic right upper quadrant pain (Fitz-Hugh–Curtis syndrome)	Fever, vaginal discharge, pelvic peritonitis causing tenderness on rectal examination, right upper quadrant tenderness (perihepatitis), pain/tenderness on vaginal examination (cervical excitation), swelling/fullness in the fornix on vaginal examination

8.44 Clinical signs in the 'acute abdomen'

Sign	Disease associations	Examination
Murphy's	Acute cholecystitis Sensitivity 50–97% Specificity 50–80%	As the patient takes a deep breath in, gently palpate in the right upper quadrant of the abdomen; the acutely inflamed gallbladder contacts the examining fingers, evoking pain with the arrest of inspiration
Rovsing's	Acute appendicitis Sensitivity 20–70% Specificity 40–96%	Palpation in the left iliac fossa produces pain in the right iliac fossa
Iliopsoas	Retroileal appendicitis, iliopsoas abscess, perinephric abscess	Ask the patient to flex the thigh against the resistance of your hand; a painful response indicates an inflammatory process involving the right psoas muscle
Grey–Turner's and Cullen's	Haemorrhagic pancreatitis, aortic rupture and ruptured ectopic pregnancy (see Fig. 8.28)	Bleeding into the falciform ligament; bruising develops around the umbilicus (Cullen) or in the loins (Grey–Turner)

EBE 8.45 Acute appendicitis

In adults, the absence of pain, tenderness or guarding in the right lower quadrant makes acute appendicitis unlikely.

Wagner JM, McKinney WP, Carpenter JL. In: Simel D, Rinne D (eds) The rational clinical examination. New York: JAMA and Archives Journals/McGraw-Hill Professional, 2008, pp. 53–63.

8.46 Investigations in gastrointestinal (GI) and hepatobiliary disease

Investigation	Indication/comment
Radiology	
Chest X-ray	Acute abdomen, perforated viscus, subphrenic abscess Pneumonia, free air beneath diaphragm, pleural effusion, elevated diaphragm
Abdominal X-ray	Intestinal obstruction, perforation, renal colic Fluid levels, air above the liver, urinary tract stones
Barium meal	Dysphagia, dyspepsia if gastroscopy is not possible Oesophageal obstruction (endoscopy preferable, especially if previous gastric surgery)
Small-bowel barium follow-through or MR enteroclysis	Malabsorption, subacute obstruction, unexplained GI bleeding Duodenal diverticulosis, Crohn's disease, lymphoma
Large-bowel barium enema or CT colonography	Altered bowel habit, iron deficiency anaemia, rectal bleeding. Useful in colon cancer screening, in the frail, sick patient and if colonoscopy is unsuccessful Colon cancer, inflammatory bowel disease, diverticular disease
Upper abdominal ultrasound scan	Biliary colic, jaundice, pancreatitis, malignancy Gallstones, liver metastases, cholestasis, pancreatic calcification, subphrenic abscess
Abdominal CT	Acute abdomen, suspected pancreatic or renal mass, tumour staging, abdominal aortic aneurysm Confirm or exclude metastatic disease and leaking from aortic aneurysm
MR cholangiopancreatography (MRCP)	Obstructive jaundice, acute and chronic pancreatitis
Pelvic ultrasound scan	Pelvic masses, inflammatory diseases, ectopic pregnancy, polycystic ovary syndrome Pelvic structures and abnormalities Ascitic fluid
Invasive	
Upper GI endoscopy	Dysphagia, dyspepsia, GI bleeding, gastric ulcer, malabsorption Gastric and/or duodenal biopsies are useful

Continued

8.46 Investigations in gastrointestinal (GI) and hepatobiliary disease – *cont'd*

Investigation	Indication/comment
Lower GI endoscopy (colonoscopy)	Rectal bleeding, unexplained GI bleeding, altered bowel habit Able to biopsy lesions, remove polyps
Video capsule endoscopy	Unexplained GI bleeding, small-bowel disease Vascular malformations, inflammatory bowel disease
Endoscopic retrograde cholangiopancreatography (ERCP)	Obstructive jaundice, acute and chronic pancreatitis Diagnostic and therapeutic role Stenting strictures and removing stones
Laparoscopy	Acute abdomen, chronic pelvic pain, suspected ovarian disease, peritoneal and liver disease Appendicitis, hepatic cirrhosis, ectopic pregnancy, ovarian cysts, endometriosis, pelvic inflammatory disease
Ultrasound or CT-guided aspiration cytology and biopsy	Liver metastases, intra-abdominal or retroperitoneal tumours
Liver biopsy	Parenchymal disease of liver Tissue biopsy by percutaneous, transjugular or laparoscopic route
Others	
Pancreatic function tests	Stool elastase Pancreolauryl test

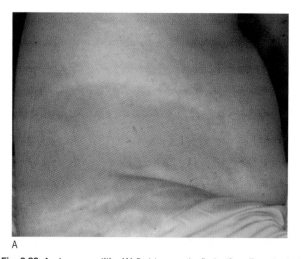
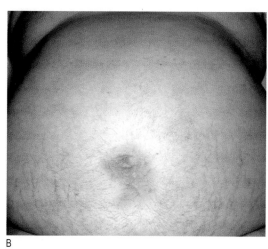

A   B

Fig. 8.28 Acute pancreatitis. (A) Bruising over the flanks (Grey–Turner's sign). **(B)** Bruising round the umbilicus (Cullen's sign).

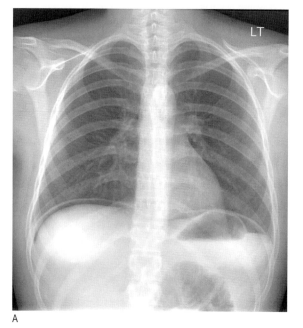
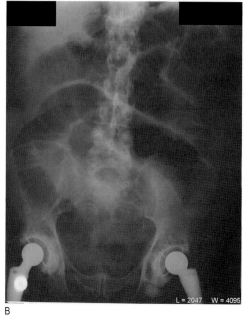

A   B

Fig. 8.29 Radiography in gastrointestinal disease. (A) Air under the diaphragm on chest X-ray due to perforated duodenal ulcer. **(B)** Dilated small bowel due to acute intestinal obstruction.

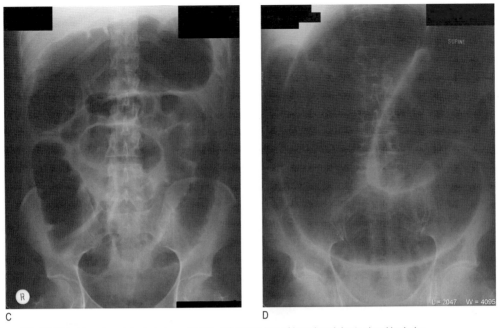

C

D

Fig. 8.29, cont'd **(C)** Dilated large bowel due to toxic megacolon. **(D)** Dilated loop of large bowel due to sigmoid volvulus.

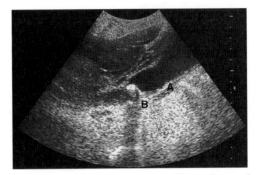

Fig. 8.30 **Ultrasound scan** showing thick-walled gallbladder **(A)** containing gallstones with posterior acoustic shadowing **(B)**.

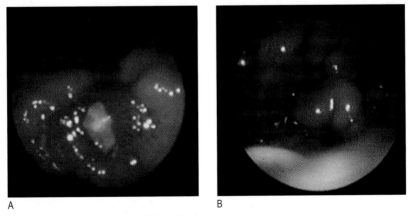

A

B

Fig. 8.31 **Gastrointestinal endoscopy. (A)** Gastric ulcer. **(B)** Gastric varices.

8

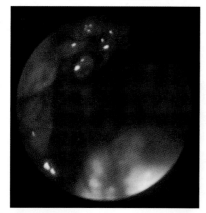

Fig. 8.32 Colonoscopy. Colon cancer.

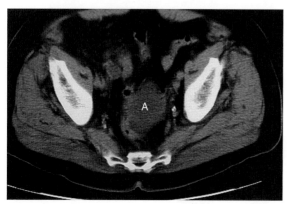

Fig. 8.33 CT of pelvis showing diverticular abscess **(A)**.

gastrointestinal haemorrhage and inflammatory bowel disease. The test has value as a population screening tool for colorectal cancer.

Urine

Test the urine for bilirubin and urobilinogen to confirm jaundice and point to its cause (Box 8.23). Urinalysis is

8.47 Severity and prognosis in cirrhosis (Child–Pugh classification)			
Score	**1**	**2**	**3**
Bilirubin (μmol/l)	<34	34–50	>50
Albumin (g/l)	>35	28–35	<28
Prothrombin time (seconds prolonged)	<4	4–6	>6
Ascites	None	Mild	Marked
Encephalopathy	None	Mild	Marked

Child A = score <7; Child B = score 7–9; Child C = score >9.

useful in diagnosing non-surgical causes of acute abdominal pain, e.g. diabetes mellitus (glucose, ketones), porphyria (porphobilinogen) and renal colic (haematuria).

Ascitic fluid

Obtain a sample of fluid for inspection and analysis from all patients with ascites (diagnostic ascitic tap or abdominal paracentesis). Use either iliac fossa at a point one-third of the distance from the anterior superior iliac spine to the umbilicus, avoiding any previous surgical scars. Insert a needle using strict aseptic technique and aspirate up to 20 ml.

Ascitic fluid is usually clear and straw-coloured. Uniformly blood-stained fluid suggests intra-abdominal malignancy. Turbid fluid may indicate a high cell count due to infection, or high protein content. Occasionally, ascitic fluid may be chylous, with a milky appearance due to a high lipid content, usually indicating lymphatic obstruction. Send the fluid for analysis of protein/albumin content, cell count and culture, cytology for malignant cells, and measurement of amylase and glucose. Measure the serum ascites albumin gradient, the difference in albumin content between serum and ascitic fluid. Values <11 g/L indicate an exudate, i.e. an inflammatory or malignant process; values >11 g/L indicate a transudate, most commonly due to cirrhosis and portal hypertension (Boxes 8.12 and 8.47).

Allan Cumming
Stephen Payne

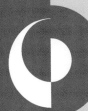

The renal system

9

RENAL EXAMINATION

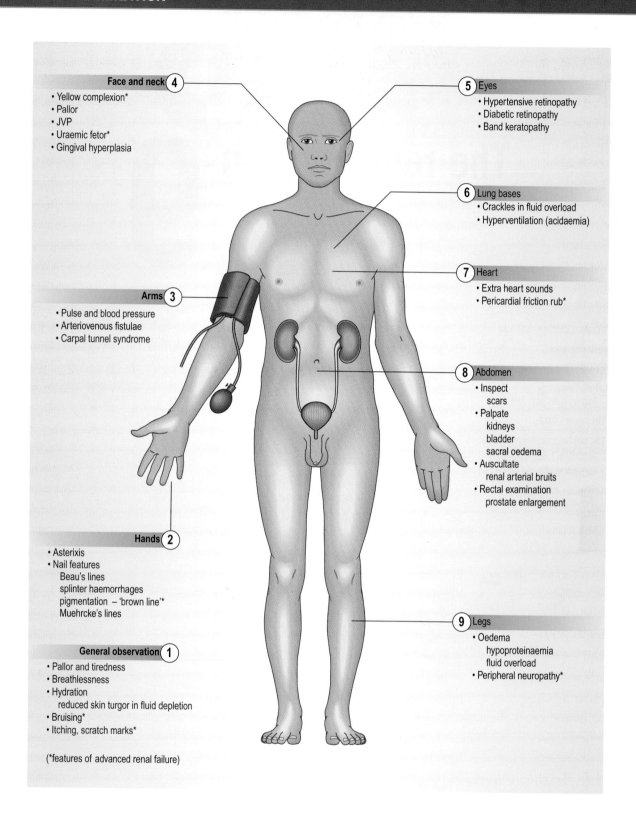

Face and neck ④
- Yellow complexion*
- Pallor
- JVP
- Uraemic fetor*
- Gingival hyperplasia

⑤ Eyes
- Hypertensive retinopathy
- Diabetic retinopathy
- Band keratopathy

⑥ Lung bases
- Crackles in fluid overload
- Hyperventilation (acidaemia)

⑦ Heart
- Extra heart sounds
- Pericardial friction rub*

Arms ③
- Pulse and blood pressure
- Arteriovenous fistulae
- Carpal tunnel syndrome

⑧ Abdomen
- Inspect
  scars
- Palpate
  kidneys
  bladder
  sacral oedema
- Auscultate
  renal arterial bruits
- Rectal examination
  prostate enlargement

Hands ②
- Asterixis
- Nail features
  Beau's lines
  splinter haemorrhages
  pigmentation – 'brown line'*
  Muehrcke's lines

General observation ①
- Pallor and tiredness
- Breathlessness
- Hydration
  reduced skin turgor in fluid depletion
- Bruising*
- Itching, scratch marks*

(*features of advanced renal failure)

⑨ Legs
- Oedema
  hypoproteinaemia
  fluid overload
- Peripheral neuropathy*

ANATOMY

The kidneys lie posteriorly in the abdomen, retroperitoneally on either side of the spine at the T12–L3 level (Fig. 9.1) and are 11–14 cm long. The right kidney lies 1.5 cm lower than the left because of the liver. The liver and spleen lie anterior to the kidneys. The kidneys move downwards during inspiration as the lungs expand.

Together, the kidneys receive ~25% of cardiac output. Each kidney contains about one million nephrons, each comprising a glomerulus, proximal tubule, loop of Henle, distal tubule and collecting duct (Fig. 9.2). Urine is formed by glomerular filtration, modified by complex processes of secretion and reabsorption in the tubules, and then enters the calyces and the renal pelvis.

The primary functions of the kidneys are:
- excretion of waste products of metabolism such as urea and creatinine
- maintaining salt, water and electrolyte homeostasis
- regulating blood pressure via the renin–angiotensin system
- endocrine functions related to erythropoiesis and vitamin D metabolism.

The renal capsule and ureter are innervated by T10–12/L1 nerve roots; pain from these structures is felt in these dermatomes (Fig. 11.28). The bladder acts as a reservoir. As it fills, it becomes ovoid, and rises out of the pelvis in the midline towards the umbilicus, behind the anterior abdominal wall. The bladder wall contains a layer of smooth muscle, the detrusor, which contracts under parasympathetic control, allowing urine to pass through the urethra (micturition). The conscious desire to micturate occurs when the bladder holds ~ 250–350 ml of urine. The male urethra runs from the bladder to the tip of the penis and has three parts: prostatic, membranous and spongiose (Fig. 9.3). The female urethra is much shorter, with the external meatus situated anterior to the vaginal orifice and behind the clitoris (Fig. 10.20). Two muscular rings acting as valves (sphincters) control micturition:
- The internal sphincter is at the bladder neck and is involuntary.
- The external sphincter surrounds the membranous urethra and is under voluntary control; it is innervated by the pudendal nerves (S2–4).

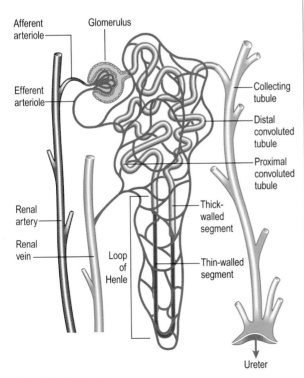

Fig. 9.1 The surface anatomy of the kidneys from the back.

Labels: Costovertebral angle, 11th rib, 12th rib, Kidney

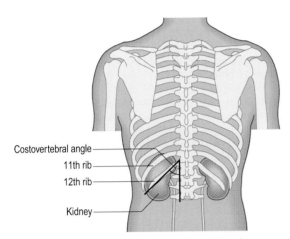

Fig. 9.2 A single nephron.

Labels: Afferent arteriole, Glomerulus, Efferent arteriole, Collecting tubule, Distal convoluted tubule, Proximal convoluted tubule, Renal artery, Thick-walled segment, Renal vein, Loop of Henle, Thin-walled segment, Ureter

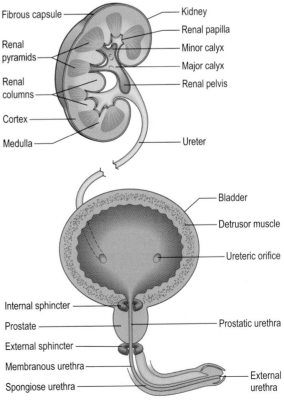

Fig. 9.3 The male urinary tract.

Labels: Fibrous capsule, Kidney, Renal papilla, Renal pyramids, Minor calyx, Major calyx, Renal columns, Renal pelvis, Cortex, Medulla, Ureter, Bladder, Detrusor muscle, Ureteric orifice, Internal sphincter, Prostate, Prostatic urethra, External sphincter, Membranous urethra, Spongiose urethra, External urethra

9

SYMPTOMS AND DEFINITIONS

Severe renal disease may be asymptomatic, or have non-specific symptoms, such as tiredness or breathlessness from renal failure or associated anaemia. Detection often follows incidental testing of blood and urine. Ask about the following symptoms, but always test urine and blood to assess renal function.

Pain

Most kidney disease is painless. However, pain may arise from the kidney capsule (loin pain), the ureter (ureteric colic) or the bladder/urethra.

Renal angle (between the 12th rib and the spine) or loin pain is due to stretching of the renal capsule or renal pelvis. Causes include infection, inflammation or mechanical obstruction. Constant loin pain, with systemic upset, fever, rigors and pain on voiding, suggests infection of the upper urinary tract and kidney (acute pyelonephritis). Chronic dull, aching loin discomfort may occur with chronic renal infection and scarring from vesicoureteric reflux, adult polycystic kidney disease (APKD) or chronic urinary tract obstruction. Chronic obstruction may, however, be painfree. Dull loin pain also occurs in renal stone disease and some forms of glomerulonephritis, e.g. IgA nephropathy. It can be difficult to distinguish between renal pain and musculoskeletal conditions, e.g. osteoarthritis of the spine.

Ureteric colic ('renal colic') is caused by acute obstruction with distension of the renal pelvis and ureter by a stone, blood clot or, rarely, a necrotic renal papilla.

- **S**ite – unilateral, in the renal angle and flank area
- **O**nset – sudden
- **C**haracter – usually very severe and sustained, may vary cyclically in intensity
- **R**adiation – may radiate to the iliac fossa, the groin and the genitalia, especially the testes
- **A**ssociated features – patient is usually restless and nauseated, and often vomits
- **T**iming – may last for several hours or even days, until the obstructing body reaches the bladder, when symptoms usually resolve
- **E**xacerbating/relieving factors – analgesia with non-steroidal anti-inflammatory drugs (NSAIDs) or opioids is required
- **S**everity – variable, but often very severe and incapacitating.
- **S**imilar – distinguish from intestinal or biliary colic, appendicitis, torsion of an ovarian cyst, ruptured ectopic pregnancy. Test the urine for blood; haematuria (visible or non-visible) is usual and, if absent, casts doubt on the diagnosis (Box 9.1).

Patients with loin pain–haematuria syndrome complain of chronic unilateral or bilateral loin discomfort of varying severity. Characteristically they have non-visible haematuria and episodic visible haematuria.

Dysuria (voiding pain) is pain during or immediately after passing urine, often described as a 'burning' sensation felt at the urethral meatus or suprapubically.

EBE **9.1 Renal colic**

In a patient with acute flank pain, loin tenderness together with microscopic haematuria strongly suggests ureterolithiasis.

Eskelinen M, Ikonen J, Lipponen P. Usefulness of history-taking, physical examination and diagnostic scoring in acute renal colic. Eur Urol 1998;34:467–473.

Strangury describes slow and painful discharge of small volumes of urine related to involuntary bladder contractions.

Frequency is a desire to pass urine more often than usual.

The most common cause of the above symptoms is infection and/or inflammation of the bladder (cystitis). Prostatitis and urethritis produce similar symptoms. Prostatitis may cause perineal and rectal pain at the same time. Pain localised to the penis indicates local pathology, e.g. an inflammatory stricture, stone or, rarely, tumour.

Testicular and epididymal pain may be felt primarily in the groin and lower abdomen. Tenderness and swelling of the testis may be due to acute epididymo-orchitis; in pubertal boys and young men consider torsion of the testis, and be careful to distinguish these conditions from a strangulated inguinal hernia (p. 187).

Voiding symptoms

Lower urinary tract symptoms may be:

- during the storage phase of micturition
- during the voiding phase of micturition
- after micturition
- with incontinence.

Storage symptoms

- Frequency – micturating more often with no increase in the total urine output.
- Urgency – a sudden strong need to pass urine. Urgency is due to either overactivity in the detrusor muscle or abnormal stretch receptor activity from the bladder (sensory urgency). Incontinence may occur.
- Nocturia – waking more than twice at night to void.

Storage symptoms are usually associated with bladder, prostate or urethral problems, e.g. lower urinary tract infection, tumour, urinary stones or obstruction from prostatic enlargement, or are a consequence of neurological disease.

Voiding phase symptoms

Hesitancy is difficulty or delay in initiating urine flow. In men over 40 this is commonly due to bladder outlet obstruction by prostatic enlargement (Box 9.2). Assess the intrusiveness of this by the International Prostate Symptom Score (IPSS) (Boxes 9.3 and 9.4). In women these symptoms suggest urethral obstruction from stenosis or in association with genital prolapse (Boxes 9.5 and 9.6).

9.2 Features of bladder outlet obstruction due to prostatic hyperplasia

- Slow flow
- Hesitancy
- Incomplete emptying (the need to pass urine again within a few minutes of micturition)
- Dribbling after micturition
- Frequency and nocturia (due to incomplete bladder emptying)
- A palpable bladder

EBE 9.3 The International Prostate Symptom Score

The International Prostate Symptom Score (IPSS) reliably assesses the severity of voiding phase symptoms in men >40 years.

Barry MJ, Fowler FJ, O'Leary MP et al. The American Urological Association symptom index for benign prostatic hyperplasia. J Urol 1992;148: 1549–1557.

9.4 International Prostate Symptom Score (IPSS)

Symptom	Not at all	Less than 1 time in 5	Less than half the time	About half the time	More than half the time	Almost always	Score
Incomplete emptying							
Over the past month, how often have you had a sensation of not emptying your bladder completely after you finish urinating?	0	1	2	3	4	5	
Frequency							
Over the past month, how often have you had to urinate again less than 2 hours after you finished urinating?	0	1	2	3	4	5	
Intermittency							
Over the past month, how often have you found you stopped and started again several times when you urinated?	0	1	2	3	4	5	
Urgency							
Over the last month, how difficult have you found it to postpone urination?	0	1	2	3	4	5	
Weak stream							
Over the past month, how often have you had a weak urinary stream?	0	1	2	3	4	5	
Straining							
Over the past month, how often have you had to push or strain to begin urination?	0	1	2	3	4	5	
Nocturia							
Over the past month, how many times did you most typically get up to urinate from the time you went to bed until the time you got up in the morning?	0	1	2	3	4	5	
Quality of life due to urinary symptoms	Delighted	Pleased	Mostly satisfied	Mixed: about equally satisfied and dissatisfied	Mostly dissatisfied	Unhappy	Terrible
If you were to spend the rest of your life with your urinary condition the way it is now, how would you feel about that?	0	1	2	3	4	5	6

Total IPSS score: 0–7, mildly symptomatic; 8–19, moderately symptomatic; 20–35, severely symptomatic.

9

9.5 Functional assessment of the lower urinary tract

Frequency/volume chart

- Use to monitor micturition patterns, including nocturia, and fluid intake
- The patient collects his urine, measures each void, and charts it against time over 3–5 days

Urine flow rate

- The patient voids into a special receptacle that measures the rate of urine passage
- A low flow does not differentiate between poor detrusor contractility and bladder outlet obstruction

Urodynamic tests

- Invasive tests, necessitating insertion of bladder and rectal catheters to measure total bladder pressure and abdominal pressure and to allow bladder filling
- Filling studies determine detrusor activity and compliance
- Low detrusor pressures with low urine flow suggest detrusor function problems
- High detrusor pressures with a low flow suggest bladder outlet obstruction

9.6 Causes of urinary incontinence

- Pelvic floor weakness following childbirth
- Pelvic surgery or radiotherapy
- Detrusor overactivity
- Bladder outlet obstruction
- Urinary tract infection
- Degenerative brain diseases and stroke
- Neurological diseases, e.g. multiple sclerosis
- Spinal cord damage

After micturition

Dribbling and incomplete emptying are caused by bladder neck obstruction, but if they are associated with storage symptoms, may indicate abnormal detrusor function.

Incontinence

Involuntary release of urine may occur with a need to void (urge incontinence), result from an increase in intra-abdominal pressure (stress incontinence) or be a combination of both (mixed incontinence) (Box 9.6). Urge incontinence occurs when the detrusor is overactive. Stress incontinence occurs in women due to weakness of the pelvic floor, usually following childbirth. Continual incontinence implies a fistula between the bladder and either the urethra or the vagina due to complications of obstetric delivery, pelvic surgery, radiotherapy, tumour or trauma. Such fistulas are a major public health problem for women in many underdeveloped countries due to inadequate obstetric care and a high incidence of impacted labour. Enuresis is incontinence during sleep, and common in childhood. In adults

it suggests bladder outlet obstruction or abnormalities of the wakening mechanism.

Abnormalities in urine volume and composition

Healthy adults produce 2–3 litres of urine per day, equivalent to their fluid intake minus insensible fluid losses through the skin and respiratory tract (500–800 ml/day).

Polyuria

Polyuria is an abnormally large volume of urine, and is most commonly due to excessive fluid intake. Rarely, this is a manifestation of psychiatric disease (psychogenic polydipsia). Polyuria also occurs when the kidneys cannot concentrate urine. Causes may be extrarenal, e.g. diuretic drugs; hyperglycaemia with glycosuria causing an osmotic diuresis; lack of arginine vasopressin (AVP) from the pituitary gland in cranial diabetes insipidus, or failure of aldosterone secretion by the adrenal gland in Addison's disease. Renal causes occur when the kidney tubules fail to reabsorb water appropriately in response to AVP. This occurs in nephrogenic diabetes insipidus, usually due to genetic mutation in the tubular AVP receptor. It may also reflect chronic tubulointerstitial damage, reflux nephropathy, analgesic nephropathy and drugs, e.g. lithium.

Oliguria

Oliguria is a reduction in urine volume to <800 ml/day. It may be appropriate with a very low fluid intake, but may also indicate loss of kidney function. The minimum urine volume needed to excrete the daily solute load varies with diet, physical activity and metabolic rate, but is at least 400 ml/day. Acute renal failure is usually associated with oliguria, although 20% of patients have non-oliguric acute renal failure.

Anuria

Anuria is the total absence of urine production. Exclude urinary tract obstruction, which may be lower (bladder neck or urethral obstruction causing acute urinary retention) or upper, e.g. a ureteric stone in a patient with a single functioning kidney.

Pneumaturia

Pneumaturia, passing gas bubbles in the urine, is rare. It may be associated with faecuria, when faeces are voided. It suggests a fistula between the bladder and the colon, from a diverticular abscess, cancer or Crohn's disease.

Haematuria

Haematuria is red blood cells in the urine arising from the kidneys or urinary tract. This may be visible (to the naked eye) or non-visible (detected on urinalysis or microscopy). Non-visible haematuria occurs in renal or urinary tract disease, especially if associated with proteinuria, hypertension, raised serum creatinine or reduced estimated glomerular filtration rate. Visible haematuria may be due to urinary tract infection with its associated symptoms but should be investigated, if painless, by upper urinary tract imaging and cystoscopy, as it may be due to cancer of the kidney, bladder

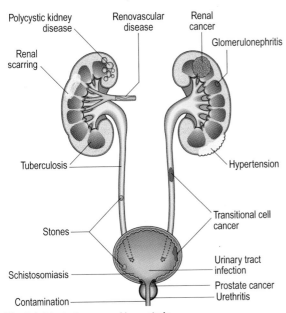

Fig. 9.4 Principal sources of haematuria.

Labels: Polycystic kidney disease, Renovascular disease, Renal cancer, Glomerulonephritis, Renal scarring, Tuberculosis, Hypertension, Stones, Transitional cell cancer, Schistosomiasis, Urinary tract infection, Prostate cancer, Contamination, Urethritis

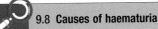

9.8 Causes of haematuria

Painless

- Glomerulonephritis
- Tumours of the kidney, ureter, bladder or prostate*
- Tuberculosis*
- Schistosomiasis*
- Hypertensive nephrosclerosis
- Interstitial nephritis (unless very acute/severe)
- Acute tubular necrosis
- Renal ischaemia (renovascular disease)
- Distance running or other severe exercise
- Coagulation disorders, anticoagulant therapy

Associated with pain

- Urinary tract infection
- Renal stones with obstruction
- Loin pain-haematuria syndrome

May be either

- Urinary tract infection
- Reflux nephropathy and renal scarring
- Adult polycystic kidney disease
- Renal stones without obstruction

*Painless provided there is no acute obstruction of the urinary tract.

9.7 Abnormalities of urine colour

Orange-brown

- Conjugated bilirubin
- Rhubarb, senna
- Concentrated normal urine, e.g. very low fluid intake
- Drugs: sulfasalazine

Red-brown

- Blood, myoglobin, free haemoglobin, porphyrins
- Beetroot, blackberries
- Drugs: rifampicin, rifabutin, clofazimine, entacapone

Brown-black

- Conjugated bilirubin
- Drugs: L-dopa, metronidazole, nitrofurantoin, chloroquine, primaquine
- Homogentisic acid (in alkaptonuria or ochronosis)

Blue-green

- Drugs/dyes, e.g. propofol, fluorescein, triamterene

9.9 Causes of proteinuria

Renal disease

- Glomerulonephritis
- Diabetes mellitus
- Amyloidosis
- Systemic lupus erythematosus
- Drugs, e.g. gold, penicillamine
- Malignancy, e.g. myeloma
- Infection

Non-renal disease

- Fever
- Severe exertion
- Severe hypertension
- Burns
- Heart failure
- Orthostatic proteinuria*

*Occurs when a patient is upright but not lying down; the first morning sample will not show proteinuria.

9.10 Causes of transient proteinuria

- Cold exposure
- Vigorous exercise
- Febrile illness
- Abdominal surgery
- Heart failure

or prostate. Investigate all patients >40 years with haematuria (visible or non-visible), because the incidence of these conditions increases with age.

Distinguish haematuria from contamination of the urine by blood from the female genital tract during menstruation. Free haemoglobin in the urine due to haemolysis, myoglobin in rhabdomyolysis and other abnormalities of urine colour may mimic haematuria (Box 9.7) but can be differentiated by urinalysis and urine microscopy (Fig. 9.4 and Box 9.8).

Proteinuria

Proteinuria is excess protein in urine and indicates kidney disease (Boxes 9.9 and 9.10). It is usually asymptomatic and detected by urinalysis. Albumin (from plasma) is the main component, although in certain conditions, e.g. myeloma, chronic lymphatic leukaemia or amyloidosis, globulins and immunoglobulin light chains (Bence Jones protein) may predominate. Suspect these conditions if the urine dipstick test is negative but other tests suggest proteinuria, since the stick reagents are albumin-specific.

Proteinuria up to 2 g/24 h is non-specific. Values greater than this indicate a glomerular abnormality, most commonly glomerulonephritis or diabetic nephropathy. Radioimmunoassay techniques can detect albumin excretion rates as low as 30 mg/day. Micro-albuminuria (30–300 mg/day) occurs early in diabetic nephropathy, and is a risk factor for myocardial infarction, stroke and venous thromboembolism.

Proteinuria may occur in normal patients with febrile illness. Orthostatic proteinuria is proteinuria <1 g/l which disappears when lying down and is occasionally found in healthy young subjects; protein is not detected in the first urine passed after sleeping recumbent overnight, but is present during the day.

Severe proteinuria may produce frothy urine. If it lowers the plasma albumin concentration enough to reduce the plasma oncotic pressure, the patient develops generalised oedema: the nephrotic syndrome.

Pruritus (itch) is a prominent symptom of advanced chronic kidney disease (CKD stage 4–5).

THE HISTORY

Presenting complaint

Ask about the reason(s) for seeking medical attention. then ask about the key symptoms above, including pain, symptoms related to micturition, any change in urine volume or appearance (Box 9.11).

Other symptoms include tiredness, breathlessness, poor appetite, sleep disturbance, restless legs, particularly at night, muscle twitching due to hypocalcaemia and, in end-stage renal disease, vomiting, diarrhoea, confusion and altered consciousness.

Growth retardation is common with CKD in childhood.

Past history

Ask about any previous history of renal system disease. Also ask about:

- hypertension (which may cause or result from renal disease)
- diabetes mellitus (associated with diabetic nephropathy and renovascular disease)
- vascular disease at other sites (which makes renovascular disease more likely)
- past history of urinary tract stones or surgery
- recurrent infections (particularly urinary infections which may be associated with renal scarring, and upper respiratory infections which may be associated with glomerulonephritis and/or vasculitis)
- anaemia (which may be due to CKD).

> **9.11 Urinary incontinence: points to cover in the history**
> - Age at onset and frequency of wetting
> - Occurrence during sleep (enuresis)
> - Any other urinary symptoms
> - Provocative factors, e.g. coughing, sneezing, exercising
> - Past medical, obstetric and surgical histories
> - Number of pads used. Are they damp, wet or soaked?
> - Impact on daily living

Drug history

Renal failure affects drug metabolism and pharmacokinetics, and drugs may adversely affect renal function.

Take a full drug history, paying particular attention to drugs which accumulate in renal failure, such as digoxin, lithium, aminoglycosides, opioids and water-soluble beta-blockers, e.g. atenolol. Drugs which may affect renal function include angiotensin-converting enzyme inhibitors, angiotensin receptor antagonists and NSAIDs. These drugs do not impair the function of normal kidneys, but further reduce glomerular filtration when the kidneys are underperfused. Ask about over-the-counter NSAIDs, which can dramatically reduce renal function in the context of systemic infection or hypovolaemia. Aminoglycosides, amphotericin, lithium, ciclosporin, tacrolimus and, in overdose, paracetamol are toxic to normal kidneys. Some drugs cause kidney failure indirectly: for example, cocaine and ecstasy can cause rhabdomyolysis and myoglobinuria leading to acute renal failure.

Family history

The most common inherited conditions are APKD (autosomal dominant) and Alport's syndrome (X-linked dominant) (Box 9.12). APKD is associated with subarachnoid haemorrhage from intracranial berry aneurysms; Alport's syndrome is associated with high-tone sensorineural deafness. Some patients with type 1 diabetes mellitus have a genetically increased susceptibility to diabetic nephropathy which may be revealed by the family history.

Social history

Find out about your patients' ideas, concerns and expectation (ICE: p. 8). End-stage renal disease requiring dialysis and/or transplantation has major implications for lifestyle, employment and relationships. Similarly, incontinence has major implications for daily living.

Smoking is a risk factor for atheromatous renal vascular disease, for nephropathy in diabetic patients and for urothelial cancers. Excess alcohol consumption is associated with hypertensive renal damage and increased incidence of IgA nephropathy.

Take a dietary history in patients with renal stones: include intake of water, calcium, e.g. milk and dairy products, and oxalate, e.g. chocolate, rhubarb, spinach and soya. Assess dietary protein intake in patients with CKD to make sure it is not excessive. Ask about salt (sodium) intake in patients with hypertension and CKD.

Some renal conditions are found in particular ethnic groups: for example, Balkan nephropathy (interstitial nephritis and urinary tract tumours, probably caused by fungal toxins in grain), systemic lupus erythematosus (SLE) with nephritis in the Far East, and severe hypertension or diabetes mellitus with renal failure in patients of African origin.

9.12 Some hereditary and congenital conditions affecting the kidneys and urinary tract

Name	Principal findings	Commonly associated abnormalities	Most common form of inheritance
Adult polycystic kidney disease	Bilateral enlarged kidneys, sometimes massive, with nodular surface	Liver cysts Intracranial berry aneurysms Mitral or aortic valve abnormalities	Autosomal dominant
Alport's syndrome	Haematuria, proteinuria, renal failure	Nerve deafness Lens and retinal abnormalities	X-linked dominant
Medullary sponge kidney	Tubular dilatation; renal stones	Other congenital abnormalities, e.g. hemihypertrophy, cardiac valve abnormalities, Marfan's syndrome	Congenital, rarely familial
Nail–patella syndrome	Proteinuria Renal failure (30%)	Nail dysplasia, patellar dysplasia or aplasia	Autosomal dominant
Cystinosis	Tubular dysfunction; renal failure	Rickets, growth retardation, retinal depigmentation and visual impairment	Autosomal recessive
Tuberous sclerosis complex	Renal cysts Renal angiolipomata	Seizures, mental retardation, facial angiofibromata, retinal lesions	Autosomal dominant
Prune-belly syndrome	Dilated bladder and urinary tract; urinary infection and renal failure	Absent abdominal wall musculature	Sporadic mutation

9.13 Kidney stones: predisposing factors

Environmental and dietary

- Low urine volumes: high ambient temperature, low fluid intake
- Diet: high protein intake, high sodium, low calcium
- High sodium excretion
- High oxalate excretion
- High urate excretion
- Low citrate excretion

Other medical conditions

- Hypercalcaemia of any cause
- Ileal disease or resection (leads to increased oxalate absorption and urinary excretion)
- Renal tubular acidosis type I (distal), e.g. in Sjögren's syndrome

Congenital and inherited conditions

- Familial hypercalciuria
- Medullary sponge kidney
- Cystinuria
- Renal tubular acidosis type I (distal)
- Primary hyperoxaluria

Occupational history

Living and working in hot conditions with more concentrated urine may predispose to renal stone formation (Box 9.13). Exposure to organic solvents may cause glomerulonephritis. Aniline dye and rubber workers have an increased incidence of urothelial cancer. Long-term exposure to lead and cadmium may cause renal damage.

THE PHYSICAL EXAMINATION

Physical examination may be normal, even with significant kidney disease.

Examination sequence

Assess the patient's general appearance and conscious level. Is he well or ill?

- Look for fatigue, pallor, breathlessness, uraemic complexion, cushingoid appearance and hirsutism.
- Measure the temperature.
- Look at the eyes for the conjunctival pallor of anaemia and across the cornea – for band keratopathy, and at the edge of the cornea – limbic calcification.
- Note any bruising or excoriation.
- Examine the hands for nail changes.
- Ask the patient to hold out the arms and fully extend the hands. Look for a coarse flapping tremor (asterixis) developing after a few seconds (Fig. 7.10).
- Smell the patient's breath for uraemic fetor.
- Assess hydration by checking skin turgor, eyeball tone, JVP and presence of oedema (p. 61).

Abnormal findings

CKD may be associated with a lemon-yellow coloration of the skin (uraemic complexion; Fig. 9.5), and bruising and excoriation secondary to pruritus (Fig. 9.6). These patients are often anaemic and have a urine-like smell on the breath (uraemic fetor). Nail changes include a brownish discoloration of the distal nail bed (Fig. 9.7), leukonychia (white nails), Muehrcke's nails (leukonychia striata; band-like pale discolorations) and Beau's lines (transverse grooves or furrows on the nail plate) in chronic hypoalbuminaemia (Fig. 4.15C).

In untreated end-stage renal disease there may be altered consciousness and asterixis (p. 148).

Note any surgically created arteriovenous (AV) fistula at the wrist or elbow which allows vascular access for haemodialysis.

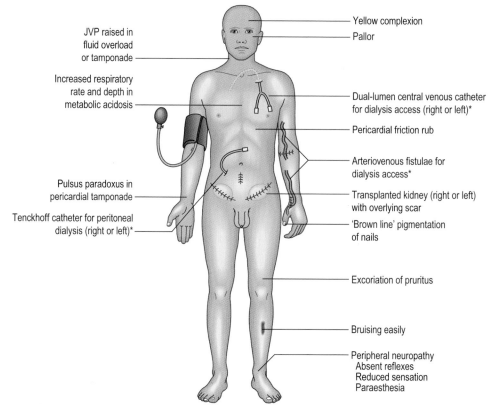

Yellow complexion

Pallor

JVP raised in
fluid overload
or tamponade

Increased respiratory
rate and depth in
metabolic acidosis

Dual-lumen central venous catheter
for dialysis access (right or left)*

Pericardial friction rub

Arteriovenous fistulae for
dialysis access*

Pulsus paradoxus in
pericardial tamponade

Transplanted kidney (right or left)
with overlying scar

Tenckhoff catheter for peritoneal
dialysis (right or left)*

'Brown line' pigmentation
of nails

Excoriation of pruritus

Bruising easily

Peripheral neuropathy
Absent reflexes
Reduced sensation
Paraesthesia

Fig. 9.5 Physical signs in chronic kidney disease. *Features of renal replacement therapy. JVP, jugular venous pressure.

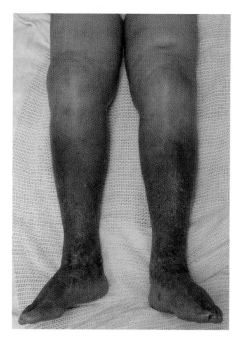

Fig. 9.6 Pruritus/excoriation in chronic kidney disease.

Drug treatment may cause abnormalities: for example, cushingoid features with steroid therapy, hirsutism and gum hypertrophy related to ciclosporin, and warts and skin cancers due to immunosuppression in patients with a renal transplant.

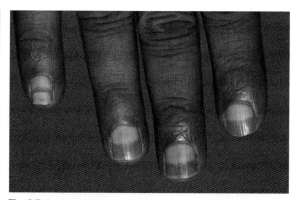

Fig. 9.7 Brown nail banding.

Abdominal examination

Examination sequence

Ask the patient to lie flat with his head on a pillow with his arms by his side to relax the abdominal muscles. Expose the abdomen fully.

Inspection

■ Look for distension (from the enlarged kidneys of APKD, or occasionally in obstructive uropathy) and suprapubically from bladder distension.

■ Look in the loins for scars of renal tract surgery and in the iliac fossae for those of transplant surgery. You may see a catheter for peritoneal dialysis or small scars left by one in the midline and hypochondrium.

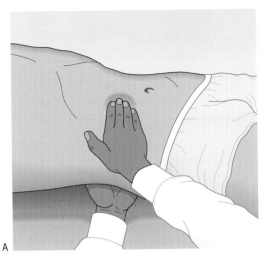

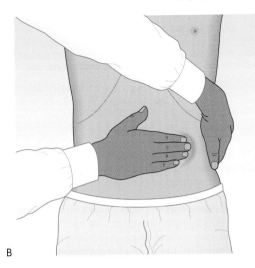

9

Fig. 9.8 **Palpation of the kidney. (A)** Right kidney. **(B)** Left kidney.

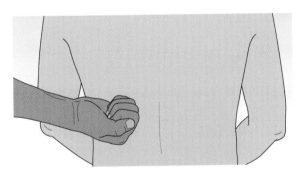

Fig. 9.9 **Assessing tenderness over the renal angles.**

Palpation

- Use the fingers of your right hand. Start in the right lower quadrant and palpate each area systematically (Fig. 8.3).
- To detect lesser degrees of kidney enlargement; place your left hand behind the patient's back below the lower ribs and your right hand anteriorly over the upper quadrant just lateral to the rectus muscle (Fig. 9.8).
- Firmly, but gently, push your hands together as the patient breathes out. Ask the patient to breathe in deeply; feel for the lower pole of the kidney moving down between your hands. If this happens, gently push the kidney back and forwards between your two hands to demonstrate its mobility. This is ballotting, and confirms that this structure is the kidney.
- If the kidney is palpable, assess its size, surface and consistency.
- Ask the patient to sit up. Palpate the renal angle (between the spine and 12th rib posteriorly) firmly but gently. If this does not cause the patient discomfort, firmly (but with moderate force only) strike the renal angle once with the ulnar aspect of your closed fist after warning the patient what to expect (Fig. 9.9) and note any discomfort.

Percussion

Percussion of the kidneys is unhelpful.

- Percuss for the bladder over a resonant area in the upper abdomen in the midline and then down towards the symphysis pubis. A change to a dull percussion note indicates the upper border of the bladder.

Auscultation

- Auscultate for bruits arising from the renal arteries. Listen carefully over both loins posteriorly and in the epigastrium, using the stethoscope diaphragm. Renal artery bruits cannot be distinguished from those in adjacent vessels, e.g. the mesenteric arteries, but any abdominal bruits, diminished or absent femoral artery pulses and bruits increase the probability of coexistent atheromatous renal artery disease.
- Test for ascites (p. 184), which may be found in nephrotic syndrome or in patients having peritoneal dialysis.
- In men examine the external genitalia and perform a rectal examination (pp. 236 and 187) to assess the prostate for benign or malignant change.
- In women, perform a vaginal examination to exclude pelvic malignancy and to assess prolapse and the integrity of the pelvic floor (p. 223).

Abnormal findings

The kidneys are normally mobile and move as much as 3 cm inferiorly during inspiration. It is usually easier to feel the right kidney, as it is lower than the left. Minor degrees of kidney enlargement are difficult to assess. In very thin subjects the lower pole of a normal right kidney may be palpable, but even very large kidneys may be impossible to feel in obese subjects. A markedly enlarged liver is difficult to differentiate from the right kidney, especially if APKD is associated with cystic disease of the liver.

Enlargement of one kidney may result from compensatory hypertrophy due to renal agenesis, hypoplasia or atrophy, or surgical removal of the other kidney. It may also be due to a renal tumour or hydronephrosis. Enlargement of both kidneys occurs in APKD, amyloidosis and in acute glomerulonephritis. A transplanted kidney is palpable as a smooth mass in either iliac fossa with an overlying scar.

Polycystic kidneys have a distinctive irregular nodular surface and vary in size from moderately enlarged to filling the whole of one side of the abdomen. Kidneys containing tumours are usually firm and irregular, and sometimes tethered to surrounding structures. Enlarged obstructed or hypertrophic kidneys have a smooth surface. Tenderness over the kidneys is most often due to acute pyelonephritis or acute urinary obstruction. A distended bladder is a smooth firm mass arising from the pelvis, which disappears after urethral catheterisation (Box 9.14).

Cardiovascular examination

Examination sequence

- Measure the pulse and blood pressure (do not use an arm with an AV fistula for blood pressure measurement; Fig. 9.10).
- Assess the JVP (Fig. 6.19).
- Palpate the apex beat (p. 117).
- Auscultate for:
  - a mid-systolic 'flow' murmur
  - third or fourth heart sounds
  - pericardial friction rub.
- Look for pitting oedema in the ankles, the sacrum, and the back of the thighs in recumbent patients (Fig. 9.11).

Abnormal findings

Blood pressure is often elevated in renal disease, but may be low with a postural drop in patients with tubulo-interstitial disease who lose sodium and water inappropriately because of impaired tubular reabsorption. Pulsus paradoxus (p. 111) may be present with pericardial tamponade due to uraemic pericarditis, along with a raised JVP and low blood pressure. In the nephrotic syndrome, although oedema is present, the JVP is not usually raised and there are no added heart sounds, as the intravascular volume is often normal or reduced.

The apex beat may be displaced in fluid overload and heart failure, or heaving in patients with left ventricular hypertrophy or secondary to hypertension. 'Flow' murmurs are common in patients with 'renal' anaemia, particularly if the cardiac output is increased because of an AV fistula. Added heart sounds occur in fluid overload and/or heart failure, and a pericardial friction rub may be present due to uraemic pericarditis.

Peripheral oedema usually signifies fluid retention and expanded extracellular fluid volume; the

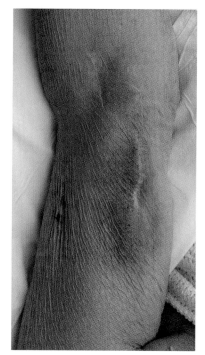

Fig. 9.10 Arteriovenous fistula showing sites of needle cannulation for haemodialysis.

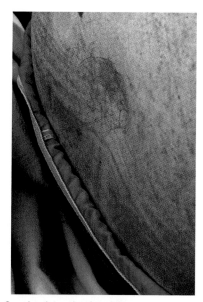

Fig. 9.11 Sacral oedema showing pitting.

exceptions are in hypoalbuminaemia (decreased capillary oncotic pressure) and the use of vasodilator drugs, e.g. calcium channel blockers (increased capillary hydrostatic pressure).

Respiratory examination

- Measure the respiratory rate (p. 143).
- Percuss the chest to detect pleural effusions.
- Auscultate for bilateral basal lung crackles indicating fluid overload or heart failure.

Abnormal findings

In CKD, respiratory compensation for the associated metabolic acidosis may lead to an increased respiratory rate and deep sighing respirations (Küssmaul respiration; p. 144). Pleural effusions may be present due to fluid overload or hypoalbuminaemia.

Nervous system

- Assess level of consciousness (Box 19.14).
- Test sensation and the tendon reflexes (p. 261).
- Examine the optic fundi (p. 291).

Abnormal findings

Altered consciousness or even coma is a feature of very advanced CKD, as is peripheral neuropathy. Retinal infarcts are seen in vasculitis or SLE, and retinopathy is an important finding in diabetes mellitus and hypertension.

PUTTING IT ALL TOGETHER

In renal disease, blood-and urine tests and appropriate imaging are essential for definitive diagnosis. Although some kidney conditions are primary, e.g. many forms of glomerulonephritis, others are secondary to systemic conditions, e.g. diabetes, autoimmune disorders and systemic vasculitis, adverse drug reactions, malignancies such as lymphoma, and infections including septicaemia.

INVESTIGATIONS

Urinalysis

Examine the urine in all patients (Boxes 9.15 and 9.16). Urine abnormalities may reflect:

- abnormally high levels of a substance in the blood exceeding the capacity for normal tubular reabsorption, e.g. glucose, ketones, conjugated bilirubin and urobilinogen (Fig. 9.12)
- altered kidney function, e.g. proteinuria, failure to concentrate urine
- abnormal contents, e.g. blood entering at any point from the kidney to the urethra.

Normal fresh urine is clear but varies in colour. Phosphates and urates may precipitate out of normal clear urine left to stand and make it cloudy. Cloudy fresh urine is usually due to the presence of leukocytes (pyuria), often with bacteria. An unusually strong fishy smell suggests urinary infection. Some foods, e.g. asparagus, impart a characteristic smell to the urine (Box 9.17).

Other investigations

Measure the 24-hour urine volume to confirm oliguria or polyuria. In critically ill patients, hourly urine flow is a good dynamic indicator of organ perfusion (Box 9.4; Boxes 9.18 and 9.19).

9.15 Uses of urinalysis

Use	Indication	Of value in:
Screening	Random	Diabetes mellitus Asymptomatic bacteriuria
	Selective	Antenatal care Hypertensive patients
Diagnosis	Primary renal disease	Glomerulonephritis
	Secondary renal disease	Bacterial endocarditis
	Non-renal disorders	Diabetes mellitus
Monitoring	Disease progression	Diabetic nephropathy
	Drug toxicity	Gold therapy
	Drug compliance	Rifampicin therapy
	Illicit drug use	Opioids, benzodiazepines

9.16 Urine dipstick test*

Investigation	Comment
Specific gravity	Reflects urine solute concentration. Varies between 1.002 and 1.035; ↑ when kidneys actively reabsorb water, e.g. fluid depletion or renal failure due to ↓ perfusion. Abnormally low values indicate failure to concentrate urine
pH	Normally 4.5–8.0. In renal tubular acidosis pH never falls <5.3 despite acidaemia
Glucose	Small amounts may be excreted by normal kidneys
Ketones	Test is specific for acetoacetate and does not detect other ketones, e.g. β-OH butyrate, acetone. Ketonuria occurs in diabetic ketoacidosis, starvation, alcohol use and very-low-carbohydrate diets
Protein	Readings > 'trace' (300 mg/L) indicate significant proteinuria. Proteinuria >2 g/day suggests glomerular disease
Blood	The test does not differentiate between haemoglobin and myoglobin. If you suspect rhabdomyolysis, measure myoglobin with specific laboratory test
Bilirubin and urobilinogen	Bilirubin not normally present. Urobilinogen may be up to 33 μmol/L in health. Abnormalities of bilirubin and urobilinogen require investigation for possible haemolysis or hepatobiliary disease
Leukocyte esterase	Indicates presence of leukocytes in urine. Seen in urinary tract infection or inflammation, stone disease and urothelial cancers
Nitrite	Most Gram-ve bacteria convert urinary nitrate to nitrite. A positive result indicates bacteriuria, but a negative result does not exclude its presence

*Use freshly passed urine (Fig. 9.12).

9

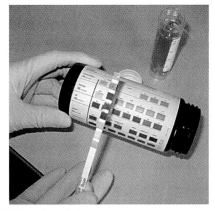

Fig. 9.12 Stix testing of urine.

EBE 9.17 **Urinary tract infection in women**

In a woman with one or more relevant symptoms (dysuria, frequency, haematuria, back pain), the probability of (culture-positive) urinary tract infection is ~50%. This increases to ~80% with a positive dipstick urinalysis for nitrite and leukocyte esterase.

Bent S, Nallamothu BK, Simel DL et al. Does this woman have an acute uncomplicated urinary tract infection? In: Simel D, Rinne D (eds) The rational clinical examination. New York: JAMA and Archives Journals/McGraw-Hill Professional, 2008, pp. 675–685.

9.18 Biochemical and serological investigations

Investigation	Indication/comment
Plasma urea/creatinine	Levels generally ↑ as GFR ↓, but values are affected by diet and muscle mass and do not measure renal function accurately
Creatinine clearance	A good measurement of GFR, but requires a 24-hr urine collection and a blood sample
Estimated glomerular filtration rate (eGFR)	Calculate the eGFR from an equation. Normal eGFR is ~100 ml/min/1.73 m^2 Chronic kidney disease (CKD) is classified on the basis of the eGFR as follows:

Stage	Description	GFR ml/min/1.73 m^2
CKD1	Kidney damage with normal or ↑ GFR	≥90
CKD2	Kidney damage with mild ↓ GFR	60–89
CKD3	Moderate ↓ GFR	30–59
CKD4	Severe ↓ GFR	15–29
CKD5	End-stage kidney disease (dialysis-requiring)	<15

Investigation	Indication/comment
Plasma electrolytes	↑ Potassium (↓ excretion) occurs in acute, and advanced chronic kidney disease ↓ Bicarbonate (↓ H$^+$ excretion) common in acute and chronic kidney disease ↓ Calcium (impaired renal vitamin D$_3$ activation) and ↑ phosphate (↓ excretion) in chronic kidney disease ↑ Urate common in chronic kidney disease (but seldom associated with gout)
Urine osmolality	The definitive measurement of renal concentrating ability in unexplained hyponatraemia. If the plasma osmolality is low, the urine osmolality should be lower still (<150 mosmol/kg); in the absence of hypovolaemia, any other finding is consistent with syndrome of inappropriate antidiuretic hormone (ADH) secretion. In patients with unexplained polyuria, test the concentrating ability of the kidneys by an overnight fluid deprivation test. In healthy subjects, urinary osmolality should rise to >800 mosmol/kg; any other finding suggests lack of ADH or renal tubular unresponsiveness to ADH
Alkaline phosphatase and parathyroid hormone	↑ In secondary hyperparathyroidism related to ↓ calcium and ↑ phosphate levels
Antinuclear factor and antineutrophil cytoplasmic antibodies (ANCA)	Systemic lupus erythematosus and vasculitis may affect the kidney

9.19 Imaging and biopsy investigations

Investigation	Indication/Comment
Plain abdominal X-ray	Assesses renal outline/size, stones (>90% are radio-opaque), gas in the urinary collecting system
Ultrasound scan	Assesses kidney size/shape/position; evidence of obstruction; renal cysts or solid lesions; stones; ureteric urine flow; gross abnormality of bladder, post-micturition residual volume Used to guide kidney biopsy
Doppler ultrasound of renal vessels	Assesses renovascular disease, renal vein thrombosis Arterial resistive index may indicate obstruction
IV urography	Haematuria; renal colic; renal mass; renal, ureteric or bladder stones; cysts; tumours; hydronephrosis NB In many hospitals IVU has been replaced by CT and other imaging forms
CT urogram	Stone disease; renal mass; ureteric obstruction; tumour staging; renal, retroperitoneal or other tumour masses or fibrosis
Angiography/CT or MR angiography	Hypertension ± renal failure, renal artery stenosis; angioplasty and/or stenting
Isotope scan	Suspected renal scarring, e.g. reflux nephropathy; diagnosis of obstruction Assessment of GFR in each kidney - measures renal uptake and excretion of radio-labelled chemicals
Renal biopsy	Used to diagnose parenchymal renal disease

9

Elaine Anderson
Colin Duncan
Jane Norman
Stephen Payne

The reproductive system

10

10 THE BREAST EXAMINATION

ANATOMY

The breasts are modified sweat glands. Pigmented skin covers the areola and the nipple, which is erectile tissue. The openings of the lactiferous ducts are on the apex of the nipple. The nipple is in the fourth intercostal space in the mid-clavicular line, but accessory breast/nipple tissue may develop anywhere down the nipple line (axilla to groin) (Figs 10.2 and 10.3). The adult breast is divided into the nipple, the areola and four quadrants, upper and lower, inner and outer, with an axillary tail projecting from the upper outer quadrant (Fig. 10.4).

The size and shape of the breasts are influenced by age, hereditary factors, sexual maturity, phase of the menstrual cycle, parity, pregnancy, lactation and general state of nutrition. Fat and stroma surrounding the glandular tissue determine the size of the breast, except during lactation, when enlargement is mostly glandular. The breast responds to fluctuations in oestrogen and progesterone levels. Swelling and tenderness are more common in the premenstrual phase. The amount of glandular tissue reduces and fat increases with age, so that the breasts are softer and more pendulous. Lactating breasts are swollen and engorged with milk, and are best examined after breastfeeding.

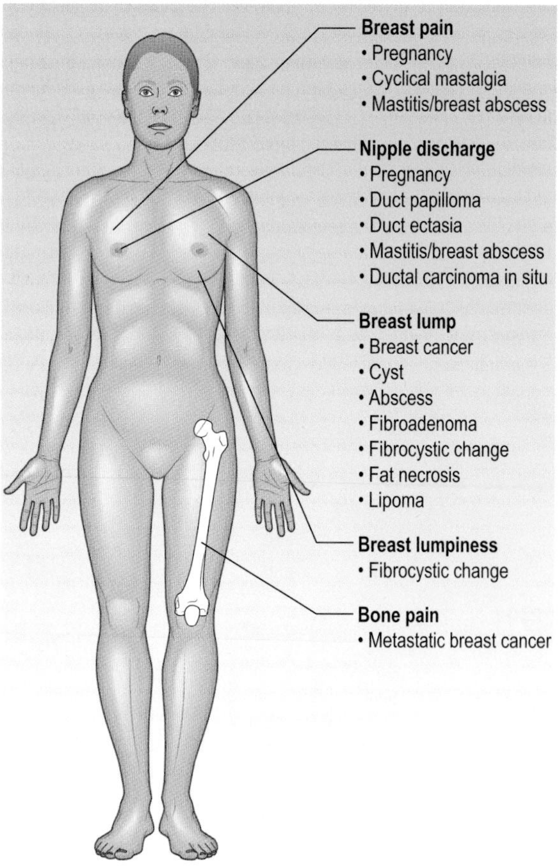

SYMPTOMS AND DEFINITIONS

Breast lump

Breast cancer

Cancers are solid masses with an irregular outline. They are usually, but not always, painless, firm and hard, contrasting in consistency with the surrounding breast tissue. The cancer may extend directly into the overlying tissues such as skin, pectoral fascia and pectoral muscle, or metastasise to regional lymph nodes or the systemic circulation. In the UK, this cancer affects 1 in 9 women. The incidence increases with age, but manage any mass

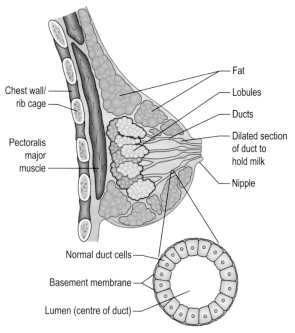

Fig. 10.2 Accessory breast tissue in the axilla.

Breast pain
- Pregnancy
- Cyclical mastalgia
- Mastitis/breast abscess

Nipple discharge
- Pregnancy
- Duct papilloma
- Duct ectasia
- Mastitis/breast abscess
- Ductal carcinoma in situ

Breast lump
- Breast cancer
- Cyst
- Abscess
- Fibroadenoma
- Fibrocystic change
- Fat necrosis
- Lipoma

Breast lumpiness
- Fibrocystic change

Bone pain
- Metastatic breast cancer

Fig. 10.1 Conditions affecting the breast.

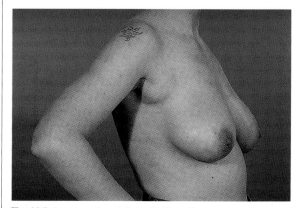

Chest wall/rib cage

Pectoralis major muscle

Fat

Lobules

Ducts

Dilated section of duct to hold milk

Nipple

Normal duct cells

Basement membrane

Lumen (centre of duct)

Fig. 10.3 Cross-section of the female breast.

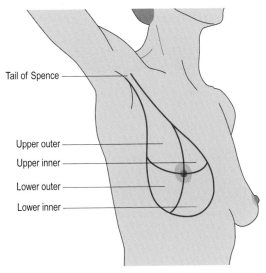

Fig. 10.4 The adult right breast.

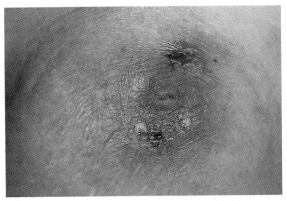

Fig. 10.5 Mamillary fistulae at the areolocutaneous border.

10

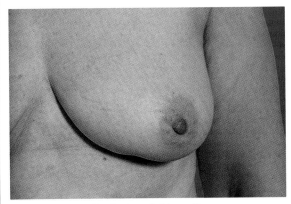

Fig. 10.6 Skin dimpling due to underlying malignancy.

as potentially malignant until proven otherwise. Cancer of the male breast is uncommon and can have a strong genetic factor.

Fibrocystic changes

Fibrocystic changes are rubbery, bilateral and benign, and most prominent premenstrually, but investigate any new focal change in young women which persists after menstruation. These changes and irregular nodularity of the breast are common, especially in the upper outer quadrant in young women.

Fibroadenomas

These smooth, mobile, discrete and rubbery lumps are the second most common cause of a breast mass in women under 35 years old. These are benign overgrowths of parts of the terminal duct lobules.

Breast cysts

These are smooth fluid-filled sacs, most common in women aged 35–55 years. They are soft and fluctuant when the sac pressure is low but hard and painful if the pressure is high. Cysts may occur in multiple clusters. Most are benign, but investigate any cyst with bloodstained aspirate or a residual mass following aspiration, or which recurs after aspiration.

Breast abscesses

There are two types:
- lactational abscesses in women who are breastfeeding, usually peripheral
- non-lactational abscesses, which occur as an extension of periductal mastitis and are usually found under the areola, often associated with nipple inversion. They usually occur in young female smokers. Occasionally, a non-lactating abscess may discharge spontaneously through a fistula, classically at the areolocutaneous border (Fig. 10.5).

 10.1 Characteristics of mastalgia

Cyclical mastalgia
- Related to the menstrual cycle; usually worse in the latter half of the cycle and relieved by the period

Non-cyclical mastalgia
- No variation

Breast pain

Most women suffer cyclical mastalgia at some stage (Box 10.1). Chest wall pain may be confused with breast pain.

Skin changes

Simple skin dimpling

The skin remains mobile over the cancer (Fig. 10.6).

Indrawing of the skin

The skin is fixed to the cancer.

Lymphoedema of the breast

The skin is swollen between the hair follicles and looks like orange peel (peau d'orange; Fig. 10.7). The most

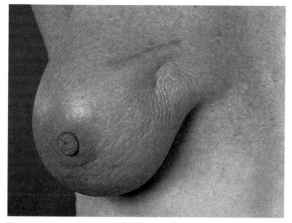

Fig. 10.7 Peau d'orange of the breast.

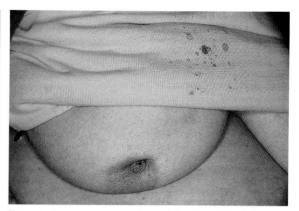

Fig. 10.9 Breast cancer presenting as indrawing of the nipple. Note the bloody discharge on the underclothing.

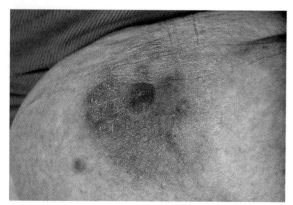

Fig. 10.8 Paget's disease of the nipple.

10.2 Nipple inversion	
Benign	
• Symmetrical	• Slit-like
Malignant	
• Asymmetrical • Distorting	• Nipple pulled to the side

common causes are infection or tumour and it may be accompanied by redness, warmth and tenderness. Investigate any 'infection' which does not respond to one course of antibiotics to exclude an inflammatory cancer. These are aggressive tumours with a poor prognosis.

Eczema of the nipple and areola

This may be part of a generalised skin disorder. If it affects the true nipple, it may be due to Paget's disease of the nipple (Fig. 10.8), or invasion of the epidermis by an intraductal cancer.

Nipple changes

Nipple inversion

Retraction of the nipple is common and is often benign; however it can be the first subtle sign of malignancy when it is usually asymmetrical (Fig. 10.9 and Box 10.2).

Nipple discharge

A small amount of fluid may be expressed from multiple ducts by massaging the breast. It may be clear, yellow, white or green in colour. Investigate persistent single duct discharge or blood-stained (macroscopic or microscopic) discharge to exclude duct ectasia, periductal mastitis, intraduct papilloma or intraduct cancer.

Galactorrhoea

Galactorrhoea is a milky discharge from multiple ducts in both breasts due to hyperprolactinaemia. It often causes hyperplasia of Montgomery's tubercles, small rounded projections covering areolar glands.

Gynaecomastia

Gynaecomastia is enlargement of the male breast and often occurs in pubertal boys. In chronic liver disease gynaecomastia is caused by high levels of circulating oestrogens which are not metabolised by the liver. Many drugs can cause breast enlargement (Box 10.3 and Fig. 10.10).

THE HISTORY

Benign and malignant conditions cause similar symptoms but benign changes are more common. Not all patients have symptoms. Women may have an abnormality on screening mammography; asymptomatic women may present with concerns about their family history. Breast cancer may present with symptoms of metastatic disease. Men may present with gynaecomastia. Explore the patient's ICE (p. 8). Women are often worried that they have breast cancer.

Presenting complaint

- How long have symptoms been present?
- What changes have occurred?
- Is there any relationship to the menstrual cycle?
- Does anything make it better or worse?

Evaluate potential risk factors (Box 10.4) and menopausal status. Use a pain chart to establish the timing of symptoms (Fig. 10.11).

THE PHYSICAL EXAMINATION

Offer a chaperone and record that person's name; if the patient declines, note this. Male doctors should always have a chaperone. Ask the patient to undress to the waist and sit upright on a well-illuminated chair or on the side of a bed.

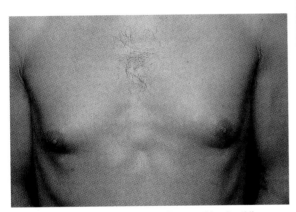

Fig. 10.10 Drug-induced gynaecomastia caused by cimetidine.

10.3 Causes of gynaecomastia

Drugs, including

- Cannabis
- Oestrogens used in treatment of prostate cancer
- Spironolactone
- Cimetidine
- Digoxin

Decreased androgen production

- Klinefelter's syndrome

Increased oestrogen levels

- Chronic liver disease
- Thyrotoxicosis
- Some adrenal tumours

10.4 Indicators of breast cancer risk*

- Female
- Increasing age
- Family history, especially if associated with:
  - Early age of onset
  - Multiple cases of breast cancer
  - Ovarian cancer
  - Male breast cancer
- Early menarche
- Nulliparity or late age of first child
- Late menopause
- Prolonged hormone replacement therapy use
- Postmenopausal obesity
- Mantle irradiation for Hodgkin's disease, especially at young age (<30 years)

*The role of the oral contraceptive pill as a major risk factor for breast cancer is still debated.

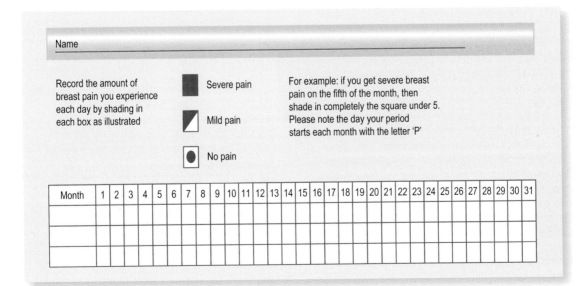

Fig. 10.11 Daily breast pain chart.

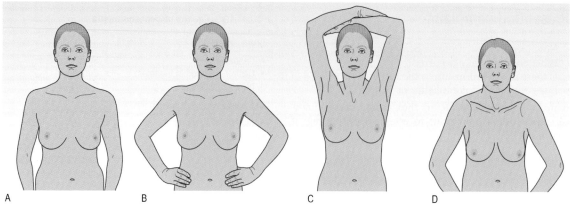

A   B   C   D

Fig. 10.12 Positions for inspecting the breasts. (A) Hands resting on thighs. **(B)** Hands pressed on to hips. **(C)** Arms above head. **(D)** Leaning forward with breasts pendulous.

Examination sequence

- Ask her to rest her hands on her thighs to relax the pectoral muscles (Fig. 10.12A).
- Face the patient and look at the breasts for:
  - asymmetry
  - local swelling
  - skin changes
  - nipple changes.
- Ask the patient to press her hands firmly on her hips to contract the pectoral muscles and inspect again (Fig. 10.12B).
- Ask her to raise her arms above her head and then lean forward to expose the whole breast and exacerbate skin dimpling (Fig. 10.12C and D).
- Ask her to lie with her head on one pillow and her hand under her head on the side to be examined (Fig. 10.13).
- Hold your hand flat to her skin and palpate the breast tissue, using the palmar surface of your middle three fingers. Compress the breast tissue firmly against her chest wall.
- View the breast as a clock face. Examine each 'hour of the clock' from the outside towards the nipple, including under the nipple (Fig. 10.14). Compare the texture of one breast with the other. Examine all the breast tissue. The breast extends from the clavicle to the upper abdomen and from the midline to the anterior border of latissimus dorsi (posterior axillary fold). Define the characteristics of any mass (Box 3.11).
- Elevate the breast with your hand to uncover dimpling overlying a tumour which may not be obvious on inspection.
- Is the mass fixed underneath? With the patient's hands on her hips, hold the mass between your thumb and forefinger. Ask her to contract and relax the pectoral muscles alternately by pushing into her hips. As the pectoral muscle contracts, note whether the mass moves with it and if it is separate when the muscle is relaxed. Infiltration suggests malignancy.
- Examine the axillary tail between your finger and thumb as it extends towards the axilla.
- Palpate the nipple by holding it gently between your index finger and thumb. Try to express any discharge. Massage the breast towards the nipple to uncover any discharge. Note the colour and consistency of any discharge, along with the

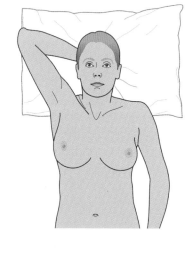

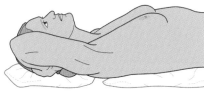

Fig. 10.13 Position for examination of the right breast.

number and position of the affected ducts. Test any nipple discharge for blood using urine-testing sticks.
- Palpate the regional lymph nodes, including the supraclavicular group. Ask the patient to sit facing you, and support the full weight of her arm at the wrist with your opposite hand. Move the flat of your other hand high into the axilla and upwards over the chest to the apex. This can be uncomfortable for patients, so warn them beforehand and check for any discomfort. Compress the contents of the axilla against the chest wall. Assess any palpable masses for:
  - size
  - consistency
  - fixation.
- Examine the supraclavicular fossa, looking for any visual abnormality. Palpate the neck from behind and systematically review all cervical lymphatic chains (p. 54).

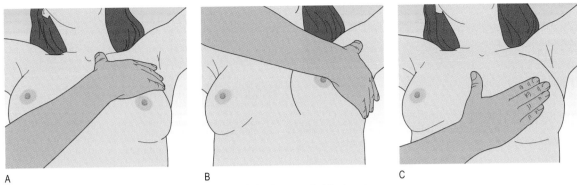

A   B   C

Fig. 10.14 Clinical examination of the breast: palpating clockwise to cover all of the breast.

10

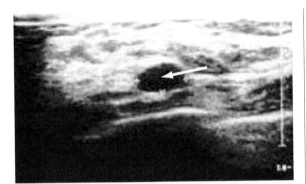

Fig. 10.15 Ultrasound of a breast cyst, showing a characteristic smooth-walled hypoechoic lesion (arrow).

10.5 Investigation of breast lumps

Investigation	Indication/comment
Ultrasound	Lump
Mammography	Not in women under 35 unless there is a strong suspicion of cancer
Magnetic resonance imaging	Dense breasts/ruptured implant
Fine-needle aspiration	Aspirate lesion using a 21 or 23 G needle
Core biopsy	To differentiate invasive or in situ cancer
Large-core vacuum-assisted core biopsy	
Open surgical biopsy	

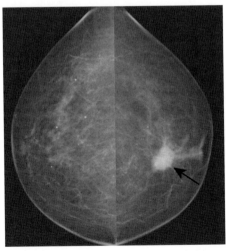

Fig. 10.16 Digital mammogram, demonstrating a spiculate opacity characteristic of a cancer.

INVESTIGATIONS

Accurate diagnosis of breast lesions depends on clinical assessment, backed up by mammography and/or breast ultrasound and pathological diagnosis, either by fine-needle aspiration cytology or core biopsy ('triple assessment') (Box 10.5 and Figs 10.15 and 10.16). Up to 5% of malignant lesions require excision biopsy for the diagnosis to be made. Magnetic resonance imaging is useful to investigate possible implant rupture, extent of cancer in a mammographically dense breast and as a screening tool in those with genetic markers – BRCA1 or 2. In the UK there are specific guidelines for the appropriate referral of patients with breast symptoms to specialist units where this assessment is carried out.

THE GYNAECOLOGICAL EXAMINATION

ANATOMY

The uterus

Pear-shaped, about 6–8 cm long, 4–6 cm wide and stabilised by the broad ligament, the uterus lies between the bladder and rectum and consists of muscular myometrium surrounding a cavity lined by endometrium (Figs 10.17 and 10.18). Ovarian hormones stimulate the endometrium to proliferate; secretion and breakdown (menstruation) follow.

The Fallopian tubes

Approximately 10 cm long, the Fallopian tubes run from the lateral border of the uterine fundus to the ovary. The distal ampulla is mobile and ends with finger-like fimbria (Fig. 10.19).

The ovaries

Oval, sitting behind and above the uterus close to the pelvic side-wall, and 1–2 × 2–3 cm, the ovaries increase in size during the follicular phase of the menstrual cycle when a dominant follicle develops.

The cervix

Connecting the uterine body to the upper vagina, this fibrous tube 2 × 3 cm has the external cervical os visible on its surface. Inside the cervix, where the single-layer epithelium changes to multilayered epithelium, is the transition zone where malignant transformation occurs (Fig. 10.20).

The vagina

The vagina is a rugged tube 10–15 cm in length with the cervix invaginating the top, forming lateral fornices on either side and anterior and posterior fornices. Two centimetres into the vagina is a ring of tissue, the remnant hymen (Fig. 10.20).

The external female genitalia

The vulva consists of labia majora – fat pads covered with hair. The labia minora are hairless skin flaps at each side of the vulval vestibule, which contains the urethral opening and the vaginal orifice. The fourchette, the posterior part of the clitoris, is anterior and usually obscured by a prepuce or hood. The perineum is the fibrous tissue; muscle and skin separate the vestibule from the anus (Fig. 10.21).

SYMPTOMS AND DEFINITIONS

Menstrual cycle

The first day of one period (menstrual bleeding) to the first day of the next lasts 22–35 days (average 28 days) with bleeding for 3–6 days. Record bleeding for 4–5 days during a cycle of 25–29 days as 4–5/25–29.

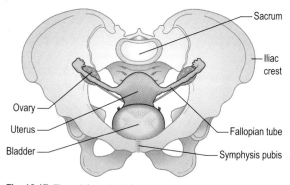

Fig. 10.17 The pelvis and pelvic organs.

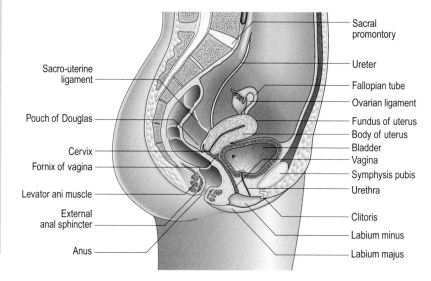

Fig. 10.18 Lateral view of the female internal genitalia, showing the relationship to the rectum and bladder.

Abnormal uterine bleeding

Heavy menstrual bleeding affects 20% of premenopausal women over 35 (Box 10.6). Average blood loss is 35 ml but is subjective. Ask how many sanitary pads and tampons the patient uses and how often she changes them overnight. Flooding, where menstrual blood soaks through protection, passing blood clots or anaemia implies heavy bleeding.

Intermenstrual bleeding and postcoital bleeding suggest cervical pathology.

Amenorrhoea is absent periods. Primary amenorrhoea is when a girl has not started her periods by 16 years old and secondary amenorrhoea is no periods for 3 months or more in a woman who has previously menstruated. The commonest cause of secondary amenorrhoea is pregnancy. Otherwise, secondary amenorrhoea is due to hypothalamic–pituitary–ovarian axis dysfunction and affects 5–7% of woman in their reproductive years (Box 10.7).

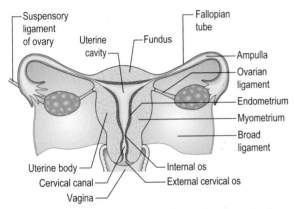

Fig. 10.19 Section through pear-shaped, muscular uterus showing the cervix, body (corpus) and fundus and the Fallopian tubes showing the ligamentous attachments of the ovary. The uterine mucosa is the endometrium. The cervical canal has an internal and an external os.

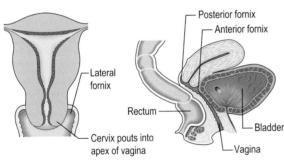

Fig. 10.20 Sagittal and coronal sections of the uterus showing vaginal fornices.

EBE 10.6 Postmenopausal bleeding
Postmenopausal bleeding occurs in 1.5% of women. It must be investigated, since 10% have endometrial cancer.
SIGN guidelines 61. Investigation of postmenopausal bleeding. Available online at: http://www.sign.ac.uk/guidelines/fulltext/61/section2.html.

10.7 Gynaecological symptoms and definitions	
Menarche	Age at first period (average in UK 12 years)
Menopause	Age at last menstrual period. Only determined retrospectively after 1 year with no periods
Perimenopause (climacteric)	The time before the menopause (2–5 years) when periods become irregular and flushes and sweats occur
Heavy menstrual bleeding	Excess blood loss (80 ml+) during a period, previously called menorrhagia
Intermenstrual bleeding	Bleeding between periods, suggesting hormonal, endometrial or cervical pathology
Postcoital bleeding	Bleeding after intercourse, suggesting cervical pathology
Postmenopausal bleeding	Bleeding more than 1 year after menopause
Primary amenorrhoea	No periods by age 16
Secondary amenorrhoea	No periods for 3 months in a woman who has previously menstruated
Oligomenorrhoea	Periods with a cycle more than 35 days

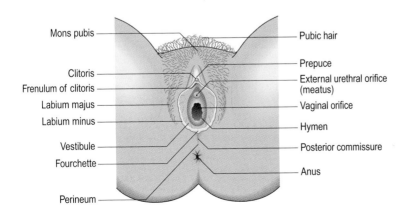

Fig. 10.21 The external female genitalia.

10

Urinary incontinence

Inappropriate and involuntary voiding of urine severely affects 10% of women, and its prevalence increases with age. Stress incontinence occurs on exertion, coughing, laughing or sneezing and is associated with pelvic floor weakness. Urge incontinence, an overwhelming desire to urinate when the bladder is not full, is due to detrusor muscle dysfunction.

Prolapse

The pelvic contents may bulge into (Fig. 10.22) or beyond (Fig. 10.23) the vagina in 30% of women. Women feel something 'coming down', particularly when standing or straining. It is associated with previous childbirth (Box 10.8).

Pain

Pain in either iliac fossa may be due to ovarian cysts, cyst conditions, e.g. haemorrhage, rupture or torsion, or diseased Fallopian tubes. Infection, pelvic adhesions and endometriosis can cause generalised pain (Boxes 10.9 and 10.10).

Vaginal discharge

This may be normal and variable during the menstrual cycle. Prior to ovulation it is clear, abundant and stretches like egg white; after ovulation it is thicker, does not stretch and is less abundant. Abnormal vaginal discharge occurs with infection. The most common non-sexually transmitted infection (caused by *Candida* species) gives a thick, white, curdy discharge often associated with marked vulval itching. Bacterial vaginosis is a common, non-sexually acquired infection, usually caused by *Gardnerella vaginalis*, producing a watery, fishy-smelling discharge. The pH of normal vaginal secretions is usually <4.5 but in bacterial vaginosis it is >5. Sexually transmitted infections (STIs) can cause discharge, vulval ulceration or pain, dysuria, lower abdominal pain and general malaise. They may also be asymptomatic.

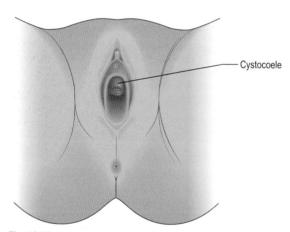

Fig. 10.22 Anterior vaginal wall prolapse.

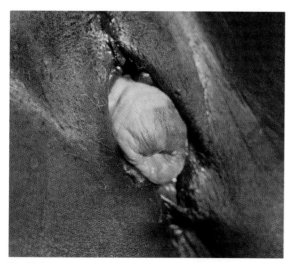

Fig. 10.23 External prolapse of the uterus.

10.8 Definitions related to prolapse

Cystocoele	Bulge of the anterior vaginal wall containing the bladder
Rectocoele	Bulge of the posterior vaginal wall containing the rectum
Enterocoele	Bulge of the distal wall posteriorly containing small bowel and peritoneum
Urethrocoele	Prolapse of the urethra into the vagina, often occurring with a cystocoele
Uterine prolapse	Grade 1 is descent halfway to the hymen, grade 2 is to the hymen and grade 3 is past the hymen within the vagina
Procidentia	External prolapse of the uterus (grade 4)
Vault prolapse	Bulge of the roof of the vagina after hysterectomy

10.9 Pelvic pain definitions

Primary dysmenorrhea	Ongoing pain during a period that is most intense just before and during a period, caused by uterine contraction
Secondary or progressive dysmenorrhea	Worsening pain that deteriorates during a period, suggesting pathology such as endometriosis or chronic infection
Ovarian torsion	Twisting of an ovarian cyst on its vascular pedicle, causing acute ischaemia
Dyspareunia	Pain with intercourse, suggesting endometriosis or pelvic adhesions
Vaginismus	Pain on penetration secondary to involuntary contraction of the pelvic floor
Mittelschmertz	Pain associated with follicle rupture during ovulation

10.10 Characteristics of pelvic pain

	Uterine pain	Ovarian pain	Adhesions or pelvic infection	Endometriosis
Site	Midline	Left or right iliac fossa	Generalised lower abdomen; more on one side	Variable
Onset	Builds up before period	Sudden, intermittent	Builds up, acute on chronic	Builds up, sudden
Character	Cramping	Gripping	Shooting, gripping	Shooting, cramping
Radiation	Lower back and upper thighs	Groin; if free fluid, to shoulder		
Associated	Bleeding from vagina	Known cyst, pregnancy, irregular cycle	Discharge, fever, past surgery	Infertility
Timing	With menstruation	May be cyclical	Acute, may be cyclical	Builds up during period
Exacerbating		Positional	Movement, examination	Intercourse Cyclical
Severity	Variable in spasms	Intense	Intense in waves	Varies

10

Pelvic masses

These can cause abdominal distension and pressure effects or be asymptomatic. The most common is a pregnant uterus. Uterine leiomyoma (fibroids) or ovarian cysts are other causes.

Dyspareunia

This is pain during intercourse, which may be felt around the entrance to the vagina (superficial) or within the pelvis. Pain due to involuntary spasm of muscles at the vaginal entrance (vaginismus) may make intercourse impossible. Persistent deep dyspareunia suggests underlying pelvic pathology. Dyspareunia can occur due to vaginal dryness following the menopause.

THE HISTORY

Presenting complaint

Ensure you understand what the woman's main problems are, how these developed, how they affect her from day to day and how she copes. She may have no specific problems and have come for a routine cervical smear. Find out her ICE (p. 8) and any previous investigations and management.

Clarify the presenting complaint and take a general gynaecological history. Always consider that she may be pregnant and ask about her last menstrual period (LMP) and whether this was normal. Ask about past and present contraceptive use as well as plans for fertility and any weight changes (Box 10.11).

People often find it difficult talking about sexual matters. It is important that you are at ease and ask questions in a straightforward and non-judgemental manner (p. 9). Do not perform a pelvic examination in someone who has not been sexually active (Box 10.12).

Past history

Ask about the patient's cervical smears, when taken and the results, along with any treatment required for abnormalities. Note any abdominal surgery, pelvic infection or previous sexually transmitted disease. Document each pregnancy, its outcome and any interventions.

Drug history

Ask about contraception. Document current or previous use of hormone replacement therapy or hormonal preparations, e.g. tamoxifen. Antibiotic use can be associated with vaginal candidiasis and some antipsychotic drugs can cause hyperprolactinaemia. Other prescribed medications may reduce the effectiveness of the contraceptive pill, e.g. women on some antiepileptic drugs require a high-dose combined oral contraceptive (Box 10.13).

Family history

Ovarian cancer can be familial and a family history of diabetes is associated with some reproductive abnormalities, such as polycystic ovarian syndrome (PCOS). Hereditary bleeding disorders can present with heavy menstrual bleeding.

Social history

Smoking, occupation and lifestyle affect many gynaecological conditions, e.g. obesity and PCOS reduce fertility.

Sexual history

The patient may find these questions embarrassing so put her at ease and be comfortable yourself about these issues. Explain why you need to ask these questions and be non-judgemental. Ask clear unambiguous questions (Box 10.12).

The sexual partners of women with STIs should be informed and treated to prevent further transmission of the infection or reinfection of the treated person. Confidentiality is paramount, so do not give information to a third party.

10.11 Menstrual history checklist

Ask about:	Information to obtain	Comment
Menarche	Age at which periods began	Not essential in older women with children
Last menstrual period	Date of the first day of the last period	If the period is late, exclude pregnancy. If the patient is menopausal, record the age at which periods stopped
Length of period	Number of days the period lasts	Normal 3–6 days
Amount of bleeding	How heavy the bleeding is each month (light, normal or heavy). Any episodes of flooding or passed clots?	If heavy, how many sanitary pads and tampons are used? Does the patient get up at night to change her sanitary protection? How many times?
Regularity of periods	Number of days between each period. Is the pattern regular or irregular?	Normal 22–35 days. Around the menopause, cycles lengthen until they stop altogether
Erratic bleeding	Bleeding between periods or after intercourse	May indicate serious underlying disease
Pain	Association with menstruation. Does the pain precede or occur during the period?	Common in early adolescence; usually no underlying pathology. Painful periods starting in older women may be associated with underlying disease
Pregnancies	Record any births, miscarriages or abortions	Some women may not disclose an abortion or baby given up for adoption
Infertility	Is the patient trying to become pregnant?	How long has she been trying to conceive?
Contraception	Record current and previous methods. Note that the patient's partner may have had a vasectomy or she may be in a same-sex relationship	Hormonal and intrauterine contraception can affect menstrual bleeding patterns
Lifestyle	Ask about weight, dieting and exercise	Rapid or extreme weight loss and excessive exercise often cause oligoamenorrhoea. Obesity causes hormonal abnormalities, menstrual changes and infertility. Acne and hirsutism may be signs of an underlying hormonal disorder

10.12 Taking a sexual history

- Are you currently in a relationship?
- How long have you been with your partner?
- Is it a sexual relationship?
- Have you had any (other) sexual partners in the last 12 months?
- How many were male? How many female?
- When did you last have sex with:
  - Your partner?
  - Anyone else?
- Do you use barrier contraception – sometimes, always or never?
- Have you ever had a sexually transmitted infection?
- Are you concerned about any sexual issues?

10.13 Methods of contraception

- Condoms
- Combined oral contraceptive pill (or combined transdermal patch)
- Progestogen-only pill ('mini pill')
- Depot progestogen injection (Depo-Provera)
- Progestogen implant (Implanon)
- Copper intrauterine device (IUD or coil)
- Progestogen-releasing intrauterine system (IUS or Mirena)
- Female barrier method: diaphragm, cervical cap or female condom
- Natural methods: rhythm method, Persona, lactational amenorrhoea
- Sterilisation: vasectomy or female sterilisation

THE PHYSICAL EXAMINATION

General examination

Assess the woman's demeanour and for signs of anaemia or evidence of weight change. In amenorrhoeic patients note any hirsuitism, acanthosis nigricans (Fig. 5.13A) or galactorrhoea. Measure blood pressure and body mass index.

Offer a female chaperone, record her name and whether the patient declines. The examination area should be private, with the equipment to hand and an adjustable light source. The woman should have an empty bladder and remove her clothing from the waist down along with any sanitary protection. Leave her in privacy to do this.

Abdominal examination

Note any masses arising from the pelvis, tenderness, ascites or inguinal lymph nodes (p. 53).

Pelvic examination

Explain what you are going to do, why it is necessary (Box 10.14) and obtain verbal consent. Use a vaginal

10.14 Reasons to carry out a vaginal examination

- To take a cervical smear
- To assess the size of a pregnant uterus (<12 weeks' gestation)
- In the presence of:
  - Suspected infection
  - Menstrual bleeding problems
  - Lower abdominal pain or dyspareunia
  - Urogenital prolapse
  - Early pregnancy problems
  - A mass arising from the pelvis

speculum to see the cervix and the vaginal walls, to carry out a cervical smear and to take swabs. Specula are metal or plastic and come in various sizes and lengths. Metal specula may be sterilised and reused. Plastic specula are always disposable. A metal speculum is cold, so warm it under the hot tap. Most women find a speculum examination mildly uncomfortable, so put a small amount of lubricating gel on the tip of each blade, even if you are carrying out a cervical smear.

Ask the patient to lie on her back on the couch, covered with a modesty sheet to the waist, with her knees bent and knees apart (Fig. 10.24).

Wash your hands and put on medical gloves.

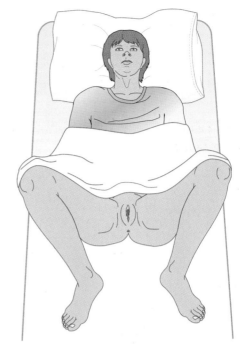

Fig. 10.24 Position for pelvic examination.

Examination sequence

- Look at the perineum for any deficiency associated with childbirth; note abnormal hair distribution and cliteromegaly (associated with hyperandrogenism) (Fig. 5.22). Note any skin abnormalities, discharge or swellings of the vulva, such as the Bartholin's glands on each side of the fourchette (Fig. 10.25).
- Ask the woman to cough and look for any prolapse or incontinence.
- Gently part the labia using your left hand (Fig. 10.26). With your right hand gently insert a lightly lubricated bivalve speculum (Figs 10.27 and 10.28A), with the blades vertical, fully into the vagina, rotating the speculum 90° so that the handles point anteriorly and the blades are now horizontal (Fig. 10.28B). A woman who has been pregnant will need a larger or longer speculum if the cervix is very posterior. If the woman finds the examination difficult, ask her to try and insert the speculum herself.
- Slowly open the blades and see the cervix between them. If you cannot see it, reinsert the speculum at a more downward angle as the cervix may be behind the posterior blade. Note any discharge or vaginal or cervical abnormalities.

  To assess prolapse:
- Ask the woman to lie on her left side and bring her knees up to her chest.
- Place a small amount of lubricating jelly on the blade of the speculum.
- Insert the blade to hold back the posterior wall.
- Ask the women to cough and look for uterine descent and the bulge of a cystocoele (Fig. 10.29).
- Repeat, using the speculum to hold back the anterior vaginal wall to see a rectocoele or enterocoele.

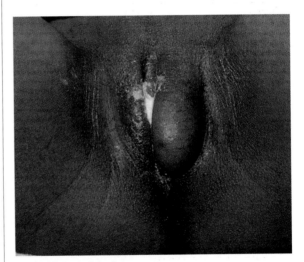

Fig. 10.25 Bartholin's abscess.

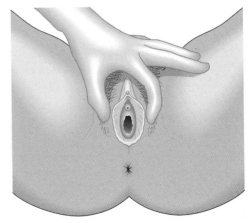

Fig. 10.26 Inspection of the vulva.

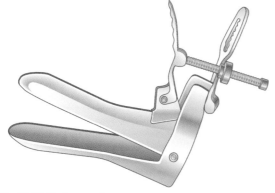

Fig. 10.27 Bivalve speculum.

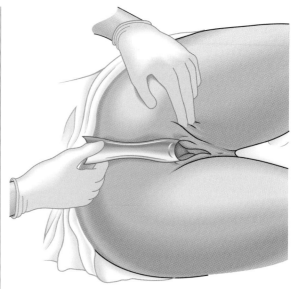

Fig. 10.29 Examination in the left lateral position using a Sims speculum.

A Using a spatula

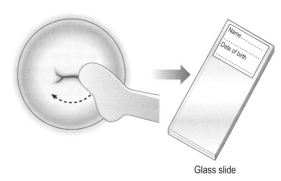

Glass slide

B Liquid-based cytology

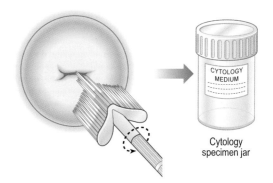

Cytology specimen jar

Fig. 10.30 Taking a cervical smear.

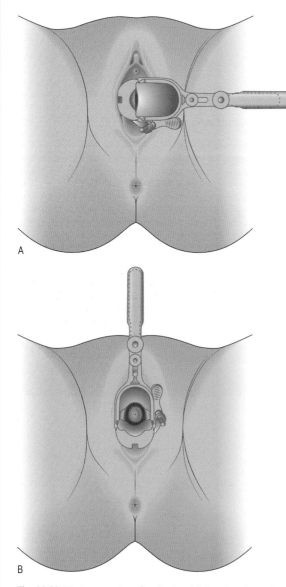

A

B

Fig. 10.28 Bivalve speculum examination. **(A)** Insertion of speculum. **(B)** Visualisation of cervix after rotation through 90°.

Taking a cervical smear

There are two ways of taking a smear:

- using a microscope slide
- using liquid-based cytology.

Liquid-based cytology allows smears to be processed more efficiently and gives a smaller percentage of inadequate smears. Always label the microscope slide (in pencil) or the vial of cytological medium with the woman's details before examining her so you do not mix up specimens (Fig. 10.30).

Examination sequence

- Label the cytological medium or slide and fill in the request form before starting the examination.
- Clearly visualise the entire cervix.
- For a conventional smear, insert the longer blade of the spatula into the cervical os.
- Rotate the spatula through 360°.
- Spread once across the glass slide.
- Place the slide immediately into fixative (methylated spirits) for 3–4 minutes.
- Remove it and leave it to dry in air.
- Insert the centre of the plastic broom into the cervical os.
- Rotate the broom five times through 360° (Fig. 10.30).
- Push the brush 10 times against the bottom of the specimen container.
- Twirl five times through 360° to dislodge the sample.
- Firmly close the lid.

Bimanual examination

- Apply lubricating gel to your right index and middle finger.
- Gently insert them into the vagina and feel for the firm cervix. The uterus is usually anteverted (Fig. 10.31A) and you feel its firmness anterior to the cervix. If the uterus is retroverted (15%) and lying over the bowel, feel the firmness posterior to the cervix (Fig. 10.31B).
- Push your fingers into the posterior fornix and lift the uterus while pushing on the abdomen with your left hand.
- Place your left hand above the umbilicus and bring it down, palpating the uterus between both hands and note its size, regularity and any discomfort (Fig. 10.32).
- Move your fingers to the lateral fornix and, with your left hand above and lateral to the umbilicus, bring it down to assess any adnexal masses between your hands on each side (Fig. 10.33).
- If stress incontinence occurs when the patient coughs, try lifting the anterior vaginal wall with your fingers and asking her to cough again. This stops genuine stress incontinence.

Normal findings

The cervix os may be a slit after childbirth. Vaginal squamous epithelium and the endocervical columnar epithelium meet on the cervix. The position of this squamocolumnar junction varies throughout reproductive life and so the cervix can look very different in individual women. The transition zone may be seen on the cervix. This is called an ectropion and looks red and friable; there may be small cysts called nabothian follicles.

The uterus should feel regular and be mobile and the size of a plum. The Fallopian tubes cannot be felt and normal ovaries are only palpated in very slim women.

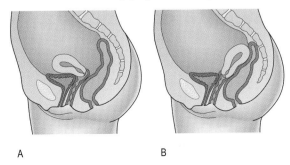

A   B

Fig. 10.31 Coronal section showing: (A) Anteverted uterus. **(B)** Retroverted uterus.

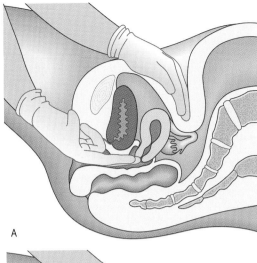

A

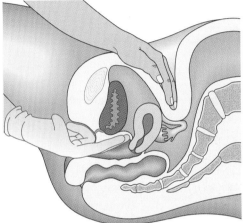

B

Fig. 10.32 Bimanual examination of the uterus. (A) Use your vaginal fingers to push the cervix back and upwards, and feel the fundus with your abdominal hand. **(B)** Then move your vaginal fingers into the anterior fornix and palpate the anterior surface of the uterus, holding it in position with your abdominal hand.

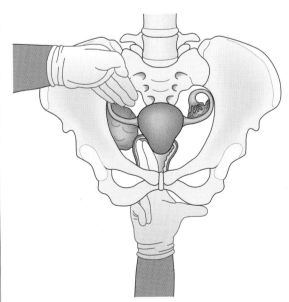

Fig. 10.33 Palpating an adnexal mass.

10

Abnormal findings

Vulval changes include specific skin disease and infections such as herpes, thrush or malignancy. Visual abnormalities of the cervix such as ulceration or bleeding suggest cervical pathology, including polyps or malignancy. Tender nodules in the posterior fornix suggest endometriosis, and both endometriosis and pelvic adhesions cause fixation of the uterus. Acute pain when touching the cervix (cervical excitation) suggests an acute pelvic condition such as infection, cyst accident or tubal rupture.

Fibroids can cause uterine irregularity and enlargement. The size is related to that of the uterus in pregnancy. A tangerine-sized uterus is 6 weeks, an apple 8 weeks, an orange 10 weeks and a grapefruit 12 weeks.

It is hard to tell whether a large midline mass is ovarian or uterine. Push the mass upwards with your left hand and feel the cervix with your right hand. A mass which moves without the cervix suggests an ovarian mass.

INVESTIGATIONS

See Figures 10.33-35. Always consider carrying out a pregnancy test even if the woman says she cannot be pregnant (Box 10.15).

10.15 Investigations in gynaecological disease

Full blood count	Heavy menstrual bleeding
White blood cell count	Pelvic infection
C-reactive protein	Pelvic infection
Renal and liver function tests	Pelvic masses
Gonadotrophins, sex steroids, prolactin	Ovarian dysfunction
High vaginal swab	Pelvic and vaginal infections
Midstream urine	Urinary infection
Endocervical swab	Chlamydia or gonorrhoea
Biopsy	Vulva, vagina and cervix
Pipelle biopsy	Endometrial biopsy
Transabdominal or transvaginal ultrasound	Assess pelvic organs
X-ray	Assess tubal patency
Hysteroscopy	Intrauterine pathology
Laparoscopy	Pelvic visualisation and intervention
Urodynamic studies	Stress and urge incontinence
Colposcopy	Assess cervix for premalignant changes

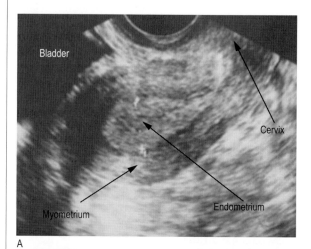

A

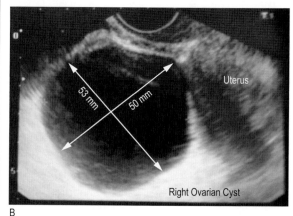

B

Fig. 10.35 Pelvic ultrasound: (A) Transvaginal scan of the uterus. **(B)** Scan of ovarian cyst.

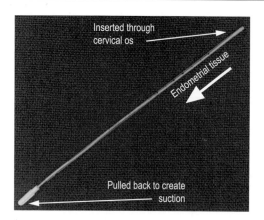

Fig. 10.34 Pipelle for endometrial biopsy.

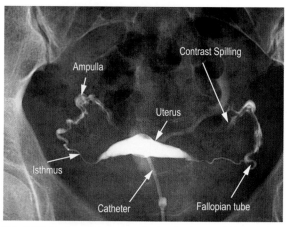

Fig. 10.36 Hysterosalpingogram showing the uterus and bilateral tubal patency.

THE OBSTETRIC EXAMINATION

ANATOMY

The size of the uterus increases as pregnancy advances (Fig. 10.37). At 20 weeks, the uterine fundus is at the umbilicus; by 36 weeks it reaches the xiphisternum. The distance from the pubic symphysis to the top of the uterine fundus is the symphyseal fundal height (SFH). If the baby is growing well, the SFH in centimetres approximates to the duration of pregnancy in weeks.

SYMPTOMS AND DEFINITIONS

Last menstrual period

This is the first date of the LMP.

Estimated date of delivery (EDD)

This is the date that the baby is 'due' to deliver, 40 weeks from the first day of the LMP.

To calculate the EDD: add 1 year and 7 days and subtract 3 months from the date of the LMP. So, if the date of the LMP was 28 August 2013, the EDD is 4 June 2014.

However, only a very small proportion of babies deliver on the exact EDD; the majority deliver from 37 to 42 weeks' gestation. The EDD is most accurately estimated from ultrasound measurement of fetal crown, rump length or head circumference in the first trimester of pregnancy.

Parity

The number of previous births is written in the format 'para $x + y$'. x is the number of live births and any births over 24 weeks' gestation. y is the number of births before 24 weeks of pregnancy of babies who did not show any signs of life, all ectopic pregnancies, miscarriages and terminations of pregnancy before 24 weeks' gestation. For example, a woman who has had one baby

by caesarean section at 39 weeks, a termination of pregnancy at 12 weeks and an ectopic pregnancy at 8 weeks is para 1 + 2. A woman is 'parous' if she has had one or more live births or births over 24 weeks (Box 10.16).

Gestation

The number of weeks that the woman has been pregnant is the gestation. It is counted from the LMP and expressed in weeks plus days, e.g. 24 + 6. Pregnancy is dated from the LMP for convenience. Fertilisation and implantation do not occur until after ovulation. Ovulation occurs 14 days before the next LMP. For example, a woman with a 28-day cycle ovulates on day 14 but a woman with a 32-day cycle ovulates on day 18.

The 40 weeks of a pregnancy are divided into first, second and third trimesters.

The lie

This describes the longitudinal axis of the fetus related to the longitudinal axis of the mother's uterus. Most fetuses have a longitudinal lie in the third trimester (Fig. 10.38).

The presentation

This is the part of the fetus's body which is expected to deliver first. With a longitudinal lie there is either a cephalic or a breech presentation (Fig. 10.38).

Oligoamnios and polyhydramnios

These terms describe too little or excess amounts of amniotic fluid respectively.

Miscarriage

Miscarriage is the expulsion of the fetus before viability.

Live birth

Live birth is the spontaneous birth of a live baby, regardless of the length of time the baby lives for.

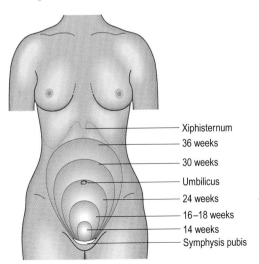

Xiphisternum
36 weeks
30 weeks
Umbilicus
24 weeks
16–18 weeks
14 weeks
Symphysis pubis

Fig. 10.37 Approximate fundal height with changing gestation.

10.16 Examples of parity	
A women who:	**Para**
is not pregnant, has had a single live birth, one miscarriage and one termination	1 + 2
has had two previous pregnancies resulting in a live birth and a stillbirth	2 + 0
is pregnant with a singleton pregnancy, has had live twins and a previous ectopic	1 + 1
is not pregnant, has had a twin pregnancy resulting in two live births	1 + 0

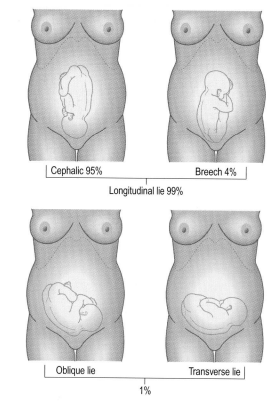

Cephalic 95%   Breech 4%

Longitudinal lie 99%

Oblique lie   Transverse lie

1%

Fig. 10.38 The lie and presentation of the fetus.

Stillbirth

The birth of a potentially viable baby who shows no signs of life is a stillbirth. In the UK it includes all births at 24 weeks' gestation and above; in Australia it includes all births at 20 weeks' gestation and above.

Viability

This describes the potential for a baby to survive after birth.

Puerperium

The 6-week period after the mother has given birth is the puerperium.

Linea nigra

Linea nigra is dark discoloration of the midline of the abdominal skin.

Striae gravidarum

Striae gravidarum are stretch marks and are normal.

Liquor

Liquor is amniotic fluid.

Fetal movements

Fetal movements are initially felt by pregnant women at 16–20 weeks' gestation. Their frequency increases until about 32 weeks to an average of 30 movements per hour and this level remains unchanged until delivery. The 'classic' fetal movement is a kick, but any perceived fetal activity counts as movement. Movements may decrease if the mother is given sedative drugs, and may not be felt if the placenta is anterior. They also may decrease with intrauterine compromise which may precede stillbirth.

Physiological symptoms

Physiological symptoms are common. Breast tenderness, often the earliest symptom of pregnancy, may occur even before a missed period. Mild dyspnoea may be due to increased respiratory drive early in pregnancy or diaphragmatic compression by the growing uterus late in pregnancy. Heartburn increases in prevalence as pregnancy advances, affecting up to three-quarters of all pregnant women by the third trimester. Constipation, urinary frequency, nausea and vomiting (which usually resolve by 16–20 weeks) and aches and pains, especially backache, carpal tunnel syndrome and pubic symphyseal discomfort, also occur.

Secondary amenorrhoea is the most obvious symptom of early pregnancy.

Bleeding in pregnancy

Bleeding in pregnancy before 24 weeks may herald a miscarriage; after 24 weeks it is called an antepartum haemorrhage.

Pre-eclampsia

Pre-eclampsia is a multifactorial syndrome associated with high blood pressure, proteinuria and placental compromise and is a significant cause of maternal and fetal morbidity. It is often asymptomatic and is detected by blood pressure monitoring and urinalysis.

Pruritus

Pruritus (itching) occurs in one-quarter of pregnant women and may rarely be associated with liver cholestasis.

Breathlessness

Breathlessness is common in pregnancy but, if associated with chest pain, consider pulmonary embolism (p. 155).

Maternal mortality

This is the death of a woman while pregnant or within 42 days of delivery, miscarriage or termination. Death can be from any cause but must be related to or aggravated (directly or indirectly) by the pregnancy or its

- Date and gestation of delivery
- Indication for and mode of delivery, e.g. spontaneous vaginal delivery, operative vaginal delivery (forceps or ventouse) or caesarean section
- Singleton or multiple pregnancy
- Any pregnancy complications (take a full history)
- Duration of first and second stage of labour
- Weight and sex of the baby
- Health at birth, mode of infant feeding
- Postnatal information about mother and baby

10.18 Examples of single-gene disorders that can be detected antenatally

Autosomal dominant

- Huntington's chorea
- Myotonic dystrophy

Autosomal recessive

- Cystic fibrosis
- Sickle cell disease
- Thalassaemia

X-linked

- Duchenne muscular dystrophy
- Haemophilia

management. Deaths from accidents or incidental causes are not included. Late maternal deaths are those occurring between 42 days and 1 year. Deaths in pregnant women from conditions that are not unique to pregnancy are remaining constant in the UK and are commoner than maternal deaths due to complications arising directly as a result of pregnancy, delivery or its management.

THE HISTORY

Take a full history at the first visit (the 'booking' visit) and establish the LMP (Box 10.17). At subsequent visits explore any new symptoms, symptoms relevant to ongoing conditions, and whether the patient feels the baby move. Remember that pregnant women can have illnesses that are not directly related to pregnancy.

Past history

Record information about each previous pregnancy (Box 10.17).

Note all past medical and surgical events. Pregnancy may adversely affect many diseases. Some conditions, e.g. asthma, may improve during pregnancy but worsen postnatally. Many illnesses adversely affect pregnancy outcome, and indirectly may cause maternal death.

Drug history

Ask about any prescribed medication, over-the-counter drugs, 'natural' remedies and illegal drugs. Find out at what gestation these drugs were taken. Advise the patient to stop smoking and abstain from alcohol. Check that she is taking 400 µg of folic acid until 12 weeks' gestation to reduce the incidence of neural tube defects, including spina bifida.

Family history

To explore possible inherited conditions, find out the full family history of both the pregnant woman and the father (Boxes 10.18 and 10.19).

Social history

Lower socioeconomic status is linked with increased perinatal and maternal mortality. Ask the patient who

10.19 Age-related risk of Down's syndrome (trisomy 21)

Maternal age	Risk
20	1 in 1500
30	1 in 900
35	1 in 400
40	1 in 100
45	1 in 30

10.20 Checklist for the obstetric history

- Age
- Parity
- Menstrual history, last menstrual period, gestation, expected date of delivery
- Presenting complaint
- Past obstetric history
- Past medical and surgical history
- Drug history
- Family history
- Social history

EBE 10.21 Antenatal booking visits

Subsequent visits: 10 visits are recommended in an uncomplicated first pregnancy, seven for subsequent pregnancies.

National Collaborating Centre for Women's and Children's Health (2008) Antenatal care. Routine care for the healthy pregnant woman. Available online at: http://www.nice.org.uk/nicemedia/live/11947/40145/40145.pdf.

her partner is, how stable the relationship is, and if she is not in a relationship, who will give her support during and after her pregnancy. Was the pregnancy planned or not? If unplanned, find out how she feels about it. Encourage her to exercise regularly and to avoid certain foods, such as tuna (high mercury content), soft cheeses (risk of *Listeria*) and liver (high vitamin A content). Domestic violence can start or escalate in pregnancy and is associated with an increased risk of maternal death.

Occupational history

Ask what her job entails and whether she plans to return to it. Use this opportunity to give her advice on the safety (or otherwise) of continuing work. Occupations

10

which involve exposure to ionising radiation have specific risks to the fetus or pregnant woman and her job profile may require modification. There is no definitive evidence of a link between heavy work and preterm labour or pre-eclampsia.

THE PHYSICAL EXAMINATION

Antenatal examinations

Booking visit

Do not perform a routine full physical examination (including breast and vaginal examination) in healthy pregnant women. It is unnecessarily intrusive and has a low sensitivity for disease identification. Calculate body mass index and fully examine any woman with poor general health. Take the blood pressure (p. 113) (Box 10.21).

Examination sequence

- Before examining the patient, measure her height and weight and ask her to empty her bladder. She should lie with her head on a low pillow, her abdomen exposed from the symphysis pubis to the xiphisternum.
- Examine women in late pregnancy in the left lateral position, 15° to the horizontal, to avoid vena caval compression, which can cause hypotension for the mother and hypoxia for the fetus.
- Note her general demeanour. Is she at ease or distressed by physical pain?
- Measure blood pressure.
- Note any scars, particularly from previous caesarean section, as well as a linea nigra and striae gravidarum. Note the swelling of the uterus arising from the pelvis and any other swellings.

Uterine examination

- Ask the patient to tell you about any tenderness and constantly observe her facial and verbal responses.

- Place the flat of your hand on the uterine swelling. Gently flex your fingers to palpate the upper and lateral edges of its firm mass. Note any tenderness, rebound or guarding outside the uterus. Palpate lightly to avoid triggering myometrial contraction which makes fetal parts difficult to feel. Avoid deep palpation of any tender areas of the uterus. Note any contractions.
- Face the woman's head. Place both your hands on either side of the fundus and feel the fetal parts. Estimate if the liquor volume is normal. Assess how far from the surface the fetal parts are. If you can only feel them on deep palpation, this implies large amounts of fluid (Fig. 10.39A).
- With your right hand on the woman's left side, feel down both sides of the uterus. The side which is fuller suggests the fetal back is on that side (Fig. 10.39B).
- Now face the woman's feet. Place your hands on either side of the uterus, with your left hand on the woman's left side, and feel the lower part of the uterus to try and identify the presenting part. Ballott the head by pushing it gently from one side to the other and feel its hardness move between your fingers (Fig. 10.39C).
- After 20 weeks measure the SFH in centimetres. With a tape measure, fix the end at the highest point on the fundus (not always in the midline) and measure to the top of the symphysis pubis. To avoid bias, place the blank side of the tape facing you, lift the tape and read the measurement on the other side.
- In late pregnancy or labour, assess whether more than 50% of the presenting part has entered the bony pelvis. This is usually the head and it is then said to be engaged (Fig. 10.40).
- Percussion of the pregnant abdomen is unnecessary.
- Listen for the fetal heart if you cannot feel fetal movements. A hand-held Doppler machine can be used from 14 weeks. From 28 weeks you can use a Pinard stethoscope over the anterior shoulder of the fetus. Face the mother's feet and place your ear against the smaller end. Take your hand away and keep the stethoscope in place using only your head. Listen for the fetal heart which sounds distant, like listening to a clock through a pillow (Fig. 10.41).
- Do not perform a vaginal examination routinely in pregnancy unless there is a specific indication.

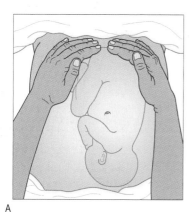
A

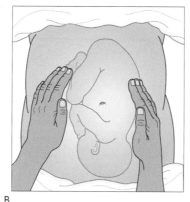
B

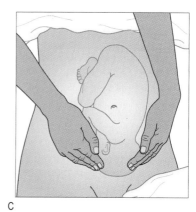
C

Fig. 10.39 Abdominal examination. (A) Palpate the fundal area to identify which pole of the fetus (breech or head) is occupying the fundus. **(B)** Slip your hands gently down the sides of the uterus to identify which side the firm back and knobbly limbs of the fetus are positioned. **(C)** Turn to face the patient's feet and slide your hands gently on the lower part of the uterus.

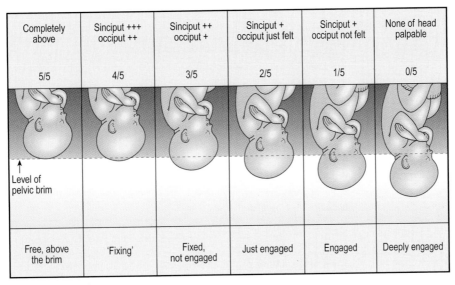

Completely above	Sinciput +++ occiput ++	Sinciput ++ occiput +	Sinciput + occiput just felt	Sinciput + occiput not felt	None of head palpable
5/5	4/5	3/5	2/5	1/5	0/5
Free, above the brim	'Fixing'	Fixed, not engaged	Just engaged	Engaged	Deeply engaged

Fig. 10.40 Descent of the fetal head.

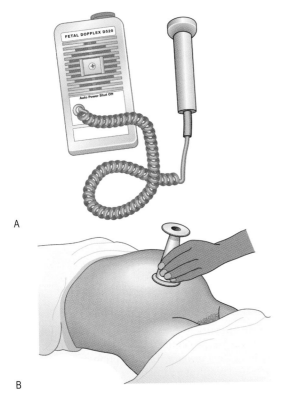

A

B

Fig. 10.41 Auscultation of the fetal heart. (A) Doppler fetal heart rate monitor. **(B)** Pinard fetal stethoscope. The fetal rate varies between 110 and 160 bpm and should be regular.

EBE 10.22 **Gestational diabetes**
The sensitivity of glycosuria in the detection of gestational diabetes is less than 30%.
NICE. Antenatal care. Routine care for healthy pregnant women. 2008. Available online at: www.nice.org.uk/CG062.

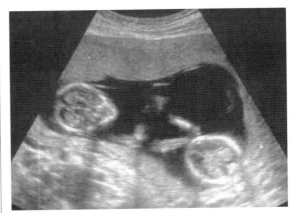

Fig. 10.42 Ultrasound scan taken at 12 weeks, showing a twin pregnancy.

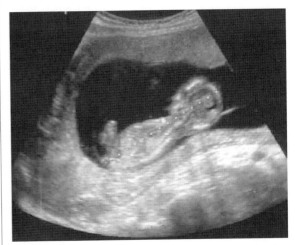

Fig. 10.43 Ultrasound scan showing fetal crown–rump measurement.

10.23 Antenatal investigations

Urinary glucose	Every visit: if persists, consider glucose tolerance test
Urinary protein	Every visit: trace or +, check midstream specimen of urine; ++ or more, consider pre-eclampsia
Full blood count	Booking, 28 weeks, 36 weeks: treat if haemoglobin level falls <105 g/L
Haemoglobin electrophoresis	Booking: sickle cell and thalassaemias. Routine for patients of mixed ethnicity
Blood grouping and antibody screen	Booking and as advised by laboratory. Rhesus and Kell most common cause of isoimmunisation
Rubella	Booking
Hepatitis B and C	Booking
Human immunodeficiency virus (HIV)	Booking (unless patient opts out)
Syphilis testing	Booking
Plasma glucose	28 weeks
Urine specimen for culture	As required
Combined biochemical screening and nuchal translucency measurement for trisomy 21	11–14 weeks: detects 80–90% of pregnancies affected by trisomy 21
First-trimester ultrasound scan	6–13 weeks: confirms viability, gestational age within 1 week, multiple pregnancy, adnexal mass
Detailed ultrasound scan	18–22 weeks: detects 90% of major congenital abnormalities
Ultrasound scan for placental site	Antepartum haemorrhage after 24 weeks: more reliable as gestation advances when lower segment forms – 1 in 4 patients have a low placenta at 20 weeks; all patients with a previous caesarean section
Ultrasound scan for growth	Clinical suspicion of poor growth, usually after 24 weeks
Amniocentesis	15 weeks for fetal karyotype: 0.5–1% risk of miscarriage
Chorionic villus biopsy	10 weeks onwards for fetal karyotype, single-gene disorders 2% risk of miscarriage

Normal findings

Abdominal organs are displaced during pregnancy so swelling may be difficult to identify, e.g. ovarian cyst, and pain and tenderness may not be in usual sites. The kidneys and liver cannot be palpated and listening for bowel sounds may be difficult in late pregnancy. In tall or thin patients, the SFH may be less than expected; in obese patients, it may be larger. Ultrasound scanning is now routinely used to assess fetal development (Figs 10.42 and 10.43).

Abnormal findings

After 25 weeks' gestation a difference of 3 or more between the number of completed weeks of pregnancy and the SFH in centimetres may suggest that the baby is small or large for dates. Investigate this with ultrasound. From 36 weeks a lie other than longitudinal is abnormal and requires further investigation or treatment. Do not routinely listen to the fetal heart unless the mother requests this.

INVESTIGATIONS

Perform dipstick urinalysis at each visit, looking for glycosuria or proteinuria. One + or more of protein may indicate a urinary tract infection or pre-eclampsia. Glycosuria requires a formal test for gestational diabetes (Boxes 10.22 and 10.23).

THE MALE GENITAL EXAMINATION

ANATOMY

The male genitalia include the testes, epididymes and seminal vesicles, penis, scrotum and prostate gland (Fig. 10.44).

The testes develop intra-abdominally near the embryonic kidneys and migrate through the inguinal canal into the scrotum, by birth. They have their own blood, lymphatic and nerve supply, so testicular problems may cause abdominal pain and tumours or inflammation may result in enlargement of the para-aortic lymph nodes. The testes lie within the scrotum separated from each other by a muscular septum; the left testis lies lower than the right. Each testis is oval and 3.5–4 cm long and covered by a fibrous layer, the tunica albuginea, which forms the posterior wall of the tunica vaginalis. This is a prolongation of the

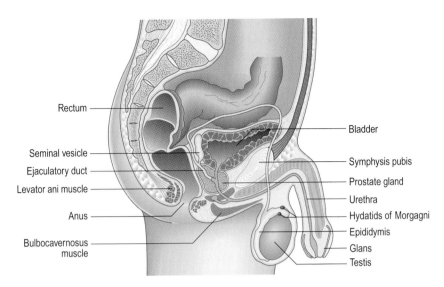

Rectum

Seminal vesicle

Ejaculatory duct

Levator ani muscle

Anus

Bulbocavernosus muscle

Bladder

Symphysis pubis

Prostate gland

Urethra

Hydatids of Morgagni

Epididymis

Glans

Testis

Fig. 10.44 Anatomy of the male genitalia. The male genitalia include the external organs, seminal vesicles and the prostate gland.

10

peritoneal tube that developmentally follows the testis down into the scrotum; if it persists, it is called the processus vaginalis and may be associated with an indirect inguinal hernial sac or cause a congenital hydrocoele. Along the posterior border of each testis the epididymis is formed by efferent tubules draining the seminiferous tubules through the rete testis. Multiple veins in the pampiniform plexus form one vein at the deep inguinal ring.

The testes produce sperm and hormones, predominantly testosterone. Sperm are produced from the germinal epithelium. They mature in the epididymis and pass down the vas deferens to the seminal vesicles for storage. They are ejaculated from the urethra, together with prostatic fluid, at orgasm. Testosterone is produced from the Leydig cells. Sperm and testosterone production commences at puberty, which occurs between 10 and 15 years of age (Fig. 15.18).

The penis has two cylinders of endothelial-lined spaces surrounded by smooth muscle, the corpora cavernosa (Fig. 10.45). These are bound with the bulbospongiosus surrounding the urethra and expanding into the glans penis. The penile skin is reflected over the glans, forming the prepuce (foreskin). The penis carries urine and semen. Sexual arousal causes a parasympathetically mediated increased blood flow into the corpora cavernosa with erection to enable vaginal penetration. Continued stimulation causes sympathetic-mediated contraction of the seminal vesicles and prostate, closure of the bladder neck and ejaculation. Following orgasm, reduction in blood inflow causes detumescence (Fig. 10.44).

The scrotum is a pouch lying posterior to the penis which contains the testes. It has thin pigmented, ridged or wrinkled skin enclosing the dartos muscle (Fig. 10.46). The dartos is highly contractile and helps to regulate the temperature of the scrotal contents. The testes are held in the scrotum as sperm production is most efficient at temperatures lower than the body.

The prostate and seminal vesicles produce a fructose-rich fluid as an energy substrate for sperm. After age 40

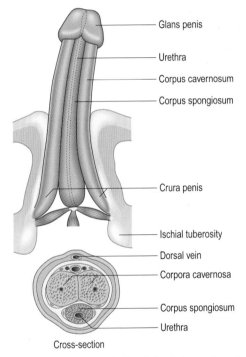

Glans penis

Urethra

Corpus cavernosum

Corpus spongiosum

Crura penis

Ischial tuberosity

Dorsal vein

Corpora cavernosa

Corpus spongiosum

Urethra

Cross-section

Fig. 10.45 Anatomy of the penis. The shaft and glans penis are formed from the corpus spongiosum and the corpus cavernosum.

the prostate develops a trilobar structure because of benign enlargement. Two lateral lobes and a variable median lobe protrude into the bladder and may cause urethral and bladder outflow obstruction. Prostate cancer develops in the peripheral tissue of the lateral lobes and sometimes may be detected by digital rectal examination. Only the posterior aspect and the lateral lobes of the prostate can be felt by rectal examination (p. 188).

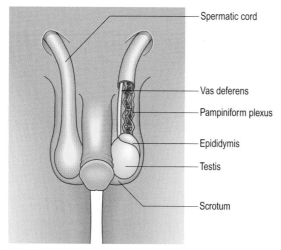

Fig. 10.46 The scrotum and its contents.

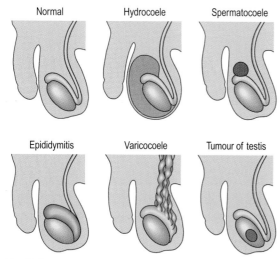

Fig. 10.47 Swellings of the scrotum.

SYMPTOMS AND DEFINITIONS

Scrotum

Lumps

Hydrocoeles

These are swellings due to fluid in the tunica vaginalis (Fig. 10.47). They are usually idiopathic but may be secondary to inflammatory conditions or tumours.

Epididymal cysts

Swellings of the epididymis which are completely separate from the body of the testis are epididymal cysts. They are isolated, adherent to the epididymis alone and virtually never malignant. Painful swellings at the superior pole of the testis, or adjacent to the head of the epididymis, are usually due to torsion of a paramesonephric duct remnant, the hydatids of Morgagni.

Varicocoeles

These are varicosities of the spermatic vein which feel like a 'bag of worms' in the scrotum.

Testicular tumours

These cause painless hard swellings of the body of the testis. Around 15% of tumours may occur close to the rete testis and may cause epididymal swelling and pain.

Epididymitis

Inflammation of the epididymus produces painful epididymal swelling, most often caused by STIs in young men, or coliform urinary infection in the elderly.

A single testis

This may be due to incomplete testicular descent of the 'missing' testis through the inguinal canal or an ectopic testis in the groin. Ask about previous surgery for a testicular tumour or testicular maldescent. Unilateral testicular atrophy may result from mumps infection, torsion of the testis, vascular compromise after inguinal hernia repair or from a late orchidopexy for undescended testis.

Bilateral testicular atrophy

This suggests primary, or secondary, hypogonadism or primary testicular failure. Look for hormonal abnormalities, or signs of anabolic steroid usage, and check the development of secondary sexual characteristics (Fig. 15.19).

Penile and urethral abnormalities

Urethritis

Inflammation of the urethra may cause dysuria (pain on micturition) or a urethral discharge. The most common causes are non-specific urethritis and gonococcal infection.

Phimosis

Narrowing of the preputial orifice which prevents retraction of the foreskin is called phimosis. This may produce balanitis (recurrent infection of the glans penis), posthitis (infection of the prepuce) or both (balanoposthitis).

Paraphimosis

This is an inability to pull the foreskin forward, after retraction, because of a constriction ring in the prepuce which jams behind the corona of the glans (Fig. 10.48).

Peyronie's disease

Peyronie's disease is a fibrotic condition of the shaft of the penis, of unknown aetiology, producing curvature, narrowing or shortening of the corpora cavernosa with erection.

Priapism

This persistent rigidity in the corpora cavernosa is characterised by longitudinal rigidity with a flaccid glans.

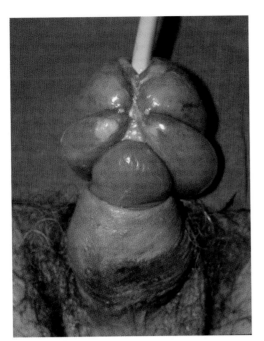

Fig. 10.48 Paraphimosis. Oedema of the foreskin behind an encircling constriction ring due to the foreskin not being replaced – in this case, after catheterisation.

10.24 Types of male sexual dysfunction

Change in libido
Unable to achieve an erection
Unable to maintain an erection
Problems achieving orgasm
Premature ejaculation
Failure to ejaculate

Causes include leukaemia and sickle cell disease, pelvic malignancy and drugs.

Genital ulcer

A break in the mucosa or skin anywhere on the genitals is an ulcer. Painful ulcers are usually caused by herpes simplex; painless ulcers occur in reactive arthritis (p. 321), lichen simplex and (rarely) syphilis.

Sexual dysfunction

There are different problems and causes of sexual dysfunction, including psychological issues, alcohol, systemic disease (especially diabetes mellitus), peripheral vascular disease and drugs (Box 10.24).

Prostate abnormalities

Prostatitis

Inflammation of the prostate gland causes boggy, tender enlargement of the prostate. Usual causes are STI in younger men and *Escherichia coli* in older men.

Benign hyperplasia

This is common in men >60 years and associated with urinary symptoms (Box 9.2). The median sulcus is preserved and the prostate may feel smooth and rubbery.

Prostate cancer

This may be asymptomatic or produce urinary symptoms. It feels stony hard or causes firm nodularity in the palpable lateral lobes.

Bladder problems

See p. 198.

THE HISTORY

10

Presenting complaint

Ensure you understand what the man's main genital or urinary problems are, the timescale of their development and how they affect his lifestyle. Be sensitive to his concerns but clarify the exact nature of any sexual activity (Ch. 9 and p. 9).

Take a general urological history, including a history about genital swelling, problems with micturition or discharge; be precise in asking about the site of any pain apparently emanating from the urinary tract. Ask about past, or intended, conceptions and about the man's sexual function, when appropriate.

Past history

Ask about previous urological procedures, including neonatal surgery, hypertension and urinary infections. Relevant general surgical procedures, particularly pelvic operations, previous vasectomy and STIs and their complications, are important.

Drug history

Ask about previous urological drug treatments and obtain a full list of all medications and drugs taken recreationally. In particular note drugs such as α-adrenoreceptor blockers, which may cause retrograde ejaculation; antihypertensive agents, which may cause erectile dysfunction; vasoactive drugs, e.g. alprostadil, which may result in a prolonged erection, and antidepressants, which may affect sexual function.

Family history

Undescended testis and Peyronie's disease may have a hereditary basis so check for any family history of these problems. BRCA2 gene abnormalities, causing breast cancer in female members of the family, may increase the risk of prostate cancer in men carrying this mutation.

Social history

Smoking, alcohol and recreational drugs can affect fertility and sexual function. Erectile dysfunction is a common early symptom of diabetes or heart disease. Bladder cancer, and its recurrence, is more common in smokers.

THE PHYSICAL EXAMINATION

Ensure privacy. Explain what you are going to do, why it is necessary and offer a chaperone. Record the chaperone's name; if the offer is refused, record the fact. Allow the patient privacy to undress.

Have a warm, well-lit room with a moveable light source. Apply alcohol gel and put on gloves.

Ask the patient to stand and expose the area from his lower abdomen to the top of his thighs unless you are examining the inguinoscrotal area. In this case ask him to lie on his back initially.

The skin

Examination sequence

- Look in turn at the groin, skin creases, perineum and scrotal skin for redness, swellings or ulcers. Note the hair distribution.
- If you see any swellings in the groin palpate these and define them using SPACESPIT (Box 3.11).

Abnormal findings

There may be alopecia or infestation. Patients who shave their pubic hair may have dermatitis (inflammation of the dermis) or folliculitis (infection around the base of the hairs) causing an irritating red rash. Intertrigo (infected eczema) occurs in the skin creases and lymphadenopathy may be due to local or general causes.

Scrotal oedema can be caused by systemic or local disease. Heart and liver dysfunction may cause significant genital oedema, as may the nephrotic syndrome and lymphoedema due to para-aortic lymphadenopathy.

The penis

Examination sequence

- Look at the shaft and check the position of the urethral opening to exclude hypospadias (urethra opening partway along the shaft of the penis) (p. 363).
- Palpate the shaft for fibrous plaques (usually on the dorsum). Palpate any other lesions to define them.
- Retract the prepuce and inspect the glans for red patches or vesicles.
- Always draw the foreskin forward after examination to avoid a paraphimosis.
- Take a urethral swab if your patient has a discharge or is having sexual health screening.

Normal findings

Enlarged follicles may mimic warts. Numerous uniform pearly penile papules around the corona of the glans are normal.

Abnormal findings

Warts, sebaceous cysts, or a hard plaque of Peyronie's disease may occur on the shaft and phimosis, adhesions, inflammation or swellings on the foreskin or glans.

The scrotum

Examine the scrotum with the man standing. Then ask him to lie down if you find a swelling you can't 'get above'.

Ask the patient whether he has any genital pain. If the patient is cold or apprehensive the dartos muscle contracts and you will not be able to palpate the scrotal contents properly.

Examination sequence

- Inspect the scrotum for redness, swelling or ulcers, lifting it to inspect the posterior surface.
- Note the position of the testes and any paratesticular swelling and tenderness.
- Palpate the scrotum gently using both hands. Check that both testes are present. If they are not, examine the inguinal canal and perineum, checking for ectopic testes.
- With each testis in turn, place the fingers of both your hands behind the testis to immobilise it and use your index finger and thumb to palpate the body of the testis methodically. Feel the anterior surface and medial border with your thumb and the lateral border with your index finger (Fig. 10.49).
- Check the size and consistency of the testis. Note any nodules or irregularities. Measure the testicular size in centimetres from one to the other.
- Palpate the spermatic cord with your right hand. Gently pull the testis downward and place your fingers behind the neck of the scrotum. Feel the spermatic cord and within it the vas, like a thick piece of string.
- Decide whether a swelling arises in the scrotum or from the inguinal canal. If you can feel above the swelling, it originates from the scrotum; if you can't, the swelling usually originates in the inguinal region (Fig. 10.50).
- Place the bright end of a torch against a scrotal swelling (transillumination) (Fig. 15.5). Fluid-filled cysts allow light transmission and the scrotum glows bright red. This is an inconsistent sign which does not differentiate a hydrocoele from other causes of intrascrotal fluid, such as a large epididymal cyst. With thick-walled cysts transillumination may be absent (Fig. 15.5).

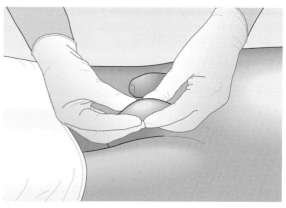

Fig. 10.49 Palpation of the testis.

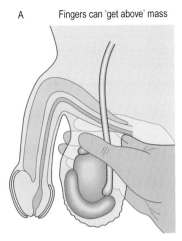

A   Fingers can 'get above' mass

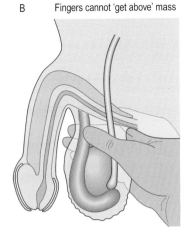

B   Fingers cannot 'get above' mass

Fig. 10.50 Testing for scrotal swellings. (A) It is possible to 'get above' a true scrotal swelling. **(B)** This is not possible if the swelling is caused by an inguinal hernia that has descended into the scrotum.

10

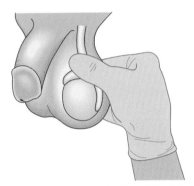

Fig. 10.51 Palpation of the epididymis. The epididymis is readily felt only at the top of the testis.

Normal findings

The right testicle is usually closer to the inguinal canal than the left but testes may be highly mobile (retractile). A normal testis is 5 cm long. The normal epididymis is barely palpable except for its head (Fig. 10.51), which feels like a pea separate from the superior pole of the body of the testicle.

Abnormal findings

Sebaceous cysts are common in the scrotal skin. If you can get above a scrotal swelling, it is a true scrotal swelling. If not, it may be a varicocoele or inguinal hernia which has descended into the scrotum. A varicocoele feels like a 'bag of worms' in the cord and should disappear when the patient lies down. If it does not, then consider a retroperitoneal mass compressing the testicular veins. A bulky or painful mass in the scrotum when you cannot palpate the testis needs an ultrasound scan to clarify the nature of the intrascrotal structures.

A retracted testicle accompanied by acute pain and swelling occurs in testicular torsion (Fig. 10.52).

The prostate

Ask the patient to lie in the left lateral position.

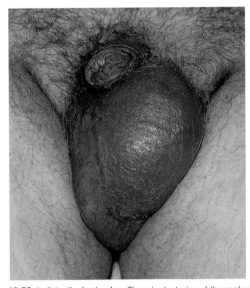

Fig. 10.52 Left testicular torsion. There is shortening of the cord with retraction of the testis and global swelling of the scrotal contents. Refer the patient urgently to a surgeon for scrotal exploration.

Examination sequence

- Perform a rectal examination (p. 188).
- Palpate the prostate anteriorly through the rectal wall.
- Note any tenderness and assess the consistency. Is it hard, or boggy?
- Feel for any nodules.
- Withdraw your finger. Give the patient tissues to clean himself and privacy in which to get dressed.

Normal findings

The prostate is normally smooth, rubbery, non-tender and about the size of a walnut. It has defined margins with an indentation, or sulcus, between the two lateral lobes. Sometimes the seminal vesicles are felt above the prostate.

10.25 Investigations in male genital disease

Investigation	Indication/comment
Urinalysis	Protein and blood +++ in urinary tract infection and epididymitis
Serum prostate-specific antigen	Raised in prostate cancer but increases with age, prostatic volume, following prostatic trauma and in seminal or urinary tract infection
Serum beta-human chorionic gonadotrophin, alpha-fetoprotein and leukocyte alkaline phosphatase	Raised in some types of testicular cancer and in bony metastases
Serum follicle-stimulating hormone (FSH) and luteinising hormone (LH)	In azoospermia FSH and LH levels may be low due to pituitary dysfunction. FSH may be normal in obstructive azoospermia or maturation arrest and will be elevated in primary testicular failure
Serum prolactin	Raised prolactin suggests a pituitary tumour when libido is reduced
Serum testosterone and sex hormone-binding globulin (SHBG)	Low in lack of virilisation or sometimes in erectile dysfunction
Midstream urine	Urinary tract infection, testicular pain, epididymitis
Urinary chlamydial polymerase chain reaction	Sexually transmitted infection (STI), urethral discharge or epididymitis
Urethral swab	Suspected STI
Semen analysis/culture	In infertility to assess volume, number and quality of sperm in the ejaculate. Two separate samples should be analysed. Culture semen only when pus cells are found or haemospermia persists
Genital ultrasound examination	Hydrocoele, acute scrotal pain, testicular or penile mass
Colour Doppler imaging	To assess blood flow in suspected testicular torsion, priapism and erectile dysfunction
Transrectal ultrasound examination	Increases the sensitivity and specificity of digital rectal examination in suspected prostate cancer. Defines the anatomy of the prostate and the seminal vesicles in infertility or persisting haemospermia
CT scanning	To find the site of an undescended testis and to stage testicular cancer
MR scanning	To stage prostate cancer and delineate the seminal vesicles

Abnormal findings

Tenderness or soft 'bogginess' suggests prostatitis or prostatic abscess.

Prostate cancer may be felt as a discrete nodule, a craggy mass or obliteration of the midline sulcus or may be fixed to the lateral pelvic side wall.

INVESTIGATIONS

See Box 10.25.

Richard Davenport
Hadi Manji

The nervous system
11

NERVOUS SYSTEM EXAMINATION

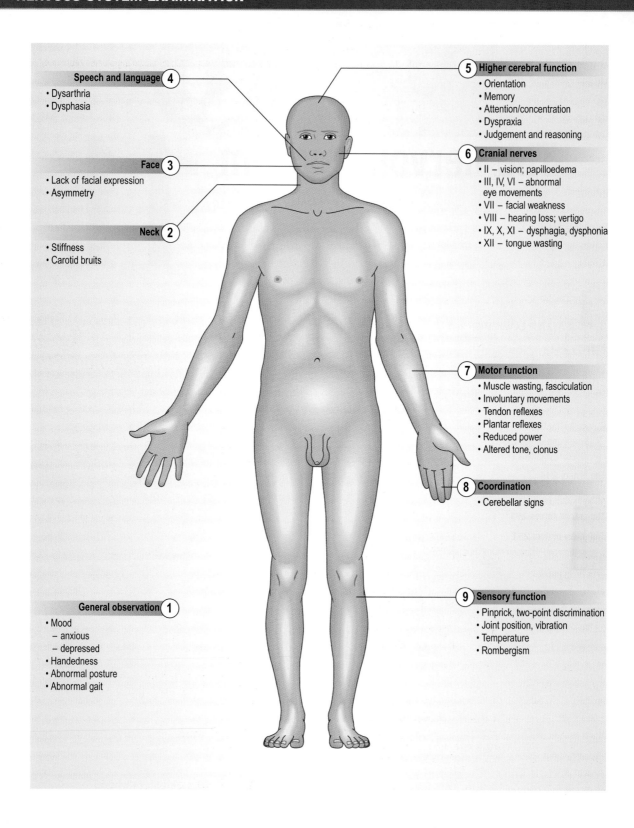

Speech and language ④
- Dysarthria
- Dysphasia

Face ③
- Lack of facial expression
- Asymmetry

Neck ②
- Stiffness
- Carotid bruits

⑤ **Higher cerebral function**
- Orientation
- Memory
- Attention/concentration
- Dyspraxia
- Judgement and reasoning

⑥ **Cranial nerves**
- II – vision; papilloedema
- III, IV, VI – abnormal eye movements
- VII – facial weakness
- VIII – hearing loss; vertigo
- IX, X, XI – dysphagia, dysphonia
- XII – tongue wasting

⑦ **Motor function**
- Muscle wasting, fasciculation
- Involuntary movements
- Tendon reflexes
- Plantar reflexes
- Reduced power
- Altered tone, clonus

⑧ **Coordination**
- Cerebellar signs

General observation ①
- Mood
  - anxious
  - depressed
- Handedness
- Abnormal posture
- Abnormal gait

⑨ **Sensory function**
- Pinprick, two-point discrimination
- Joint position, vibration
- Temperature
- Rombergism

ANATOMY

The nervous system consists of the brain and spinal cord (central nervous system, CNS) and peripheral nerves (peripheral nervous system, PNS). The PNS includes the autonomic nervous system, responsible for control of involuntary functions.

The neurone is the functional unit of the nervous system. Each neurone has a cell body and axon terminating at a synapse, supported by astrocytes and microglial cells. Astrocytes provide the structural framework for the neurones, control their biochemical environment and form the blood–brain barrier. Microglial cells are blood-derived mononuclear macrophages with immune and scavenging functions. In the CNS, oligodendrocytes produce and maintain a myelin sheath around the axons. In the PNS myelin is produced by Schwann cells.

The brain consists of two cerebral hemispheres, each with four lobes (frontal, parietal, temporal and occipital), the brainstem and the cerebellum. The brainstem comprises the midbrain, pons and medulla. The cerebellum lies in the posterior fossa, with two hemispheres and a central vermis attached to the brainstem by three pairs of cerebellar peduncles. Between the brain and the skull are three membranous layers: dura mater next to the bone, arachnoid and pia mater next to the nervous tissue. The subarachnoid space between the arachnoid and pia is filled with cerebrospinal fluid (CSF).

The spinal cord contains afferent and efferent fibres arranged in discrete bundles which are responsible for the transmission of motor and sensory information. Peripheral nerves have myelinated and unmyelinated axons. The sensory cell bodies of peripheral nerves are situated in the dorsal root ganglia. The motor cell bodies are in the anterior horns of the spinal cord (Fig. 11.1).

SYMPTOMS AND DEFINITIONS

Common neurological symptoms are headache, weakness, numbness, disturbance/loss of consciousness, imbalance, abnormal movements and memory loss. The history is crucial as many neurological diseases, e.g. migraine or epilepsy, have no clinical signs. Some symptoms, e.g. loss of consciousness or amnesia, demand an eye-witness history.

Headache

Headache is the most common neurological symptom and may be either primary or secondary to other pathology (Box 11.1). The most common causes of headache are migraine and tension-type headache (Box 11.2).

Transient loss of consciousness (TLOC)

Syncope is loss of consciousness due to inadequate cerebral perfusion and is the commonest cause of TLOC. Vasovagal syncope (a 'faint') is the most common type and is usually precipitated by stimulation of the

11.1 Primary and secondary headache syndromes

Primary

Migraine
Tension-type headache
Trigeminal autonomic cephalalgias (including cluster headache)
Primary stabbing, cough, exertional or sex headaches
Primary thunderclap headache
New daily persistent headache

Secondary (symptomatic) to:

Head or neck trauma
Head or neck vascular disease, e.g. subarachnoid haemorrhage, vertebral artery dissection, temporal arteritis
Non-vascular intracranial disease
Recreational drug use
Medication overuse e.g. analgesia
Infection
Non-traumatic disorders of head, neck, eyes, ears, nose, teeth, mouth, sinuses
Cranial neuralgias, e.g. trigeminal neuralgia

11.2 Onset and causes of headache

Acute single episode (thunderclap)	Subarachnoid haemorrhage Idiopathic intracranial hypotension Cerebral vein thrombosis Acute meningitis, encephalitis
Acute recurrent	Migraine Tension-type headache Cluster headache
Subacute progressive	Raised intracranial pressure (tumour, abscess, hydrocephalus, idiopathic intracranial hypertension) Infections (meningitis, encephalitis) Temporal arteritis
Chronic	Chronic daily headache syndrome Chronic migraine Medication overuse headache Cervicogenic headache Drugs, e.g. nitrates, dipyridamole

parasympathetic nervous system, e.g. pain, prolonged standing. Exercise-related syncope suggests a cardiac cause (Box 11.3). An epileptic seizure can cause TLOC. These are caused by paroxysmal electrical discharges from the brain involving the whole brain (generalised seizures: Box 11.4) or part of the brain (focal seizures: Box 11.5). The history from the patient and witnesses wherever possible helps distinguish syncope from epilepsy (Box 11.6).

Stroke and transient ischaemic attack (TIA)

A stroke is a focal (occasionally global) neurological deficit of rapid onset due to a vascular cause. Hemiplegia following middle cerebral artery occlusion is a

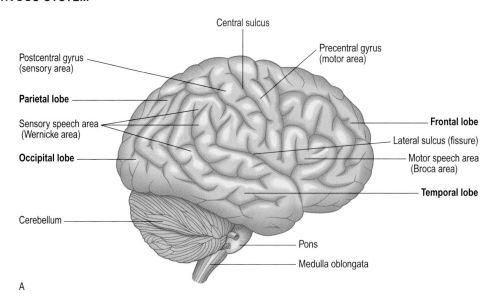

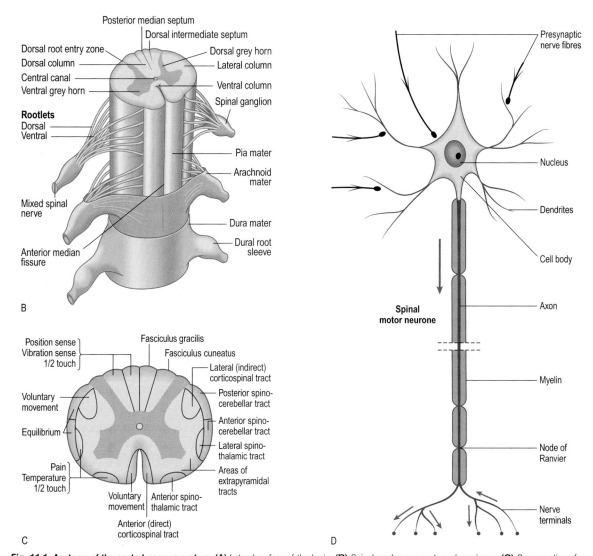

Fig. 11.1 Anatomy of the central nervous system. (A) Lateral surface of the brain. **(B)** Spinal cord, nerve roots and meninges. **(C)** Cross-section of the spinal cord. **(D)** Spinal motor neurone. The terminals of presynaptic neurones form synapses with the cell body and dendrites of the motor neurones.

11.3 Causes of transient loss of consciousness (TLOC)

Syncope	Vasovagal (faint) Carotid sinus Situational, e.g. cough, micturition
Cardiac syncope	Arrhythmias Structural disease, e.g. aortic stenosis, hypertrophic cardiomyopathy, pulmonary embolus
Epileptic seizures	Usually generalised tonic-clonic
Postural hypotension	Drugs e.g. antihypertensive, L-dopa Autonomic failure
Functional or psychiatric	Hyperventilation/panic attack Psychogenic non-epileptic seizures (pseudoseizures/dissociative attacks)

11.4 The typical pattern of a generalised tonic-clonic seizure

Focal onset (aura)

- Not present in idiopathic generalised syndromes, usually precedes convulsion by seconds to minutes if present

Tonic phase

- Loss of consciousness and fall
- Whole body stiffening
- Tonic cry
- Cyanosis

Clonic phase

- Neat rhythmical jerking of limbs and trunk which accelerates/decelerates
- Tongue biting

Postictal phase

- Initially deep sleep with snoring, unresponsive
- Confusion/aggression on recovery of consciousness
- Headache
- Amnesia

11.5 Features of focal seizures

- Spreading motor or sensory symptoms (in seconds)
- Autonomic symptoms, including epigastric sensations
- Psychic symptoms, including memory disturbance (flashbacks, déjà-vu, jamais vu), fear, terror, rage, pleasure, depression, cognitive disturbance, e.g. forced thinking, dreamy states, depersonalisation, illusions and hallucinosis
- Abnormal behaviour (automatism), e.g. lip smacking
- Consciousness may or may not be affected, but complete loss of consciousness is unusual

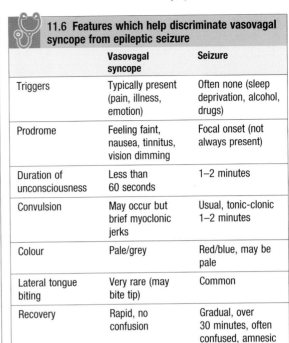

11.6 Features which help discriminate vasovagal syncope from epileptic seizure

	Vasovagal syncope	Seizure
Triggers	Typically present (pain, illness, emotion)	Often none (sleep deprivation, alcohol, drugs)
Prodrome	Feeling faint, nausea, tinnitus, vision dimming	Focal onset (not always present)
Duration of unconsciousness	Less than 60 seconds	1–2 minutes
Convulsion	May occur but brief myoclonic jerks	Usual, tonic-clonic 1–2 minutes
Colour	Pale/grey	Red/blue, may be pale
Lateral tongue biting	Very rare (may bite tip)	Common
Recovery	Rapid, no confusion	Gradual, over 30 minutes, often confused, amnesic

11.7 Stroke and vascular territory

Site of lesion	Clinical features	Side
Anterior cerebral circulation (via internal carotid artery)	Middle cerebral artery: hemiparesis (face and arm > leg), hemianaesthesia Dysphasia (dominant hemisphere), dyspraxia (non-dominant hemisphere), visual field defect Anterior cerebral artery: leg weakness	Contralateral to lesion
Posterior cerebral circulation (via vertebrobasilar supply)	Visual field defect (hemianopia) Ataxia, diplopia, nystagmus, dysarthria, dysphagia, facial weakness/numbness, loss of consciousness Sensory symptoms	Ipsilateral to lesion

11

typical example, but symptoms are dictated by the vascular territory involved (Box 11.7). In industrialised countries, about 80% of strokes are ischaemic, the remainder haemorrhagic, but haemorrhagic stroke is much more prevalent in Asian populations. A TIA is the same, but with symptoms resolving within 24 hours;

TIAs are an important risk factor for impending stroke, and demand urgent assessment and treatment. Spinal strokes are exceedingly rare.

Dizziness and vertigo

Patients use 'dizziness' to describe many sensations. Recurrent 'dizzy spells' affect ~30% of those >65 years and can be due to postural hypotension, cerebrovascular disease, cardiac arrhythmia or hyperventilation induced by anxiety and panic. Vertigo (the illusion of movement) specifically indicates a problem in the vestibular

11

apparatus (peripheral) or, much less commonly, the brain (central). TIAs do not cause isolated vertigo.

Functional symptoms

Many neurological symptoms are not due to physical disease. These symptoms are often called 'functional' but other terms used include psychogenic, hysterical, somatisation or conversion disorders. Presentations include blindness, limb weakness and collapsing attacks.

THE HISTORY

Presenting complaint

Neurological symptoms may be difficult for patients to describe, so clarify exactly what the patient tells you. Words such as 'blackouts', 'dizziness', 'weakness' and 'numbness' may indicate a different symptom from what you first imagined, so ensure you understand what the patient means. Clarifying or reviewing the history with the patient and/or witness is essential and provides diagnostic clues.

Time relationships

The onset, duration and pattern of symptoms over time often provide clues to the diagnosis, e.g. headache (Box 11.2) or vertigo (Box 13.5).

- When did the symptoms start (or when was the patient last well)?
- Are they persistent or intermittent?
- If persistent, are they getting better, worse, or staying the same?
- If intermittent, how long do they last?
- Was the onset sudden, e.g. subarachnoid haemorrhage, or gradual, e.g. migraine headache?

Precipitating, exacerbating or relieving factors

- What was the patient doing when the symptoms occurred?
- Does anything make the symptoms better or worse, e.g. time of day, menstrual cycle, position?

Associated symptoms

Associated symptoms might aid diagnosis, e.g. headache may be associated with other symptoms such as nausea, vomiting, photophobia (aversion to light), suggesting meningism, or phonophobia (aversion to sound), suggesting migraine.

Headache

Use SOCRATES to define the nature of the headache (Box 2.10); the onset and periodicity may provide aetiological clues (Box 11.2).

Transient loss of consciousness

If patients are unaware of their symptoms, obtain a witness account. This is more valuable than an unfocused neurological examination. Ask the witness about symptoms before, during and after the TLOC – were there any warning symptoms, any colour changes, did the patient lie still or move, what was the patient like immediately afterwards?

Stroke and TIA

Ask if the symptoms started suddenly, and how long they lasted. Were symptoms accompanied by headache?

Dizziness and vertigo

Distinguish vertigo (the illusion of movement, most commonly spinning) from lightheadedness, which rarely localises and is a non-specific symptom. Was the dizziness brought on by certain movements, e.g. rising from a chair, rolling over in bed?

Past history

Forgotten symptoms may be important, e.g. a history of recovered visual loss (optic neuritis) in a patient now presenting with numbness suggests multiple sclerosis. Birth history and development may be important in some situations, e.g. epilepsy. Contact parents or family doctors to obtain such information. If considering a vascular cause for neurological symptoms, ask about important risk factors, e.g. other vascular disease, hypertension, family history and smoking.

Drug history

Always consider drugs, including prescribed, over-the-counter and complementary therapies, as they may cause many neurological symptoms (Box 11.8). Adverse reactions may be idiosyncratic, dose-related or caused by chronic use.

Family history

Many neurological disorders are caused by single-gene defects. Others have an important polygenic influence, e.g. multiple sclerosis. Some conditions have a variety of inheritance patterns, e.g. Charcot–Marie–Tooth disease. Neurological disease may also be caused by mitochondrial DNA abnormalities (Box 11.9).

Social history

Alcohol is the most common neurological toxin and damages both the CNS (ataxia, seizures, cognitive symptoms) and the PNS (neuropathy). Poor diet with vitamin deficiency compounds these problems. Other recreational drugs may damage the nervous system, e.g. cocaine and ecstasy can cause seizures and strokes, and smoking contributes to vascular and malignant disease. Always consider sexually transmitted or blood-borne

11.8 Neurological symptoms/syndromes due to drugs

Ataxia

- Phenytoin
- Carbamazepine
- Lithium

Epileptic seizures

- Tricyclic antidepressants
- Phenothiazines
- Clozapine

Headaches

- Glyceryl trinitrate
- Dipyridamole
- Nifedipine
- Sildenafil

Myopathy

- Statins
- Corticosteroids

Parkinsonism

- Neuroleptics
- Prochlorperazine
- Metoclopramide

Peripheral neuropathy

- Chemotherapy (vincristine, platinum drugs, thalidomide)
- Metronidazole
- Amiodarone
- Antiretroviral drugs (stavudine, dideocytabine)

Tremor

- β-agonists e.g. salbutamol, terbutaline
- Lithium
- Sodium valproate

11.9 Examples of inherited neurological disorders

Autosomal dominant

- Myotonic dystrophy
- Neurofibromatosis types I and II
- Charcot–Marie–Tooth 1a
- Spinocerebellar ataxias (SCA)
- Tuberous sclerosis
- Huntington's disease
- Fascioscapulohumeral muscular dystrophy (FSH)

Autosomal recessive

- Wilson's disease
- Friedreich's ataxia

X-linked recessive

- Duchenne and Becker muscular dystrophy
- Fragile X syndrome

Mitochondrial DNA

- Myoclonic epilepsy with ragged red fibres (MERRF)
- Mitochondrial encephalomyopathy with lactic acidosis and stroke-like episodes (MELAS)
- Leber's hereditary optic neuropathy (LHON)
- Chronic progressive external ophthalmoplegia (CPEO)
- Kearns–Sayre syndrome (KSS)

11

infection, e.g. human immunodeficiency virus (HIV) or syphilis, especially in high-risk groups.

Social circumstances are relevant. How are patients coping with their symptoms? Do they drive? If so, should they? What are the physical and emotional support circumstances? Always ask what they think or fear might be wrong with them, as neurological symptoms cause much anxiety. Patients commonly research their symptoms on the internet; searches of common benign neurological symptoms, e.g. numbness, usually list the most alarming (and unlikely) diagnoses (multiple sclerosis, motor neurone disease, tumours) first.

Occupational history

Occupational factors are relevant to several neurological disorders. For example, toxic peripheral neuropathy due to exposure to heavy or organic metals, e.g. lead, causes a motor neuropathy; manganese causes a parkinsonian syndrome.

THE PHYSICAL EXAMINATION

Neurological assessment begins with your first contact with the patient and continues during the history. Note facial expression, demeanour, dress, posture, gait and speech. Mental state examination (p. 21) and general examination (Ch. 3) are integral parts of the neurological examination.

Assessment of conscious level

Consciousness has two main components:

- The state of consciousness depends largely on integrity of the ascending reticular activating system, which extends from the brainstem to the thalamus.
- The content of consciousness refers to how aware the person is and depends on the cerebral cortex, the thalamus and their connections.

Do not use ill-defined terms such as stuporose or obtunded. Use the Glasgow Coma Scale (Box 19.14), a reliable and reproducible tool, to record conscious level.

Meningeal irritation

Meningism (inflammation or irritation of the meninges) can lead to increased resistance to passive flexion of the neck (neck stiffness) or the extended leg (Kernig's sign). Patients may lie with flexed hips to ease their symptoms. Meningism suggests infection (meningitis) or blood within the subarachnoid space (subarachnoid haemorrhage), but can occur with non-neurological infections, e.g. urinary tract infection. Absence of meningism does not exclude pathology within the subarachnoid space. In meningitis, a finding of neck stiffness has relatively low sensitivity but higher specificity.

Examination sequence

- Position the patient supine with no pillow.
- Expose and fully extend both the patient's legs.

Neck stiffness

- Support the patient's head with the fingers of your hands at the occiput and the ulnar border of your hands against the paraspinal muscles of the patient's neck (Fig. 11.2A).
- Flex the patient's head gently until his chin touches his chest.
- Ask the patient to hold that position for 10 seconds. If neck stiffness is present, the neck cannot be passively flexed and you may feel spasm in the neck muscles.
- Flexion of the knees in response to neck flexion is Brudzinski's sign.

Kernig's sign

- Flex one of the patient's legs at the hip and knee, with your left hand placed over the medial hamstrings.
- Use your right hand to extend the knee while the hip is maintained in flexion. Look at the other leg for any reflex flexion (Fig. 11.2B). Kernig's sign is positive when extension is resisted by spasm in the hamstrings. Kernig's sign is absent in local causes of neck stiffness, e.g. cervical spine disease or raised intracranial pressure (Boxes 11.10 and 11.11).

Disorders of movement

The principal motor pathway has CNS (corticospinal or pyramidal tract – upper motor neurone) and PNS (anterior horn cell – lower motor neurone) components. Other parts of the nervous system, e.g. basal ganglia and cerebellum, have important modulating effects on movement. It is essential to distinguish upper from lower motor neurone signs (Box 11.12).

Upper motor neurone lesions

If the lesion affects the CNS pathways, the lower motor neurones are under the uninhibited influence of the spinal reflex. The motor units then have an exaggerated response to stretch with increased tone (spasticity), clonus and brisk reflexes. There is weakness but not wasting (although atrophy may develop with longstanding lesions). Primitive reflexes, e.g. plantar extensor response (Babinski sign), may be present.

Lower motor neurone lesions

The group of muscle fibres innervated by a single anterior horn cell forms a 'motor unit'. A lower motor neurone lesion causes weakness and wasting in these muscle fibres, reduced tone (flaccidity), fasciculation and reduced or absent reflexes.

EBE 11.10 **Meningitis**

The absence of all three signs of fever, neck stiffness and an altered mental state virtually eliminates the diagnosis of meningitis.

A positive Kernig's or Brudzinski's sign is highly specific for bacterial meningitis but absence of these signs cannot exclude meningitis. McGee S. Evidence based physical diagnosis. St Louis, MO: Saunders/Elsevier, 2007, p. 279.

EBE 11.11 **Subarachnoid haemorrhage**

In patients with acute headache, predictive features of subarachnoid haemorrhage are: age > 40 years, onset with exertion, neck stiffness or pain, raised blood pressure, loss of consciousness and vomiting.

Perry JJ, Stiell IG, Sivilotti MLA et al. High risk clinical characteristics for subarachnoid haemorrhage in patients with acute headache: prospective cohort study. BMJ 2010;341:1035.

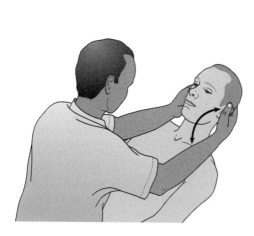

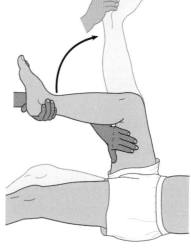

A   B

Fig. 11.2 Testing for meningeal irritation. (A) Neck rigidity. **(B)** Kernig's sign.

11.12 Features of motor neurone lesions

	Upper motor neurone lesion	Lower motor neurone lesion
Inspection	Usually normal (wasting in longstanding lesions)	Wasting, fasciculation
Tone	Increased with clonus	Normal or decreased, no clonus
Weakness	Preferentially affects extensors in arms, flexors in leg	Usually more focal, in distribution of nerve root or peripheral nerve
Deep tendon reflexes	Increased	Decreased/absent
Plantar response	Extensor	Flexor

11.13 Common gait abnormalities

Gait disturbance	Description	Causes
Parkinsonian	Stooped Shuffling (reduced stride length) Loss of arm swing Postural instability Freezing	Parkinson's disease Other parkinsonian syndromes
Gait apraxia	Small shuffling steps (marche à petit pas) Difficulty in starting to walk/freezing Better 'cycling' on bed than walking	Cerebrovascular disease Hydrocephalus
Spastic paraparesis	Stiff 'walking through mud' or scissors gait	Spinal cord lesions
Myopathic	Waddling (proximal weakness) Bilateral Trendelenburg signs	Muscular dystrophies Acquired myopathies
Foot drop	Foot slapping	Neuropathies L5 radiculopathy
Central ataxia	Wide based 'drunken' Tandem gait poor	Cerebellar disease
Sensory ataxia	Wide-based Positive Romberg sign	Neuropathies Spinal cord disorders
Functional gait	Variable, often bizarre, inconsistent Knees flexed, buckling Dragging immobile leg behind them	Conversion disorder

Stance and gait

Stance and gait depend upon intact visual, sensory, corticospinal, extrapyramidal and cerebellar pathways, together with functioning lower motor neurones and spinal reflexes. Non-neurological gait disorders are discussed in Chapter 14. Certain abnormal gait patterns are recognisable, suggesting diagnoses (Box 11.13 and Fig. 3.2).

Examination sequence

Stance

■ Ask the patient to stand with his (preferably bare) feet close together and eyes open.
■ Swaying, lurching, or inability to stand with the feet together with the eyes open suggest a cerebellar ataxia.
■ Ask the patient to close his eyes (Romberg's test) but be prepared to steady/catch the patient. Repeatedly falling is a positive result.

Gait

■ Time the patient walking a measured 10 metres, with a walking aid if needed, turning through 180° and returning.
■ Note stride length, arm swing, steadiness (including turning), limping or other difficulties.
■ Listen for the slapping sound of a foot drop gait.
■ Ask the patient to walk first on tip toes, then on the heels. Ankle dorsiflexion weakness (foot drop) is much more common than plantar flexion weakness, and makes walking on the heels difficult or impossible.
■ Ask the patient to walk heel to toe in a straight line (tandem gait). This emphasises any gait ataxia.

Abnormal findings

• Unsteadiness on standing with the eyes open is common in cerebellar disorders.
• Instability which only occurs, or is markedly worse, on eye closure (Romberg's sign) indicates proprioceptive sensory loss in the feet (sensory ataxia).

• Hemiplegic gait (unilateral upper motor neurone lesion) is characterised by extension at the hip, knee and ankle and circumduction at the hip, such that the foot on the affected side is plantar flexed and describes a semicircle as the patient walks. The upper limb will be flexed.
• Bilateral upper motor neurone damage causes a scissor-like gait due to spasticity.
• Cerebellar dysfunction leads to a broad-based, unsteady (ataxic) gait, which usually makes walking heel to toe in a straight line impossible.
• In parkinsonism, initiation of walking may be delayed; the steps are short and shuffling with loss/reduction of arm swing. A pill-rolling tremor may be apparent. The stooped posture and impairment of postural reflexes can result in a festinant (rapid, short-stepped, hurrying) gait. As a doorway or other obstacle approaches, the person may freeze. Turning involves many short steps, with the risk of falls.
• Proximal muscle weakness may lead to a waddling gait with bilateral Trendelenburg signs (p. 344).
• Bizarre gaits, such as dragging a leg behind the patient, are often functional, but some diseases, e.g. Huntington's disease, produce unusual gaits.

11

11

Speech

Symptoms and definitions

Dysarthria is slurred speech caused by articulation problems due to a motor deficit.

Dysphonia is loss of volume caused by laryngeal disorders.

Dysphasia is disturbance of language resulting in abnormalities of speech production and/or understanding and may also involve other language symptoms, e.g. writing and reading, unlike dysarthria and dysphonia.

Examination sequence

- Listen to the patient's spontaneous speech, noting volume, rhythm and clarity.
- Ask the patient to repeat phrases such as 'yellow lorry' to test lingual (tongue) sounds and 'baby hippopotamus' for labial (lip) sounds, then a tongue twister, e.g. 'the Leith police dismisseth us'.
- Ask the patient to count steadily to 30 to assess fatigue.
- Ask the patient to cough and to say 'Ah'; observe the soft palate rising bilaterally.

Abnormal findings

Dysarthria Disturbed articulation may result from lesions of the tongue, lips or mouth, ill-fitting dentures or disruption of the neuromuscular pathways.

Bilateral upper motor neurone lesions of the corticobulbar tracts cause a pseudobulbar dysarthria, characterised by a contracted, spastic tongue and difficulty pronouncing consonants, and may be accompanied by a brisk jaw jerk and emotional lability.

Bulbar palsy results from bilateral lower motor neurone lesions affecting the same group of cranial nerves. The nature of the speech disturbance is determined by the specific nerves and muscles involved. Weakness of the tongue results in difficulty with lingual sounds, while palatal weakness gives a nasal quality to the speech.

Cerebellar dysarthria may be slow and slurred, similar to alcohol intoxication.

Myasthenia gravis is the most common cause of fatiguing speech.

Parkinsonism may cause dysarthria and dysphonia, with a low-volume, monotonous voice in which the words run into each other.

Dysphonia This usually results from either vocal cord pathology, as in laryngitis, or damage to the vagal (X) nerve supply to the vocal cords (recurrent laryngeal nerve). Inability to abduct one of the vocal cords leads to a 'bovine' (and ineffective) cough (p. 139).

Dysphasias

Anatomy

The language areas are located in the dominant cerebral hemisphere, which is the left in almost all right- and most left-handed people.

Broca's area (inferior frontal region) is concerned with word production and language expression.

Wernicke's area (superior posterior temporal lobe) is the principal area for comprehension of spoken language. Adjacent regions of the parietal lobe are involved in understanding written language and numbers.

The arcuate fasciculus connects Broca's and Wernicke's areas.

Examination sequence

Dysphasia

- During spontaneous speech, listen to the fluency and appropriateness of the content, particularly for paraphasias and neologisms.
- Show the patient a common object, e.g. coin or pen, and ask its name.
- Give a simple three-stage command, e.g. pick up this piece of paper, fold it in half and place it under the book.
- Ask the patient to repeat a simple sentence, e.g. 'Today is Tuesday'.
- Ask the patient to read a passage from a newspaper.
- Ask the patient to write a sentence; examine his handwriting.

Abnormal findings

Expressive (motor) dysphasia results from damage to Broca's area. It is characterised by reduced verbal output with non-fluent speech and errors of grammar and syntax. Comprehension is intact.

Receptive (sensory) dysphasia occurs with dysfunction in Wernicke's area. There is poor comprehension, and although speech is fluent, it may be meaningless and contain paraphasias (incorrect words) and neologisms (nonsense or meaningless new words).

Global dysphasia is a combination of expressive and receptive difficulties due to involvement of both areas.

Dysphasia (a focal sign) is frequently misdiagnosed as confusion (non-focal sign). Always consider dysphasia before assuming confusion, as this fundamentally alters the differential diagnosis and investigation plan.

Dominant parietal lobe lesions affecting the supramarginal gyrus may cause dyslexia (difficulty comprehending written language), dyscalculia (problems with simple addition and subtraction) and dysgraphia (impairment of writing).

Cortical function

Thinking, emotions, language, behaviour, planning and initiating movements, and perceiving sensory information are functions of the cerebral cortex and are central to awareness of, and interaction with, the environment. Certain cortical areas are associated with specific functions, so particular patterns of dysfunction can help localise the site of pathology (Fig. 11.3A). Assessment of higher cortical function is difficult and time-consuming. There are various tools. For the bedside, the Mini-Mental State Examination (p. 26) is quick to administer, whereas a global tool such as the Addenbrooke's Cognitive Examination helps detect early cognitive changes but takes much longer to administer (Box 11.14).

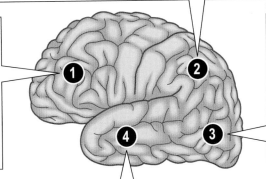

2 Parietal lobe

Dominant side		**Non-dominant side**	
FUNCTION Calculation Language Planned movement Appreciation of size, shape, weight and texture	LESIONS Dyscalculia Dysphasia Dyslexia Apraxia Agnosia Homonymous hemianopia	FUNCTION Spatial orientation Constructional skills	LESIONS Neglect of non-dominant side Spatial disorientation Constructional apraxia Dressing apraxia Homonymous hemianopia

1 Frontal lobe

FUNCTION Personality Emotional response Social behaviour LESIONS Disinhibition Lack of initiative Antisocial behaviour Impaired memory Incontinence Grasp reflexes Anosmia

3 Occipital lobe

FUNCTION Analysis of vision LESIONS Homonymous hemianopia Hemianopic scotomas Visual agnosia Impaired face recognition (prosopagnosia) Visual hallucinations (lights, lines and zig-zags)

4 Temporal lobe

Dominant side		**Non-dominant side**	
FUNCTION Auditory perception Speech, language Verbal memory Smell	LESIONS Dysphasia Dyslexia Poor memory Complex hallucinations (smell, sound, vision) Homonymous hemianopia	FUNCTION Auditory perception Music, tone sequences Non-verbal memory (faces, shapes, music) Smell	LESIONS Poor non-verbal memory Loss of musical skills Complex hallucinations Homonymous hemianopia

A

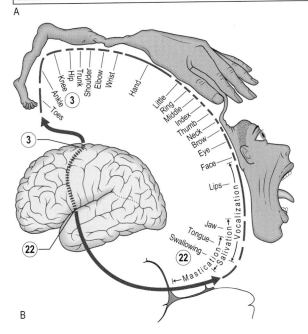

B

Fig. 11.3 Cortical function. (A) Features of localised cerebral lesions.
(B) Somatotropic homunculus.

EBE 11.14 Dementia screening

The revised Addenbrooke's Cognitive Examination is a validated dementia screening test, sensitive to early cognitive dysfunction.

Mioshi E, Dawson K, Mitchell J et al. The Addenbrooke's Cognitive Examination Revised (ACE-R): a brief cognitive test battery for dementia screening. Int J Geriatr Psychiatry 2006;21:1078–1085.

Frontal lobe

Anatomy

The posterior part of the frontal lobe is the motor strip (precentral gyrus) which controls voluntary movement. The motor strip is organised somatotopically (Fig. 11.3B). The area anterior to the precentral gyrus is concerned with personality, social behaviour, emotions, cognition and expressive language, and contains the frontal eye fields and cortical centre for micturition (Fig. 11.4).

11

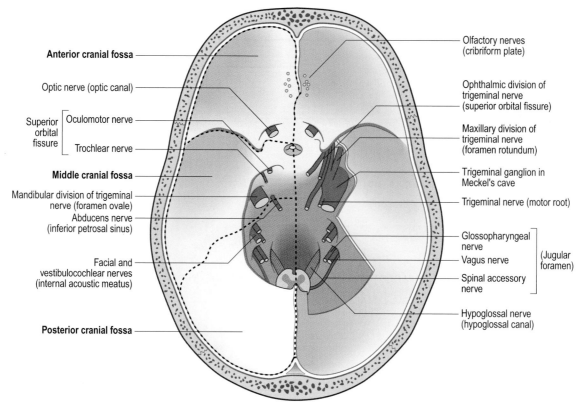

Fig. 11.4 Base of the cranial cavity: showing the dura mater, with the cranial nerves and their exits from the skull. On the right side, part of the tentorium cerebelli and the roof of the trigeminal cave have been removed.

Abnormal findings

Frontal lobe damage may cause:

- personality and behaviour changes, e.g. apathy or disinhibition
- loss of emotional responsiveness or emotional lability
- cognitive impairments, e.g. memory, attention and concentration
- dysphasia (dominant hemisphere)
- conjugate gaze deviation to the side of the lesion
- urinary incontinence
- primitive reflexes, e.g. grasp
- focal motor seizures (motor strip).

Temporal lobe

Anatomy

The temporal lobe contains the primary auditory cortex, Wernicke's area and parts of the limbic system. The latter is crucially important in memory and smell appreciation. The temporal lobe also contains the lower fibres of the optic radiation and the area of auditory perception.

Abnormal findings

Temporal lobe dysfunction may cause:

- memory impairment
- focal seizures with psychic symptoms (Box 11.5)

- contralateral upper quadrantanopia
- receptive dysphasia (dominant hemisphere).

Parietal lobe

Anatomy

The postcentral gyrus (sensory strip) is the most anterior part of the parietal lobe and is the principal destination of conscious sensations. The upper fibres of the optic radiation pass through it. The dominant hemisphere contains aspects of language function and the non-dominant lobe is concerned with spatial awareness.

Abnormal findings

Damage to the parietal lobes is often associated with re-emergence of primitive reflexes. Features of parietal lobe dysfunction include:

- cortical sensory impairments
- contralateral lower quadrantanopia (Fig. 12.3 (part 5))
- dyslexia, dyscalculia, dysgraphia
- apraxia (an inability to carry out complex tasks despite having an intact sensory and motor system)
- focal sensory seizures (postcentral gyrus)
- visuospatial disturbance (non-dominant parietal lobe).

Occipital lobe

Anatomy

The occipital lobe blends with the temporal and parietal lobes, and forms the posterior part of the cerebral cortex. Its main function is analysis of visual information.

Abnormal findings

- Visual field defects: hemianopia (loss of part of a visual field) or scotoma (blind spot)
- Visual agnosia: the inability to recognise visual stimuli
- Disturbances of visual perception, e.g. macropsia (seeing things larger) or micropsia (smaller)
- Visual hallucinations.

THE CRANIAL NERVES

Anatomy

The 12 pairs of cranial nerves (with the exception of the olfactory (I) pair) arise from the brainstem (Fig. 11.4). Cranial nerves II, III, IV and VI relate to the eye (Ch. 12) and the VIII nerve to hearing and balance (Box 11.17, Ch. 13).

The olfactory (I) nerve

The olfactory nerve conveys the sense of smell.

Anatomy

Bipolar cells in the olfactory bulb form olfactory filaments with small receptors projecting through the cribriform plate high in the nasal cavity. These cells synapse with second-order neurones, which project centrally via the olfactory tract to the medial temporal lobe and amygdala.

Examination sequence

Bedside testing of smell is of limited clinical value, and rarely performed, although objective 'scratch and sniff' test cards are available, e.g. the University of Pennsylvania Smell Identification Test (UPSIT).

Abnormal findings

Hyposmia or anosmia (reduction or loss of the sense of smell) may result from ear, nose and throat disease, damage to the olfactory filaments after head injury or local compression or invasion by basal skull tumours. Disturbance of smell may also occur in the presymptomatic stages of Parkinson's and Alzheimer's diseases. Patients often also note hypogeusia/ageusia (altered taste) with anosmia.

Parosmia is when pleasant odours are perceived as unpleasant; it may occur with head trauma, sinus infection or as an adverse effect of drugs. Olfactory hallucinations may occur in Alzheimer's disease and focal epilepsies.

The optic (II), oculomotor (III), trochlear (IV) and abducens (VI) nerves

See Chapter 12.

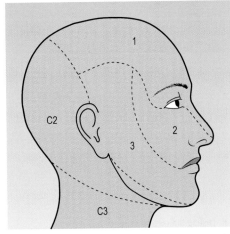

Fig. 11.5 The sensory distribution of the three divisions of the trigeminal nerve. (1) Ophthalmic division. (2) Maxillary division. (3) Mandibular division.

The trigeminal (V) nerve

Anatomy

The V nerve provides sensation to the face, mouth and part of the dura, and motor supply to the muscles of mastication.

The cell bodies of the sensory fibres are located in the trigeminal (Gasserian) ganglion, which lies in a cavity (Meckel's cave) in the petrous temporal dura (Fig. 11.4). There are three major branches of the nerve (Fig. 11.5):

- ophthalmic (V_1): sensory
- maxillary (V_2): sensory
- mandibular (V_3): sensory and motor.

The ophthalmic branch leaves the ganglion and passes forward to the superior orbital fissure via the wall of the cavernous sinus. In addition to the skin of the upper nose, upper eyelid, forehead and scalp, V_1 supplies sensation to the eye (cornea and conjunctiva) and the mucous membranes of the sphenoidal and ethmoid sinuses and upper nasal cavity.

The maxillary branch (V_2) passes from the ganglion via the cavernous sinus to leave the skull by the foramen rotundum. It contains sensory fibres from the mucous membranes of the upper mouth, roof of pharynx, gums, teeth and palate of the upper jaw and the maxillary, sphenoidal and ethmoid sinuses.

The mandibular branch (V_3) exits the skull via the foramen ovale and supplies the floor of the mouth, common sensation, i.e. not taste, to the anterior two-thirds of the tongue, the gums and teeth of the lower jaw, mucosa of the cheek and the temporomandibular joint in addition to the skin of the lower lips and jaw area, but not the angle of the jaw (Fig. 11.5).

- From the trigeminal ganglion, the V nerve passes to the pons. From here, pain and temperature pathways descend to the C2 segment of the spinal cord, so ipsilateral facial numbness may occur with cervical cord lesions.

The motor fibres of V run in the mandibular branch (V_3) and innervate the temporalis, masseter, medial and lateral pterygoids (muscles of mastication).

11

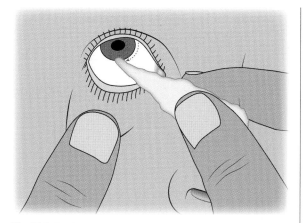

Fig. 11.6 Testing the corneal reflex.

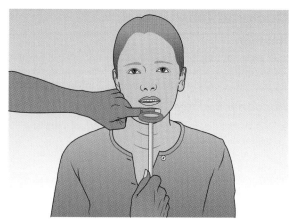

Fig. 11.7 Eliciting the jaw jerk.

Examination sequence

There are four functions: sensory, motor and two reflexes.

Sensory

- Ask the patient to close his eyes and say 'yes' each time he feels you lightly touch them using a cotton wool tip. Do this in the areas of V_1, V_2 and V_3.
- Repeat using a fresh neurological pin, e.g. Neurotip, to test superficial pain.
- Compare both sides. If you identify an area of reduced sensation, map it out. Does it conform to the distribution of the trigeminal nerve or branches? Remember the angle of the jaw is not served by the trigeminal nerve, but V_1 does extend towards the vertex (Fig. 11.5).
- 'Nasal tickle' test: use a wisp of cotton wool to 'tickle' the inside of each nostril and ask the patient to compare: it is an unpleasant sensation easily appreciated by the patient.

Motor (signs rare)

- Inspect for wasting of the muscles of mastication (most apparent in temporalis).
- Ask the patient to clench his teeth; feel the masseters, estimating their bulk.
- Place your hand under the jaw to provide resistance; ask the patient to open his jaw. Note any deviation.

Corneal reflex

- Explain to the patient what you are going to do, and ask him to remove contact lenses, if relevant.
- Gently depress the lower eyelid while the patient looks upwards.
- Lightly touch the lateral edge of the cornea with a wisp of damp cotton wool (Fig. 11.6):
- Look for both direct and consensual blinking.

Jaw jerk

- Ask the patient to let his mouth hang loosely open.
- Place your forefinger in the midline between lower lip and chin.
- Percuss your finger gently with the tendon hammer in a downwards direction (Fig. 11.7), noting any reflex closing of the jaw. An absent, or just present, reflex is normal.

Abnormal findings

Sensory symptoms include facial numbness and pain (trigeminal neuralgia). Unilateral loss of sensation in one or more branches of the V nerve may result from direct injury in association with facial fractures (particularly V_2) or local invasion by cancer. Lesions in the cavernous sinus often cause loss of the corneal reflex and V_1 or V_2 cutaneous sensory loss. Cranial nerves III, IV and VI may also be involved (Ch. 12). Trigeminal neuralgia causes severe, lancinating pain typically in distribution of V_2 or V_3, and is often due to neurovascular compression. Reactivation of herpes varicella zoster virus (chickenpox) can affect any sensory nerve, but typically either a thoracic dermatome or V_1 (Fig. 11.8). Clinically significant weakness of the muscles of mastication is unusual, but may occur in myasthenia, with fatigable chewing. A brisk jaw jerk occurs in pseudobulbar palsy.

The facial (VII) nerve

The facial nerve supplies the muscles of facial expression, and carries parasympathetic secretomotor fibres to the lacrimal, submandibular and sublingual salivary glands (via nervus intermedius). It receives taste sensation from the anterior two-thirds of the tongue (via the chorda tympani branch), and also provides the efferent supply to several reflexes (Fig. 11.9).

Anatomy

From its motor nucleus in the lower pons, fibres of the VII nerve pass back to loop around the VI nucleus before emerging from the lateral pontomedullary junction in close association with the VIII nerve; together they enter the internal acoustic meatus (Figs 11.4 and 11.9). At the lateral end of the meatus the VII nerve continues in the facial canal within the temporal bone, exiting the skull via the stylomastoid foramen. Passing through the parotid gland, it gives off its terminal branches. In its course in the facial canal it gives off branches to the stapedius muscle and its parasympathetic fibres, as well as being joined by the taste fibres of the chordae tympani (Fig. 11.10).

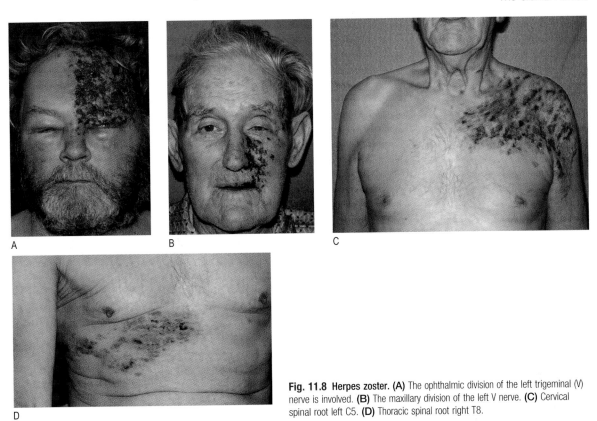

A

B

C

D

Fig. 11.8 Herpes zoster. (A) The ophthalmic division of the left trigeminal (V) nerve is involved. **(B)** The maxillary division of the left V nerve. **(C)** Cervical spinal root left C5. **(D)** Thoracic spinal root right T8.

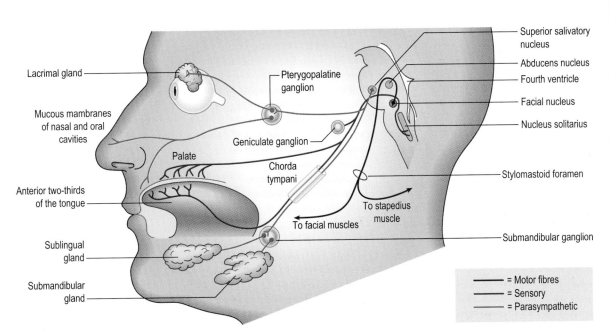

Lacrimal gland

Mucous mambranes of nasal and oral cavities

Pterygopalatine ganglion

Superior salivatory nucleus

Abducens nucleus

Fourth ventricle

Facial nucleus

Nucleus solitarius

Geniculate ganglion

Palate

Chorda tympani

Anterior two-thirds of the tongue

Stylomastoid foramen

To stapedius muscle

To facial muscles

Sublingual gland

Submandibular ganglion

Submandibular gland

— = Motor fibres
— = Sensory
— = Parasympathetic

Fig. 11.9 Component fibres of the facial nerve and their peripheral distribution.

11

Examination sequence

Examination is usually confined to motor function; taste is rarely tested.

Motor function

- Inspect the face for asymmetry or differences in blinking or eye closure on one side. Note that minor facial asymmetry is common and rarely pathological.
- Watch for spontaneous or involuntary movement.
- Ask the patient to raise the eyebrows and observe for symmetrical wrinkling of the forehead (Fig. 11.11A).
- Demonstrate baring your teeth and ask the patient to mimic you. Look for asymmetry (Fig. 11.11B).
- Test power by saying: 'Screw your eyes tightly shut and stop me from opening them,' then 'Blow out your cheeks with your mouth closed' (Fig. 11.11C and D).

Abnormal findings

In a unilateral lower motor neurone VII nerve lesion, there is weakness of both upper and lower facial muscles. Bell's palsy is a common condition presenting with acute lower motor neurone VII nerve paralysis, often preceded by mastoid pain. It may be associated with impairment of taste and hyperacusis (high-pitched sounds appearing unpleasantly louder than normal). Bell's phenomenon occurs when the patient is unable to close his eye. As he tries, the eyeball rolls upwards,

exposing the conjunctiva below the cornea (Fig. 11.12A). Ramsay Hunt syndrome occurs in herpes zoster infection of the geniculate (facial) ganglion. This produces a severe lower motor neurone facial palsy, ipsilateral loss of taste and buccal ulceration, and a painful vesicular

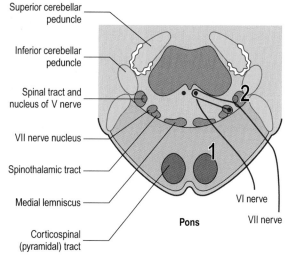

Fig. 11.10 Lesions of the pons. Lesions at (1) may result in ipsilateral VI and VII nerve palsies and contralateral hemiplegia; at (2) ipsilateral cerebellar signs and impaired sensation on the ipsilateral side of the face and on the contralateral side of the body may occur.

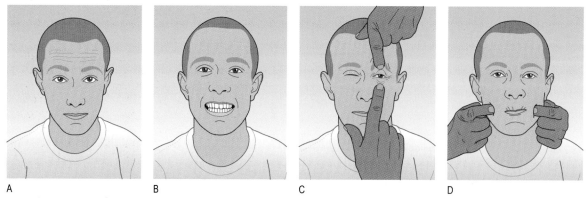

A B C D

Fig. 11.11 Testing the motor function of the facial nerves. (A) Ask the patient to raise his eyebrows. **(B)** Ask him to show his teeth. **(C)** Ask him to close eyes against resistance. **(D)** Ask him to blow out his cheeks.

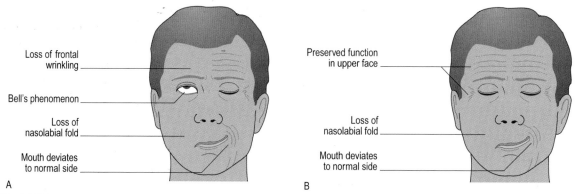

A B

Fig. 11.12 Types of facial weakness. (A) Right-sided lower motor neurone lesion (within facial nerve or nucleus); Bell's phenomenon is also shown. **(B)** Right-sided upper motor neurone lesion.

eruption in the external auditory meatus. Other causes of a lower motor neurone VII lesion include cerebellopontine angle tumours, e.g. acoustic neuroma, trauma and parotid tumours. Synkinesis (most commonly twitching of the corner of the mouth on ipsilateral blinking) is a sign of aberrant reinnervation, and may be seen in recovering lower motor neurone VII lesions.

In unilateral VII nerve upper motor neurone lesions, weakness is marked in the lower facial muscles with relative sparing of the upper face. This is because there is bilateral cortical innervation of the upper facial muscles. The nasolabial fold may be flattened and the corner of the mouth droop, but eye closure is usually preserved (Fig. 11.12B). Involuntary emotional movements, e.g. spontaneous smiling, have different pathways and may be preserved in the presence of paresis.

Bilateral facial palsies are less common, but occasionally occur, e.g. Guillain–Barré syndrome, sarcoidosis, Lyme disease and HIV infection. Distinct from VII nerve palsies, Parkinson's disease can cause loss of spontaneous facial movements, including a slowed blink rate, and involuntary facial movements (levodopa-induced dyskinesias) may complicate advanced disease.

The vestibulocochlear (VIII) nerve

See Chapter 13.

The glossopharyngeal (IX) and vagus (X) nerves

The IX and X nerves have an intimate anatomical relationship. Both contain sensory, motor and autonomic components. The glossopharyngeal (IX) nerve mainly carries sensation from the pharynx and tonsils, and sensation and taste from the posterior one-third of the tongue. The vagus (X) nerve carries important sensory information but also innervates upper pharyngeal and laryngeal muscles. The main functions of IX and X are swallowing, phonation/articulation and sensation from the pharynx/larynx.

Anatomy

Both nerves arise as several roots from the lateral medulla and leave the skull together via the jugular foramen (Fig. 11.4). The IX nerve passes down and forward to supply the stylopharyngeus muscle, the mucosa of the pharynx, the tonsils and the posterior one-third of the tongue, and sends parasympathetic fibres to the parotid gland. The X nerve courses down in the carotid sheath into the thorax, giving off several branches, including pharyngeal and recurrent laryngeal branches, which provide motor supply to the pharyngeal, soft palate and laryngeal muscles. The main nuclei of these nerves in the medulla are the nucleus ambiguus (motor), the dorsal motor vagal nucleus (parasympathetic) and the solitary nucleus (visceral sensation) (Fig. 11.13).

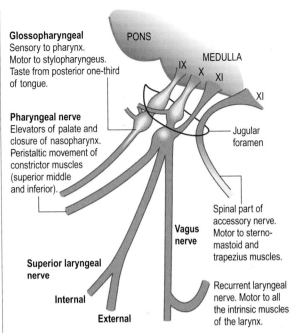

Fig. 11.13 The lower cranial nerves: glossopharyngeal (IX), vagus (X) and accessory (XI).

Glossopharyngeal
Sensory to pharynx.
Motor to stylopharyngeus.
Taste from posterior one-third of tongue.

PONS
MEDULLA
IX X XI
XI
Jugular foramen

Pharyngeal nerve
Elevators of palate and closure of nasopharynx. Peristaltic movement of constrictor muscles (superior middle and inferior).

Vagus nerve

Spinal part of accessory nerve. Motor to sternomastoid and trapezius muscles.

Superior laryngeal nerve

Internal

External

Recurrent laryngeal nerve. Motor to all the intrinsic muscles of the larynx.

Examination sequence

- Assess the patient's speech for dysarthria or dysphonia.
- Ask him to say 'Ah'; look at the movements of the palate and uvula using a torch. Normally, both sides of the palate elevate symmetrically and the uvula remains in the midline.
- Ask the patient to puff out his cheeks with the lips tightly closed. Listen for air escaping from the nose. For the cheeks to puff out, the palate must elevate and occlude the nasopharynx. If palatal movement is weak, air will escape audibly through the nose.
- Ask the patient to cough; assess the strength of the cough.
- Testing pharyngeal sensation and the gag reflex is unpleasant and has poor predictive value for aspiration. Instead, and in fully conscious patients only, use the swallow test. Administer 3 teaspoons of water and observe for absent swallow, cough or delayed cough, or change in voice quality after each teaspoon. If there are no problems, watch for the same reactions while the patient swallows a glass of water.

Abnormal findings

Isolated unilateral IX nerve lesions are rare. Unilateral X nerve damage leads to ipsilateral reduced elevation of the soft palate, which may cause deviation of the uvula (away from the side of the lesion) when the patient says 'Ah'. Damage to the recurrent laryngeal branch of the X nerve due to lung cancer, thyroid surgery, mediastinal tumours and aortic arch aneurysm causes dysphonia and a 'bovine' cough (p. 139). Bilateral X nerve lesions cause dysphagia and dysarthria. Less severe cases can result in nasal regurgitation of fluids and nasal air escape when the cheeks are puffed out (dysarthria and nasal escape are often evident during history taking: Box 11.15).

The accessory (XI) nerve

The accessory nerve has two components:
- a cranial part closely related to the vagus nerve
- a spinal part which provides fibres to the upper trapezius and the sternocleidomastoid muscles,

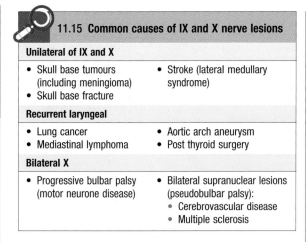

11.15 Common causes of IX and X nerve lesions

Unilateral of IX and X

- Skull base tumours (including meningioma)
- Skull base fracture
- Stroke (lateral medullary syndrome)

Recurrent laryngeal

- Lung cancer
- Mediastinal lymphoma
- Aortic arch aneurysm
- Post thyroid surgery

Bilateral X

- Progressive bulbar palsy (motor neurone disease)
- Bilateral supranuclear lesions (pseudobulbar palsy):
  - Cerebrovascular disease
  - Multiple sclerosis

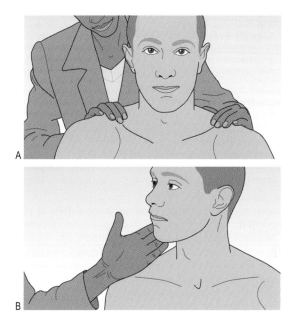

Fig. 11.14 Testing the trapezius and left sternocleidomastoid muscles. **(A)** Trapezius. **(B)** Left sternocleidomastoid.

responsible for elevating (shrugging) the shoulders, and head turning/flexing.

The spinal component is discussed here.

Anatomy

The spinal nuclei arise from the anterior horn cells of C1–5. Fibres emerge from the spinal cord, ascend through the foramen magnum, and exit via the jugular foramen (Fig. 11.4), passing posteriorly.

Examination sequence

- Face the patient and inspect the sternocleidomastoid muscles for wasting or hypertrophy; palpate them to assess their bulk.
- Stand behind the patient to inspect the trapezius muscle for wasting or asymmetry.
- Ask the patient to shrug the shoulders, then apply downward pressure with your hands to assess the power (Fig. 11.14A).
- Test power in the left sternocleidomastoid by asking the patient to turn the head to the right while you provide resistance with your hand placed on the right side of the patient's chin (Fig. 11.14B). Reverse the procedure to check the right sternocleidomastoid.

Abnormal findings

Isolated XI nerve lesions are uncommon but the nerve may be damaged during surgery in the posterior triangle of the neck, penetrating injuries or local invasion by tumour. Wasting of the upper fibres of trapezius may be associated with displacement of the upper vertebral border of the scapula away from the spine, while the lower border is displaced towards it. Wasting and weakness of the sternocleidomastoids are characteristic of myotonic dystrophy, and head drop may be seen in myasthenia, motor neurone disease and some myopathies.

The hypoglossal (XII) nerve

The XII nerve innervates the tongue muscles; the nucleus lies in the dorsal medulla beneath the floor of the fourth ventricle.

Anatomy

The nerve emerges anteriorly and exits the skull in the hypoglossal canal, passing to the root of the tongue (Fig. 11.4).

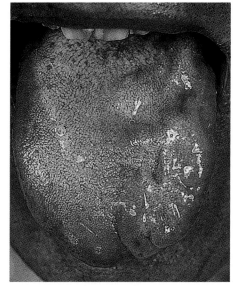

Fig. 11.15 Left hypoglossal nerve lesion.

Abnormal findings

Unilateral lower motor XII nerve lesions lead to tongue wasting on the affected side and deviation to that side on protrusion (Fig. 11.15). Bilateral lower motor neurone damage results in global wasting, the tongue lies thin and shrunken and fasciculation may be evident. Normal rippling or undulating movements may be mistaken for fasciculation, especially if the tongue is protruded; these usually settle when the tongue is at rest in the mouth. When associated with lesions of IX, X and XI nerves, typically in motor neurone disease, these features are called bulbar palsy.

11.16 Comparison of bulbar and pseudobulbar palsy

	Bulbar palsy	Pseudobulbar palsy
Motor lesion	Lower motor neurone	Upper motor neurone
Speech	Dysarthria	Dysarthria and dysphonia
Swallowing	Dysphagia	Dysphagia
Tongue	Weakness, wasting and fasciculation	Spastic, slow moving
Jaw jerk	Absent	Present/brisk
Emotional lability	Absent	May be present

11.17 Summary of all 12 cranial nerves

Nerve	Examination	Abnormalities/symptoms
I	Sense of smell, each nostril	Anosmia/parosmia
II	Visual acuity Visual fields Pupil size and shape Pupil light reflex Fundoscopy	Partial sight/blindness Scotoma; hemianopia Anisocoria Impaired or lost Optic disc and retinal changes
III	Accommodation reflex	Impaired or lost
III, IV and VI	Eye position and movements	Strabismus, diplopia, nystagmus
V	Facial sensation Corneal reflex Muscles of mastication Jaw jerk	Impaired, distorted or lost Impaired or lost Weakness of chewing movements Increased in upper motor neurone lesions
VII	Muscles of facial expression Taste over anterior two-thirds of tongue	Facial weakness Ageusia
VIII	Whisper and tuning fork tests Vestibular tests	Impaired hearing/deafness Nystagmus and vertigo
IX	Pharyngeal sensation	Not routinely tested
X	Palate movements	Impaired unilaterally or bilaterally
XI	Trapezius and sternomastoid	Weakness of neck movement
XII	Tongue appearance and movement	Dysarthria and chewing/swallowing problems

Unilateral upper motor XII nerve lesions are uncommon; bilateral lesions lead to a tongue with increased tone (spastic), and the patient has difficulty flicking the tongue from side to side. Bilateral upper motor lesions of IX–XII nerves may also affect the V and VII, and are called pseudobulbar palsy. They usually result from vascular disease, motor neurone disease or occasionally multiple sclerosis (Box 11.16). Tremor of the resting or protruded tongue may occur in Parkinson's disease, although jaw tremor is more common. Other orolingual dyskinesias (involuntary movements of the mouth and tongue) are often drug-induced, e.g. tardive dyskinesias due to neuroleptics.

Examination sequence

- Ask the patient to open his mouth. Look at the tongue at rest for wasting, fasciculation or involuntary movement.
- Ask the patient to put out his tongue. Look for deviation or involuntary movement.
- Ask the patient to move the tongue quickly from side to side.
- Test power by asking the patient to press the tongue against the inside of each cheek in turn while you press from the outside with your finger.
- Assess speech by asking the patient to say 'yellow lorry'.
- Assess swallowing with a water swallow test (p. 255).

THE MOTOR SYSTEM

Assess the motor system under the following headings:
- inspection and palpation of muscles
- assessment of tone
- testing movement and power
- examination of reflexes
- testing coordination.

Inspection and palpation of the muscles

Anatomy

Motor fibres, together with input from other systems involved in the control of movement, including extrapyramidal, cerebellar, vestibular and proprioceptive afferents, converge on the cell bodies of lower motor neurones in the anterior horn of the grey matter in the spinal cord (Fig. 11.16).

Examination sequence

- Completely expose the patient while keeping the patient's comfort and dignity.
- Look for asymmetry, inspecting both proximally and distally. Note deformities, e.g. clawing of the hands or pes cavus.
- Examine for wasting or hypertrophy, fasciculation and involuntary movement.

Abnormal findings

Muscle bulk Lower motor neurone lesions may cause muscle wasting. This is not seen in acute upper motor neurone lesions, although disuse atrophy may develop with longstanding lesions. A motor neurone lesion in childhood may impair growth (causing a smaller limb or hemiatrophy) or cause limb deformity, e.g. pes cavus. Muscle disorders usually result in proximal wasting (the notable exception is myotonic dystrophy, in which it is distal, often with associated temporalis wasting). Certain occupations, e.g. professional sports players, may lead to physiological muscle hypertrophy.

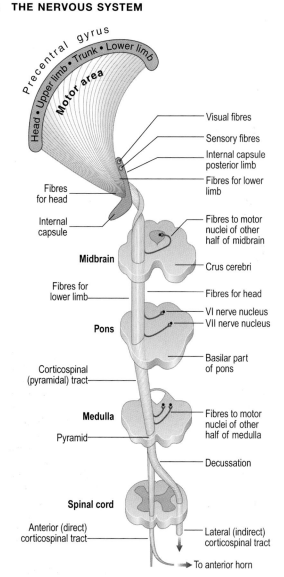

Fig. 11.16 Principal motor pathways.

Pseudohypertrophy may occur in muscular dystrophy but the muscles are weak. If you suspect wasting, ask the patient and/or partner whether they have also noticed this, as minor asymmetry in muscle bulk is often normal.

Fasciculation Fasciculation is irregular twitches under the skin overlying resting muscles caused by individual motor units firing spontaneously. This occurs in lower motor neurone disease, usually in wasted muscles. Fasciculation is seen, not felt, and you may need to observe carefully for several minutes to be sure that this is not present. Physiological fasciculation is common, especially in the calves, but is not associated with weakness or wasting. Myokymia is rapid bursts of repetitive motor unit activity often occurring in an eyelid or first dorsal interosseus, and is rarely pathological.

Myoclonic jerks These are sudden shock-like contractions of one or more muscles which may be focal or diffuse and occur singly or repetitively. Healthy people commonly experience these when falling asleep (hypnic jerks). They may also occur pathologically in association with epilepsy, diffuse brain damage and dementia.

Tremor Tremor is an oscillatory movement about a joint or a group of joints resulting from alternating contraction and relaxation of muscles. Tremors are classified according to their frequency, amplitude, position (at rest, on posture or on movement) and body part affected.

Physiological tremor is a fine (low-amplitude), fast (high-frequency) postural tremor seen with anxiety. A similar tremor occurs in hyperthyroidism and with excess alcohol or caffeine intake, and is a common adverse effect of β-agonist bronchodilators.

Essential tremor is the most common pathological cause of an action tremor, typically affecting the upper limbs and head, with postural and action components. It may be improved by alcohol, and often demonstrates an autosomal dominant pattern of inheritance.

Parkinson's disease causes a slow, coarse tremor, worse at rest but reduced with voluntary movement. It is more common in the upper limbs, usually asymmetrical, and does not affect the head.

Isolated head tremor is usually dystonic, and may be associated with abnormal neck postures such as torticollis (twisting to one side), anterocollis (neck flexion) or retrocollis (neck extension).

Intention tremor is absent at rest but maximal on movement, and is usually due to cerebellar damage. It is assessed with the finger-to-nose test (p. 264).

Functional tremors: movement disorders, including tremor, are common functional symptoms. They are often inconsistent, with varying frequencies and amplitudes, and may be associated with other signs.

Other involuntary movements

These are classified according to their appearance.

Dystonia is caused by sustained muscle contractions, leading to twisting, repetitive movements and sometimes tremor. It may be focal, e.g. torticollis, a twisting neck, or global.

Chorea describes brief, random, purposeless movements which may affect various body parts, but commonly the arms.

Athetosis is a slower, writhing movement, more similar to dystonia than chorea.

Ballism refers to violent flinging movements sometimes affecting only one side of the body (hemiballismus).

Tics are repetitive, stereotyped movements which can be briefly suppressed by the patient.

Tone

Tone is the resistance felt by the examiner when moving a joint passively.

Examination sequence

- Ask the patient to lie supine on the examination couch, and to relax and 'go floppy'. Enquire about any painful joints or limitations of movement before proceeding.
- Passively move each joint tested through as full a range as possible, both slowly and quickly in all anatomically possible directions. Be unpredictable with these movements, both in direction and speed, to prevent the patient actively moving with you; you want to assess passive tone.

Upper limb

- Hold the patient's hand as if shaking hands, using your other hand to support his elbow. Assess tone at the wrist and elbow.
- Activation is a technique used to exaggerate subtle increase in tone, and is particular useful for assessing extrapyramidal tone increase. Ask the patient to describe circles in the air with the contralateral limb while assessing tone. A transient increase in tone with this manoeuvre is normal.

Lower limb

- Roll the leg from side to side, then briskly lift the knee into a flexed position, observing the movement of the foot (Fig. 11.17A and B). Typically the heel moves up the bed, but increased tone may cause it to lift off the bed due to failure of relaxation.

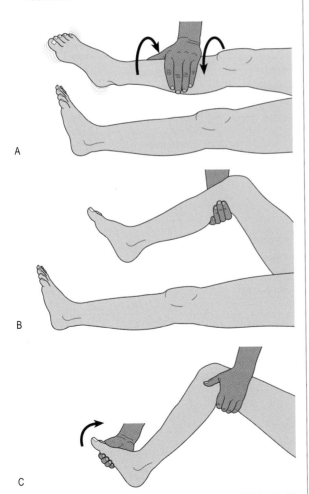

A

B

C

Fig. 11.17 Testing for tone. (A) Rock the leg to and fro. **(B)** Quickly lift the leg at the knee and observe the movement of the heel. **(C)** Test for ankle clonus.

Ankle clonus

- Support the patient's leg, with both the knee and ankle resting in 90° flexion.
- Briskly dorsiflex and partially evert the foot, sustaining the pressure (Fig. 11.17C). Clonus is felt as repeated beats of dorsiflexion/plantar flexion.

Abnormal findings

Hypotonia (decreased muscle tone) or hypertonia (increased) suggest a lower or upper motor neurone lesion respectively.

Hypotonia This may occur in lower motor neurone lesions and is usually associated with muscle wasting, weakness and hyporeflexia. It may be a feature of cerebellar disease or in the early phases of cerebral or spinal shock, when the paralysed limbs are atonic prior to developing spasticity. Reduced tone can be difficult to elicit.

Hypertonia There are two types of hypertonia: spasticity and rigidity.

Spasticity is velocity-dependent resistance to passive movement: it is detected with quick movements and is a feature of upper motor neurone lesions. It is usually accompanied by weakness, hyperreflexia, an extensor plantar response and sometimes clonus. In mild forms it is detected as a 'catch' at the beginning or end of passive movement. In severe cases it limits the range of movement and may be associated with contracture. In the upper limbs it may be more obvious on attempted extension; in the legs it is more evident on flexion.

Rigidity is a sustained resistance throughout the range of movement and is most easily detected when the limb is moved slowly. In parkinsonism this is classically described as 'lead pipe rigidity'. In the presence of a parkinsonian tremor there may be a regular interruption to the movement, giving it a jerky feel ('cog wheeling').

Clonus is a rhythmic series of contractions evoked by sudden stretch of the muscle and tendon. Unsustained (<6 beats) clonus may be physiological. When sustained, it indicates upper motor neurone damage and is accompanied by spasticity. It is best elicited at the ankle; knee (patella) clonus is rare, and not routinely tested.

Power

Strength varies with age, occupation and fitness. Grade muscle power using the Medical Research Council scale (Box 11.18). In practice, most cases of weakness are

	11.18 Medical Research Council scale for muscle power
0	No muscle contraction visible
1	Flicker of contraction but no movement
2	Joint movement when effect of gravity eliminated
3	Movement against gravity but not against examiner's resistance
4	Movement against resistance but weaker than normal
5	Normal power

11

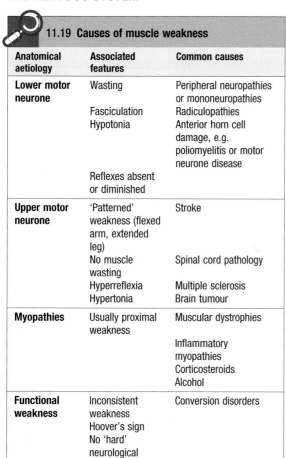

11.19 Causes of muscle weakness

Anatomical aetiology	Associated features	Common causes
Lower motor neurone	Wasting	Peripheral neuropathies or mononeuropathies
	Fasciculation	Radiculopathies
	Hypotonia	Anterior horn cell damage, e.g. poliomyelitis or motor neurone disease
	Reflexes absent or diminished	
Upper motor neurone	'Patterned' weakness (flexed arm, extended leg)	Stroke
	No muscle wasting	Spinal cord pathology
	Hyperreflexia	Multiple sclerosis
	Hypertonia	Brain tumour
Myopathies	Usually proximal weakness	Muscular dystrophies
		Inflammatory myopathies
		Corticosteroids
		Alcohol
Functional weakness	Inconsistent weakness Hoover's sign No 'hard' neurological signs	Conversion disorders

11.20 Definitions of paralysis

Term	Definition
Paresis	Partial paralysis
Plegia	Complete paralysis
Monoplegia	Involvement of a single limb
Hemiplegia	Involvement of one-half of the body
Paraplegia/diplegia	Paralysis of the legs
Tetraplegia	Paralysis of all four limbs

11.21 Nerve and muscle supplies of commonly tested movements

Movement	Muscle	Nerve/root
Shoulder abduction	Deltoid	Axillary C5
Elbow flexion	Biceps Brachioradialis	Musculocutaneous C5, 6 Radial C6
Elbow extension	Triceps	Radial C7
Wrist extension	Extensor carpi radialis longus	Posterior interosseus nerve (radial) C6
Finger extension	Extensor digitorum communis	Posterior interosseous (radial) C7
Finger flexion	Flexor pollicis longus (thumb) Flexor digitorum profundus (index and middle fingers)	Anterior interosseus (median) C8
	Flexor digitorum profundus (ring and little fingers)	Ulnar C8
Finger abduction	First dorsal interosseous	Ulnar T1
Thumb abduction	Abductor pollicis brevis	Median T1
Hip flexion	Iliopsoas	Iliofemoral nerve L1, 2
Hip extension	Gluteus maximus	Sciatic L5/S1
Knee flexion	Hamstrings	Sciatic S1
Knee extension	Quadriceps	Femoral L3/4
Ankle dorsiflexion	Tibialis anterior	Deep peroneal L4, L5
Ankle plantar flexion	Gastrocnemius and soleus	Tibial S1/2
Great toe extension (dorsiflexion)	Extensor hallucis longus	Deep peroneal L5
Ankle eversion	Peronei	Superficial peroneal L5/S1
Ankle inversion	Tibialis posterior	Tibial nerve L4, 5

grade 4. Plus or minus signs, e.g. 4+ or 4–, are helpful. Record what the patient can actually do in terms of daily activities, e.g. whether he can stand, walk, raise both arms above the head. Lesions at different sites may produce different clinical patterns of weakness (Boxes 11.19 and 11.20).

Examination sequence

- Do not test every muscle in most patients; the commonly tested muscles are listed in Box 11.21.
- Ask about pain which may interfere with testing.
- Test upper limb power with the patient sitting on the edge of the couch. Test lower limb power with the patient reclining.
- Ask the patient to undertake a movement. First assess whether he can overcome gravity, e.g. instruct the patient 'Lift your right leg off the bed' to test hip flexion. Then apply resistance to this movement testing across a single joint, e.g. apply resistance to the thigh in hip flexion, not the lower leg.
- Ask the patient to lift his arms above his head.
- Ask him to 'play the piano', checking movements of the outstretched arms (asymmetric loss of fine finger movement may be a very early sign of cortical or extrapyramidal disease).

- Observe the patient getting up from a chair and walking. Assess individual muscles depending on the history.
- Observe the patient with his arms outstretched and supinated (palms up) and eyes closed for 'pronator drift', when one arm starts to pronate (Box 11.22). Asking the patient to squeeze your fingers with his hand assesses the patient's ability to obey commands, not power.
- To test truncal strength, ask the patient to sit up from the lying position, or rise from a chair, without using the arms.

Abnormal findings

Upper motor neurone lesions produce weakness of a relatively large group of muscles, e.g. a limb or more than one limb. Lower motor neurone damage can cause paresis of an individual and specific muscle so more detailed examination of individual muscles is required (Ch. 14). Look for patterns of weakness which may suggest a diagnosis (Box 11.20). Patients may find it difficult to sustain maximum power for reasons other than weakness, most commonly pain. You need only show that the patient can achieve maximum power briefly. Very few organic diseases cause power to fluctuate; the fatigable weakness of myasthenia is the chief exception. Wildly fluctuating or sudden 'giveway' weakness suggests a functional explanation. Hoover's sign is often present in functional leg weakness, and is helpful diagnostically and therapeutically (you can show patients that the leg is not actually weak using this sign).

Deep tendon reflexes

Anatomy

A tendon reflex is the involuntary contraction of a muscle in response to stretch. It is mediated by a reflex arc consisting of an afferent (sensory) and an efferent (motor) neurone with one synapse between (a monosynaptic reflex). Muscle stretch activates the muscle spindles, which send a burst of afferent signals that lead to direct efferent impulses, causing muscle contraction. These stretch reflex arcs are served by a particular spinal cord segment which is modified by descending upper motor neurones.

Abnormal findings

Hyperreflexia (abnormally brisk reflexes) is a sign of upper motor neurone damage. Diminished or absent jerks are most commonly due to lower motor neurone lesions. In healthy elderly people the ankle jerks may be reduced or lost (Box 11.23), and in the Holmes–Adie syndrome, myotonic pupils (Fig. 12.26B and p. 290) are associated with loss of some deep tendon reflexes. Isolated loss of a reflex suggests a mononeuropathy or radiculopathy, e.g. loss of ankle jerk with L5/S1 lumbosacral disc prolapse compressing the S1 nerve root. Reflex patterns are helpful in localising neurological lesions, but you should know the nerve roots which serve the commonly tested reflexes (Box 11.24). There are several reflex-grading systems, but interobserver agreement is poor; record reflexes as present (and if so, whether normal, increased or decreased) or absent. Never conclude a reflex is absent until you have used reinforcement; this is a technique when concurrent

---

EBE **11.22 An early feature of upper motor neurone lesion**

Pronator drift is an early feature of an upper motor neurone lesion and the test has good specificity and sensitivity.

Anderson NE. The forearm and finger rolling tests. Pract Neurol 2010;10:39–42.

EBE **11.23 Ankle jerks**

Reduced or lost ankle jerks may be normal in elderly people.

Vrancken AFJE, Kalmijn S, Brugman F et al. The meaning of distal sensory loss and absent ankle reflexes in relation to age: a meta-analysis. J Neurol 2006;253:578–589.

11.24 Monosynaptic (deep tendon) reflexes and root innervation

Reflex (muscle)	Nerve root
Biceps	C5
Supinator (brachioradialis)	C6
Triceps	C7
Knee (quadriceps)	L3, 4
Ankle (gastrocnemius, soleus)	S1

---

motor activity in other muscles may augment (reinforce) the reflex tested.

An 'inverted' biceps reflex is caused by combined spinal cord and root pathology localising to a specific spinal level. It is most common at the C5/6 level. When elicited, the biceps reflex is absent or reduced but finger flexion occurs. This is because the lesion at the C5/6 level affects the efferent arc of the biceps jerk (C5 nerve root), causing it to be reduced or lost, and also the spinal cord increasing reflexes below this level (including the finger jerks). It is most commonly seen in cervical spondylotic myeloradiculopathy.

A positive Hoffmann's reflex (thumb flexion elicited by flicking the distal phalanx of the middle finger) and finger jerks suggest hypertonia, but can occur in healthy individuals, and are not useful signs in isolation. In cerebellar disease the reflexes may be pendular, and muscle contraction and relaxation tend to be slow, but these are not sensitive or specific cerebellar signs.

Examination sequence

- Ask the patient to lie supine on the examination couch with the limbs exposed. He should be as relaxed and comfortable as possible, as anxiety and pain can cause an increased response.
- Flex your wrist and allow the weight of the tendon hammer head to determine the strength of the blow. Strike the tendon, not the muscle or bone.
- Record the response as:
  - increased
  - normal
  - diminished
  - present only with reinforcement
  - absent.

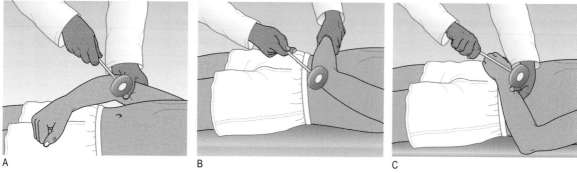

A   B   C

Fig. 11.18 **Testing the deep tendon reflexes of the upper limb. (A)** Eliciting the biceps jerk, C5. **(B)** Triceps jerk, C7. **(C)** Supinator jerk, C6.

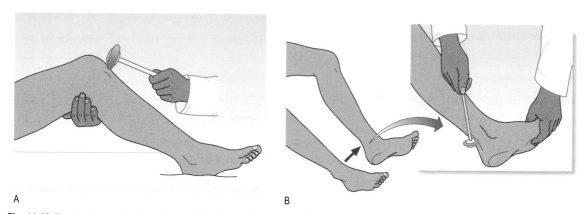

A   B

Fig. 11.19 **Testing the deep tendon reflexes of the lower limb. (A)** Eliciting the knee jerk (note that the legs should not be in contact with each other), L3, L4. **(B)** Ankle jerk of recumbent patient, S1.

Principal reflexes

- Ensure that both limbs are positioned identically with the same amount of stretch.
- Compare each reflex with the other side; check for symmetry of response (Figs 11.18 and 11.19).
- Use reinforcement whenever a reflex appears absent. For knee and ankle reflexes, ask the patient to interlock the fingers and pull one hand against the other on your command, immediately before you strike the tendon (Jendrassik's manœuvre; Fig. 11.20).
- To reinforce upper limb reflexes, ask the patient to clench the teeth or to make a fist with the contralateral hand. The patient should relax between repeated attempts. Strike the tendon immediately after your command to the patient.

Hoffmann's reflex

- Place your right index finger under the distal interphalangeal joint of the patient's middle finger.
- Use your right thumb to flick the patient's finger downwards.
- Look for any reflex flexion of the patient's thumb (Fig. 11.21A).

Finger jerk

- Place your middle and index fingers across the palmar surface of the patient's proximal phalanges.
- Tap your own fingers with the hammer.
- Watch for flexion of the patient's fingers (Fig. 11.21B).

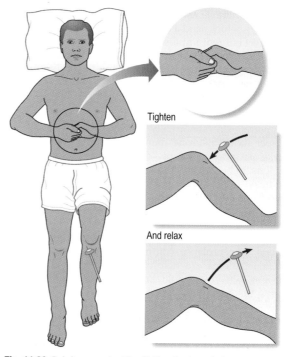

Tighten

And relax

Fig. 11.20 Reinforcement while eliciting the knee jerk.

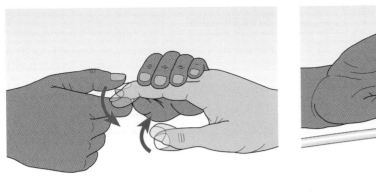

A   B

Fig. 11.21 Testing the deep tendon reflexes of the hand. (A) Hoffmann's sign. **(B)** Eliciting a finger jerk.

Superficial reflexes

This group of reflexes is polysynaptic and elicited by cutaneous stimulation rather than stretch. With the exception of the plantar response, they are not part of the routine examination, and have poor sensitivity and specificity. The cremasteric reflex applies only in males.

Abnormal findings

An abnormal plantar response is extension of the large toe (extensor plantar or Babinski response). This is a sign of upper motor neurone damage and is usually associated with other upper motor neurone signs, e.g. spasticity, clonus and hyperreflexia. Fanning of the toes is normal and not pathological.

Superficial abdominal reflexes (T8–12) are lost in upper motor neurone lesions but are also affected by lower motor neurone damage affecting T8–12. They are usually absent in the obese, the elderly or after abdominal surgery.

The cremasteric reflex in males (L1 and L2) may be absent on the side of spinal cord or root lesions, but this is of little clinical significance.

Examination sequence

Plantar response (S1–2)

- Run a blunt object (orange stick) along the lateral border of the sole of the foot towards the little toe (Fig. 11.22).
- Watch both the first movement of the great toe and the other leg flexor muscles. The normal response is flexion of the great toe with flexion of the other toes.
- A true Babinski sign:
  - involves activation of the extensor hallucis longus tendon (not movement of the entire foot, a common 'withdrawal' response to an unpleasant stimulus)
  - coincides with contraction of other leg flexor muscles
  - is reproducible.

Abdominal reflexes (T8–12)

- The patient should be supine and relaxed.
- Use an orange stick and briskly, but lightly, stroke the upper and lower quadrants of the abdomen in a medial direction (Fig. 11.23).

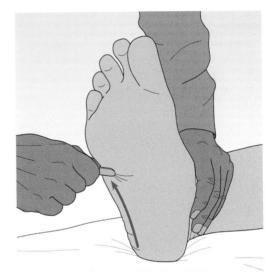

Fig. 11.22 Eliciting the plantar reflex.

- The normal response is contraction of the underlying muscle, with the umbilicus moving laterally and up or down depending upon the quadrant tested.

Cremasteric reflex (L1–2): males only

- Explain what you are going to do and why it is necessary.
- Abduct and externally rotate the patient's thigh.
- Use an orange stick to stroke the upper medial aspect of the thigh.
- Normally the testis on the side stimulated will rise briskly.

Primitive reflexes

These are present in normal neonates and young infants but disappear as the nervous system matures. People with congenital or hereditary cerebral lesions and a few healthy individuals retain these reflexes, but their return after early childhood is often associated with brain damage or degeneration. The primitive reflexes (snout, grasp, palmomental and glabellar tap) have little localising value and in isolation are of little significance, but

11

11

in combination suggest diffuse or frontal cerebral damage (Box 11.25). Unilateral grasp and palmomental reflexes may occur with contralateral frontal lobe pathology. The glabellar tap is an unreliable sign of Parkinson's disease.

11.25 Primitive reflexes
Snout reflex
• Lightly tap the lips. An abnormal response is lip pouting
Grasp reflex
• Firmly stroke the palm from the radial side. In an abnormal response, your finger is gripped by the patient's hand
Palmomental reflex
• Apply firm pressure to the palm next to the thenar eminence with a tongue depressor. An abnormal response is ipsilateral puckering of the chin
Glabellar tap
• Stand behind the patient and tap repeatedly between his eyebrows with the tip of your index finger. Normally the blink response stops after three or four taps

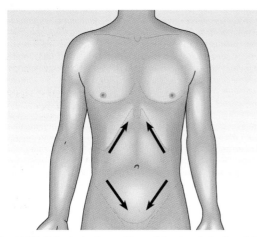

Fig. 11.23 Abdominal reflexes. Sites and direction of stimuli to elicit the reflexes.

Coordination

Performing complex movements smoothly and efficiently depends upon intact sensory and motor function and an intact cerebellum.

Anatomy

The cerebellum lies in the posterior fossa and consists of two hemispheres with a central vermis. Afferent and efferent pathways convey information to and from the cerebral motor cortex, basal ganglia, thalamus, vestibular and other brainstem nuclei and the spinal cord. In general, midline structures, e.g. vermis, influence body equilibrium, while each hemisphere controls ipsilateral coordination.

Examination sequence

Test cerebellar function by testing limb coordination, then for dysarthria (p. 248), nystagmus (p. 289), stance and gait (p. 247).

Finger-to-nose test
- Ask the patient to touch her nose with the tip of her index finger and then touch your finger tip. Hold your finger just within the patient's arm's reach (you should make the patient use her arm outstretched).
- Ask her to repeat the movement between nose and target finger as quickly as possible.
- Make the test more sensitive by changing the position of your target finger. Timing is crucial – move your finger just as the patient's finger is about to leave her nose, otherwise you will induce a false-positive finger-to-nose ataxia.
- Some patients are so ataxic that they may injure their eye/face with this test. If so, use your two hands as the targets (Fig. 11.24).

Heel-to-shin test
- With the patient lying supine, ask him to place his heel on his opposite knee, and then slide his heel up and down the shin between knee and ankle (Fig. 11.25).

Rapid alternating movements
- Demonstrate repeatedly patting the palm of your hand with the palm and back of your opposite hand as quickly and regularly as possible.

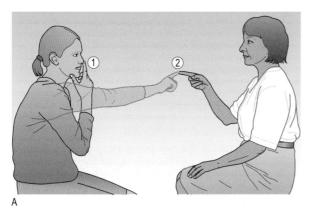
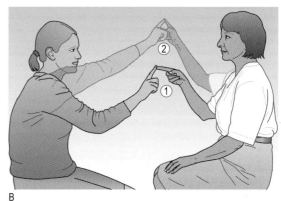

A B

Fig. 11.24 Finger-to-nose test. (A) Ask the patient to touch the tip of her nose and then your finger. **(B)** Move your finger from one position to another, towards and away from the patient, as well as from side to side.

- Ask the patient to copy your actions.
- Repeat with the opposite hand.
- Alternatively, ask the patient to tap a steady rhythm rapidly with his hand on the other hand or table, and 'listen to the cerebellum'; ataxia makes this task difficult, with a slower, irregular rhythm than normal.

Rebound phenomenon (rarely useful)

- Ask the patient to stretch his arms out and maintain this position.
- Push the patient's wrist quickly downward and observe the returning movement.

Abnormal findings

The finger-to-nose test may reveal a tendency to fall short or overshoot the examiner's finger (dysmetria or past-pointing). In more severe cases there may be a tremor of the finger as it approaches the target finger and the patient's own nose (intention tremor). The movement may be slow, disjointed and clumsy (dyssynergia). The heel-to-shin test is the equivalent test for the lower limbs. It is abnormal if the heel wavers away from the line of the shin. Weakness may produce false-positive finger-to-nose or heel-to-shin tests, so demonstrate that power is normal first.

Dysdiadochokinesis (impairment of rapid alternating movements) is evident as slowness, disorganisation and irregularity of movement. Dysarthria (p. 248) and nystagmus (p. 281) also occur with cerebellar disease. Much less reliable signs of cerebellar disease include: the rebound phenomenon, when the displaced outstretched arm may fly up past the original position (the normal response is to return to the original position); pendular reflexes; and hypotonia.

In disorders predominantly affecting midline cerebellar structures, e.g. tumours of the vermis and alcoholic cerebellar damage, the above tests may be normal, and truncal ataxia may be the only finding. In the most severe cases, this may mean the patient cannot sit unsupported. Tandem gait (heel–toe walking) may be impaired in less severe cases. Cerebellar dysfunction occurs in many conditions, and the differential diagnosis varies with age and speed of presentation (Box 11.26).

Apraxia

Dyspraxia or apraxia is difficulty or inability to perform a task, despite no impairment of the necessary individual functions. It is a sign of higher cortical dysfunction, usually localising to the non-dominant frontal or parietal lobes.

Examination sequence

- Ask the patient to perform an imaginary act, e.g. drinking a cup of tea, combing the hair, folding a letter and placing it in an envelope. Ask the patient to copy movements you make with your fingers, e.g. pointing.
- Ask the patient to copy a geometrical figure (interlocking pentagons or cube).
- Ask the patient to put on a pyjama top or dressing gown, one sleeve of which has been pulled inside out.

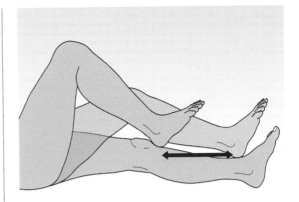

Fig. 11.25 Performing the heel-to-shin test with the right leg.

11.26 Acquired and genetic causes of ataxia

Toxic	Drugs, e.g. phenytoin, lithium, amiodarone Toxins, e.g. alcohol, heavy metals
Vascular	Stroke (ischaemic or haemorrhagic)
Neoplastic	Metastases Primary brain tumours Paraneoplastic cerebellar degeneration (anti-Hu antibody, associated with cancers of lung, breast, ovary)
Inflammatory	Inflammatory, e.g. multiple sclerosis Sarcoidosis
Infective/ transmissible	Viral, e.g. mumps, herpes zoster, human immunodeficiency virus Bacterial, e.g. syphilis, Whipple's disease Variant Creutzfeldt–Jakob disease
Degenerative	Multiple system atrophy
Structural and traumatic	Arnold–Chiari malformation Traumatic brain injury
Metabolic, nutritional	Hypothyroidism Vitamin B_1, B_{12} or E deficiency
Genetic	Friedreich's ataxia (autosomal recessive, age of onset <25 years) Spinocerebellar ataxias (SCA, autosomal dominant, age of onset >25 years) Episodic ataxias 1 and 2 (channelopathies)

Abnormal findings

The patient may be unable to initiate a task or perform it in an odd or bizarre fashion.

Constructional apraxia (difficulty drawing a figure) is a feature of parietal disturbance.

Dressing apraxia, often associated with spatial disorientation and neglect, is usually due to non-dominant hemisphere parietal lesions.

THE SENSORY SYSTEM

Detailed examination of sensation is time-consuming and unnecessary unless the patient volunteers sensory symptoms or you suspect a specific pathology, e.g. spinal cord compression or mononeuropathy.

11

Anatomy

Proprioception (joint position sense) and vibration are conveyed in large, myelinated fast-conducting fibres in the peripheral nerves and in the posterior (dorsal) columns of the spinal cord. Pain and temperature sensation are carried by small, slow-conducting fibres of the peripheral nerves and the spinothalamic tract of the spinal cord. The posterior column remains ipsilateral from the point of entry up to the medulla, but most pain and temperature fibres cross to the contralateral spinothalamic tract within one or two segments of entry to the spinal cord. All sensory fibres relay in the thalamus before sending information to the sensory cortex in the parietal lobe (Fig. 11.26).

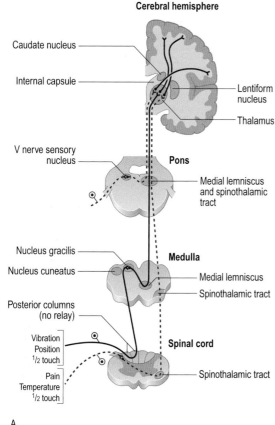

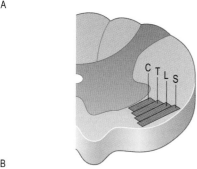

Fig. 11.26 The sensory system. (A) Main sensory pathways.
(B) Spinothalamic tract: layering of the spinothalamic tract in the cervical region. C represents fibres from cervical segments which lie centrally; fibres from thoracic, lumbar and sacral segments (labelled T, L and S respectively) lie progressively more laterally.

Symptoms and definitions

Sensory symptoms are numerous (Box 11.27), and it is important to discern what the patient is describing. Clarify that by 'numbness' the patient means lack of sensation rather than weakness or clumsiness. Neuropathic pain (pain due to disease or dysfunction of the PNS or CNS) is often severe and refractory to standard analgesia. Reduced ability to feel pain may be accompanied by scars from injuries or burns.

The sensory modalities

In addition to the modalities conveyed in the principal ascending pathways (touch, pain, temperature, vibration and joint position sense), sensory examination includes tests of discriminative aspects of sensation which may be impaired by lesions of the sensory cortex. Only assess these cortical sensory functions if the main pathway sensations are intact.

Consider abnormalities on sensory testing according to whether the lesion(s) is in the peripheral nerve(s), dorsal root(s), spinal cord, or intracranial.

Peripheral nerve and dorsal root

Many diseases affect peripheral nerves, generally resulting in peripheral neuropathies or polyneuropathies (Box 11.28). Peripheral neuropathies tend to affect the lower limbs first (length-dependent). Symptoms affecting the upper limbs first suggest a demyelinating rather than axonal neuropathy or a disease process in the spinal cord. In many cases, touch and pinprick sensation are lost in a 'stocking and glove' distribution (Fig. 11.27A).

In large-fibre neuropathies, vibration and joint position sense are disproportionately affected. Patients may report staggering when they close their eyes during hair washing (Romberg's sign: p. 247). When joint position sense is affected in the arms, pseudoathetosis may be demonstrated by asking the patient to close his eyes and hold his hands outstretched: the fingers will make involuntary, slow wandering movements, mimicking athetosis. Interpretation of sensory signs requires knowledge of the relevant anatomy of sensory nerves and dermatomes (Box 11.29, Fig. 11.28 and Fig. 11.32).

11.27 Neuropathic symptoms	
Paraesthesia	Tingling, or pins and needles Spontaneous or provoked Not unduly unpleasant or painful
Dysaesthesia	Unpleasant paraesthesia
Hypoaesthesia	Reduced sensation to a normal stimulus
Analgesia	Numbness or loss of sensation
Hyperaesthesia	Increased sensitivity to a stimulus
Allodynia	Painful sensation resulting from a non-painful stimulus
Hyperalgesia	Increased sensitivity to a painful stimulus

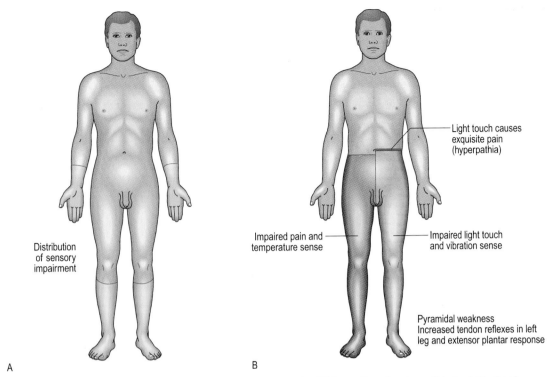

Light touch causes
exquisite pain
(hyperpathia)

Distribution
of sensory
impairment

Impaired pain and
temperature sense

Impaired light touch
and vibration sense

Pyramidal weakness
Increased tendon reflexes in left
leg and extensor plantar response

A

B

Fig. 11.27 Patterns of sensory loss. (A) In length dependent peripheral neuropathy. **(B)** Brown-Séquard syndrome. Note the distribution of corticospinal, posterior column and lateral spinothalamic tract signs. The cord lesion is in the left half of the cord.

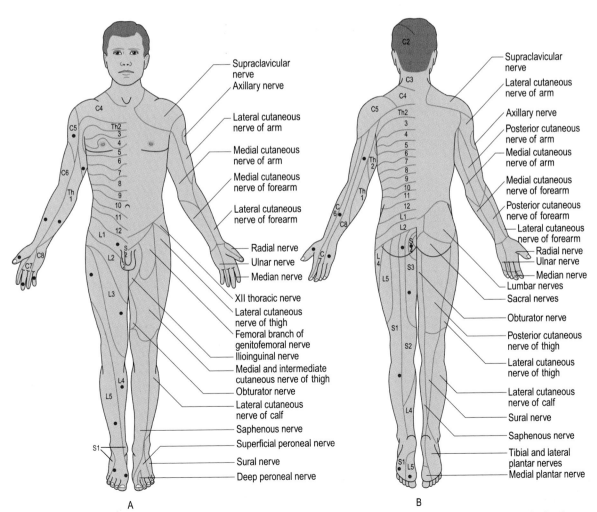

Supraclavicular
nerve
Axillary nerve

Lateral cutaneous
nerve of arm

Medial cutaneous
nerve of arm

Medial cutaneous
nerve of forearm

Lateral cutaneous
nerve of forearm

Radial nerve
Ulnar nerve
Median nerve

XII thoracic nerve
Lateral cutaneous
nerve of thigh
Femoral branch of
genitofemoral nerve
Ilioinguinal nerve
Medial and intermediate
cutaneous nerve of thigh
Obturator nerve
Lateral cutaneous
nerve of calf
Saphenous nerve
Superficial peroneal nerve
Sural nerve
Deep peroneal nerve

Supraclavicular
nerve
Lateral cutaneous
nerve of arm
Axillary nerve
Posterior cutaneous
nerve of arm
Medial cutaneous
nerve of arm
Medial cutaneous
nerve of forearm
Posterior cutaneous
nerve of forearm
Lateral cutaneous
nerve of forearm
Radial nerve
Ulnar nerve
Median nerve
Lumbar nerves
Sacral nerves
Obturator nerve
Posterior cutaneous
nerve of thigh
Lateral cutaneous
nerve of thigh
Lateral cutaneous
nerve of calf
Sural nerve
Saphenous nerve
Tibial and lateral
plantar nerves
Medial plantar nerve

A

B

Fig. 11.28 Dermatomal and sensory peripheral map innervation. Points (blue) for testing cutaneous sensation of limbs. By applying stimuli at the points marked, both the dermatomal and main peripheral nerve distributions are tested simultaneously.

11

11.28 Causes of polyneuropathy

Genetic	Charcot–Marie–Tooth (CMT) Hereditary neuropathy with liability to pressure palsies (HNPP) Hereditary sensory ± autonomic neuropathies (HSN, HSAN) Familial amyloid polyneuropathy Refsum's disease
Drugs and toxins	Amiodarone Antibiotics (dapsone, isoniazid, metronidazole) Antiretrovirals (stavudine, dideoxycitabine) Nitrous oxide (recreational use) Toxins (phenytoin, alcohol, lead, arsenic, mercury, solvents)
Vitamin deficiencies	B_1, B_6, B_{12} Note: excess B_6 also causes neuropathy
Infections	Human immunodeficiency virus (HIV) Leprosy Lyme (radiculoneuropathy) *Brucella* (radiculoneuropathy) Diphtheria
Inflammatory	Acute inflammatory demyelinating neuropathy (Guillain–Barré syndrome) Chronic inflammatory demyelinating neuropathy (CIDP) Vasculitis (polyarteritis nodosa, granulomatosis with polyangiitis, rheumatoid arthritis, systemic lupus erythematosus)
Systemic medical conditions	Diabetes mellitus Renal failure Sarcoidosis
Malignant disease	Paraneoplastic (antibody-mediated) Infiltration
Others	Paraproteinaemias Amyloidosis

EBE 11.29 Vibration sense

Absent, or reduced, vibration sense at the ankle may occur in healthy people >60 years.

Vrancken AFJE, Kalmijn S, Brugman F et al. The meaning of distal sensory loss and absent ankle reflexes in relation to age: a meta-analysis. J Neurol 2006;253:578–589.

Spinal cord

Traumatic and compressive spinal cord lesions cause loss or impairment of sensation in a dermatomal distribution below the level of the lesion. A zone of hyperaesthesia may be found immediately above the level of sensory loss.

Anterior spinal artery syndrome usually results in loss of spinothalamic sensation and motor function, with sparing of dorsal column sensation. A similar dissociated pattern of pain and temperature loss and sparing of dorsal column sensation occurs in syringomyelia.

When one-half of the spinal cord is damaged, the Brown-Séquard syndrome may occur. This is characterised by ipsilateral motor weakness and loss of vibration and joint position sense, with contralateral loss of pain and temperature (Fig. 11.27B).

Intracranial

Brainstem lesions are often vascular, and you must understand the relevant anatomy to determine the site of the lesion (Fig. 11.29). Lower brainstem lesions may cause ipsilateral numbness on one side of the face (V nerve nucleus) and contralateral body numbness (spinothalamic tract).

Thalamic lesions may cause a patchy sensory impairment on the opposite side with unpleasant, poorly localised pain, often of a burning quality.

Cortical parietal lobe lesions typically cause sensory inattention but may also affect joint position sense, two-point discrimination, stereognosis (tactile recognition) and localisation of point touch. Two-point discrimination and touch localisation are not helpful signs and are not performed routinely.

Examination sequence

Light touch
- While the patient looks away or closes his eyes, use a wisp of cotton wool (or lightly apply your finger) and ask the patient to say yes to each touch.
- Time the stimuli irregularly and make a dabbing rather than a stroking or tickling stimulus.
- Compare each side for symmetry.

Superficial pain
- Use a fresh neurological pin, e.g. Neurotip, not a hypodermic needle. Dispose of the pin after each patient to avoid transmitting infection.
- Explain and demonstrate that the ability to feel a sharp pinprick is being tested.
- Map out the boundaries of any area of reduced, absent or increased sensation and compare with Figure 11.28. Move from reduced to higher sensibility: i.e. from hypoaesthesia to normal, or normal to hyperaesthesia.

Temperature
- Touch the patient with a cold metallic object, e.g. tuning fork, and ask if it feels cold. More sensitive assessment requires tubes of hot and cold water at controlled temperatures but is seldom performed.

Vibration
- Place a vibrating 128 Hz tuning fork over the sternum.
- Ask the patient, 'Do you feel it buzzing?'
- Place it on the tip of the great toe (Fig. 11.30).
- If sensation is impaired, place the fork on the interphalangeal joint and progress proximally, to the medial malleolus, tibial tuberosity and anterior iliac spine, depending upon the response.
- Repeat the process in the upper limb. Start at the distal interphalangeal joint of the forefinger, and if sensation is impaired, proceed proximally.
- If in doubt as to the accuracy of the response, ask the patient to close his eyes and to report when you stop the fork vibrating with your fingers.

Joint position sense

- With the patient's eyes open, demonstrate the procedure.
- Hold the distal phalanx of the patient's great toe at the sides. Tell the patient you are going to move his toe up or down, demonstrating as you do so (Fig. 11.31).
- Ask the patient to close his eyes and to identify the direction of small movements in random order.
- Test both great toes (or middle fingers). If impaired, move to more proximal joints in each limb.

Stereognosis and graphaesthesia

- Ask the patient to close his eyes.
- Place a familiar object, e.g. coin or key, in his hand and ask him to identify it (stereognosis).
- Use the blunt end of a pencil or orange stick and trace letters or digits on the patient's palm. Ask the patient to identify the figure (graphaesthesia).

Sensory inattention (only test if sensory pathways are otherwise intact)

- Ask the patient to close his eyes.
- Touch his arms/legs in turn and ask which side has been touched.
- Now touch both sides simultaneously and ask whether the left, right or both sides were touched.

THE PERIPHERAL NERVES

Peripheral nerves may be damaged individually (mononeuropathy) or multiply (peripheral neuropathy or mononeuritis multiplex). Certain nerves (median nerve at the wrist, common peroneal nerve at the knee) are prone to trauma or compression.

Median nerve

This may be compressed as it passes between the flexor retinaculum and the carpal bones at the wrist (carpal tunnel syndrome); it is the most common entrapment neuropathy and initially produces sensory symptoms (Box 11.30).

Examination sequence

- Test for altered sensation over the hand involving the thumb, index and middle fingers and the lateral half of the ring finger – splitting of the ring finger (Fig. 11.32A and Fig. 14.29).
- Look for wasting of the thenar eminence.
- Test thumb abduction with the patient's hand held palm up on a flat surface. Ask the patient to move the thumb vertically against your resistance (abductor pollicis brevis).
- Test opposition by asking the patient to touch the thumb and ring finger together while you attempt to pull them apart (opponens pollicis).

Radial nerve

This may be compressed as it runs through the axilla, or injured in fractures of the humerus. It typically causes wrist drop.

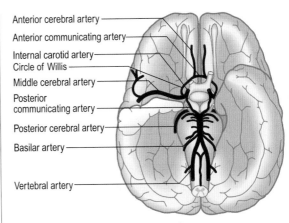

Anterior cerebral artery
Anterior communicating artery
Internal carotid artery
Circle of Willis
Middle cerebral artery
Posterior communicating artery
Posterior cerebral artery
Basilar artery
Vertebral artery

Fig. 11.29 Arteries at the base of the brain.

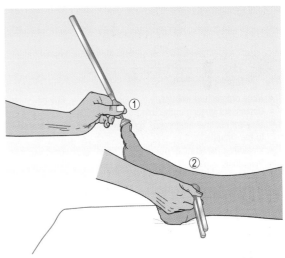

Fig. 11.30 Testing vibration sensation. At the big toe (1) and the ankle (2).

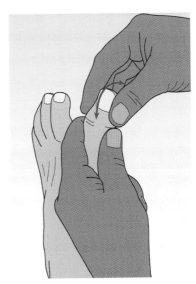

Fig. 11.31 Testing for position sense in the big toe.

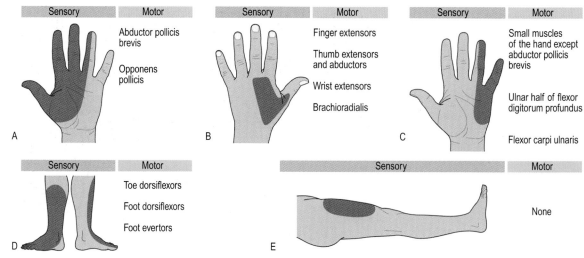

Fig. 11.32 **Sensory and motor deficits in nerve lesions. (A)** Median. **(B)** Radial. **(C)** Ulnar. **(D)** Common peroneal. **(E)** Lateral cutaneous of the thigh.

11.30 Common features of carpal tunnel syndrome

- More common in women
- Unpleasant tingling in the hand
- May not observe anatomical boundaries, radiating up the arm to the shoulder
- Weakness uncommon, but affects thumb abduction if occurs
- Symptoms commonly occur at night, wakening patient from sleep
- The patient may hang the hand and arm out of the bed for relief
- Thenar muscle wasting (in longstanding cases)
- Associated with pregnancy, diabetes and hypothyroidism

Examination sequence

- Test for weakness of arm and forearm extensors (triceps and the wrist and fingers).
- Look for sensory loss over the dorsum of the hand (Fig. 11.32B) and loss of triceps tendon jerk.

Ulnar nerve

This is most often affected at the elbow by external compression or injury, e.g. dislocation.

Examination sequence

- Look for wasting of interossei (dorsal guttering).
- Test for weakness of finger abduction with the patient's fingers on a flat surface, and ask him to spread the fingers against resistance from your fingers.
- Test adduction by placing a card between the patient's fingers and pulling it out using your own fingers.
- Assess for sensory loss on the ulnar side of the hand, splitting the ring finger (Fig. 11.32C).

- Examine the elbow (the commonest place of entrapment). Note any scars or other signs of trauma.
- Examine the range of movement and feel for the nerve in the ulnar groove.

Common peroneal nerve

This typically presents with foot drop. It may be damaged in fibular head fractures, or compressed particularly in immobile patients, or as a result of repetitive kneeling or squatting.

Examination sequence

- Test for weakness of ankle dorsiflexion and eversion. Inversion will be preserved.
- Test for sensory loss over the dorsum of the foot (Fig. 11.32D).

Lateral cutaneous nerve of thigh

This purely sensory nerve may be compressed as it passes under the inguinal ligament, producing paraesthesiae in the lateral thigh (meralgia paraesthetica) (Fig. 11.32E).

Examination sequence

- Test for disturbed sensation over the lateral aspect of the thigh.

PUTTING IT ALL TOGETHER

Having completed the history and examination, decide whether the symptoms are due to neurological disease. Determine the site(s) of damage (where is the lesion?). Try to localise the lesion to a single area of the nervous system, although some conditions may cause multiple symptoms and signs due to several lesions, e.g. multiple sclerosis. Consider the likely underlying pathology: what is the lesion?

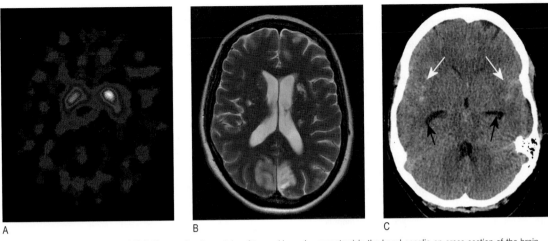

Fig. 11.33 Scanning of the head: (A) DaT scan showing uptake of tracer (dopamine receptors) in the basal ganglia on cross-section of the brain. **(B)** MR scan showing ischaemic stroke T2 imaging demonstrates bilateral occipital infarction and bilateral hemisphere lacunar infarction. **(C)** Unenhanced CT scan showing subarachnoid blood in both sylvian fissures (white arrows) and early hydrocephalus, with temporal horns of the lateral ventricles visible (black arrows).

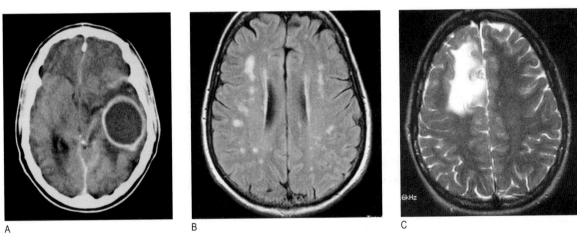

Fig. 11.34 Scanning of the head. (A) CT scan showing a cerebral abscess. **(B)** MR scan showing multiple sclerosis with white demyelinating plaques. **(C)** MR scan showing a glioma involving the right cerebral hemisphere.

Draw up a differential diagnosis and then consider which (if any) investigations are pertinent.

Do not place undue emphasis on an isolated sign that fails to fit with the history, e.g. an apparently isolated extensor plantar response in a patient with typical migraine – it is likely this is a false-positive sign rather than indicating underlying pathology.

Remember that medically unexplained symptoms are common but distinguishing them from organic disease is difficult, even for experts (p. 27).

INVESTIGATIONS

Lumbar puncture

See Box 11.31 and Figures 11.33-35. Lumbar puncture is a key investigation in a number of acute and chronic neurological conditions (Box 11.32). Always measure the CSF opening pressure (in a lying position, not sitting). CSF is routinely examined for cells, protein content, and glucose (in comparison to simultaneously taken blood glucose); it is also stained and cultured for bacteria. Other specific tests may be carried out, e.g. analysis for oligoclonal bands, meningococcal and pneumococcal antigens, polymerase chain reaction (PCR) for certain viruses or cytology for malignant cells.

Neurophysiological tests

Electroencephalography (EEG) records the spontaneous electrical activity of the brain, using scalp electrodes. It is used in the investigation of epilepsy, encephalitis or dementia. Modifications to the standard EEG improve sensitivity, including sleep-deprived studies, prolonged video telemetry and invasive EEG monitoring.

11.31 Investigations in nervous system disease

Investigation	Indication/comment	Investigation	Indication/comment
Urine tests		Urea/creatinine	Encephalopathy Peripheral neuropathy
Glucose	Diabetic peripheral neuropathy	Electrolytes	Seizures Encephalopathy Diabetes insipidus/syndrome of inappropriate antidiuretic hormone secretion (SIADH)
Ketones	Diabetic coma (ketoacidosis)		
Bence Jones protein	Myeloma		
Porphobilinogen	Porphyria		
Blood tests		Glucose	Coma Stroke Neuropathies
Haemoglobin	Syncope, seizures, stroke		
Mean corpuscular volume	Vitamin B_{12} deficiency, alcohol excess, iron deficiency	Serum lipids and cholesterol	Stroke
White cell count	Infection, e.g. meningitis	Calcium	Epilepsy Tetany
Blood culture	Meningitis, endocarditis, stroke		
Erythryocyte sedimentation rate/C-reactive protein	Cranial arteritis	Drug/toxin screen	Coma Epilepsy Peripheral neuropathy
Vitamin B_{12} and folate	Peripheral neuropathy, dementia		
Clotting/thrombophilia screen and antiphospholipid antibody	Young onset stroke	Caeruloplasmin/serum copper	Wilson's disease
		Creatine phosphokinase	Muscular dystrophy, myopathy
Venereal Disease Research Laboratory–*Treponema pallidum* haemagglutination assay (VDRL–TPHA)	Neurosyphilis	DNA (nuclear and mitochondrial) analysis	Huntington's disease Hereditary ataxias and neuropathies Mitochondrial disorders
		Neurophysiology	
Human immunodeficiency virus	Numerous central/peripheral nervous system syndromes	Electroencephalogram (EEG)	Epilepsy Encephalopathy/encephalitis Sleep disorders
Antinuclear factor and dsDNA	Demyelination		
Rheumatoid factor	Peripheral neuropathy	Electromyogram (EMG)	Myopathy Muscular dystrophy Motor neurone disease
Acetylcholine receptor and muscle-specific kinase (MuSK) antibodies	Myasthenia gravis		
		Single-fibre EMG	Myasthenia gravis
Voltage-gated calcium channel antibodies	Lambert–Eaton myasthenic syndrome	Nerve conduction studies	Entrapment neuropathy Peripheral neuropathy
Voltage-gated potassium channel antibodies/ anti-NMDA receptor antibodies	Limbic encephalitis Psychosis, seizures Abnormal movements	Visual evoked potentials	Multiple sclerosis
		12-lead ECG	Epilepsy/syncope Stroke Muscular dystrophy
Paraneoplastic antibodies	Paraneoplastic neurological syndromes (cerebellar ataxia, sensory neuropathies, limbic encephalitis)	**Radiology**	
		Chest X-ray	Source of cerebral metastases Tuberculosis Sarcoidosis
Serum immunoglobulins and protein electrophoresis	Neuropathy	CT brain scan	Trauma: fractures, intracranial haematoma Stroke and subarachnoid haemorrhage Tumours, tuberculoma
Thyroid function test	Tremor Carpal tunnel syndrome		
Growth hormone, adrenocorticotrophic hormone, follicle-stimulating hormone/luteinising hormone, prolactin, thyroid-stimulating hormone	Pituitary tumour	CT angiography/venography	Subarachnoid/intracranial haemorrhage Intracranial venous sinus thrombosis
Liver function tests	Ataxia/seizures/neuropathy due to alcohol	MR brain scan	Multiple sclerosis Infection Metastases Infiltrative malignancy

11.31 Investigations in nervous system disease – *cont'd*

Investigation	Indication/comment	Investigation	Indication/comment
MRI of the spine	Tumours Prolapsed intervertebral disc Syringomyelia Vascular malformations	**Invasive**	
		Nerve biopsy	Peripheral neuropathies
		Muscle biopsy	Muscular dystrophies or myopathies
Single photon emission CT (SPECT: DaTscan) scan	Parkinsonian syndromes	Brain biopsy	Mass lesions of uncertain cause (most commonly tumours)
Ultrasound of carotid arteries	Atherosclerotic stenosis	Needle aspiration of brain	Cerebral abscess
Transcranial ultrasound	Hydrocephalus (in infants)	Needle aspiration of spine	Tuberculosis
Transthoracic/ transoesophageal echocardiogram	Stroke: source of embolism	Lumbar puncture	Meningitis, encephalitis Multiple sclerosis Malignant infiltration
Catheter angiography	Aneurysms Arteriovenous malformations		

11

11.32 Cerebrospinal fluid (CSF) findings in some common disorders

Condition	Pressure	Appearance	Cells/μl	Protein (g/l)	Glucose	Microbiology
Normal	15–180 mm	Crystal clear	<5 lymphocytes	0.1–0.4	>60% of blood glucose	Sterile
Acute bacterial meningitis	Usually increased/normal	Cloudy/turbid	100–50 000 polymorphs (lymphocytes in early stages)	Increased	Reduced	Gram stain of organism + culture
Tuberculous meningitis	Usually increased/normal	Clear/cloudy	25–500 lymphocytes (polymorphs in early stages)	Increased	Reduced	Auramine/ Ziehl–Neelsen stain + culture, PCR
Viral meningitis	Usually normal/ slight increase	Crystal clear	5–200 lymphocytes (occasional polymorphs in early stages)	Normal/slightly increased	Normal/ occasionally reduced	PCR
Tumour	Normal/increased	Crystal clear/ occasionally cloudy	0–500 lymphocytes + malignant cells	Increased	Normal/ reduced	Sterile
Subarachnoid haemorrhage	Increased	Blood-stained or xanthochromic supernatant	Red cells + normal/slightly raised white cells	Increased	Normal	Sterile
Multiple sclerosis	Normal/increased	Crystal clear	0–50 lymphocytes	Normal/ increased oligoclonal bands	Normal	Sterile

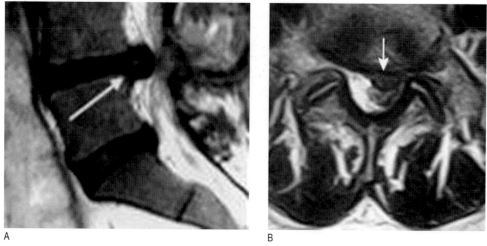

A   B

Fig. 11.35 T2 magnetic resonance images showing a large left paracentral L4–5 disc protrusion (arrowed) compressing the L5 nerve root. **(A)** Sagittal section. **(B)** Axial section.

Electromyography (EMG) involves needle electrodes inserted into muscle. Electrical activity is displayed on an oscilloscope and an audio monitor, allowing the neurophysiologist to see and hear the pattern of activity. Neurogenic and myogenic pathology may cause characteristic EMG abnormalities.

Nerve conduction studies involve applying electrical stimuli to nerves and measuring the speed of impulse conduction. They are used for both motor and sensory nerves, and are helpful in diagnosing peripheral nerve disorders such as nerve compressions or polyneuropathies.

John Olson
Rebecca Ford

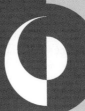

The visual system

12

12

ANATOMY

Eyelids, conjunctiva and lacrimal system

The eyelids protect the eye from injury and excessive light, distribute tears and contribute to facial expression. Levator palpebrae superioris muscle (oculomotor (III) nerve), and Müller's muscle (sympathetic autonomic system) open the lid. Active lid closure is mediated by the orbicularis oculi muscle (facial (VII) nerve).

Secretions from three glands contribute to a healthy tear film: mucin from goblet cells in the conjunctiva, aqueous tears from the lacrimal gland in the superotemporal orbit and accessory lacrimal glands in the conjunctiva and oil from meibomian glands in the eyelids.

The conjunctiva is a thin mucous membrane lining the eyelids and reflected at the superior and inferior fornices on to the surface of the eye. Basal tear production carries nutrients and immune system proteins to the cornea. Tears wash away foreign bodies and express emotion in crying. The lacrimal ducts drain into the superior fornix. Tears drain through the lacrimal canaliculi via the puncta at the medial edge of each eyelid, then into the lacrimal sac in the anterior part of the medial wall of the orbit, and from there into the nasolacrimal duct which opens into the nasal inferior meatus.

The eye

The eye focuses an image on to the neurosensory retina. The globe comprises three layers:

- an outer fibrous layer, five-sixths of which is the sclera and one-sixth the cornea. The regular orientation of collagen fibres renders the cornea transparent and it has two-thirds of the focusing power of the eye. The cornea is continuous posteriorly with the sclera, the tough, opaque white outer wall of the eyeball

- a middle vascular pigmented layer, the uveal tract, comprising the choroid posteriorly and the iris/ciliary body complex anteriorly
- an inner neurosensory layer, the retina (Fig. 12.1).

Key structures within the globe

The anterior chamber lies between the cornea and the iris and is filled with aqueous humour produced by the ciliary body in the posterior chamber. This flows through the pupil before draining through the trabecular meshwork of the angle of the anterior chamber.

The lens is a transparent, biconvex structure behind the iris and in front of the vitreous. It is suspended by the suspensory ligaments of the ciliary body.

The vitreous is a transparent gel behind the lens. Posteriorly, it is firmly attached to the margins of the optic disc, and anteriorly, to the retina at the ora serrata.

Sensation from the cornea, conjunctiva and intraocular structures is conveyed by the ophthalmic branch (V_1) of the trigeminal nerve (Ch. 11).

The optic (II) cranial nerve

The visual pathway consists of the retina, optic chiasm, optic tracts, lateral geniculate bodies, optic radiations and visual cortex.

The retina consists of an outer pigmented layer, and an inner neurosensory layer which is continuous with the optic nerve. The retinal pigment epithelium lies adjacent to the highly vascular choroid. Around 90% of ocular blood supply passes through the choroid, supplying the posterior two-thirds of the retina, the optic nerve and the fovea. The retinal vessels supply the relatively inert inner one-third of the retina. The neurosensory retina consists of photoreceptors, ganglion cells and interconnecting bipolar cells.

- Rod photoreceptors are responsible for night vision and detection of peripheral movement.

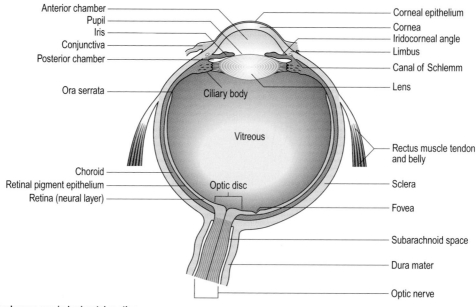

Fig. 12.1 The human eye in horizontal section.

- Cone photoreceptors are responsible for colour and central vision.
- Photoreceptors synapse with the vertically oriented bipolar cells of the retina, which in turn synapse with the ganglion cells of the optic nerve (Fig. 12.2).

The optic nerve is purely sensory and cannot regenerate. The optic nerve fibres myelinate on leaving the eye through the optic disc and enter the cranium through the optic canal. The two optic nerves join at the optic chiasm, where the nasal fibres, responsible for the temporal visual field, decussate. Leaving the chiasm, the visual pathway is renamed the 'optic tract'. The optic tracts terminate in the lateral geniculate bodies of the thalamus. However, some fibres leave the tract to form the afferent limb of the pupillary reflex.

Optic radiations pass through the cerebral hemisphere in the posterior part of the internal capsule and the parietal and temporal lobes to terminate in the occipital cortex (Fig. 12.3).

The occipital lobe analyses visual information and damage produces a homonymous hemianopia or scotoma (a discrete visual defect). The occipital lobe has a dual blood supply from the posterior and middle cerebral arteries. The middle cerebral artery supplies the posterior tip of the occipital lobe responsible for central vision from the macula. A lesion, affecting only the posterior tip of the occipital lobe, may produce central homonymous hemianopia with sparing of peripheral vision. A lesion, affecting only the anterior occipital lobe, may cause homonymous hemianopia involving peripheral vision but sparing central macular vision. Damage to secondary visual areas causes visual agnosia (inability to recognise visual stimuli) and distorted perceptions of visual images, such as macropsia (seeing things larger) or micropsia (smaller than reality) and visual hallucinations.

The oculomotor (III), trochlear (IV) and abducens (VI) cranial nerves innervate the six external ocular muscles controlling eye movement and, through parasympathetic nerves, also affect pupillary size (Fig. 12.4).

The oculomotor (III) nerve passes just below the free edge of the tentorium in relation to the posterior communicating artery and enters the dura surrounding the cavernous sinus. It enters the orbit through the superior oblique fissure, and innervates the superior, medial and inferior recti, the inferior oblique and levator palpebrae superioris muscles. These muscles open the upper lid (levator palpebrae superioris) and move the globe

12

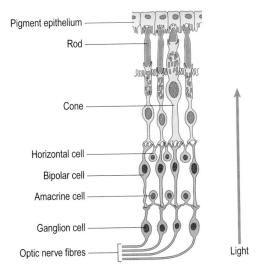

Pigment epithelium

Rod

Cone

Horizontal cell

Bipolar cell

Amacrine cell

Ganglion cell

Optic nerve fibres

Light

Fig. 12.2 The cellular organisation of the retina.

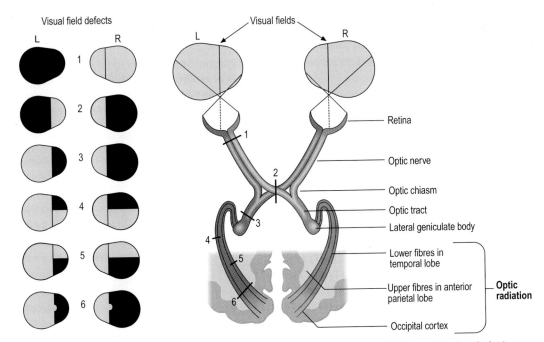

Visual field defects

L   R

Visual fields

L   R

Retina

Optic nerve

Optic chiasm

Optic tract

Lateral geniculate body

Lower fibres in temporal lobe

Upper fibres in anterior parietal lobe

Occipital cortex

Optic radiation

Fig. 12.3 Visual field defects. (1) Total loss of vision in one eye because of a lesion of the optic nerve. **(2)** Bitemporal hemianopia due to compression of the optic chiasm. **(3)** Right homonymous hemianopia from a lesion of the optic tract. **(4)** Upper right quadrantanopia from a lesion of the lower fibres of the optic radiation in the temporal lobe. **(5)** Lower quadrantanopia from a lesion of the upper fibres of the optic radiation in the anterior part of the parietal lobe. **(6)** Right homonymous hemianopia with sparing of the macula due to lesion of the optic radiation in the occipital lobe.

A

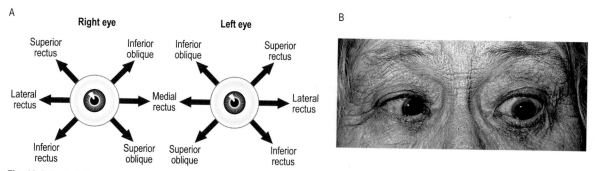

Fig. 12.4 Control of eye movement. (A) Fields of action of pairs of extraocular muscles. This diagram will help you to work out which eye muscle is paretic. For example, a patient whose diplopia is maximum on looking down and to the right has either an impaired right inferior rectus or a weak left superior oblique. **(B)** Left sixth-nerve palsy causing weakness of the lateral rectus muscle. The patient is shown here attempting to look to the left.

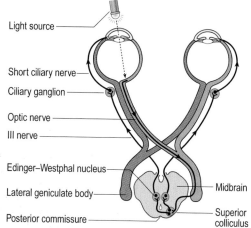

Fig. 12.5 Pathway of pupillary constriction and the light reflex (parasympathetic).

upwards (superior rectus, inferior oblique), downwards (inferior rectus) and medially (medial rectus). Through the parasympathetic fibres arising from the Edinger–Westphal nerves, the nerve indirectly supplies the sphincter muscles of the iris, causing constriction of the pupil, and the ciliary muscle which focuses the lens for near vision (accommodation) (Fig. 12.5).

The trochlear (IV) nerve fibres decussate before leaving the midbrain posteriorly (the left nucleus innervates the right trochlear nerve and vice versa). The nerve enters the orbit in the superior orbital fissure, supplying the superior oblique muscle, which causes downward movement of the globe when the eye is adducted.

The abducens (VI) nerve has a long course around the brainstem before it pierces the dura to enter the cavernous sinus. The nerve is in direct relation to the internal carotid artery before it passes through the superior orbital fissure to the lateral rectus muscle. Lateral rectus abducts the eye (Fig. 12.6).

The pupils admit light into the eyeball and are round, regular, equal in size and symmetrical in their responses. The autonomic nervous system and integrity of the iris determine the size of the resting pupil. The afferent limb of the pupillary reflex involves the optic nerve, chiasm (where some fibres decussate) and the optic tract, bypassing the lateral geniculate nucleus to terminate in the III nerve (Edinger–Westphal) nucleus. The efferent limb involves the inferior division of the III nerve,

passing through the ciliary ganglion in the orbit to the constrictor muscle of the iris. Sympathetic stimulation causes pupillary dilatation and upper and lower eyelid retraction. With parasympathetic stimulation (the fibres travel with the III nerve), the opposite occurs.

SYMPTOMS AND DEFINITIONS

Ocular pain

Pain is common and ranges from irritation to the excruciating pain of scleritis. Note if the affected eye is red or not to make the diagnosis.

Ocular pain with a 'white eye'

If the patient feels 'something in the eye', the problem involves the eye surface. The most common cause is a dry eye secondary to blepharitis (inflammation of the eyelid margins) with disruption of meibomian glandular secretions. Paradoxically, patients often complain of watery eyes due to reflex overproduction of tears from the lacrimal gland. Blepharitis may be associated with systemic skin conditions, e.g. atopic eczema, acne rosacea or seborrhoeic dermatitis. Severe dry eyes are a feature of Sjögren's syndrome. Preceding visual disturbance associated with headache or eye pain suggests migraine. Cluster headaches may present as ocular pain. In subacute episodes of angle closure (raised intraocular pressure), patients describe seeing haloes around lights. Pain on eye movement usually indicates either optic neuritis or scleritis. The eye in optic neuritis is white; in scleritis it is red.

Ocular pain with a 'red eye'

Circumciliary injection (redness around the corneal limbus) reflects involvement of the anterior ciliary arteries supplying the cornea, iris and ciliary body (uveitis). Diffuse redness suggests scleritis or conjunctivitis.

Entropion (an inverted eyelid) leads to painful corneal erosion (Fig. 12.7) and ectropion (everted eyelid) causes dryness in the exposed eye. Foreign bodies on the eye surface are usually associated with an at-risk activity, e.g. grinding metal without eye protection.

Severe unilateral pain with a cloudy cornea, circumciliary injection and an oval non-reactive pupil indicates acute angle closure glaucoma with high intraocular

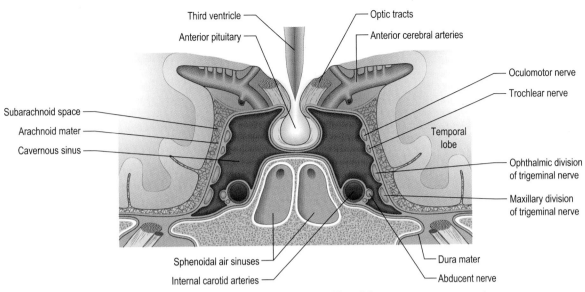

Third ventricle

Anterior pituitary

Optic tracts

Anterior cerebral arteries

Oculomotor nerve

Trochlear nerve

Subarachnoid space

Arachnoid mater

Cavernous sinus

Temporal lobe

Ophthalmic division of trigeminal nerve

Maxillary division of trigeminal nerve

Sphenoidal air sinuses

Internal carotid arteries

Dura mater

Abducent nerve

Fig. 12.6 Sagittal section illustrating neuroanatomy and lesions of the III, IV and VI cranial nerves.

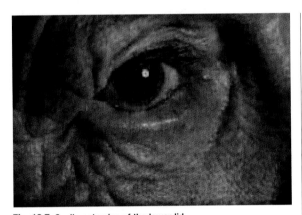

Fig. 12.7 Senile entropion of the lower lid.

pressure. Long-sighted people with shallow anterior chambers and the elderly, in whom lens thickening makes the anterior chamber shallower, are at risk. Pupillary dilatation may precipitate acute angle closure. Corneal oedema clouds the underlying iris, which may become ischaemic and fixed in mid-dilation. The pain is severe and may be associated with systemic symptoms. Treat both eyes to prevent recurrence.

Acute iritis produces a small, irregularly shaped pupil (Fig. 12.8A) and redness around the limbus. The inflamed iris becomes stuck to the underlying lens. The pain is not as severe as in angle closure glaucoma and photophobia may be prominent. Rarely, iritis presents bilaterally.

Corneal ulceration may be due to herpes simplex virus (Box 12.1), but in contact lens wearers, dry eyes or debilitated patients suspect bacterial infection. Depending on severity, redness may vary from circumciliary injection to diffuse redness associated with spontaneous lacrimation.

Pain on moving a red eye indicates scleritis (Fig. 12.8B) and may be the first manifestation of systemic vasculitis. The redness is frequently bilateral and involves the whole sclera or a sector of the sclera, unlike the circumciliary injection of iritis or angle closure glaucoma. Episcleritis is uncomfortable rather than painful and appears less dramatic than scleritis.

Conjunctivitis is an uncomfortable inflammation of the conjunctivae. There is always associated discharge or watering. The inner eyelid is inflamed and red, unlike scleritis or episcleritis (Fig. 12.8C). Bacterial conjunctivitis is associated with a yellow/green purulent discharge. Chlamydial and viral infection causes a clear discharge and preauricular lymphadenopathy. Persistent watery discharge with itchy eyes and no lymphadenopathy suggests an allergic cause.

Visual disturbance

Visual acuity

The curvature of the optic lens alters to adapt the focal length to suit the varying distance of the entering light rays and produce a clear, focused image. Common refractive errors are:

- Hypermetropia (long-sightedness): rays of light from a distant object are focused behind the retina. It is common in infants, and young people can compensate for hypermetropia by contracting the ciliary muscle, increasing the refractive power of the lens (Fig. 12.9).
- Myopia (short-sightedness): rays from a distant object are focused in front of the retina. Simple myopia usually starts in childhood and worsens during the growing years (Fig. 12.10).
- Presbyopia (impaired power of accommodation for near objects) occurs as the lens ages and is less able to change its curvature. It is very common in those >45 years.
- Astigmatism is when the cornea is irregularly curved, preventing light rays being brought to a common focus on the retina.

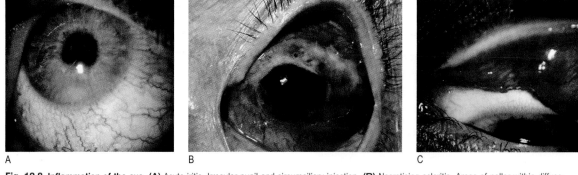

A   B   C

Fig. 12.8 Inflammation of the eye. (A) Acute iritis. Irregular pupil and circumciliary injection. **(B)** Necrotising scleritis. Areas of pallor within diffuse areas of redness, indicating ischaemia. **(C)** Giant papillary conjunctivitis seen on everting upper lid. A form of allergic conjunctivitis induced by contact lens wear.

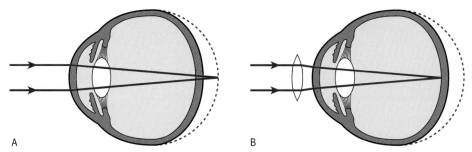

A   B

Fig. 12.9 The hypermetropic (long-sighted) eye. (A) The eye is too short and the image on the retina is not in focus. **(B)** The use of a convex (plus) lens brings the image on the retina into focus.

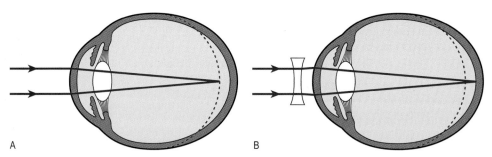

A   B

Fig. 12.10 The myopic (short-sighted) eye. (A) The eye is too long and the image on the retina is not in focus. **(B)** The use of a concave (minus) lens brings the image on the retina into focus.

12.1 Causes of corneal ulceration

Cause	History	Examination
Bacterial	Previous corneal disease Dry eyes, contact lenses	Ulcer affecting central cornea
Herpes simplex	Previous episode, general	Dendritic pattern most common manifestation
Herpes zoster	Ophthalmic shingles affecting external nose	Crusting vesicles affecting ophthalmic division of trigeminal nerve
Acanthamoeba	Contact lens users washing lens with tap water	Severe ocular pain and photophobia
Fungal	Ocular trauma with vegetable matter or immunocompromised patient	Feathery indistinct white lesion or non-responding 'bacterial ulcer'
Neurotrophic	Previous brainstem stroke (V nerve palsy), or previous herpes simplex virus or herpes zoster virus infection	Absent or reduced corneal sensation
Alkali burn	Injury with chemicals	Loss of adjacent conjunctival vessels suggests poor prognosis
Corneal abrasion	Trauma	A linear scratch suggests a foreign body under eyelid
Marginal keratitis	Blepharitis	Ulcer affecting peripheral cornea
Exposure	Lid malposition, especially nocturnal lagophthalmos in VII nerve palsy	Ulcer within exposed / open part of eye

Diplopia (double vision)

This may be uniocular or binocular. Binocular diplopia is caused by imbalance of eye movements; uniocular is due to intraocular disease.

Blurred vision

Distinguish true blurring of the whole visual field from a scotoma (a discrete defect). Generalised blurring is due to an ocular problem, ranging from uncorrected refractive error, e.g. myopia, hypermetropia, astigmatism or presbyopia, to opacities in the cornea, lens, aqueous chamber or vitreous gel.

Sudden-onset visual loss

This may be temporary or permanent, unilateral or bilateral. Patients may not notice gradual visual loss in one eye but only notice and complain when they close their unaffected eye.

Transient visual loss or disturbance is caused by the aura of migraine or unilateral amaurosis fugax (transient retinal ischaemia). The aura of classical migraine usually takes the form of coloured lines, often scintillating, and is always homonymous (present in both visual fields), although patients may mistakenly attribute it to one eye. Unlike amaurosis fugax, it is still seen with the eyes shut. In contrast, retinal migraine causes unilateral visual loss and may be difficult to differentiate from amaurosis fugax.

Amaurosis fugax produces a negative unilateral visual phenomenon which is black or grey. This is short-lasting (minutes) and appears like a shutter coming down, up or from the side, before resolving in a similar fashion. It may be confused with migraine aura or the homonymous hemianopia of transient occipital lobe ischaemia. Visual impairment following exercise or a hot bath is characteristic of demyelinating optic neuritis (Uthoff's phenomenon). Permanent, sudden visual loss is usually due to vascular occlusion. Establish whether the symptoms are uniocular or homonymous (Box 12.2). Permanent homonymous visual loss, in the absence of hemiparesis or dysphasia, usually indicates occipital lobe infarction.

Gradual-onset visual loss

Gradual onset of visual loss is commonly caused by cataract or atrophic age-related macular degeneration. Both cause glare from bright lights. Slowly progressive visual loss, accompanied by optic atrophy, occurs when the optic nerve or chiasm is compressed by tumours within the orbit or skull base, e.g. meningioma or pituitary adenoma.

Distortion of vision

Distortion is caused by disruption of the photoreceptors at the macula, most commonly macular degeneration in the elderly. Untreated, central visual loss is rapid and irreversible. Scarring of the outer surface of the vitreous (epiretinal membrane) may pucker the normally smooth surface of the macula and follow any insult to the vitreous, including haemorrhage, inflammation or trauma.

Flashes and floaters

Flashes and floaters are caused by vitreous degeneration, especially in those >65 years and in myopia (short sight). As the vitreous degenerates, the gel liquefies and fluid escapes through perforations in the outer surface of the vitreous overlying the macula. The fluid peels the vitreous off the retina and the remaining contents swirl about on eye movement. The vitreous is attached to the retina in places, and as it detaches, retinal traction may produce flashes and lead to retinal tears. Retinal tears allow fluid from the vitreous cavity to enter the potential space between the retina and the retinal pigment epithelium, causing retinal detachment (Fig. 12.11). The patient notices visual loss starting peripherally and moving centrally.

Haloes

Haloes are coloured lights seen around bright lights due to corneal oedema which acts as a prism. They occur with angle closure glaucoma.

Oscillopsia

Oscillopsia, when objects appear to oscillate, causes mild blurring to rapid and periodic jumping, and is common in acquired nystagmus affecting primary gaze.

Nystagmus

Nystagmus is an involuntary oscillation of the eyes that is often rhythmical, with both eyes moving synchronously. It may be vertical, horizontal, rotary or multidirectional.

Anisocoria

Anisocoria is inequality of the pupil sizes.

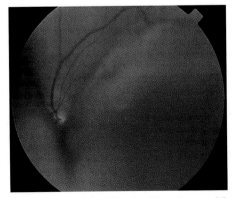

Fig. 12.11 Retinal detachment. Elevation of the retina around the 'attached' optic disc. The retina may be so elevated that it is visible on viewing the red reflex.

12.2 Causes of sudden-onset, uniocular, permanent visual loss

- Retinal artery occlusion
- Anterior ischaemic optic neuropathy
- Retinal vein occlusion
- Traumatic optic neuropathy

12

THE HISTORY

Presenting complaint

The time course of the presenting complaint is crucial to diagnosis. For example, vascular causes are sudden in onset, whereas slow, inexorable progression of symptoms is seen in compression of the optic pathway by a tumour. Symptoms which worsen over about 2 weeks, last 2–3 weeks and then resolve suggest demyelination. Always clarify terms used by patients; for example, diplopia and blurring are easily confused.

Past history

Information about previous ocular and systemic illnesses can help the diagnosis (Box 12.3). Old family photographs can help assess the onset of pupil abnormalities and features such as proptosis.

12.3 Past history and the eye

History	Association
Diabetes mellitus	Diabetic retinopathy, diabetic macular oedema, ocular ischaemia, III or VI nerve palsy, retinal vein occlusion
Thyroid disease	Exophthalmos (proptosis in autoimmune thyroid eye disease), ophthalmoplegia, red eye
Hypertension	Retinal vein occlusion, arteriosclerosis, hypertensive retinopathy (accelerated), non-arteritic anterior ischaemic optic neuropathy
Cerebrovascular or ischaemic heart disease, peripheral vascular disease	Retinal vein occlusion, retinal artery occlusion, non-arteritic anterior ischaemic optic neuropathy, ocular ischaemia, occipital lobe infarction
Atrial fibrillation	Embolic retinal artery occlusion, occipital lobe infarction
Tuberculosis	Uveitis
Multiple sclerosis	Optic neuritis, VI nerve palsy, bilateral internuclear paresis
Hayfever, asthma, eczema	Allergic eye disease
Myeloma, hyperviscosity syndrome, leukaemia	Retinal vein occlusion
Inflammatory bowel disease, rheumatoid arthritis	Episcleritis, scleritis
Ankylosing spondylitis	Recurrent anterior uveitis
Persistent ear, nose and throat symptoms	Granulomatosis with polyangiitis
Glaucoma	Retinal vein occlusion
Cataract surgery	Retinal detachment

Drug history

List the patient's current medications (Box 12.4).

Family history

Ask about family history, especially in children. Genetic diseases include retinitis pigmentosa, and the incidence of multiple sclerosis is increased in those with a positive family history. Many patients with thyroid eye disease have a family history of autoimmune disease.

Social history

Cigarette smoking is the most important cause of vascular disease affecting the eye and is a major risk factor for age-related macular degeneration. A history of hayfever or allergies to animals suggests an allergic eye disorder. Recreational drug use may be associated with visual loss, particularly cocaine-induced vascular occlusions. Take a sexual history in all patients with ocular inflammation or unexplained neuro-ophthalmic symptoms as uveitis may be the first manifestation of human immunodeficiency virus (HIV) infection or neurosyphilis (Box 12.5).

Occupational history

Ultraviolet keratitis may be experienced by arc welders who do not use appropriate eye protection, but also occurs with unprotected recreational use of tanning beds or exposure to bright sunlight without sunglasses, e.g. snow blindness.

12.4 Drugs and the eye

Visual condition	Drug
Keratopathy	Amiodarone
Cataract	Corticosteroid
Anterior uveitis	Rifabutin, cidofovir
Angle closure glaucoma	Anticholinergics
Retinal toxicity	Chloroquine, chlorpromazine, phenothiazine, tamoxifen, interferon
Optic neuropathy	Amiodarone, sildenafil, ethambutol, isoniazid
Demyelination	Infliximab
Nystagmus	Anticonvulsants

12.5 Causes of acute anterior uveitis (iritis)

- Idiopathic
- HLA B27 association
- Sarcoidosis
- Herpes simplex keratitis
- Post-cataract surgery
- Tuberculosis
- Neurosyphilis
- Trauma

THE PHYSICAL EXAMINATION

General examination

Assess cranial nerves II, III, IV and VI and their central connections:

Inspection

Examination sequence

Carefully and systematically look at:

- head position
- position of eyelids when looking straight ahead and on eye movement
- proptosis (forward bulging of the eyeball) (Box 12.6)
- lid lag:
  - Examine the seated patient from the right.
  - Hold your finger from a point 45° above the horizontal to a point below this plane.
  - Watch how the upper eyelid moves with the downward movement of the eye.
  - Normally, there is perfect coordination as the upper lid follows the downward movement of the eye. In lid lag, as occurs in thyroid eye disease, sclera can be seen above the iris (Fig. 12.12).
- periorbital appearance (Box 12.7)
- lacrimal apparatus
- eyelid margin
- conjunctiva:
  - Look for redness or chemosis (oedema) of the white of the eye.
  - Evert the eyelid to examine the upper subtarsal conjunctiva.
  - Ask the patient to look down, hold the upper lid lashes, press gently on the upper border of the tarsal plate with a cotton bud and gently pull the eyelashes up.
  - Look for the giant papillae of allergic eye disease or a hidden foreign body (Fig. 12.13).
- sclera
- cornea:
  - To test for corneal ulceration, gently touch a fluorescein strip on to the conjunctiva, where it will leave a yellow mark.
  - Ask the patient to blink to distribute the dye on the cornea. The yellow dye reveals epithelial defects which may be obvious to the naked eye.
  - Use your ophthalmoscope with a +10 lens to visualise smaller defects. A light with a cobalt blue filter highlights any defects (Fig. 12.14).
  - Resting appearance of the pupils (p. 285).

12.6 Causes of proptosis

- Thyroid eye disease (exophthalmos)*
- Caroticocavernous fistula
- Orbital cellulitis
- Orbital haematoma
- Granulomatosis with polyangiitis
- Orbital tumours, including lymphoma, metastasis, meningioma, glioma
- Pseudoproptosis (pathological myopia, shallow orbits, contralateral enophthalmos)

*Most common cause.

Abnormal findings

Posture Congenital and longstanding paralytic squint often causes an abnormal head posture with the head turned or tilted to minimise the diplopia.

Eyelids A narrow palpebral fissure (the gap between upper and lower eyelids) suggests ptosis (drooping eyelid) (Box 12.8) or blepharospasm (tonic spasm in the orbicularis oris muscle). Eyelid retraction or proptosis makes the sclera visible above the cornea, ectropion visible below.

Causes of ptosis include:

- involutional: stretching of the levator muscle aponeurosis with age is the commonest cause
- congenital
- III nerve palsy: causes unilateral ptosis that is often complete. The pupil is large because of loss of

12

12.7 Causes of periorbital oedema

- Allergic eye disease
- Thyroid eye disease
- Orbital cellulitis
- Nephrotic syndrome
- Heart failure
- Angio-oedema

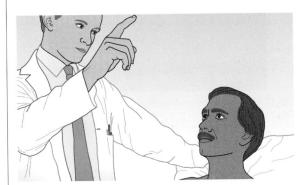

Fig. 12.12 Testing for lid lag.

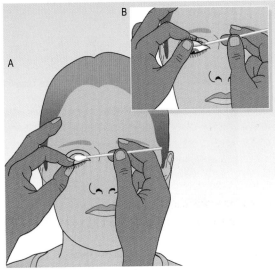

Fig. 12.13 Everting the upper eyelid to look at the conjunctiva.

parasympathetic innervation of the iris. Unopposed action of IV and VI cranial nerves results in the eye looking inferolaterally. Urgently investigate an acute III nerve palsy, especially if painful, as this may indicate a posterior communicating artery aneurysm

- Horner's syndrome (damage to sympathetic ocular innervation): paralyses Müller's muscle and lower lid retractors, producing a partial ptosis and a pseudoenophthalmos. Miosis (small pupil) is present due to lack of sympathetic innervation to the iris
- myasthenia gravis causes bilateral variable ptosis due to fatigability of the levator muscle. The patient may be unable to 'bury the eyelashes' (orbicularis muscle, VII nerve innervation), which suggests a neuromuscular junction disorder, a myopathy or a

meningeal disorder, as it is anatomically impossible for a single lesion to affect both III and VII ipsilateral cranial nerves (Fig. 12.15).

Periorbital oedema may be associated with chemosis (conjunctival oedema).

Lacrimal apparatus The lacrimal gland may become swollen through:

- inflammation, e.g. sarcoidosis
- infection, e.g. mumps
- malignancy, lymphoma, cancer.

12.8 Causes of ptosis

Mechanical	
• Chronic orbital inflammation • Degenerative • Eyelid tumour • Intraocular surgery	• Long-term use of contact lenses • Trauma

Myogenic	
• Chronic progressive external ophthalmoplegia • Congenital myogenic ptosis secondary to levator dysgenesis	• Myotonic dystrophy • Oculopharyngeal dystrophy

Neuromuscular junction
• Myasthenia gravis

Neurogenic: congenital	
• Congenital Horner's syndrome	• Congenital III nerve palsy

Neurogenic: acquired	
• Acquired Horner's syndrome • III cranial nerve palsy	• Synkinetic neurogenic ptosis, e.g. Marcus Gunn

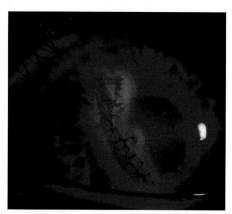

Fig. 12.14 Dendritic conjunctival ulcer. Fluorescein staining showing branching dendritic ulcer.

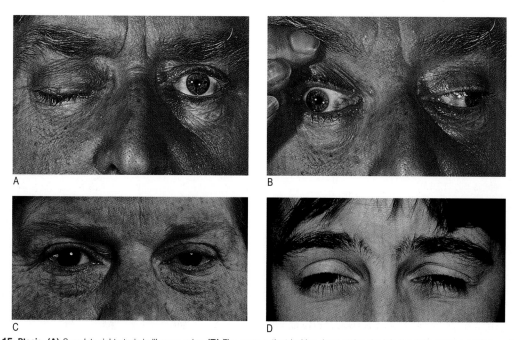

Fig. 12.15 Ptosis. (A) Complete right ptosis in III nerve palsy. **(B)** The same patient looking down and to the left; the right eye has rotated medially, demonstrating that the trochlear (IV) nerve is intact. **(C)** Left Horner's syndrome. **(D)** Myasthenia gravis. The patient is attempting to open his eyelids. Raised forehead browlines (frontalis overactivity) reflect the effort of attempting to open the eyelids.

Nasolacrimal duct blockage produces watering and sticky discharge, and may cause dacrocystitis (acute inflammation of the lacrimal sac). It is common in neonates and usually resolves spontaneously.

Eyelid margin Blepharitis (inflammation of the eyelid margin) may be associated with systemic skin involvement. Look for:

- 'ace of clubs' appearance of rosacea (erythema on forehead, cheeks and chin)
- flexural dermatitis of atopic eczema
- dandruff or seborrhoeic dermatitis.

Common lumps on the eyelids include:

- stye (eyelash microabscess)
- chalazion (pea-like swellings of the tarsal glands)
- basal cell cancer.

Conjunctiva Circumciliary injection (redness around the corneal limbus) reflects involvement of the anterior ciliary arteries supplying the cornea, iris and ciliary body (uveitis). Diffuse redness suggests scleritis or conjunctivitis.

Sclera Thin sclera is transparent, revealing the bluish choroid beneath, and occurs in scleromalacia, osteogenesis imperfecta and Ehlers–Danlos syndrome. The sclerae are yellow in jaundice (Fig. 8.8).

Scleritis causes a dark-red colour, tenderness and pain on eye movement. Systemic vasculitis causes white patches within red areas, suggesting impending necrosis.

Cornea The corneal epithelium may be affected by dryness, trauma or infection. Peripheral corneal arcus (lipid deposition) is seen with hyperlipidaemia (Fig. 6.8C). In Wilson's disease, copper is deposited round the cornea, causing Kayser–Fleischer rings (Fig. 12.16). Calcium may be deposited in chronic ocular inflammation and chronic hypercalcaemia (band keratopathy).

Pupils

Examination sequence

Visual acuity

- Ask patients to put on their distance glasses, if they use them. Only use reading glasses when testing near vision.
- Ensure good ambient lighting.
- Place a Snellen chart 6 metres from the patient (Fig. 12.17).
- Cover one of the patient's eyes with a card and ask him to read from the top down until he can no longer distinguish the letters.
- Repeat with the other eye.
- Snellen visual acuity is expressed as 6 (the distance at which the chart is read) over the number corresponding to the lowest line read. This indicates the distance at which someone with normal vision should be able to read that line, i.e. Snellen visual acuity of 6/60 indicates that at 6 metres patients can only see letters they should be able to read 60 metres away. Normal vision is 6/6. In the UK, a visual acuity of 6/12 or better is required for a driving licence.
- If the patient cannot read down to line 6 (6/6 vision), place a pinhole directly in front of his glasses to correct refractive errors. This allows only central rays of light to enter the eye and can correct for about 4 D of refractive error (Fig. 12.18).

- If patients cannot see the top line of the chart at 6 metres, bring them forward till they can and record that vision, e.g. 1/60 – can see top letter at 1 metre.
- If patients still cannot see the top letter at 1 metre, check whether they can count fingers, see hand movements or just see light.
- For children who can't yet read, use different-sized objects instead of letters.
- Repeat the process above for near vision, with the patient wearing any reading glasses. Use a test card, held at a comfortable reading distance, to assess near vision. N5 is the smallest size that most normal eyes can see (N8 is the size of normal newsprint).

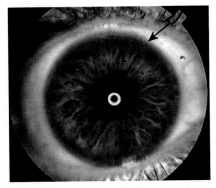

Fig. 12.16 Kayser–Fleischer ring (arrowed).

60
T
36
O Y
24
H U V
18
A T Y M
12
X O W U H
9
X U V T X O
6
A W I M H Y T
5
X V U W T O M A

Fig. 12.17 Snellen visual acuity chart.

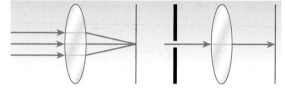

Fig. 12.18 Pinhole. Normally, the lens focuses rays of light on to a discrete point on the retina. The pinhole partially negates the role of the lens by only allowing rays from directly in front to pass through.

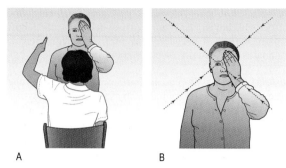

A   B

Fig. 12.20 Testing the visual fields by confrontation.

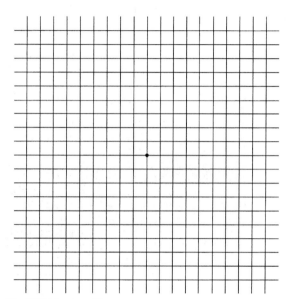

Fig. 12.19 Amsler grid.

Macular function

Examination sequence

- Use an Amsler grid (Fig. 12.19) to record visual defects, including central scotomas, quadrantanopias and hemianopias, and distortion of the central 10° of vision.
- Ask the patient:
  - to cover one eye
  - to hold the grid at a comfortable reading distance
  - to fix on the central black spot with the eye being tested
  - to keep the eye still and look at the grid using the 'sides of his vision'
  - to outline with a finger the areas where the lines are broken, distorted or missing.

Visual fields

The normal visual field extends 160° horizontally and 130° vertically. Fixation is the very centre of a patient's visual field. The physiological blind spot is located 15° temporal to the point of visual fixation and represents the optic nerve head. At the bedside, test visual fields by confrontation (Figs 12.20 and 12.21): an automated visual field analyser provides a more accurate assessment.

Examination sequence

- Sit directly facing the patient, about 1 metre away.
- Ask the patient to keep looking at your eyes.

Homonymous defects

- Keep your eyes open and ask the patient to do the same.
- Hold your hands out to their full extent. Wiggle a fingertip and ask the patient to point to it as soon as he sees it move.
- Do this at 10 and 2 o'clock, and then 8 and 4 o'clock (to screen the four outer quadrants of the patient's visual field – superotemporal, superonasal, inferotemporal, inferonasal).

Sensory inattention

- Test both eyes together.
- Both you and the patient should keep your eyes open.
- Test both left and right fields at the same time.
- Note whether the patient reports seeing only one side move and which quadrant or side is affected.

Peripheral visual fields

- Test each eye separately.
- Ask the patient to cover one eye and look directly into your opposite eye.
- Shut your eye that is opposite the patient's covered eye.
- Test each quadrant separately with a wiggling finger or white-tipped hatpin. Hold the target equidistant between you and the patient.
- Start peripherally and move the target along the diagonal towards the centre of vision until the patient detects it.
- Repeat for the other quadrants.
- Compare your visual field with the patient's.

Central visual field

- Test each eye separately using a red hatpin.
- Shut your eye that is opposite the patient's covered eye.
- Ask the patient to cover one eye and look directly at your open eye.
- Hold the hatpin in the centre of the visual field, as close to fixation as possible.
- Ask the patient what colour the hatpin is. A 'pale' or 'pink' response implies colour desaturation, usually because of a lesion affecting the optic nerve.
- Compare the four quadrants of the visual field centrally; each time ask about colour desaturation. Note that the visual field for red may be smaller than for white.

Blind spot

This is a physiological scotoma corresponding to absence of photoreceptors where the optic nerve leaves the eye.

- Test one eye at a time
- Ask the patient to cover one eye and look directly at you.
- Shut your eye that is opposite the patient's covered eye.
- Hold the hatpin at the fixation point; you and the patient focus on each other's eye.
- Move the hatpin temporally and horizontally until it disappears from your visual field. Maintaining the same temporal horizontal position, move it anteriorly or posteriorly until it also disappears from the patient's visual field.
- Compare the size of the patient's blind spot to yours.

Tubular visual fields

These are often asymptomatic.

- Test visual fields by confrontation at 1 metre and 2 metres from the patient.

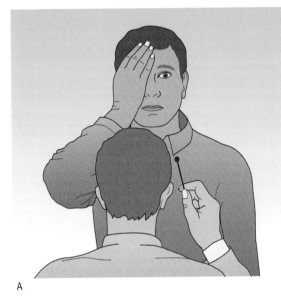

A

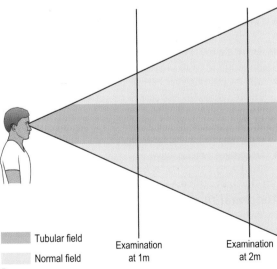

Tubular field
Normal field

Examination at 1m

Examination at 2m

B

Fig. 12.21 Visual fields. (A) Testing central visual field. **(B)** Difference between normal and tubular visual fields.

Abnormal findings

Intraocular causes of visual field defects include:

- Macular lesions, e.g. age-related macular degeneration, cause central scotomas, which may be incomplete and associated with distortion. Commonly, a patient with a central scotoma cannot see a face clearly but the rest of the visual field is unaffected.
- Peripheral retinal lesions spare central vision, causing localised scotomas, e.g. retinal detachment or scarring, or constriction of peripheral field, e.g. retinitis pigmentosa.
- Optic disc lesions cause horizontal or arcuate scotomas.

Lesions of the optic nerve within the orbit also cause central scotomas, but, unlike those of macular origin, red desaturation (red colours appear orange or pink) occurs early and there is no visual distortion.

Unilateral optic nerve lesions cause a relative afferent pupillary defect.

Distension of the nerve sheath around the optic nerve, e.g. papilloedema (Fig. 12.22), causes an enlarged blind spot. Optic atrophy occurs later.

Lesions at the optic chiasm cause bilateral temporal visual field defects (bitemporal hemianopia; Fig. 12.3). As the optic chiasm is a continuation of the optic nerve, central red desaturation may precede peripheral visual field loss.

Optic tract lesions are uncommon; they are usually suprasellar lesions, e.g. pituitary tumours, and produce asymmetrical homonymous visual field defects.

The optic radiations and occipital cortex are more commonly affected and produce:

- symmetrical visual field defects (homonymous hemianopia)
- lack of awareness of visual field loss: this suggests parietal lobe involvement
- superior homonymous quadrantanopia: this suggests temporal lobe involvement
- visual field defects: these may affect only central vision or spare the macula because of the dual blood supply of the occipital cortex
- Functional visual loss is common, particularly bilateral visual field constriction that does not expand on testing further away. This tubular constriction differentiates it from the funnel

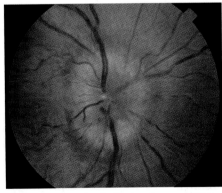

Fig. 12.22 Swollen optic disc. Papilloedema is suggested if visual acuity is unaffected, colour vision is normal and there is an enlarged blind spot.

12

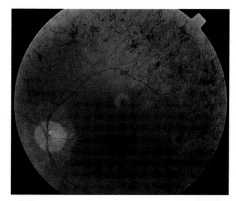

Fig. 12.23 Retinitis pigmentosa. A triad of optic atrophy, attenuated retinal vessels and pigmentary changes. Pigmentary changes typically start peripherally in association with a ring scotoma and symptoms of night blindness.

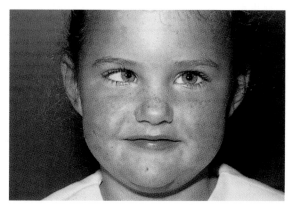

Fig. 12.24 Concomitant right convergent squint in a child.

constriction of bilateral retinal disorders, such as retinitis pigmentosa (Fig. 12.23) or bilateral homonymous hemianopia (cortical visual impairment). The normal visual field is conical and, no matter how small, its diameter doubles when the patient is tested in front of a tangent screen and then moved back from 1 metre distance to 2 metres. Patients with functional tunnel vision have an unchanged or smaller visual field (Fig. 12.21B).

Ocular alignment and eye movements

The eyes are normally parallel in all positions of gaze, except near convergence. If not, a squint (strabismus) is present. Squints are associated with:

- paresis of one or more extraocular muscles (paralytic or incomitant squint)
- defective binocular vision (non-paralytic or concomitant squint).

Acquired paralytic squints cause diplopia, in which the images are maximally separated and squint is greatest in the direction of action of the paretic muscle. Concomitant squints are the same in all positions of gaze. They usually become manifest in childhood when they are not associated with diplopia (Fig. 12.24). In children, the visual acuity of the squinting eye falls, causing amblyopia (a 'lazy' eye).

Examination sequence

Sit directly facing the patient, about 1 metre away.

Inspection
- Look for head turns or tilts in the direction of underacting muscles.
- Hold a pen torch and ask the patient to look at the light.
- Observe the position of the pen torch's reflection on the cornea. The fixating (non-deviating) eye has the pen torch's reflection in the centre; the deviating eye has an off-centre reflection. This test can be confusing if the paretic eye has better vision than the non-paretic eye and the patient fixates with it. (Hirschberg test detects any deviation in primary position.)

Ocular movements
- Hold your finger vertically at least 50 cm away from the patient, and ask him to follow it with his eyes, without moving his head.
- Move your finger steadily to one side, then up and down, then to the other and repeat, describing the letter H in the air.
- Ask whether any diplopia is horizontal, vertical, tilted or a mixture of both.
- Cover one of the patient's eyes to see if diplopia is monocular or binocular.
- If diplopia is binocular, ask which image disappears when you cover each eye; the outer image corresponds to the affected eye.
- Note the direction of gaze in which diplopia is worst and work out which muscle is affected (Fig. 12.4A).
- On horizontal movement, in the absence of proptosis, no ipsilateral sclera should be seen on extreme gaze ('burying the white'). Its presence suggests ipsilateral muscle weakness.
- On down-gaze hold the eyelids open using two fingers from your free hand.
- For each eye, look for nystagmus while examining eye movements (p. 289).

Squint (cover test)
Examine visual acuity and the visual fields as above.
- Cover one eye and ask the patient to look at the light of your pen torch.
- Closely observe the uncovered eye for any movements.
- If it moves to take up fixation, that eye was squinting.
- Repeat the sequence for the other eye.

Oculocephalic (doll's-eye) reflex
- With the patient supine, hold his head in both hands, with your thumbs holding his eyes open; if the patient is conscious, ask him to focus on your eyes.
- Rock the head gently from side to side, noting the movement of the eyes as they hold their gaze.
- An impaired reflex indicates brainstem abnormality (Fig. 12.25).

Abnormal findings

Monocular diplopia is created by 'ghosting' from structural abnormality anywhere between the cornea and fovea.

Pure horizontal diplopia usually results from involvement of the VI cranial nerve. The symptoms are worse looking to the affected side.

Orbital trauma may trap a medial rectus muscle.

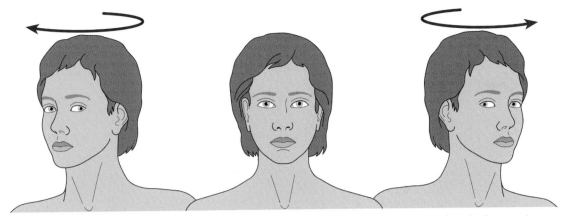

Fig. 12.25 Oculocephalic reflex. Move the head in the horizontal plane. Note that the eyes move in the opposite direction to head movement.

A demyelinating pontine lesion may be associated with ipsilateral lower motor neurone nerve palsy.

Disruption of the neuronal connection between the medial rectus and the contralateral VI nerve (median longitudinal fasciculus), e.g. in multiple sclerosis, causes underaction of the medial rectus and an internuclear ophthalmoplegia. Unlike VI nerve palsy, diplopia is worse on looking to the contralateral side.

VI nerve palsy occurs with raised intracranial pressure when the nerve is stretched as it passes upward to the cavernous sinus (Fig. 12.6).

Other causes of impaired horizontal movement include:

- pontine gaze palsies (nuclear VI nerve palsy)
- convergence spasm (impaired uniocular lateral gaze associated with bilateral miosis).
- Impaired vertical gaze can occur in:
  - orbital floor fractures, which may entrap the inferior rectus and restrict upgaze.
  - brainstem stroke, demyelination and children with hydrocephalus (when the inferior segment of the cornea lies below the lower lid – the 'setting sun' sign). IV nerve palsies cause vertical diplopia, particularly noticeable on down-gaze. The IV nerve is the only nerve to emerge from the posterior brainstem and is particularly susceptible to a blow to the occiput. Damage is often bilateral.

Thyroid eye disease is a common cause of vertical diplopia. A complaint of squint rather than diplopia suggests non-paralytic squint resulting from defective binocular vision. An amblyopic eye often diverges while monocular eye movements will be intact. The cover test is useful in children.

The oculocephalic test differentiates supranuclear lesions from cranial nerve lesions and is impaired in brainstem stroke, metabolic dysfunction or drug intoxication.

Nystagmus

Biphasic or jerk nystagmus is commonest where there is a slow drift in one direction, followed by a fast correction in the opposite direction. The direction of the fast phase or jerk is called the direction of nystagmus.

Oscillations occurring at the same speed and over the same range about a central point are pendular nystagmus.

Examination sequence

- Hold your finger an arm's length from the patient, in front of him.
- Ask the patient to look at your finger and follow it with his eyes without moving the head.
- Move your finger steadily to each side and up and down, describing an H.
- Watch the patient's eyes carefully for nystagmus and note:
  - the position in which it occurs
  - the direction in which it is most marked
  - whether it is horizontal, vertical, rotatory or multidirectional
  - whether there are fast and slow phases (jerk) or equal oscillations about a central point (pendular).

Normal findings

At extremes of lateral gaze, normal subjects may show a few nystagmoid jerks. When a person looks out of a train window at the passing scenery, a physiological opticokinetic nystagmus occurs. This can be tested using a vertically striped drum that is spun in front of the subject. The fast phase of the nystagmus is in the opposite direction to the drum's spin. It can be impaired in people with visual field defects.

Abnormal findings

Peripheral vestibular nystagmus often has horizontal, vertical and rotatory components, and is usually associated with vertigo. The amplitude of the oscillation increases with gaze towards the direction of the fast phase and is suppressed by visual fixation using Fresnel lenses.

Central vestibular nystagmus is usually unidirectional, does not alter with direction of gaze or with visual fixation, and vertigo is less prominent. Common causes include multiple sclerosis and cerebrovascular disease.

Vertical nystagmus is uncommon and indicates brainstem damage. Upbeat nystagmus, with the fast phase on looking upwards, occurs with upper brainstem lesions

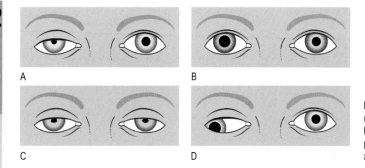

Fig. 12.26 **Pupillary defects. (A)** Right Horner's syndrome (ptosis and miosis). **(B)** Right Holmes–Adie pupil. **(C)** Argyll Robertson pupils with bilateral ptosis and small irregular pupils. **(D)** Right III nerve palsy (looking down and out, ptosis and a dilated pupil).

in multiple sclerosis, infarction and Wernicke's encephalopathy. Downbeat nystagmus may result from lesions around the craniocervical junction, e.g. Arnold–Chiari malformation or demyelination, and phenytoin or lithium intoxication. Periodic alternating nystagmus is present in the primary position but changes direction in a crescendo–decrescendo manner, often every 90 seconds with a null period of up to 10 seconds. This may be congenital, due to lesions at the craniocervical junction, or a feature of drug intoxication. Demyelination of the medial longitudinal bundle within the brainstem can cause ataxic nystagmus, where the oscillations are more marked in the abducting eye than in the adducting one. This is often associated with an internuclear ophthalmoplegia with reduced adduction.

Congenital nystagmus is usually a horizontal jerk nystagmus but can be pendular. Acquired pendular nystagmus results from cerebellar or brainstem disease, most commonly multiple sclerosis, but also from spinocerebellar degenerations and brainstem ischaemia. In functional blindness optico-kinetic nystagmus is present.

Pupils

Examination sequence

- Assess the pupils' shape and symmetry, taking account of ambient lighting.
- Ask the patient to fix his eyes on a distant point straight ahead.
- Bring a bright torchlight from the side to shine on the pupil.
- Look for constriction of that pupil (direct light reflex).
- Repeat and look for constriction of the opposite pupil (consensual light reflex).
- With his vision still fixed on a distant point, present an object about 15 cm in front of the eyes and ask the patient to focus on it (convergence). Look for pupil constriction (accommodation reflex).

Normal findings

Simple, or essential, anisocoria, a >0.4 mm difference between the pupil diameters, is common.

Abnormal findings

In diabetes mellitus, autonomic neuropathy may produce small pupils that respond poorly to pharmacological dilatation. They may mimic the Argyll Robertson pupils of syphilis (pinpoint, irregular pupils that constrict only on convergence).

An Adie pupil is usually mid-dilated and responds poorly to convergence. It results from ciliary ganglion

malfunction within the orbit. With time it may shrink in size and be confused with an Argyll Robertson pupil. It is frequently bilateral, and when associated with absent neurological reflexes, is termed the Holmes–Adie syndrome.

Optic nerve damage results in an afferent pupillary defect (Marcus Gunn pupil). Both pupils are dually innervated at the level of the midbrain. Normally, both pupils constrict to light, regardless of which eye is illuminated. If one optic nerve is damaged, whatever lighting the dominant optic nerve is exposed to determines the size of both pupils (Fig. 12.26).

A unilateral dilated pupil in a patient with deteriorating conscious level secondary to intracranial mass lesions, e.g. tumour or enlarging haematoma, occurs when brain herniation compresses the III nerve.

Colour vision

Examination sequence

- Assess red–green colour vision using Ishihara test plates (Fig. 12.27). These are coloured spots forming numbers which the patient reads out.
- The first plate is a test plate; if the patient cannot see the number, he has poor visual acuity or functional visual loss.

Abnormal findings

Red desaturation is impaired ability to identify red objects and an early indicator of optic nerve pathology.

Congenital red–green blindness is an X-linked recessive condition and affects 7% of the male population. Red–green colour vision is impaired before loss of visual acuity with optic nerve damage anywhere from the photoreceptors to the lateral geniculate nucleus of the thalamus.

Ophthalmoscopy

Examine the eye undilated first to see the pupils and iris; then, ideally, examine the eye dilated using tropicamide drops, to visualise the lens, vitreous and retina. Only the optic nerve can be reliably assessed without pupillary dilatation. If patients have particularly thick lenses, examine their eyes with their glasses in place; however, this reduces your field of view. Advise the patient not to drive or use machinery until the effect of the mydriatic has completely worn off. This may take several hours.

Examination sequence

- Hold the ophthalmoscope in your right hand and use your right eye to examine the patient's right eye. Hold the ophthalmoscope in your left hand and examine the patient's left eye with your left eye (Fig. 12.28).
- Find '0' and then rotate the 'lenses' clockwise until you obtain the number 10 (plus '10'). This should be the same colour as the '1' clockwise to '0'. If not, you have gone too far.
- Place your free hand on the patient's forehead and ask the patient to look down. Catch the upper eyelid and gently retract it against the orbital rim. Holding the eyelid against the brow enables you to approach the patient's head as closely as possible without bumping into it, and prevents the upper eyelid from obscuring your view.
- Ask the patient to fixate on a distant object straight ahead.
- From a distance of about 10 cm bring the red reflex into focus. In this way the cornea, iris and lens can be visualised and any opacity appears black against this red background.
- Now come close to the patient's head so that you are touching the hand you are resting on the patient's forehead.
- As you do so, rotate the lenses anticlockwise, progressively increasing the focal length.
- Look for black opacities in the vitreous until the retina comes into focus.

Fundal examination

- If you approach at a slight angle above the horizontal from the temporal side you should bring the optic disc into view.
- The normal disc is pink with a pigmented temporal margin (Fig. 12.29). Pallor can be difficult to judge. Confirm it by checking the relative afferent pupil response, which will be diminished with pallor (see Fig. 12.31A).
- Change the focus if you cannot see the disc clearly and assess its shape, colour and vessels.
- Follow the blood vessels as they extend from the optic disc in four directions: superotemporally, inferotemporally, superonasally and inferonasally.
- Ask the patient to look superiorly (examine horizontally), temporally (examine vertically), inferiorly (examine horizontally) and nasally (examine vertically).
- Ask the patient to look directly at the light to locate the centre of the macula. Ask her to keep her eye still while you look around the macula.

Abnormal findings

Cornea Asymptomatic corneal scars from foreign bodies, often accompanied by remnants of rust, and previous ulceration are common.

Lens There are three common forms of cataract:

- Peripheral cortical cataract is common in diabetes mellitus (Fig. 12.30). It appears as incomplete black spokes radiating from the periphery of the lens.
- Posterior subcapsular cataract, the typical 'steroid cataract', appears as a black opacity coming from the centre of the lens.
- Nuclear sclerosis ('ageing cataract') is the normally transparent lens yellowing before it becomes brown, then black. It cannot usually be detected in the red reflex, but symptoms and an inability to focus clearly on the retina confirm its presence.

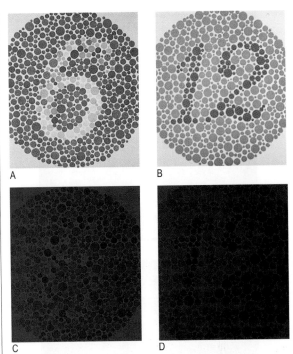

Fig. 12.27 Plates from the Ishihara series. (A and B) Normal colour vision. **(C and D)** The plates as they appear to someone with colour blindness. The person is unable to read '6' in plate A, and can just read '12' in plate B.

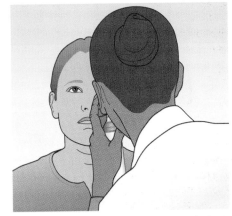

Fig. 12.28 Ophthalmoscopy: correct method. The patient's gaze is fixed on a distant point.

Vitreous The patient perceives vitreous haemorrhage as black blobs that move with eye movement (intra-gel vitreous haemorrhage). Abnormal vitreous adhesion to normal retinal vessels may cause vitreous haemorrhage, and 'flashes of light' indicate that the retina may have torn. Haemorrhage in the space between the retina and the posterior surface of the vitreous causes a subhyaloid (preretinal) vitreous haemorrhage (Fig. 12.31B).

Optic disc With a swollen and white optic nerve head (anterior ischaemic optic neuropathy), consider giant cell arteritis and polyarteritis nodosa and check markers of inflammation (raised erythrocyte sedimentation rate, C-reactive protein or platelet count) (Fig. 12.31C).

12

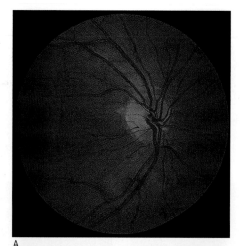

A

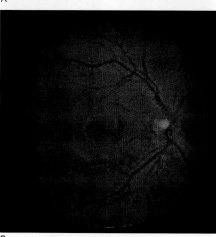

B

Fig. 12.29 Normal fundi. **(A)** Caucasian. **(B)** Asian.

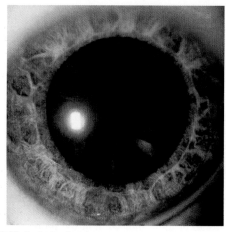

Fig. 12.30 Cortical cataract.

12.9 Common causes of arteriolar occlusion

- Accelerated hypertension
- Diabetic retinopathy
- Human immunodeficiency virus (HIV) retinopathy
- Retinal vein occlusion
- Systemic lupus erythematosus
- Systemic vasculitis

12.10 Causes of retinitis

- Cytomegalovirus
- Herpes simplex
- Herpes zoster
- Varicella zoster

visual field loss). Typically, the vertical margins are affected first.

The optic disc is a common site for new vessel formation. In the presence of an enlarged blind spot, blurring of the optic disc indicates distension of the optic nerve sheath. Reduced colour vision and a relative afferent pupillary response suggest an intrinsic optic nerve lesion.

Horizontal nerve fibre layer The nerve fibre layer runs horizontally over the retinal blood vessels. Lesions within this are therefore flat and striated, and obscure retinal blood vessels.

Arteriolar occlusion (Box 12.9) causes 'cotton-wool' spot formation (Fig. 12.31D) and flame haemorrhages (Fig. 12.31E).

Roth's spots are flame-shaped haemorrhages with a central cotton-wool spot. They are caused by immune complex deposition, and are seen in subacute bacterial endocarditis and serum sickness (see Fig. 6.8B).

Retinitis due to herpesvirus infection causes a large, rapidly progressive area of 'cotton-wool' spot formation. It can be difficult to differentiate from the cotton-wool spots of arterial occlusion and the two may coexist in HIV infection. Cotton-wool spots, however, do not enlarge over time, whereas areas of retinitis do (Box 12.10).

Retinal artery occlusion is usually embolic and causes retinal pallor because of anterior retinal layer infarction. It resembles amaurosis fugax but is permanent. The optic nerve head, the fovea and the posterior retina, including the photoreceptors, are unaffected by retinal artery occlusion, as their blood supply is from the short posterior ciliary arteries of the ophthalmic artery. This explains the cherry-red spot sign of central retinal artery occlusion, where the healthy fovea is surrounded by an oedematous retina (Fig. 12.31F). Retinal emboli may be seen at vessel bifurcations. As only the luminal contents of the vessel are normally apparent and not the wall, the embolus may appear to be paradoxically wider than the vessel it is lodged in.

Vertical bipolar layer This contains the retinal capillaries. The commonest causes of capillary disease are diabetes mellitus and retinal vein occlusion (Fig. 12.31G). Capillary occlusion is also seen with HIV and radiation retinopathies. Microaneurysm formation may occur at the site of capillary occlusion. Capillaries are too small to visualise with the naked eye. On

Pseudophakic patients with artificial intraocular lenses following cataract extraction often have falsely pale discs. Increased cup-to-disc ratio (cupped disc) is seen with chronic open-angle glaucoma (a group of diseases of the optic nerve involving loss of retinal ganglion cells, associated with raised intraocular pressure and

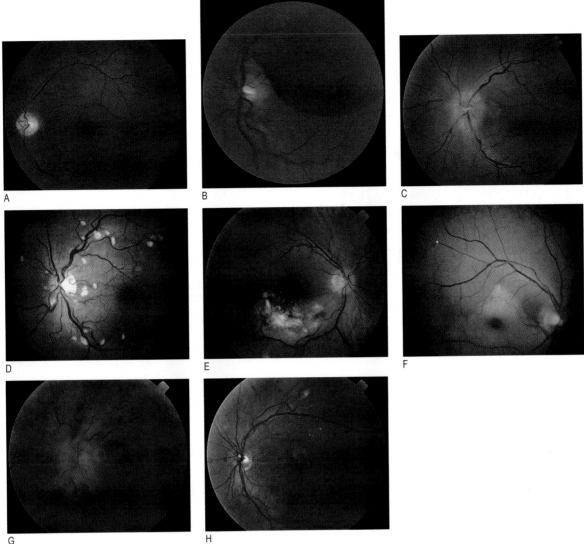

Fig. 12.31 Retinal abnormalities. (**A**) Left optic atrophy. Note the lack of a pink neuroretinal rim. (**B**) Preretinal haemorrhage. (**C**) Pale white swollen disc. This is highly suggestive of giant cell arteritis, particularly if associated with visual loss. (**D**) Arteriolar occlusion of the horizontal nerve fibre layer. Multiple cotton-wool spots in human immunodeficiency virus (HIV) retinopathy. (**E**) Cytomegalovirus retinitis. Note the large superficial retinal infiltrate associated with flame haemorrhage. (**F**) Central retinal artery occlusion. Note the milky-white pale infarcted retina surrounding healthy pink fovea ('cherry-red spot'). (**G**) Central retinal vein occlusion. Note the widespread retinal haemorrhages and swollen optic disc. (**H**) Diabetic retinopathy with multiple dot and blot haemorrhages, indicating widespread capillary occlusion, a precursor of new vessel formation.

ophthalmoscopy microaneurysms appear as round dots separate from blood vessels; they can haemorrhage and leak, leading to:

- dot haemorrhages: thin, vertical haemorrhages that may be difficult to differentiate from microaneurysms
- blot haemorrhages: larger, full-thickness bipolar layer haemorrhages that represent larger areas of capillary occlusion (Fig. 12.31H).

Intraretinal microvascular anomalies are perfused, dilated stumps of capillaries within areas of widespread capillary occlusion. Venous beading is associated with adjacent capillary bed destruction.

Microaneurysms, dot and blot haemorrhages, intraretinal microvascular anomalies and venous beading are all surrogate markers for capillary occlusion. If sufficient capillaries occlude, then new vessels will form in the potential space between the retina and the posterior vitreous surface. They differ from normal retinal vessels because they form returning loops that are distally more dilated than their proximal origins. New vessels grow into the posterior surface of the vitreous and are found at the border of perfused and non-perfused retina (Fig. 12.32). The vitreous is most strongly attached to the optic disc, and new vessels here are more likely to haemorrhage than elsewhere.

Retinal veins and arteries share a common tunica adventitia where their branches cross over. Arteriosclerosis, commonly seen with hypertension, produces arteriovenous nipping, where the thickened artery, trapped by its tunica adventitia, twists and compresses the underlying vein. Arteriosclerosis is the most common cause of retinal vein occlusion. Raised

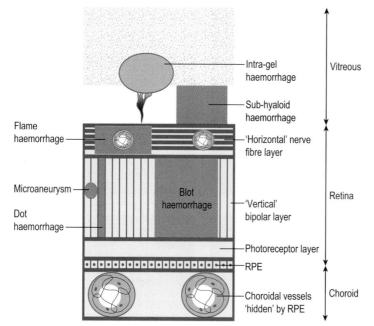

Intra-gel haemorrhage

Sub-hyaloid haemorrhage

Flame haemorrhage

'Horizontal' nerve fibre layer

Microaneurysm

Blot haemorrhage

Dot haemorrhage

'Vertical' bipolar layer

Photoreceptor layer

RPE

Choroidal vessels 'hidden' by RPE

Vitreous

Retina

Choroid

Fig. 12.32 Types of optic fundal haemorrhage, according to the retinal level. RPE, retinal pigment epithelium.

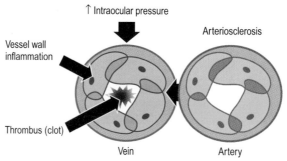

↑ Intraocular pressure

Arteriosclerosis

Vessel wall inflammation

Thrombus (clot)

Vein

Artery

Fig. 12.33 Causes of retinal vein occlusion.

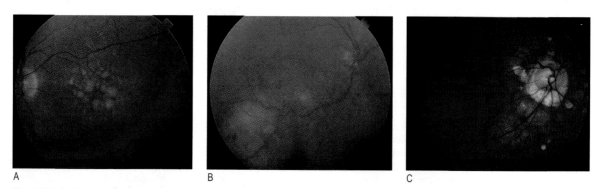

A

B

C

Fig. 12.34 Retinal pigment abnormalities. (A) Drusen maculopathy; numerous large retinal drusen affecting the central retina. **(B)** Melanoma. Large and more significantly raised pigmented lesion deep to the retinal vessels, indicating its choroid origin. **(C)** Choroiditis. Multiple white lesions (multifocus choroiditis) with additional greenish choroidal neovascular membrane and adjacent retinal haemorrhage.

12.11 Investigations in eye disease

Investigation	Indication/comment
Bedside tests	
Refraction	Short and long sight, lens disorders, cataract, corneal disorders
Corneal staining	Corneal epithelial disease
Schirmer's tear test	Dry eyes, Sjögren's syndrome
Intraocular pressure	Glaucoma
Urinalysis	Vasculitis, renal disease and diabetes mellitus
Mantoux skin test	Tuberculosis
Blood tests	
Renal function, erythrocyte sedimentation rate, C-reactive protein	Systemic disease, including vasculitis
Autoantibodies	Autoimmune disease
Angiotensin-converting enzyme activity	Sarcoidosis
Human immunodeficiency virus (HIV) and syphilis serology	Atypical uveitis or neurological signs
Prolactin	Optic neuropathy, pituitary macroadenoma
Neurophysiology	
Electrophysiology	Optic nerve and retinal disorders
Radiology	
Chest X-ray	Sarcoidosis, tuberculosis
Orbital ultrasound	Inadequate fundal view because of cataract
Digital photography	Documentation of fundal findings
Optical coherence tomography	Macular disorders and glaucoma
Fundus fluorescein angiography	Retinal disorders
CT of the brain	Intracranial tumours, compressive lesions
MR imaging of the brain	Pituitary lesion, demyelination
Invasive tests	
Lumbar puncture	Multiple sclerosis, inflammatory optic neuropathies
Temporal artery biopsy	Giant cell arteritis

12

intracapillary pressure, due to retinal vein occlusion, results in capillary rupture and retinal haemorrhage. In central retinal vein occlusion, new vessel formation may occur on the iris (rubeosis iridis). Subsequent scarring of the drainage angle leads to rubeotic glaucoma, which produces extremely painful blindness. Eyes at risk often have a relative afferent pupillary defect and profound visual loss (Fig. 12.33).

Arteriosclerotic retinal vein compression usually occurs in elderly patients or those with arteriosclerotic risk factors, e.g. smoking, hypertension, hyperlipidaemia or diabetes mellitus. Raised intraocular pressure from chronic open-angle glaucoma is also a common cause.

Retinal pigment epithelium and photoreceptors

Disease of the retinal pigmented cells produces areas of depigmentation with adjacent clumps of pigment. Age-related macular degeneration is the commonest cause of change. It is preceded by drusen formation – amorphous depositions under the retinal pigment epithelium (Fig. 12.34A). Differentiate drusen from hard exudates, in people with diabetes mellitus, by the absence of adjacent microaneurysms. Atrophic age-related macular degeneration results in areas of pigment atrophy and gradual loss of central vision. Neovascular age-related macular degeneration is more severe and is associated with rapid-onset visual distortion and central visual loss.

Choroidal naevi (hyperpigmentation of the retinal pigment epithelium) is a common asymptomatic finding. In contrast, malignant melanomas (Fig. 12.34B) are usually symptomatic and elevated, progress in size and may be associated with retinal detachment and vitreous haemorrhage.

Choroiditis (inflammation of the choroid) appears as white spots (Fig. 12.34C). When active, they have a white, poorly defined, fluffy edge with an overlying hazy vitreous, causing blurring of vision. When inactive, they have a well-defined pigmented edge. Retinal blood vessels are unaffected, and clearly visible as they cross the choroiditis. Choroiditis is associated with toxoplasmosis, sarcoidosis and tuberculosis.

INVESTIGATIONS

Specialised tests may look at the visual system itself or investigate associated systemic disorders (Box 12.11).

Janet Wilson
Fiona Nicol

The ear, nose and throat

13

13 | THE EAR

ANATOMY

The ear is the specialised sensory organ of hearing and balance.

External ear

The pinna, external auditory canal (meatus) and the lateral surface of the tympanic membrane (eardrum) (Fig. 13.1) are the only blind-ending skin-lined tract in the body. It has a self-cleansing mechanism with outward migration of desquamated cells which are incorporated with cerumen to form wax.

Middle ear

The air-filled chamber of the middle ear amplifies sound. The eardrum's vibrations are amplified by the lever of the three articulated ossicles – malleus, incus and stapes. These vibrations are focused and further amplified on the much smaller area of the oval window. The Eustachian tube allows continual restoration of atmospheric pressure in the middle ear from the postnasal space. The handle of the malleus is attached to the drum, behind which the long process of the incus may also be visible on otoscopy (Fig. 13.2). Between the malleus and incus run the taste fibres from the anterior two-thirds of the tongue, which have 'hitched a ride' with the facial nerve. The upper part of the tympanic membrane is flaccid.

Inner ear

The stapes footplate vibrates in the oval window directly stimulating fluid within the cochlear (hearing) part of the inner ear. The other part of this bony labyrinth is the sensory organ of balance. Inner-ear epithelial cells convert the movement of their 'hairs' into electrical impulses along the vestibulocochlear (VIIIth) nerve. The vestibular part of the inner ear contains:

- the lateral, superior and posterior semicircular canals. These are arranged at right angles to each other, to detect rotational motion of their fluid (endolymph) in three planes
- the utricle and the saccule, whose cell hairs project into a gel layer containing small deposits (otoliths) which are subject to gravity, head tilt and linear endolymph movement.

SYMPTOMS AND DEFINITIONS

See Box 13.1.

Pain and itching

These are common. Earache may be referred from the throat (Boxes 13.2 and 13.3).

Otorrhoea

Otorrhoea is a discharge from the ear. A chronic offensive scanty discharge may be a sign of a cholesteatoma, an invasive keratin-filled outpouching of the drum. Bleeding is most often due to the infected granulation tissue. Painful or itchy discharge implies otitis externa.

Hearing loss

Hearing loss may be due to a failure of the VIIIth nerve or its endings – sensorineural – or of the conduction mechanisms of the middle ear by fluid, fixation or drum perforations or wax obstructing the external auditory meatus. Profound loss before speech acquisition affects speech quality, often vowel-based and lacking clear articulation (Box 13.4).

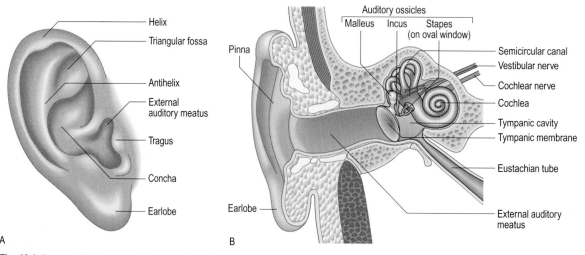

Fig. 13.1 The ear. (A) The pinna. **(B)** Cross-section of the outer, middle and inner ears.

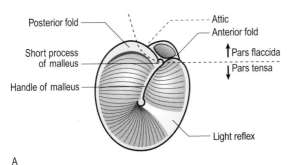

Posterior fold

Short process
of malleus

Handle of malleus

Attic
Anterior fold
↑ Pars flaccida
↓ Pars tensa

Light reflex

A

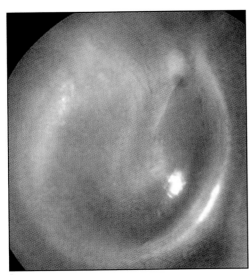

B

Fig. 13.2 Otoscopic examination of the right ear. **(A)** Main structures. **(B)** A normal tympanic membrane.

13.2 Causes of earache (otalgia)

Otological

- Acute otitis externa
- Acute otitis media
- Perichondritis
- Trauma

- Herpes zoster (Ramsay Hunt syndrome)
- Tumour

Non-otological

- Tonsillitis and pharyngitis
- Temporomandibular joint dysfunction

- Dental disease
- Cervical spine disease
- Cancer of the pharynx or larynx

EBE 13.3 Acute otitis media in children

No one criterion is a reliable indicator of acute otitis media in children. A 10-point scoring system, including pain, irritability, fever and otoscopic appearances, has been shown to have a sensitivity of 87%, specificity of 98%, positive predictive value of 91% and negative predictive value of 97%.

Casey JR, Block S, Puthoor P et al. A simple scoring system to improve clinical assessment of acute otitis media. Clin Pediatr 2011;50:623–629.

13.4 Causes of hearing loss

Conductive*

- Wax
- Otitis externa
- Middle ear effusion
- Trauma to the tympanic membrane/ossicles

- Otosclerosis
- Chronic middle ear infection
- Tumours of the middle ear

Sensorineural†

- Genetic, e.g. Alport's syndrome
- Prenatal infection, e.g. rubella
- Birth injury
- Infection:
  - Meningitis
  - Measles
  - Mumps
- Trauma

- Ménière's disease
- Degenerative (presbyacusis)
- Occupation- or other noise-induced
- Acoustic neuroma
- Idiopathic

*Disruption to the mechanical transfer of sound in outer ear, eardrum or ossicles.
†Cochlear or central damage.

13.1 Symptoms and definitions in ear disease

Symptom	Definition	Common cause
Otalgia	Pain	Otitis media or externa, referred from pharyngitis, trauma or, rarely, cancer
Pruritus	Itching	Otitis externa
Otorrhoea	Discharge	
	Purulent	Eardrum perforation with infection
Otitis externa
	Mucoid	Eardrum perforation, severe trauma causing leak of cerebrospinal fluid
	Blood-stained	Granulation tissue from infection, trauma
Hearing loss	Deafness	
Tinnitus	Noise in the absence of an objective source	Presbyacusis, noise damage
Vertigo	Hallucination of movement	Inner-ear disease
Unsteadiness		Vestibular or central disease

Tinnitus

Phantom ear noise, usually described as a 'ringing', in the absence of external stimuli, affects almost everyone at some time. Tinnitus is usually associated with hearing loss.

Vertigo

Vertigo is a sensation of movement relative to surroundings. Rotational movements are most common and

13

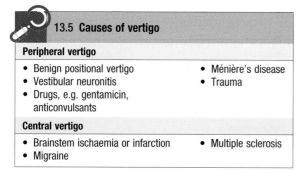

13.5 Causes of vertigo

Peripheral vertigo

- Benign positional vertigo
- Vestibular neuronitis
- Drugs, e.g. gentamicin, anticonvulsants
- Ménière's disease
- Trauma

Central vertigo

- Brainstem ischaemia or infarction
- Migraine
- Multiple sclerosis

13.7 Drugs that cause ototoxicity

Type	Examples
Antibiotics	Aminoglycosides, e.g. gentamicin
Cytotoxics	Cisplatin
Diuretics	Furosemide given intravenously after aminoglycosides
Analgesics	Aspirin
Others	Quinine

13.6 Diagnosing vertigo

	Acute labyrinthitis (vestibular neuronitis)	Benign paroxysmal positional vertigo	Ménière's disease	Central vertigo
Duration	Days	Seconds or minutes	Hours	Hours – migraine Days and weeks – MS Long-term – cerebrovascular accident
Hearing loss	–	–	++	–
Tinnitus	–	–	++	–
Aural fullness	–	–	++	–
Episodes	Rarely	Yes	Recurrent vertigo; persistent tinnitus and progressive sensorineural deafness	Migraine – recurs Central nervous system damage – usually some recovery but often persistent
Triggers	May have upper respiratory symptoms	Lying on affected ear	None	Drugs Cardiovascular disease

usually originate in the semicircular canals or, less often, centrally in the brainstem or cerebellum (Box 13.5). Ask about the following to make the diagnosis (Boxes 13.6 and 13.7):

- duration of the episodes
- positional and other precipitating factors
- associated or fluctuating hearing loss or tinnitus
- whether the ear feels 'full' during the episode
- a past history of significant head injury
- associated headaches.

Benign paroxysmal positional vertigo (BPPV) causes attacks that are particularly marked when lying on one side. It may be due to debris in the posterior semicircular canals. Idiopathic acute vestibular dysfunction (vestibular neuritis) is possibly due to reactivation of latent herpes simplex virus type 1. There is nausea, acute rotatory vertigo and horizontal spontaneous nystagmus (with a rotational component) toward the unaffected ear. The patient tends to falls towards the side of the affected ear. The condition lasts for days or weeks before resolving completely.

Ménière's disease is a rare condition that causes an episodic sensation of fullness in the ear with tinnitus, severe vertigo and headache. Between attacks, examination is normal, but hearing may be disturbed – most commonly, low-tone deafness. The diagnosis is confirmed by demonstrating excess endolymph on gadolinium-enhanced magnetic resonance imaging.

Unsteadiness

Feeling lightheaded is not a vestibular symptom, but unsteadiness may be. The rare, life-threatening causes of vertigo and unsteadiness are central, i.e. from brainstem or cerebellar changes.

Nystagmus

Nystagmus is an involuntary rhythmical oscillation of the eyes. It may be vertical, horizontal, rotatory or multi-directional. The commonest form is horizontal, jerk nystagmus with a slow (pathological) drift of both eyes in one direction, then a fast correction in the opposite direction. The direction of the fast jerk is used to define the direction of the nystagmus. A patient with horizontal jerk nystagmus visible on examination and who is steady enough to be able to walk into a consulting room has a central lesion. Pendular nystagmus (oscillations equal in rate and amplitude about a central point) occurs with central vision defects.

THE HISTORY

Past history

Ask about previous middle ear infection or trauma and systemic disorders associated with hearing loss, e.g.

granulomatosis with polyangiitis (previously known as Wegener's granulomatosis).

Family history

Some types of sensorineural deafness and of otosclerosis (conductive deafness due to fixation of the stapes footplate) are inherited.

Drug history

Principal ototoxic drugs are listed in Box 13.7.

Social history

Recreational or occupational noise exposure, especially if severe or prolonged, can cause sensorineural hearing loss. Smoking is a key risk factor for peripheral and central vascular causes of neuro-otologic symptoms.

THE PHYSICAL EXAMINATION

Examination sequence

- Note the skin, shape, size and any deformity of the pinna (Fig. 13.4A).
- Gently pull on the pinna to check for pain.
- Use the largest otoscope speculum that will comfortably fit the meatus. Explain to the patient what you are going to do.
- Hold the otoscope comfortably and rest the ulnar border of your hand against the patient's cheek (Fig. 13.3). Then, if the patient's head moves, your hand will cause less ear trauma.
- Gently pull the pinna upwards and backwards to straighten the cartilaginous external auditory meatus. Look at the canal skin through the speculum. Check for discharge, wax and foreign bodies. You should see a light reflex on a pearly grey, translucent normal tympanic membrane (Fig. 13.2B).

Abnormal findings

Congenital deformities are linked to sensorineural deafness. Low-set ears imply a first branchial arch abnormality. Trauma may produce a haematoma of the pinna (Fig. 13.4B), or mastoid bruising (if there is a skull base fracture). Basal cell and squamous cell cancers affect the fine skin of the rim of the pinna (Fig. 13.4C). Tenderness on palpation of the tragus suggests inflammation of the canal or adjacent temporomandibular joint. A very wide meatus suggests previous mastoid surgery. If the drum is not perforated, discharge is due to otitis externa (Fig. 13.5A), which may be so severe as to close off the meatus completely (furunculosis). The bony canal occasionally reveals exostoses (Fig. 13.5B).

White scars on the tympanic membrane are tympanosclerosis. Note the position and percentage of the drum involved by any perforation (Fig. 13.6A). A severe retraction pocket of the pars tensa may mimic a perforation (Fig. 13.6B), as may a cholesteatoma sac of the pars flaccida (Fig. 13.5C). The drum may look normal, or dull, or golden, or bluish. Fluid or effusion behind the drum is called otitis media with effusion (Fig. 13.7B) and a fluid level may be seen (Fig. 13.7C). Surgical treatment is by insertion of a ventilation tube or grommet (Fig. 13.6C). In acute suppurative otitis media the drum becomes gradually more inflamed (Fig. 13.7A) and may eventually perforate.

13

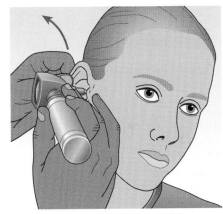

Fig. 13.3 Examination of the ear using an otoscope.

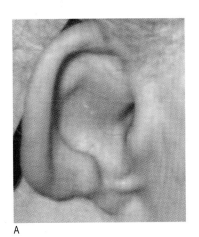

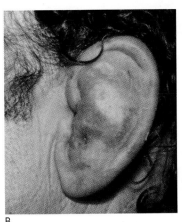

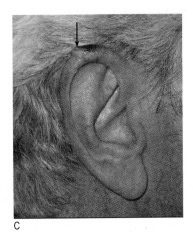

A B C

Fig. 13.4 The pinna. (A) Microtia. **(B)** Haematoma. **(C)** Squamous cancer (arrow).

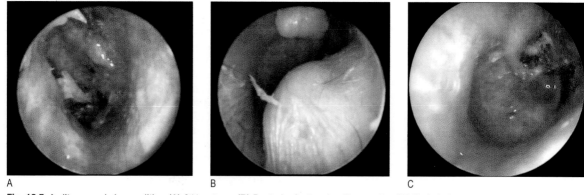

A   B   C

Fig. 13.5 Auditory canal abnormalities. (A) Otitis externa. **(B)** Exostosis of external auditory meatus. **(C)** Cholesteatoma.

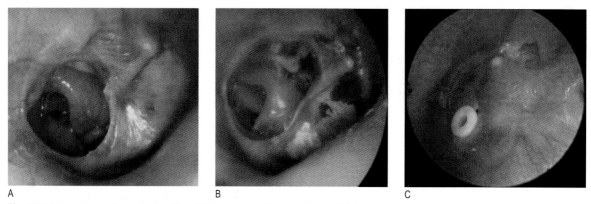

A   B   C

Fig. 13.6 Tympanic membrane abnormalities. (A) Tympanic membrane perforation. **(B)** Retraction pocket of the pars tensa. **(C)** Grommet in situ.

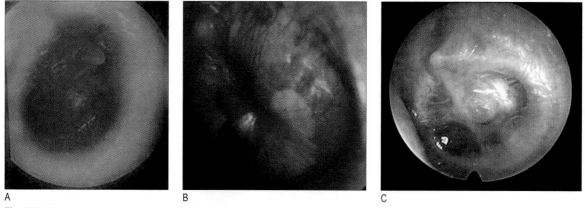

A   B   C

Fig. 13.7 Otitis media. (A) Acute otitis media. **(B)** With effusion. **(C)** Fluid level behind tympanic membrane.

Testing hearing

Whispered voice test

Examination sequence

- Stand behind the patient.
- Start with your mouth about 15 cm from the ear you are testing.

- Mask hearing in the other ear by rubbing the tragus.
- Ask the patient to repeat your words. Use a combination of multisyllable numbers and words. Start with a normal speaking voice to confirm that the patient understands the test. Lower your voice intensity to a clear whisper.
- Repeat, but this time at arm's length from the patient's ear.
  People with normal hearing can repeat words whispered at 60 cm.

Tuning fork tests

Use a 512 Hz or 256 Hz tuning fork to help differentiate between conductive and sensorineural hearing loss.

Examination sequence

Weber's test
- Hit the prongs of the fork against a padded surface to make it vibrate.
- Place the base of the vibrating tuning fork in the middle of the patient's forehead.
- Ask: 'Where do you hear the sound?'
- Record which side Weber's test lateralises to if not central (Fig. 13.8).

Normal findings
The noise is heard in the middle or equally in both ears.

Abnormal findings
The noise is louder in an ear with conductive deafness (test on yourself by putting a finger in your outer canal to block out surrounding noise). In unilateral sensorineural deafness the sound is heard better in the better-hearing ear. In symmetrical hearing loss it is heard in the middle.

Examination sequence

Rinne's test
- Place the vibrating tuning fork base on the mastoid process (Fig.13.9A). Ask the patient 'Can you hear this?', and then to indicate when she no longer hears the sound.
- Place the still-vibrating prongs 2 cm away from the external auditory meatus. Ask if she can hear it now (Fig.13.9B).

Normal findings
The sound is louder at the ear, that is, air conduction is better than bone conduction. Record this as AC > BC; this is normal (Rinne positive).

Abnormal findings
If the sound is louder on the mastoid process, bone conduction is better than air conduction. Record this as BC > AC (Rinne negative). This applies in conductive deafness.

A false-negative Rinne's test may occur if hearing is very poor on one side. Then, the sound travelling through the air is not perceived but, when the tuning fork is placed on the mastoid process of the 'poor' ear, the sound is conducted through the skull and heard in the 'good' ear.

In a mild conductive deafness, the Weber test is abnormal (lateralised) before the Rinne.

Testing vestibular function

Testing for nystagmus

Examination sequence

- With the patient seated, hold your finger an arm's length away, level with the patient's eyes.
- Ask the patient to look at, and follow, the tip of your finger. Slowly move your finger up and down and then side to side. Be careful not to get the eyes too far deviated to the side as this generates a physiological nystagmus (Box 13.8).
- Look at the patient's eyes for any oscillations and note:
  - whether they are horizontal, vertical or rotatory
  - which direction of gaze causes the most marked nystagmus
  - in which direction the fast phase of jerk nystagmus occurs
  - whether jerk nystagmus changes direction when the direction of gaze changes
  - if nystagmus is more obvious in one eye than the other (ataxic or dysconjugate nystagmus).

Dix–Hallpike positional test

Examination sequence

- Ask the patient to sit upright, close to the edge of the couch. Warn the patient about what you are going to do.
- Turn the patient's head 45° to one side.
- Rapidly lower him, so that the head is now 30° below the horizontal. Say: 'Keep your eyes open even if you feel dizzy.'
- Watch the eyes carefully for nystagmus. Repeat the test, turning the head to the other side (Fig. 13.10).

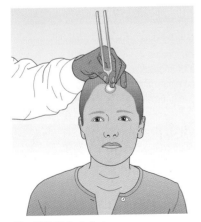

Fig. 13.8 Weber's test.

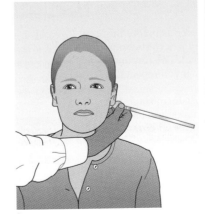

A

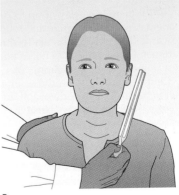

B

Fig. 13.9 Rinne's tests. **(A)** Testing bone conduction. **(B)** Testing air conduction.

13.8 Characteristics of nystagmus

Nystagmus type	Clinical pathology	Characteristics	
		Fast phase	**Maximal on looking**
Pendular	Eyes, e.g. congenital blindness, albinism	No fast phase	Straight ahead
Jerk			
Peripheral	Semicircular canal, vestibular nerve	Unidirectional Not suppressed by optic fixation Patient too dizzy to walk Dix–Hallpike fatigues on repetition	Away from affected side
Central	Brainstem, cerebellum	Bidirectional (changes with direction of gaze) Suppressed by optic fixation Patient can walk (even with nystagmus) Dix–Hallpike persists	To either side
Dysconjugate (ataxic)	Interconnections of IIIrd, IVth and VIth nerves (medial longitudinal bundle)	Typically affects the abducting eye	To either side

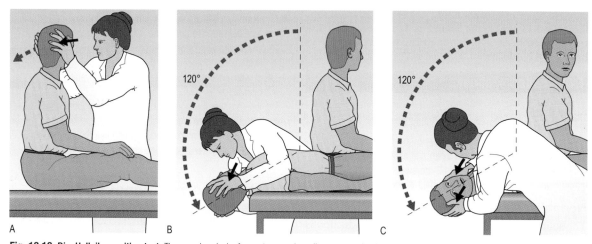

Fig. 13.10 Dix–Hallpike position test. The examiner looks for nystagmus (usually accompanied by vertigo). Both nystagmus and vertigo typically decrease (fatigue) on repeat testing.

Normal patients have no nystagmus or sensation of vertigo.

Abnormal findings

In BPPV there is a delay of up to 20 seconds before the patient experiences vertigo and rotatory jerk nystagmus towards the lower ear occurs (geotropic). The response fatigues, so there is less, or no, response if you repeat the test immediately (adaptation).

Central pathology produces immediate nystagmus, not necessarily with vertigo, and no adaptation. Lack of dizziness plus relatively coarse nystagmus is central till proved otherwise.

Unterberger's test

Examination sequence

■ Ask the patient to march on the spot with his eyes closed. The patient will rotate to the side of a damaged labyrinth.

Fistula test

Examination sequence

■ Repeatedly compress the tragus against the external auditory meatus to occlude the meatus.

If this produces a sense of imbalance or vertigo with nystagmus, it suggests an abnormal communication between the middle ear and the vestibular apparatus, e.g. erosion due to cholesteatoma.

INVESTIGATIONS

See Box 13.9.

13.9 Investigations in ear disease

Investigation	Indication/comment
Swab from external auditory meatus	Otitis media and externa
MR scan	Acoustic neuroma
Audiometry	Hearing loss A single-frequency tone at different noise levels is presented to each ear in turn through headphones in a soundproof booth. The intensity is reduced in 10-decibel steps until patients can no longer hear it. The threshold is the quietest sound they can hear
Impedance audiometry (tympanometry)	Otitis media with effusion Eustachian tube dysfunction Ossicular discontinuity The compliance of the eardrum is measured during changes in the pressure in the ear canal. Compliance should be maximal at atmospheric pressure
Vestibular testing	Unilateral vestibular hypofunction
Caloric tests	Water at 30°C and then 44°C is irrigated into the external ear canal. Electronystagmography records nystagmus. The response is reduced in vestibular hypofunction
Posturography	Vestibular hypofunction Reveals whether patients rely on vision or proprioception more than usual

13

THE NOSE AND SINUSES

ANATOMY

The nasal vault is formed from two nasal bones above, a middle pair of cartilages and two tip cartilages around the nostrils. The septum divides the nose into two nasal cavities. Posteriorly, the cavities open up, with three air baffles down each side. These are the turbinates which filter, warm and moisten the nasal airflow. The sensory olfactory epithelium is high up in the cavities (Fig. 13.11).

The paranasal sinuses – maxillary, frontal, ethmoid and sphenoid – are air-filled spaces in the skull bones. They connect through narrow openings (ostia) with the nasal cavity.

SYMPTOMS AND DEFINITIONS

Nasal obstruction

Persistent unilateral obstruction is often due to a deviated nasal septum, either congenital or secondary to trauma. Bilateral obstruction may be due to rhinitis, with or without sinusitis or polyps (Box 13.10).

Nasal discharge

Bilateral watery discharge suggests allergic or vasomotor rhinitis. Purulent discharge suggests bacterial infection, such as after the common cold, in localised sinus infection or when there is a foreign body in the nose. New onset, unilateral, crystal clear discharge following head injury suggests a cerebrospinal fluid leak.

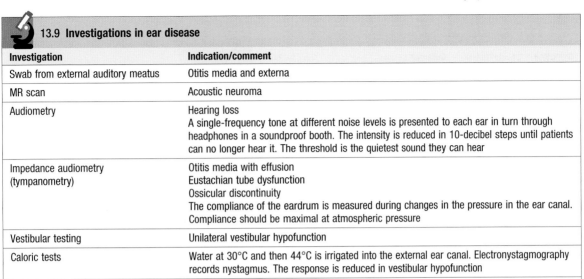

Inferior view of nose — Tip, Ala nasi, Anterior naris, Vestibule, Columella

External nose — Bridge, Ala nasi, Anterior naris, Tip, Columella

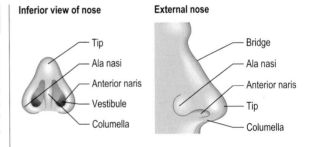

Nasal septum — Pituitary fossa, Cranial cavity, Frontal sinus, Sphenoid sinus, Bony portion of nasal septum, Septal cartilage, Little's area, Hard palate, Nasopharynx

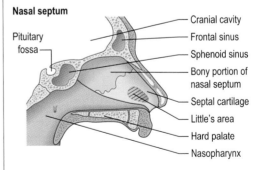

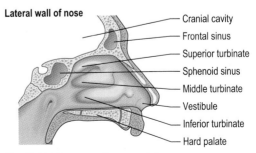

Lateral wall of nose — Cranial cavity, Frontal sinus, Superior turbinate, Sphenoid sinus, Middle turbinate, Vestibule, Inferior turbinate, Hard palate

Fig. 13.11 The nose and paranasal sinuses.

13.10 Symptoms and definitions in nasal disease

Symptom	Definition	Common cause
Nose blocked		Viral illness, deviated nasal septum, nasal polyp
Rhinorrhoea	Discharge	Watery – allergic rhinitis, cerebrospinal fluid leak Purulent – infection, foreign body
Epistaxis	Nose bleed	Trauma, infection
Sneezing		Allergy, infection
Coughing		Postnasal drip
Anosmia	Absence of smell	Head injury, viral neuropathy
Hyposmia	Reduced smell	Nasal polyps, nasal blockage
Cacosmia	Unpleasant smell	Chronic anaerobic sepsis
Nasal deformity		Trauma, rhinophyma
Pain		Sinus infection, dental infection
Septum perforation		Nose-picking, granulomatous disease, e.g. granulomatosis with polyangiitis, cocaine use, inhalation of industrial dusts, e.g. nickel, chromium

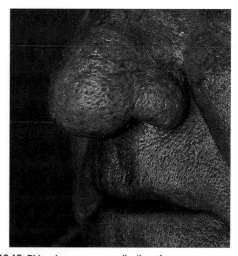

Fig. 13.12 Rhinophyma as a complication of rosacea.

EBE 13.11 Chronic rhinosinusitis

Chronic rhinosinustis is characterised by the triad of pain, obstruction and persistent purulent discharge. Nasal endoscopy may confirm the diagnosis.

Tahamiler R, Canakcioglu S, Ogreden S et al. The accuracy of symptom-based definition of chronic rhinosinusitis. Allergy 2007;62:1029–1032. Bhattacharyya N, Lee LN. Evaluating the diagnosis of chronic rhinosinusitis based on clinical guidelines and endoscopy. Otolaryngology – Head Neck Surg 2010;143:147–151.

Epistaxis

This is bleeding from inside the nose. There is a rich blood supply to an area of the anterior nasal septum (Little's area) that is easily traumatised and is a common site for bleeding. Epistaxis may be life-threatening in the elderly, notably those with impaired coagulation from disease, medication or alcohol excess.

Sneezing

This protective sudden expulsive effort clears the nasal passages of irritants. It is common in viral upper respiratory infection and allergic rhinitis.

Disturbance of smell

Anosmia (complete loss of sense of smell) may follow head injury with damage to the olfactory epithelium/olfactory nerve or can occur after a viral upper respiratory tract infection. Mechanical obstruction of the nose by nasal polyps or severe mucosal oedema and swelling in allergic rhinitis usually causes hyposmia (reduced sense of smell). Cacosmia is an unpleasant smell due to chronic sepsis in the nose or sinuses. Parosmia is a distorted sense of smell. Brief olfactory hallucinations (phantosmia) may occur in temporal lobe epilepsy.

Nasal deformity

Swelling and bruising from trauma settle over 2 weeks but nasal deformity may remain if the nasal bones have been displaced. Skin affected by acne rosacea over years causes rhinophyma (Fig. 13.12). Destruction of the nasal septum produces flattening of the bridge and a 'saddle' deformity. Causes include granulomatosis with polyangiitis, trauma, congenital syphilis and chronic abuse of cocaine (a powerful vasoconstrictor which renders the mucosa ischaemic). Widening of the nose is a feature of acromegaly and advanced nasal polyposis.

Nasal and facial pain

Nasal pain is extremely rare, except following trauma. Facial pain is caused by temporomandibular joint dysfunction, migraine, dental disease, sinusitis or trigeminal neuralgia. Cluster headache characteristically causes unilateral nasal discharge and eye watering (Box 13.11).

THE HISTORY

Past history

A past history of atopy may indicate rhinitis. One-third of patients with nasal polyps have asthma. Recurrent upper respiratory tract infections may cause sinusitis. Nasal bleeding is prolonged by hypertension and bleeding diathesis. Trauma to the face and nose may cause nasal blockage, deformity and anosmia.

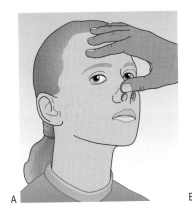
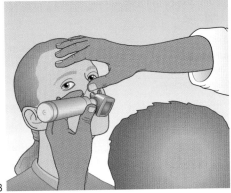

A

B

Fig. 13.13 Nasal examination.
(A) Elevating the tip of the nose to give a clear view of the anterior nares.
(B) Anterior rhinoscopy using an otoscope with a large speculum.

13

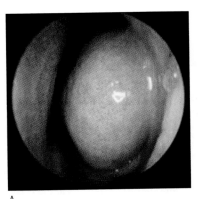
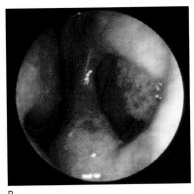
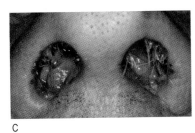

A

B

C

Fig. 13.14 Nasal abnormalities. (A) Turbinate hypertrophy. **(B)** Nasal septum perforation postsurgery. **(C)** Nasal polyps.

Drug history

Anticoagulants and non-steroidal anti-inflammatory drugs may aggravate epistaxis. 'Snorting' cocaine can cause perforation of the nasal septum (Fig. 13.14B).

Family history

Family history of atopy is relevant in rhinitis.

Social history

Ask allergic patients about their pets. Exposure to inhaled hardwood dust in certain occupations is associated with an increase of sinus cancer. Exposure to other occupational dusts or chemicals may exacerbate rhinitis. Alcohol use is important in epistaxis and rhinophyma. Smoking impedes nasal mucociliary clearance.

THE PHYSICAL EXAMINATION

Examination sequence

- Look at the external surface and appearance of the nose. Note any skin disease or deformity.

- Stand behind the patient; look down the nose from above for any external deviation.
- At rest, the nostrils face down towards the floor but the nasal cavity passes posteriorly along the upper surface of the hard palate. To look into the nose, ask your patient to hold her head in the normal position (discourage her from throwing her head back). Gently elevate the tip of her nose with the pad of your thumb to align the nostrils with the rest of the cavity.
- Look in and assess the alignment and mucosal covering of the septum (Fig. 13.13).
- In an adult use a large-size speculum on your otoscope to see the inferior turbinates. Do not try to pass instruments into a child's nose.
- Feel the nasal bones gently to distinguish bony from cartilaginous deformity. In trauma, check the integrity of the infraorbital ridges and of the range of eye movements to exclude 'orbital blowout'.
- Place a metal spatula under the nostrils and look for the condensation marks to assess airway patency or lightly occlude each nostril and ask the patient to sniff.
- Palpate for cervical lymphadenopathy (p. 53).
 Tests of olfaction are usually confined to specialist clinics.

Abnormal findings

The nasal mucosa is pale, moist and hypertrophied in allergic rhinitis (Fig. 13.14A). In chronic rhinitis, it is swollen and red. A pale grey, moist swelling blocking

Investigation	Indication/comment
Plain X-ray	Nasal bone fracture Only required if you suspect associated facial fracture
Lateral X-ray nasopharynx	Adenoidal hypertrophy Young children
Nasal endoscopy	Sinus disease
Computed tomography	Sinus disease, trauma and cancer Radiation dose to the eyes is significant, so avoid repeat imaging

the nostril may be a polyp (Fig. 13.14C). Facial swelling is unusual in sinusitis but occurs with a dental root abscess and cancer of the maxillary antrum.

In functional anosmia there is no response to a nasal irritant. Nasal irritation is mediated via the trigeminal and not the olfactory nerve.

INVESTIGATIONS

Tests of olfaction are usually only done in specialist clinics (Box 13.12).

THE MOUTH AND THROAT

ANATOMY

The mouth

The mouth extends from the lips anteriorly to the anterior pillar of the tonsils posteriorly and has two compartments: the vestibule between the buccal (cheek) mucosa and the teeth and the oral cavity internal to the teeth. In the oral cavity are the anterior two-thirds of the tongue, the floor of the mouth, the hard palate and the inner surfaces of the gums and the teeth (Fig. 13.15). The lips form a seal for the oral cavity. The tongue's normal colour varies from pink through to very dark brown. Its velvet texture is due to the filiform papillae containing taste buds (Fig. 13.16). Circumvallate papillae are groups of taste buds which mark the boundary of the anterior two-thirds and posterior third of the tongue.

The parotid, submandibular and sublingual salivary glands secrete saliva (Fig. 13.17). The parotid gland sits in front of the ear, encasing the facial nerve. The part deep to the facial nerve is called the deep lobe (p. 252). The opening of its duct is in the buccal mucosa, opposite the second upper molar. The submandibular gland lies

anterior and medial to the angle of the jaw; its duct opens into the floor of the mouth next to the frenulum of the tongue (Fig. 13.15).

The throat

The pharynx is a shared upper aerodigestive channel from the anterior faucial pillar to the laryngeal inlet. The larynx is a protective sphincter for the lower airway, known colloquially as the 'voice box' due to the importance of human phonation. It has two external cartilages, the thyroid cartilage (Adam's apple) and the cricoid cartilage, the prominence at the top of the trachea. Its sensory supply is via the superior and recurrent laryngeal branches of cranial nerve X (vagus) (p. 255). Its motor supply is mainly from the recurrent laryngeal nerve, which loops up round the aortic arch on the left and the subclavian artery on the right.

The teeth

In children the 20 deciduous teeth erupt by 3 years. There are 32 secondary teeth, erupting from ages 6 to 16 or later (Figs 13.18–13.20).

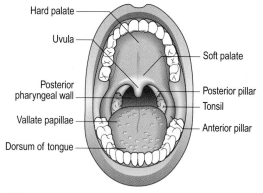

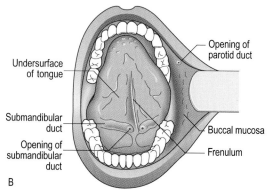

A

B

Fig. 13.15 Anatomy of the mouth and throat. (A) Examination with the mouth open. **(B)** Examination with the tongue touching the roof of the mouth.

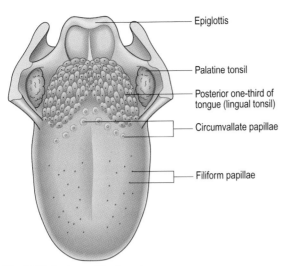

Fig. 13.16 Anatomy of the tongue.

- Epiglottis
- Palatine tonsil
- Posterior one-third of tongue (lingual tonsil)
- Circumvallate papillae
- Filiform papillae

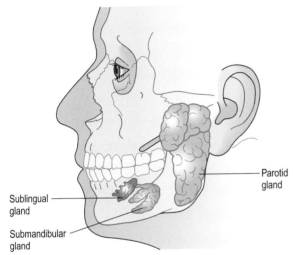

Fig. 13.17 The position of the major salivary glands.

- Parotid gland
- Sublingual gland
- Submandibular gland

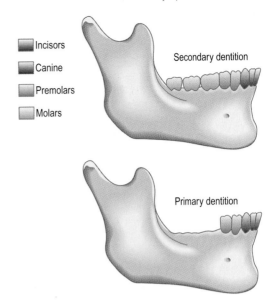

- Incisors
- Canine
- Premolars
- Molars

Secondary dentition

Primary dentition

Fig. 13.18 Primary and secondary dentition.

13

SYMPTOMS AND DEFINITIONS

See Box 13.13.

Pain

Sore mouth

Gingivitis (inflammation of the gums) may cause a narrow red line at the border of the gums (Box 13.14). Aphthous ulcers are small painful superficial ulcers on the tongue, palate or buccal mucosa. They are common, of unknown cause and heal spontaneously within a few days. The causes of oral ulcers are trauma, vitamin or mineral deficiency (anaemia), cancer or lichen planus. Unilateral painful vesicles on the palate can be caused by herpes zoster (Fig. 11.8B).

Diffuse oral infection with *Candida albicans* (candidiasis or 'thrush') may be secondary to poorly fitting dentures, the use of inhaled steroids or immunodeficiency, e.g. HIV infection or leukaemia (Box 8.4).

13.13 Symptoms and definitions in mouth and throat disease

Symptom	Definition	Common cause
Pain		Dental caries, periodontal infection
Odynophagia	Pain on swallowing	Infection, cancer of oesophagus, larynx or pharynx
Stridor	Noise from upper airway on breathing	Upper-airways obstruction, e.g. laryngeal cancer
Dysphonia	Change in the quality of the voice	Cysts, polyps, cancer, laryngitis
Dysphagia	Difficulty swallowing	Pharyngitis Oesophageal disease
Lumps		Lymphadenopathy
Halitosis	Bad breath	Poor dental hygiene
Trismus	Inability to open mouth fully	Quinsy, tetanus
Xerostomia	Dry mouth	Anticholinergic drugs, Sjögren's syndrome

13.14 The gums in systemic conditions

Condition	Description
Phenytoin treatment	Firm and hypertrophied
Scurvy	Soft and haemorrhagic
Acute leukaemia	Hypertrophied and haemorrhagic
Cyanotic congenital heart disease	Spongy and haemorrhagic
Chronic lead poisoning	Punctate blue line

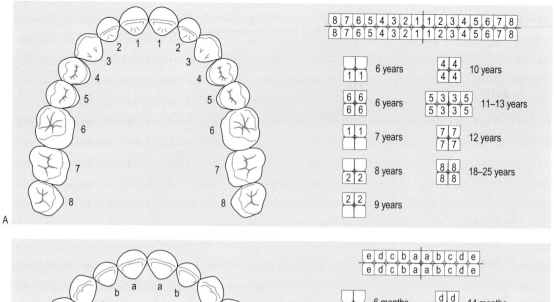

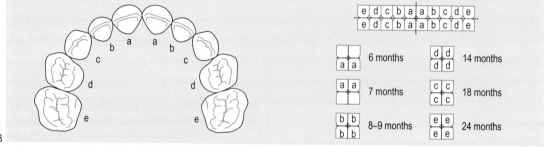

Fig. 13.19 Permanent upper arch and average eruption times. (A) The permanent teeth. **(B)** The deciduous teeth. An upper left deciduous central will be designated | a; a lower right permanent lateral incisor 2 |, a lower left permanent third molar | 8, etc.

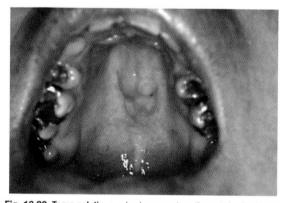

Fig. 13.20 Torus palatinus, a benign asymptomatic central palatal bony mass more common in Asian populations.

Sore throat

Throat pain often radiates to the ear because of the dual innervation of the pharynx and external auditory meatus via the vagus nerve.

Many viruses cause pharyngitis (acute inflammation of the pharynx). Acute tonsillitis may be viral or caused by *Streptococcus pyogenes* (Fig. 13.21A). There may be a pustular exudate on the tonsils and associated systemic features of fever, malaise, anorexia and cervical lymphadenopathy. You cannot distinguish viral from bacterial tonsillitis clinically.

In infectious mononucleosis (glandular fever), palatal petechiae can be seen and the tonsil may be covered in a white pseudomembrane (Fig. 13.21B). Diphtheria causes a true, grey membrane over the tonsil but is rarely seen because of immunisation.

A peritonsillar abscess (quinsy) causes extreme pain aggravated by swallowing. The patient dribbles saliva out of his mouth, there is trismus (spasm of the jaw muscles) and the uvula is displaced to the opposite side (Fig. 13.21C).

Any persistent mass or ulcer on the tonsil associated with pain may be a squamous cancer.

Globus pharyngeus is the feeling of a lump in the throat with normal examination. It generally fluctuates from day to day. Contributory factors are believed to include anxiety, habitual throat clearing or acid reflux. Rarely, globus is progressive and occurs with 'red flag' symptoms as part of the presentation of underlying malignancy (Box 13.15) (Box 8.26).

Human papillomavirus-related oropharyngeal cancer is the commonest site of primary head and neck cancer in young, sexually active non smokers.

Stridor

Stridor is a high-pitched, often harsh noise produced by airflow turbulence through partial obstruction of the upper airway. It occurs most commonly on inspiration but also on expiration or biphasically. Inspiratory stridor indicates narrowing at the vocal cords; biphasic stridor suggests tracheal obstruction, while stridor on

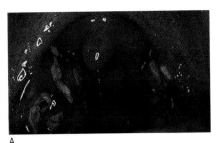

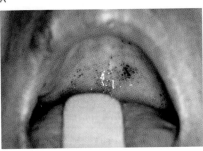

A

B

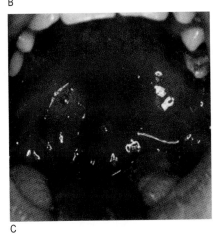

C

Fig. 13.21 Sore throat. (A) Acute tonsillitis – the presence of pus strongly suggests a bacterial (Streptococcal) aetiology. **(B)** Glandular fever showing palatal petechiae. **(C)** A left peritonsillar abscess.

13.15 Red flag symptoms

- Dysphagia
- Hoarseness
- Odynophagia
- Weight loss

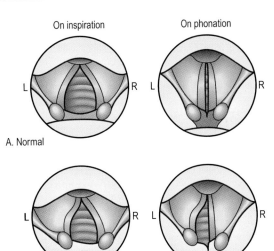

Fig. 13.22 Laryngoscopic views of the vocal cords. (A) Normal movements. **(B)** Movements in the presence of recurrent laryngeal nerve paralysis, most commonly caused by lung cancer. Note that the paralysed left cord is in the cadaveric position (between inspiration and expiration).

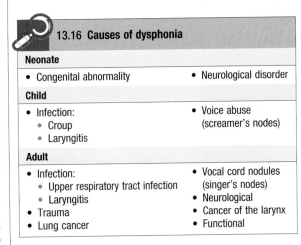

13.16 Causes of dysphonia

Neonate	
• Congenital abnormality	• Neurological disorder

Child	

• Infection:
  • Croup
  • Laryngitis
	• Voice abuse
	(screamer's nodes)

Adult	

• Infection:
  • Upper respiratory tract infection
  • Laryngitis
• Trauma
• Lung cancer
	• Vocal cord nodules
	(singer's nodes)
	• Neurological
	• Cancer of the larynx
	• Functional

expiration suggests tracheobronchial obstruction. Narrowing of smaller, peripheral airways produces wheeze heard on expiration (Fig. 13.22). Always investigate stridor. Common causes include infection/inflammation, e.g. acute epiglottitis in children and young adults and tumours of the trachea and main bronchi or extrinsic compression by lymph nodes in older adults. Rarer causes include anaphylaxis and foreign body.

Stertor, or muffled 'hot potato' speech, occurs with naso- or oropharyngeal obstruction, e.g. peritonsillar abscess (quinsy).

Dysphonia

Any disturbance of vocal cord function may cause dysphonia (Box 13.16). More than 3 weeks' continuous dysphonia requires laryngoscopy to exclude cancer. Breathy dysphonia and a weak (bovine) cough are presenting features of lung or oesophageal cancer causing recurrent laryngeal nerve palsy (Fig. 13.22 and p. 139).

Sialadenopathy

Sudden, painful unilateral salivary gland swelling is due to a stone obstructing the duct. Other causes of enlarged salivary glands are mumps, sarcoidosis, HIV-related cysts, bacterial infection (suppurative parotitis; Fig. 13.23) and cancer.

THE HISTORY

Presenting complaint

Timing of symptoms

Epiglottitis usually presents with stridor, rapidly progressive airway obstruction occurring within a few

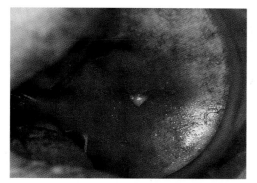

Fig. 13.23 Pus discharging from parotid duct.

hours, sore throat, fever and drooling. It may be caused by bacterial infection, e.g. *Haemophilus influenzae*, *Streptococcus pneumoniae* and group A streptococci. With the introduction of the HIB vaccine it is now relatively more common in adults than small children. Other causes are thermal injury (burns, crack cocaine smoking), radiotherapy, and caustic or foreign-body ingestion.

Acute laryngotracheobronchitis (croup) in infants usually has a longer history (24–48 hours) and the airway obstruction is less severe.

Past history

Ask about dental problems and systemic disease, particularly affecting the gastrointestinal tract as the mouth is part of this. Neurological conditions may affect the ability to masticate and swallow, and drooling or dry mouth with superimposed infection may result. Note any facial trauma or surgery.

Drug history

Many drugs, including tricyclic antidepressants and anticholinergics, cause a dry mouth. Recent and multiple courses of antibiotics increase the chance of oral candidiasis, as does any prolonged debilitating illness.

Social history

Piercings and sexually transmitted infection may affect the mouth. Oral cancer is more common in smokers and those who experience orogenital contact, chew tobacco or betel nut or have excess alcohol intake or poor oral hygiene.

THE PHYSICAL EXAMINATION

The mouth and throat

Examination sequence

- Listen to the patient's voice (Box 13.17).
- Have a good light source. Use a head mirror or head light to leave both your hands free to manipulate instruments.
- Do not try to examine the throat in a patient with stridor, as this may induce laryngospasm and total airway obstruction.

Inspection

- Ask the patient to remove any dentures. Look at his lips, then ask him to half-open his mouth. Inspect the mucosa of the vestibule, buccal surfaces and buccogingival sulci for discoloration, inflammation, ulceration or nodules, then at the bite closure.
- Ask him to open his mouth fully and touch behind the upper incisors with the tip of his tongue. Check the mucosa of the floor of mouth and the orifices of the submandibular glands.
- Ask him to stick out his tongue. Look for deviation (XIIth nerve dysfunction), mucosal change or fasciculation.
- Now ask him to deviate his tongue to one side. Retract the opposite buccal mucosa with a tongue depressor to view the lateral tongue border clearly. Repeat on the other side.
- Look at the hard palate. Note any cleft, abnormal arched palate or telangiectasia.
- Look at the oropharynx. Ask him to say 'Aaah'. Use a tongue depressor if needed.
- Look at the soft palate for any cleft or structural abnormality. Note any telangiectasia.
- Look at the tonsils. Note their symmetry, size, colour, any discharge or membrane.
- Use the tongue depressor to scrape off any white plaques gently.
- Touch the posterior pharyngeal wall gently with the tongue depressor to stimulate the gag reflex. Check for symmetrical movement of the soft palate.

Palpation

- If there is any lesion in the mouth or salivary glands, put on a pair of gloves and palpate it with one hand outside on the patient's cheek or jaw and the gloved finger of your other hand inside his mouth.
- Feel the lesion and identify its characteristics (SPACESPIT: Box 3.11; p. 53).
- If the parotid gland is abnormal or enlarged, examine the facial nerve and check if the deep lobe (tonsil area) is displaced medially.
- Palpate the length of the duct, and include the submandibular gland.
- Palpate the cervical lymph nodes systematically (Fig. 3.22).

Abnormal findings

Cold exposure causes desquamation and cracking of the lips ('chapped lips'); riboflavin deficiency causes red cracking of the lips. Inflamed painful cracking of the skin at the corners of the mouth may be due to excess saliva, chronic atrophic candidiasis or iron deficiency (Fig. 13.24). Squamous and basal cell cancers occur on the lips and are associated with smoking and sun exposure.

Neurological disease, painful mouth and a tight frenulum may all limit tongue protrusion. Normal tongue appearance includes areas of smooth mucosa (geographic tongue) or, conversely, of excessive furring. A smooth red tongue with diffuse papillary atrophy occurs in iron or vitamin B_{12} deficiency.

Macroglossia (enlarged tongue) occurs in Down's syndrome, acromegaly (Fig. 3.19A), hypothyroidism and amyloidosis. Wasting and fasciculation of the tongue are features of motor neurone disease.

Abnormal buccal pigmentation is found in Addison's disease (Fig. 5.19B), haemochromatosis or the Peutz–Jeghers syndrome (with polyposis of the small intestine) or chewing betel nut (a mild stimulant chewed in Asia which is a carcinogen).

White plaques of candidiasis on the tongue or mucosa (Fig. 13.25A) come away easily when scraped but leukoplakia (a keratotic precancerous condition) does not and requires excision biopsy (Fig. 13.25B). Cancers (usually squamous) may occur at any site in the mouth; assume any painless persistent mass is oral cancer and refer urgently for biopsy. Tonsil lesions may be lymphoma.

Oral mucous retention cysts are bluish domes a few millimetres in diameter.

Aphthous ulcers (Fig. 13.25C) are small and painful, occur in crops and usually heal within a few days. Ulcers may be the presentation of Crohn's or other inflammatory bowel diseases. Any mouth ulcers persisting for >3 weeks require biopsy to exclude oral cancer.

A stone may be felt in the submandibular (or, rarely, the parotid) duct.

Rotten teeth (dental caries) are common in patients with poor oral hygiene (Fig. 13.25D).

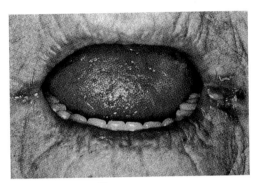

Fig. 13.24 Angular stomatitis.

The neck

Examine the neck in all patients with mouth or throat symptoms. A neck mass or rash may be the main presenting complaint (Fig. 13.26 and Box 13.18).

13

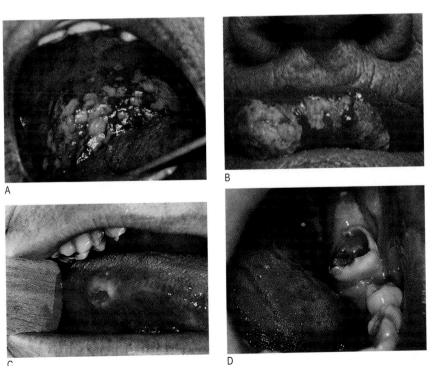

Fig. 13.25 Disorders of the tongue and teeth. (A) Oral thrush. **(B)** Leukoplakia. **(C)** Aphthous stomatitis causing a deep ulcer in a patient with inflammatory bowel disease. **(D)** Dental caries.

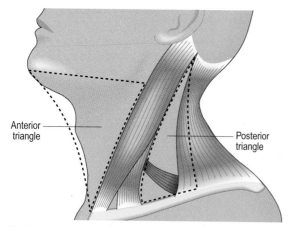

Fig. 13.26 Sites of swellings in the neck.

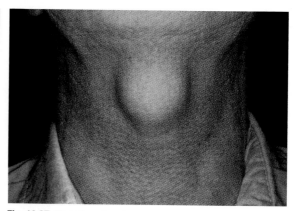

Fig. 13.27 Thyroglossal cyst.

13.18 Causes of neck lumps

Midline structures

- Thyroid isthmus swelling – most common cause in adults
- Thyroglossal cyst – lump moves when patient sticks out tongue
- Laryngeal swellings
- Submental lymph nodes
- Dermoid cysts

Lateral structures

In the anterior triangle (bounded by the midline, the anterior border of sternocleidomastoid muscle and body of mandible):
- Thyroid lobe swellings
- Pharyngeal pouch
- Submandibular gland swelling
- Branchial cyst
- Lymph nodes:
  - Malignant: lymphoma, metastatic cancer
  - Infection: any bacterial infection of head/neck (including teeth), viral infection, e.g. infectious mononucleosis, HIV, tuberculosis
- Parotid gland swelling, e.g. mumps, parotitis, stones, autoimmune disease, benign and malignant tumours

In the posterior triangle (bounded by the posterior border of sternocleidomastoid muscle, the trapezius and the clavicle):
- Lymph nodes:
  - Malignant: lymphoma, metastatic cancer
  - Infection: any bacterial infection of head/neck (including teeth) viral infection, e.g. infectious mononucleosis, HIV, tuberculosis
- Carotid artery aneurysm
- Carotid body tumour
- Cystic hygroma
- Cervical rib

Examination sequence

- With the patient sitting down, look at his neck from in front to identify any scar or visible mass or pulsation.
- From behind, palpate the neck. Work systematically around the neck, checking each of the three boundaries of the anterior and posterior triangles. Feel for midline, submental, submandibular and preauricular swellings.
- Assess the consistency, mobility and size of any swellings. Is it fluctuant (cystic) or pulsatile? Listen for bruits (p. 52).
- With a midline swelling, ask the patient to swallow (offer a glass of water if needed) and note if the swelling moves. A thyroid swelling will move superiorly on swallowing. If so, percuss for retrosternal dullness and check for dysthyroid features (p. 80).
- Ask the patient to put out his tongue and note any movement. A thyroglossal cyst will move superiorly (Fig. 13.27).

INVESTIGATIONS

See Box 13.19.

13.19 Mouth, throat and neck investigations

Investigation	Indication/comment
Full blood count	Pharyngitis
Monospot	Infectious mononucleosis
Throat swab	Acute tonsillitis and pharyngitis Patients may carry *Streptococcus pyogenes* and have a viral infection (detected by PCR), so swab does not always help direct management PCR may help identify viral causes
Endoscopy and biopsy	Cancer of larynx and pharynx, changes in vocal cords Under general anaesthetic
Ultrasound	Neck swellings
CT scan	Cancer and metastases Useful in staging

Jane Gibson
James Huntley

The musculoskeletal system

14

MUSCULOSKELETAL EXAMINATION

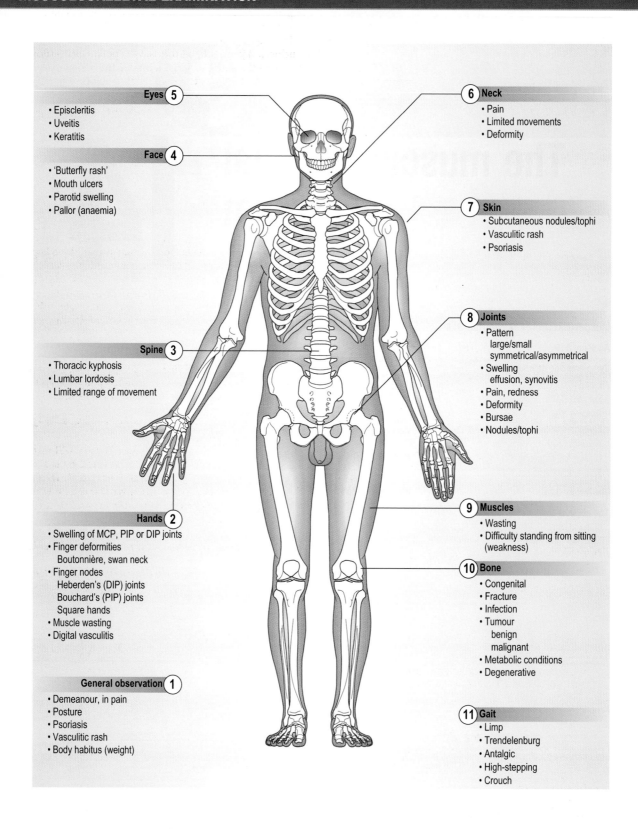

Eyes 5
- Episcleritis
- Uveitis
- Keratitis

Face 4
- 'Butterfly rash'
- Mouth ulcers
- Parotid swelling
- Pallor (anaemia)

Spine 3
- Thoracic kyphosis
- Lumbar lordosis
- Limited range of movement

Hands 2
- Swelling of MCP, PIP or DIP joints
- Finger deformities
  Boutonnière, swan neck
- Finger nodes
  Heberden's (DIP) joints
  Bouchard's (PIP) joints
  Square hands
- Muscle wasting
- Digital vasculitis

General observation 1
- Demeanour, in pain
- Posture
- Psoriasis
- Vasculitic rash
- Body habitus (weight)

6 Neck
- Pain
- Limited movements
- Deformity

7 Skin
- Subcutaneous nodules/tophi
- Vasculitic rash
- Psoriasis

8 Joints
- Pattern
  large/small
  symmetrical/asymmetrical
- Swelling
  effusion, synovitis
- Pain, redness
- Deformity
- Bursae
- Nodules/tophi

9 Muscles
- Wasting
- Difficulty standing from sitting
  (weakness)

10 Bone
- Congenital
- Fracture
- Infection
- Tumour
  benign
  malignant
- Metabolic conditions
- Degenerative

11 Gait
- Limp
- Trendelenburg
- Antalgic
- High-stepping
- Crouch

ANATOMY

Joint structure

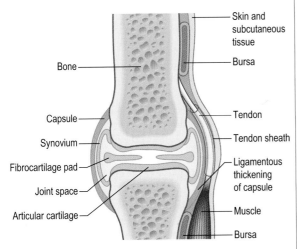

Fig. 14.1 Structure of a joint and surrounding tissues.

SYMPTOMS AND DEFINITIONS

Pain

Site

Determine whether the pain originates from a joint (arthralgia) (Box 14.1), muscle (myalgia) or other soft

14.1 Common causes of arthralgia (joint pain)

Generalised

- Infective
  - Viral, e.g. rubella, parvovirus B19, mumps, hepatitis B, chikungunya
  - Bacterial, e.g. staphylococci, tuberculosis, Borrelia
  - Fungal
- Postinfective
  - Rheumatic fever, reactive arthritis
- Inflammatory
  - Rheumatoid arthritis, systemic lupus erythematosus (SLE), ankylosing spondylitis, systemic sclerosis
- Degenerative
  - Osteoarthritis
- Tumour
  - Primary, e.g. osteosarcoma, chondrosarcoma
  - Metastatic, e.g. from lung, breast, prostate
  - Systemic tumour effects, e.g. hypertrophic pulmonary osteoarthropathy
- Crystal formation
  - Gout, pseudogout
- Trauma, e.g. road traffic accidents
- Others
  - Chronic pain disorders, e.g. fibromyalgia
  - Benign joint hypermobility syndrome

tissue. The site may be well localised and suggest the diagnosis, e.g. the first metatarsophalangeal joint in gout (Fig. 14.2), or in several joints suggesting an inflammatory arthritis.

How many joints are involved? One joint is a monoarthritis; 2–4 joints, oligoarthritis; >4 is polyarthritis (Box 14.2). Are the small or large joints of the arms or legs affected? Different patterns of joint involvement help the differential diagnosis (Fig. 14.3 and Box 14.3). Surrounding structures can be painful and include ligaments, tendons, tendon sheaths, bursae, muscle and bone (Fig. 14.1).

It may be difficult to determine the source of referred pain (Box 14.4). Almost all adults with arthritis (inflamed and swollen joints) have arthralgia (joint pain), but only a minority of patients with arthralgia have arthritis.

Onset

Pain from traumatic injury is usually immediate and is exacerbated by movement or haemarthrosis (bleeding into the affected joint). Pain from inflammatory arthritis can develop over 24 hours, or more insidiously. Crystal arthritis (gout and pseudogout) causes acute, sometimes extreme pain which develops quickly, often overnight. Joint sepsis causes pain that develops over a day or two.

Character

Bone pain is penetrating, deep or boring, and is characteristically worse at night. Localised pain suggests tumour, osteomyelitis (infection), osteonecrosis or osteoid osteoma (benign bone tumour)

Generalised bony conditions, such as osteomalacia, usually cause diffuse pain.

Muscle pain (Box 14.5) is often described as 'stiffness' and is poorly localised, deep and aggravated by use of the affected muscle(s). It is associated with muscle weakness in some conditions, e.g. polymyositis, but not in polymyalgia rheumatica. Partial muscle tears are painful; complete rupture may be less so.

Fracture pain is sharp and stabbing, aggravated by attempted movement or use, and relieved by rest and splintage.

'Shooting' pain is often caused by mechanical impingement of a peripheral nerve or nerve root: e.g. buttock

14

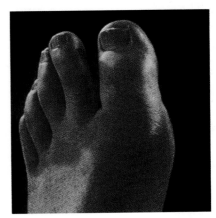

Fig. 14.2 Acute gout of the first metatarsophalangeal joint. This causes swelling, erythema, and extreme pain and tenderness (podagra).

14.2 Differential diagnosis of monoarthritis, oligoarthritis and polyarthritis

	Type	Examples
Monoarthritis (single joint involvement)	Infective	*Staphylococcus aureus, Staphylococcus epidermidis, Salmonella*, tuberculosis, *Neisseria gonorrhoeae, Escherichia coli, Haemophilus*
	Traumatic	Haemarthrosis
	Bleeding diathesis	Acute exacerbation of underlying state
	Post-traumatic	
	Degenerative	Osteoarthritis, Charcot joint
	Metabolic	Crystal arthropathies: gout, pseudogout
	Inflammatory polyarthritis presenting as monoarthritis	Rheumatoid arthritis
Oligoarthritis (involvement of 2–4 joints)	Infective	Bacterial endocarditis, *Neisseria gonorrhoeae, Mycobacterium tuberculosis*
	Degenerative	Osteoarthritis
	Inflammatory oligoarthritis	Sarcoidosis, reactive arthritis, psoriatic arthritis, ankylosing spondylitis
	Inflammatory polyarthritis presenting as oligoarthritis	Rheumatoid arthritis
Polyarthritis (involvement of ≥5 joints)	Infective	Bacterial: Lyme disease, subacute bacterial endocarditis Viral: rubella, mumps, glandular fever, chickenpox, hepatitis B and C, human immunodeficiency virus (HIV)
	Post-infective	Rheumatic fever
	Degenerative	Osteoarthritis: nodal with Heberden's/Bouchard's nodes
	Metabolic	Haemochromatosis, gout
	Inflammatory	Rheumatoid arthritis, SLE, psoriatic arthritis
	Other	Hypertrophic pulmonary osteoarthropathy

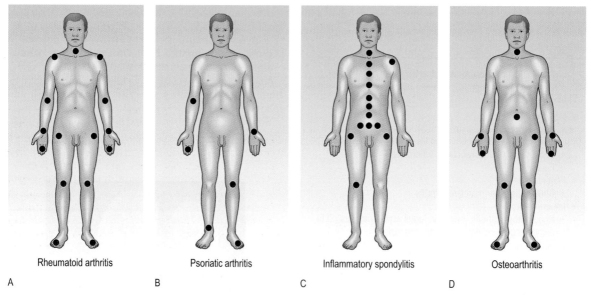

Rheumatoid arthritis	Psoriatic arthritis	Inflammatory spondylitis	Osteoarthritis
A	B	C	D

Fig. 14.3 Contrasting patterns of involvement in polyarthritis. (A) Rheumatoid arthritis (symmetrical, small and large joints, upper and lower limbs). **(B)** Seronegative psoriatic arthritis (asymmetrical, large > small joints, associated periarticular inflammation, giving dactylitis, inflammation of a whole digit, finger or toe). **(C)** Seronegative inflammatory spondylitis (axial involvement, large > small joints, asymmetrical). **(D)** Osteoarthritis (symmetrical, small and large joints).

14.3 2010 American College of Rheumatology/ European League Against Rheumatism classification criteria for rheumatoid arthritis

Joint distribution (0–5)	Score
1 large joint	0
2–10 large joints	1
1–3 small joints (large joints not counted)	2
4–10 small joints (large joints not counted)	3
>10 joints (at least one small joint)	5
Serology (0–3)	
Negative RF and negative ACPA	0
Low positive RF or low positive ACPA	2
High positive RF or high positive ACPA	3
Acute-phase reactants	
Normal CRP and normal ESR	0
Abnormal CRP or abnormal ESR	1

A score of ≥6 classifies the patient as having definite rheumatoid arthritis. This should be distinguished from a definite diagnosis as a patient may clinically have rheumatoid arthritis but not fulfil all criteria.
RF, rheumatoid factor; ACPA, anticyclic-citrullinated peptide antibodies; CRP, C-reactive protein; ESR, erythrocyte sedimentation rate.

14.4 Common patterns of referred and radicular musculoskeletal pain

Site of pathology	Perceived at
Cervical spine	
C1/C2	Occiput
C3, 4	Interscapular region
C5	Tip of shoulder, upper outer aspect of arm
C6, 7	Interscapular region or the radial fingers and thumb
C8	Ulnar side of the forearm, ring and little fingers
Thoracic spine	Chest
Lumbar spine	Buttocks, knees, legs
Shoulder	Lateral aspect of upper arm
Elbow	Forearm
Hip	Anterior thigh, knee
Knee	Thigh, hip

14.5 Causes of muscle pain (myalgia)

Infective
- Viral: Coxsackie, cytomegalovirus, echovirus, dengue
- Bacterial: *Streptococcus pneumoniae*, *Mycoplasma*
- Parasitic: Schistosomiasis, toxoplasmosis

Traumatic
- Tears, haematoma, rhabdomyolysis

Inflammatory
- Polymyalgia rheumatica, myositis, dermatomyositis

Drugs
- e.g. Alcohol withdrawal, statins, triptans

Metabolic
- Hypothyroidism, hyperthyroidism, Addison's disease, vitamin D deficiency

Neuropathic

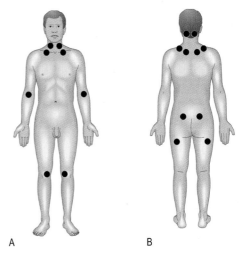

A   B

Fig. 14.4 Typical tender points in chronic pain syndrome (fibromyalgia).

pain which 'shoots down the back of the leg', caused by lumbar intervertebral disc protrusion.

Chronic joint pain in patients >40 years with progression over years is commonly caused by osteoarthritis.

Neurological involvement in diabetes mellitus, leprosy, syringomyelia and syphilis (tabes dorsalis) may cause loss of joint sensation, so pain is less than expected from examination. In these conditions, even grossly abnormal joints may be painfree (Charcot joint).

Chronic pain syndrome (fibromyalgia) causes widespread, unremitting pain with little diurnal variation that is poorly controlled by conventional analgesic/anti-inflammatory drugs. Chronic pain syndrome is defined as pain present for more than 3 months. It is due to pain pathway sensitisation and is commonly associated with sleep disorders, psychological stress and depression. Examination is normal except for the presence of typical tender points (Fig. 14.4) (p. 27).

Pain disproportionately greater than expected is seen in compartment syndrome acutely (increased pressure in a fascial compartment, which compromises perfusion and viability of the compartmental structures) and complex regional pain syndrome, chronically. This latter condition develops after injury or illness, or spontaneously, and is characterised by severe 'burning' pain, local tenderness, oedema, abnormal sweating and colour, temperature changes and localised osteoporosis.

Radiation

Pain from nerve compression radiates to the distribution of that nerve, e.g. lower leg pain in prolapsed intervertebral disc or hand pain in carpal tunnel syndrome. Neck pain radiates to the shoulder or over the top of the head. Hip pain is usually felt in the groin, but may radiate to the thigh or knee.

14

Alleviating factors/associated symptoms

Pain caused by a mechanical problem is worse on movement and eases with rest. Pain due to inflammation is worse first thing in the morning and eases with movement. Pain from a septic joint is present both at rest and with movement.

Timing (frequency, duration and periodicity of symptoms)

A history of several years of pain with a normal examination suggests chronic pain syndrome. A history of several weeks of pain, early-morning stiffness and loss of function is likely to be an inflammatory arthritis. 'Flitting' pain starting in one joint and moving to others over a period of days is a feature of rheumatic fever and gonococcal arthritis. If intermittent with resolution between episodes it is likely to be palindromic rheumatism.

Exacerbating factors

Pain from joints damaged by intra-articular derangement or osteoarthritic degeneration will worsen with exercise.

Severity

Apart from trauma, the most severe joint pain occurs in septic and crystal arthritis.

Stiffness

Establish what the patient means by stiffness. Is it:
- restricted range of movement?
- difficulty moving, but with a normal range?
- painful movement?
- localised to a particular joint or more generalised?

Stiffness may relate to the soft tissues rather than the joint itself. In polymyalgia rheumatica stiffness commonly affects the shoulder and pelvic areas. There are characteristic differences between inflammatory and non-inflammatory presentations of joint stiffness:

Inflammatory arthritis presents with early-morning stiffness that takes at least 30 minutes to wear off with activity.

Non-inflammatory, mechanical arthritis has stiffness after rest which lasts only a few minutes on movement.

Swelling

Establish the site, extent and time course of any swelling. Active inflammatory arthritis from any cause results in swelling. When vascular structures, e.g. bone and ligament, are injured, bleeding into the joint or soft tissues produces tense swelling within minutes (Fig. 14.5). This is even more rapid and severe if the patient takes anticoagulants or has an underlying bleeding disorder, e.g. haemophilia. If avascular structures, e.g. the menisci, are torn or articular cartilage is abraded, it can take hours or days to produce a significant effusion.

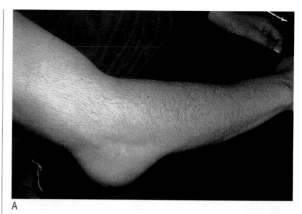

A

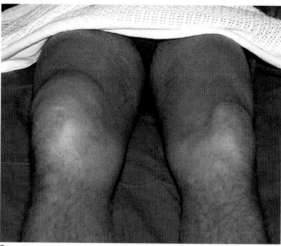

B

Fig. 14.5 Joint swelling. (A) Olecranon bursitis. **(B)** Right-knee haemarthrosis.

Erythema (redness) and warmth

Erythema is common in infective, traumatic and crystal-induced conditions and may be mildly present in inflammatory arthritis. All joints with an inflammatory or infective component will be warm.

Erythema associated with distal interphalangeal (DIP) joint swelling helps to distinguish DIP joint psoriatic arthritis from the Heberden's nodes of osteoarthritis.

Weakness

Weakness suggests joint, neurological or muscle disease. The problem may be focal or generalised.

Weakness due to joint disorders is either from pain inhibiting function or to disruption of the joint or its supporting structures. For neurological disorders producing weakness, see Chapter 11. Always consider nerve entrapment as a cause, e.g. carpal tunnel syndrome at the wrist and leg weakness due to spinal root compression caused by a prolapsed intervertebral disc or spinal stenosis. Muscle disorders can produce widespread weakness associated with pain and fatigue, e.g. in polymyositis and with a rash in dermatomyositis. Proximal muscle weakness can occur in endocrine disorders, e.g. hypothyroidism.

Locking and triggering

'Locking' is an incomplete range of movement at a joint because of an anatomical block. It may be associated with pain. Patients use 'locking' to describe a variety of problems, so clarify exactly what they mean. True locking is a block to the normal range of movement caused by mechanical obstruction, e.g. a loose body or torn meniscus, within the joint. This prevents the joint from reaching the extremes of normal range. The patient is characteristically able to 'unlock' the joint by trick manoeuvres.

Pseudo-locking is a loss of range of movement due to pain.

Triggering is a block to extension, which then 'gives' suddenly when extending a finger from a flexed position. In adults it usually affects the ring or middle fingers and results from nodular tendon thickening or fibrous thickening of the flexor sheath due to chronic low-grade trauma, e.g. occupational or associated with inflammatory arthritis. Triggering can be congenital, usually affecting the thumb.

Extra-articular features

Patients may present with features of extra-articular disease which they may not connect with musculoskeletal problems (see Box 14.7 and Fig. 14.14). The pattern of the joint condition (a/symmetric, flitting) and extent (mono-, oligo- or polyarthritis) suggests the diagnosis and directs the history.

Ask about rashes (psoriasis, vasculitis, erythema nodosum) and whether they are photosensitive (systemic lupus erythematosus: SLE).

Weight loss, low-grade fever and malaise are associated with rheumatoid arthritis and SLE. High-spiking fevers in the evening with a rash occur in adult-onset Still's disease. Headache, jaw pain on chewing (claudication) and scalp tenderness are features of temporal arteritis. Connective tissue disease may present with Raynaud's phenomenon, sicca symptoms (dryness of mouth and eyes), rash, mouth ulcers, dysphagia and gastrointestinal problems. Dyspnoea may be related to lung disease associated with rheumatoid arthritis or connective tissue disease. Abdominal pain, diarrhoea, bloody stool and mouth ulcers may suggest an arthritis associated with inflammatory bowel disease.

THE HISTORY

Presenting complaint

Record the nature and duration of pain using SOCRATES (Box 2.10), and of stiffness, swelling, weakness and locking. Instability, deformity, sensory disturbance and loss of function may also be presenting complaints.

Obtain an exact account of the mechanism of any injury and subsequent events, e.g. development of swelling.

Establish the pattern of joint involvement (Fig. 14.3). Predominant involvement of the small joints of the hands, feet or wrists suggests an inflammatory arthritis, e.g. rheumatoid arthritis or SLE. Medium or large joint swelling is more likely to be degenerative or a seronegative arthritis, e.g. osteoarthritis, psoriatic arthritis or ankylosing spondylitis (Box 14.6). Nodal osteoarthritis has a predilection for the DIP joints and carpometacarpal joint of the thumb. Ask about extra-articular features (Box 14.7).

14

14.6 Nomenclature in inflammatory arthritis

Seropositive: indicates either the presence of IgM rheumatoid factor (RF) or anti cyclic-citrullinated peptide antibodies (ACPA) in significant titres in the serum of patients with a polyarthritis. ACPA are more specific for rheumatoid arthritis (RA), are particularly associated with smoking and can be present for up to 10 years prior to the onset of clinical manifestations of RA.

Seronegative: indicates the absence of RF in the serum of patients with inflammatory arthritis. If the disease is morphologically the same as rheumatoid arthritis, it is seronegative rheumatoid arthritis. Other inflammatory arthritides, such as psoriatic arthritis, reactive arthritis and ankylosing spondylitis, are also seronegative and are the seronegative arthritides. They are more likely to be associated with HLA B27, share extra-articular features and have an asymmetric pattern of joint involvement.

14.7 Extra-articular features

Condition	Extra-articular features
Septic arthritis	Fever, malaise, source of sepsis, e.g. skin, throat, gut
Gout	Tophi, signs of renal failure or alcoholic liver disease
Reactive arthritis	Urethritis, mouth and/or genital ulcers, conjunctivitis, iritis, enthesopathy, e.g. Achilles tendinopathy/plantar fasciitis, rash (keratoderma blenorrhagica)
Ankylosing spondylitis	Enthesopathy, iritis, aortic regurgitation, pulmonary fibrosis
Psoriatic arthritis	Psoriasis, nail pitting, onycholysis
Rheumatoid arthritis	Subcutaneous rheumatoid nodules, episcleritis, dry eyes, pulmonary fibrosis, pleural effusion, small-vessel vasculitis, splenomegaly, Raynaud's phenomenon
Sjögren's syndrome	'Dry eyes' (keratoconjunctivitis sicca), xerostomia (reduced or absent saliva production), salivary gland enlargement and Raynaud's phenomenon
Systemic lupus erythematosus	Photosensitive rash, especially on face, mucocutaneous ulcers, alopecia, fever, serositis, Raynaud's phenemenon, lymphopenia
Juvenile idiopathic arthritis	Rash, fever, hepatomegaly, splenomegaly

14.8 Drugs associated with adverse musculoskeletal effects	
Drug	**Possible adverse musculoskeletal effects**
Steroids	Osteoporosis, myopathy, osteonecrosis, infection
Statins	Myalgia, myositis, myopathy
Angiotensin-converting enzyme (ACE) inhibitors	Myalgia, arthralgia, positive antinuclear antibody
Antiepileptics	Osteomalacia, arthralgia
Immunosuppressants	Infections
Quinolones	Tendinopathy, tendon rupture

14.9 Conditions linked to human leucocyte antigen HLA B27 type
• Ankylosing spondylitis
• Reactive arthritis
• Psoriatic arthritis (some forms)
• Enteropathic arthritis – associated with ulcerative colitis and Crohn's disease

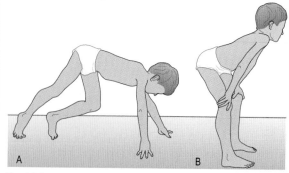

Fig. 14.6 Gower's sign. (A) Duchenne muscular dystrophy leads to great difficulty in getting up from a prone position. After rolling over the affected individual walks the hands and feet towards each other. **(B)** He then uses the hands to climb up the legs, reaching an upright position by swinging the arms and trunk sideways and upwards.

14.10 The muscular dystrophies		
	Inheritance	**Gene product**
Duchenne	X-linked	Dystrophin
Becker	X-linked	Dystrophin
Dystrophia myotonica	Autosomal dominant	Myotonin
Fascioscapulohumeral	Autosomal dominant	
Limb girdle	Autosomal recessive	

14.11 Joints involved in activities of daily living		
Activity	**Joint(s) involved**	**Function required**
Pinch grip	Thumb, index finger	Opposition and flexion of thumb (note: sensation is also required for optimal function)
Key grip	Thumb, index finger	Adduction and opposition of thumb
Gripping taps, handles, bottle tops	Hand, wrist	Grasp
Eating, cleaning teeth and face	Hand, elbow	Grasp, elbow flexion
Dressing, washing, hair care	Hand, elbow, shoulder	Pinch, grasp, elbow flexion, shoulder abduction/rotation
Toileting, cleaning perineum	Hand, wrist, elbow, shoulder	Grasp, wrist/elbow flexion, forearm supination, internal shoulder rotation

Past history

Note past episodes of musculoskeletal involvement. Identify co-morbid factors, e.g. diabetes mellitus, steroid therapy, osteoporosis, fractures, ischaemic heart disease, stroke and obesity.

Drug history

Many drugs have side-effects that may either worsen or precipitate musculoskeletal conditions (Box 14.8).

Family history

Inflammatory arthritis is more common if a first-degree relative is affected. Osteoarthritis, osteoporosis and gout are heritable in a variable polygenic fashion. Seronegative spondyloarthritis is more common in patients with HLA B27 (Box 14.9). A single-gene defect (monogenic inheritance) is found in hereditary sensorimotor neuropathy (Charcot–Marie–Tooth disease), osteogenesis imperfecta, Ehlers–Danlos syndrome, Marfan's syndrome and the muscular dystrophies (Box 14.10 and Fig. 14.6).

Environmental, occupational and social histories

Ask about current and previous occupations. Is the patient working full- or part-time, on sick leave or receiving benefits? Has the patient had to take time off work because of the condition? If so, is the patient's job at risk? Litigation may be pending in personal injury cases and occupation-related complaints, e.g. repetitive strain disorder, hand vibration syndrome and fatigue fractures. Army recruits, athletes and dancers are at particular risk of fatigue fractures.

Identify functional difficulties, including ability to hold and use items such as pens, tools and cutlery. How does the condition affect activities of daily living (Box 14.11), e.g. washing, dressing and toileting? Can patients

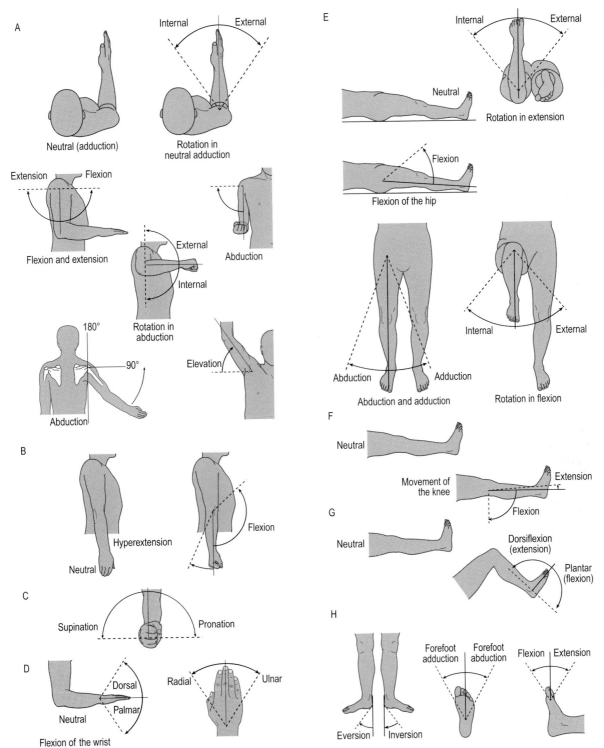

Fig. 14.7 Joint positions and movements of the upper and lower limbs.

use stairs and do they need aids to walk? Ask about functional independence, especially cooking, house-work and shopping.

Some conditions are seen in certain ethnic groups, e.g. sickle cell disease may present with bone and joint pain in African patients. Osteomalacia is more common in Asian patients. Bone and joint tuberculosis is more common in African and Asian patients.

Take a sexual history (Box 2.19), since sexually trans-mitted disease may be relevant, e.g. reactive arthritis, gonococcal arthritis, human immunodeficiency virus (HIV) infection and hepatitis B (Box 14.12).

14.12 Social factors and musculoskeletal conditions
Alcohol
• Trauma, gout, myopathy, rhabdomyolysis, neuropathy
Smoking
• Lung cancer with bony metastases, hypertrophic pulmonary osteoarthropathy, rheumatoid arthritits
Drugs of misuse
• Trauma, hepatitis B, HIV
Diet
• Vitamin deficiencies, e.g. rickets/osteomalacia (vitamin D), scurvy (vitamin C) • Anorexia nervosa, e.g. osteoporosis • Obesity, e.g. osteoarthritis, diabetes mellitus and Charcot joint

THE PHYSICAL EXAMINATION

Dynamic tests are difficult to describe in pictures and text, so ask an experienced clinician to check your technique. Practise examining as many joints as possible to become familiar with normal appearances and ranges of movement.

General principles

Ask – Look – Feel – Move.

After taking the history, follow a process of observation, palpation and movement.

Examine the overall appearance for pallor, rash, skin tightening and hair changes. Look at the skin, subcutaneous tissues and bony outline of each area. Before palpating, ask the patient which area is painful or tender. Feel for warmth, swelling, stability and deformity. Assess if a deformity is reducible or fixed. Assess active before passive movement. Do not cause the patient additional pain.

- Compare one limb with the opposite side.
- Always expose the joint above and below the one in question.
- In suspected systemic disease, examine all joints and fully examine all systems.

Use standard terminology to describe joint limb positions and movement.

- Always describe movements from the neutral position (Fig. 14.7). Commonly used terms are:
  - flexion: bending at a joint from the neutral position
  - extension: straightening a joint back to the neutral position
  - hyperextension: movement beyond the normal neutral position because of a torn ligament or underlying ligamentous laxity, e.g. Ehlers–Danlos syndrome
  - adduction: movement towards the midline of the body (finger adduction is movement towards the axis of the limb)
  - abduction: movement away from the midline.
- Describe the position of a limb because of joint/bone deformity:

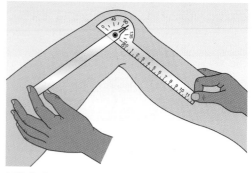

Fig. 14.8 Goniometer.

- valgus: the distal part deviates away from the midline
- varus: the distal part deviates towards the midline.

Equipment

You need a tape measure, tendon hammer, goniometer (a protractor for measuring the range of joint movement) (Fig. 14.8), stethoscope and blocks for assessing leg-length discrepancy.

General examination

Skin, nail and soft tissue

Abnormal findings

The skin and related structures are the most common sites of associated lesions. The skin and nail appearances in psoriasis may be hidden, e.g. the umbilicus, natal cleft, scalp (Figs 4.4 and 4.15). The rash of SLE is induced by ultraviolet light exposure.

Small, dark red vasculitic spots due to capillary infarcts occur in many systemic inflammatory disorders, including rheumatoid arthritis, SLE (Fig. 4.15F) and polyarteritis nodosa. These indicate active disease. Common sites are the nail folds, finger and toe tips and other pressure areas.

Raynaud's phenomenon is episodic ischaemia of the fingers precipitated by stimuli such as cold, pain and stress. There is a typical progression of colour changes: blanching (white) is followed by cyanosis (blue), and reactive hyperaemia (red). There is associated dysaesthesia (altered sensation) and pain. Raynaud's phenomenon is common in otherwise healthy individuals but is a frequent feature in systemic sclerosis and SLE (p. 131).

In systemic sclerosis, the thickened, tight skin produces a characteristic facial appearance (Fig. 3.11C). In the hands, flexion contractures, calcium deposits in the finger pulps (Fig. 14.9) and tissue ischaemia leading to ulceration may occur. The telangiectasias of systemic sclerosis are purplish, blanch with pressure and are most common on the hands and face.

Reactive arthritis has extra-articular features (Fig. 14.10A) and is associated with skin and nail changes similar to those of psoriasis, together with conjunctivitis, circinate balanitis (painless superficial ulcers on the

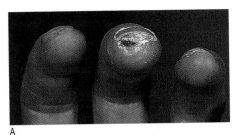

A

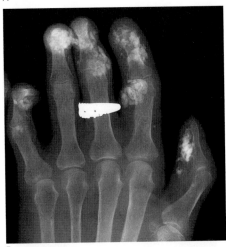

B

Fig. 14.9 Systemic sclerosis in the hand. (A) Calcium deposits ulcerating through the skin. **(B)** X-ray showing calcium deposits.

prepuce and glans; Fig. 14.10B), urethritis and superficial mouth ulcers (Fig. 14.10C).

Nodules Subcutaneous nodules in rheumatoid arthritis most commonly occur on the extensor surface of the forearm (Fig. 14.11). They are firm and non-tender, and may also be felt at sites of pressure or friction, e.g. the sacrum or Achilles tendon. Multiple small nodules can occur in the hands and are particularly associated with methotrexate therapy. Rheumatoid nodules are strongly associated with a positive rheumatoid factor and can occur at other sites, e.g. the lungs.

Bony nodules in osteoarthritis affect the hand and are smaller and harder than rheumatoid nodules. They

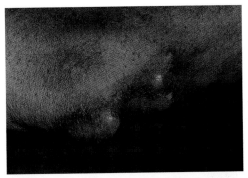

Fig. 14.11 Rheumatoid nodules and olecranon bursitis.

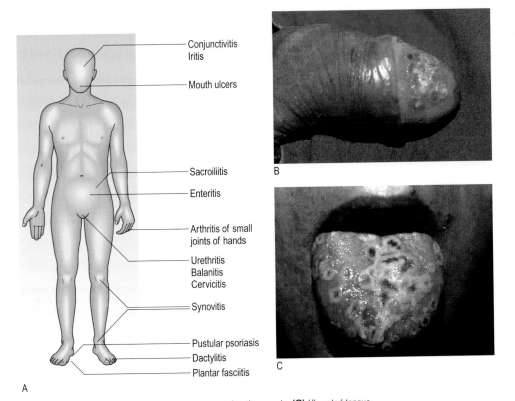

A

Fig. 14.10 Reactive arthritis. (A) Clinical features. **(B)** Lesions on the glans penis. **(C)** Ulcerated tongue.

occur on the lateral aspects of the interphalangeal (IP) joints. At the DIP joints they are called Heberden's nodes, and at the proximal interphalangeal (PIP) joints, Bouchard's nodes (Fig. 14.12).

Gouty tophi are firm, white, irregular subcutaneous crystal collections (monosodium urate monohydrate). Common sites are the olecranon bursa, helix of the ear and extensor aspects of the fingers, hands, knees and toes (Fig. 14.13). The overlying skin may ulcerate, discharge crystals and become secondarily infected.

Other extra-articular features (Fig. 14.14).

Eyes The eyes are affected in many musculoskeletal conditions.

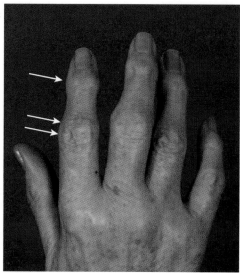

Fig. 14.12 Osteoarthritis of the hand. Heberden's (single arrow) and Bouchard's (double arrow) nodes.

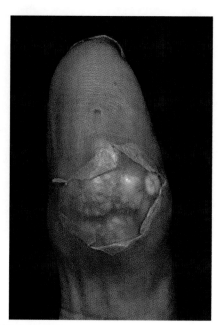

Fig. 14.13 Gouty tophus.

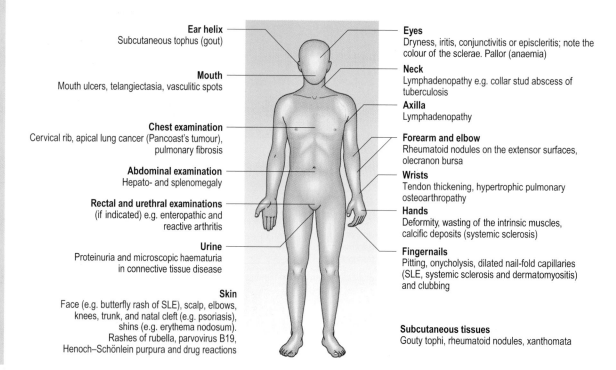

Ear helix
Subcutaneous tophus (gout)

Mouth
Mouth ulcers, telangiectasia, vasculitic spots

Chest examination
Cervical rib, apical lung cancer (Pancoast's tumour), pulmonary fibrosis

Abdominal examination
Hepato- and splenomegaly

Rectal and urethral examinations
(if indicated) e.g. enteropathic and reactive arthritis

Urine
Proteinuria and microscopic haematuria in connective tissue disease

Skin
Face (e.g. butterfly rash of SLE), scalp, elbows, knees, trunk, and natal cleft (e.g. psoriasis), shins (e.g. erythema nodosum). Rashes of rubella, parvovirus B19, Henoch–Schönlein purpura and drug reactions

Eyes
Dryness, iritis, conjunctivitis or episcleritis; note the colour of the sclerae. Pallor (anaemia)

Neck
Lymphadenopathy e.g. collar stud abscess of tuberculosis

Axilla
Lymphadenopathy

Forearm and elbow
Rheumatoid nodules on the extensor surfaces, olecranon bursa

Wrists
Tendon thickening, hypertrophic pulmonary osteoarthropathy

Hands
Deformity, wasting of the intrinsic muscles, calcific deposits (systemic sclerosis)

Fingernails
Pitting, onycholysis, dilated nail-fold capillaries (SLE, systemic sclerosis and dermatomyositis) and clubbing

Subcutaneous tissues
Gouty tophi, rheumatoid nodules, xanthomata

Fig. 14.14 Extra-articular manifestations of musculoskeletal conditions.

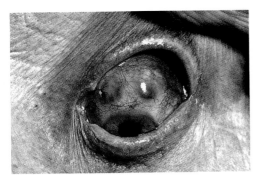

Fig. 14.15 Scleritis and scleromalacia.

Examination sequence

Perform Schirmer's tear test to diagnose keratoconjunctivitis sicca.

- Hook a small strip of notched blotting paper ~40 mm long over the lower eyelid while the patient looks upwards. The notch is ~5 mm from one end of the strip and is where the strip is bent over the eyelid.
- Ask the patient to close the eye.
- Wait for exactly 5 minutes, then remove the strip.
- Measure the distance that tears travel down the strip with a millimetre rule; >15 mm is normal, 5–15 mm equivocal and <5 mm abnormal.

Abnormal findings

Conjunctivitis is a feature of reactive arthritis. Reduced tear production with 'dry eyes' (keratoconjunctivitis sicca) contributes to conjunctivitis and blepharitis (inflammation of the eyelids). This occurs in Sjögren's syndrome and as secondary changes in rheumatoid arthritis and other connective tissue disorders. Scleritis and episcleritis (Fig. 14.15) are found in rheumatoid arthritis and psoriatic arthritis. Anterior uveitis (iritis) occurs in ~25% of patients with ankylosing spondylitis and reactive arthritis but is asymptomatic in juvenile idiopathic arthritis (JIA), so ophthalmological assessment is essential if JIA is suspected. The sclerae are blue in certain types of osteogenesis imperfecta (Fig. 3.11A) and in the scleromalacia of long-standing rheumatoid arthritis (Fig. 14.15).

The joints – the GALS screen

The GALS (gait, arms, legs, spine) screen is a rapid screen for musculoskeletal and neurological deficits, and functional ability (Fig. 14.16).

Screening questions

- Do you have any pain or stiffness in your muscles, joints or back?
- Do you have difficulty dressing yourself?
- Do you have difficulty walking up and down stairs?

If all three replies are negative, the patient is unlikely to have a significant musculoskeletal problem. If the patient answers positively, carry out a more detailed assessment.

Examination sequence

Ask the patient to undress to his underwear and stand in front of you. Demonstrate actions to the patient rather than simply telling him what to do.

Gait

Ask the patient to walk ahead in a straight line for several steps, then turn and walk back towards you. Look for smoothness and symmetry of the gait.

Arms

- Stand in front of the patient.
- Ask him to clench his fists (Fig. 14.16D), and then open his hands flat. This tests both wrists and hands.
- Inspect the dorsum of the hands and check for full finger extension at the MCP, PIP and DIP joints.
- Ask him to squeeze your index and middle fingers. This tests the strength of the power grip.
- Have him touch each fingertip with his thumb. This tests precision grip and problems in co-ordination or concentration.
- Gently squeeze the metacarpal heads (Fig. 14.16E). Tenderness suggests inflammation, e.g. rheumatoid arthritis, involving the MCP joints.
- Show him how to make a 'prayer sign', bending the wrist back as far as possible. Put the backs of the hands together in a similar fashion. This tests wrist flexion and extension.
- Ask him to put his arms straight out in front of the body. This tests elbow extension.
- Ask the patient to bend the arms up to touch the shoulders. This tests elbow flexion.
- Have him place the elbows by the side of the body and bend them 90°. Turn the palms up and down (Fig. 14.16C). This tests pronation and supination at the wrist and elbow.
- Ask him to put his hands behind the head, with the elbows going back (Fig. 14.16B). This tests abduction and external rotation of the glenohumeral joint.
- Firmly press the midpoint of each supraspinatus to detect hyperalgesia (Fig. 14.16A).

Legs

- Ask the patient to lie supine (face up) on the couch.
- If there is no contraindication, perform Thomas's test for fixed flexion deformity on both hips (p. 344, Fig. 14.47).
- Palpate each knee for warmth and swelling. Check for patellar tap. These detect inflammation and effusions.
- Flex each hip and knee with your hand on the patient's knee. Feel for crepitus in the patellofemoral joint and knee (Fig. 14.16F).
- Flex the patient's knee and hip to 90°, and passively rotate each hip internally and externally, noting pain or limited movement.
- Look at the feet for any abnormality. Examine the soles, looking for calluses and ulcers, indicative of abnormal load bearing.
- Gently squeeze the metatarsal heads for tenderness (Fig. 14.16G).

Spine

- Stand behind the patient. Assess the straightness of the spine, muscle bulk and symmetry in the legs and trunk. Look for asymmetry at the level of the iliac crests (unilateral leg shortening) and swelling or other abnormality of the gluteal,

14

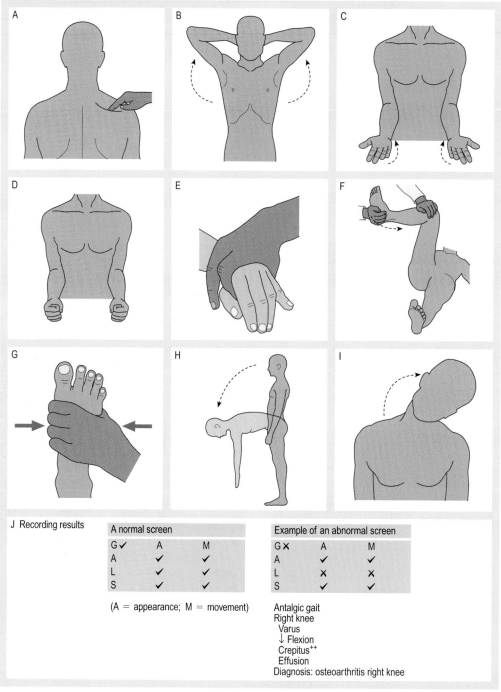

Fig. 14.16 The GALS (gait, arms, legs, spine) screen.

hamstring, popliteal and calf muscles. Look at the Achilles tendons and hindfoot regions for swelling or deformity.

- Stand beside the patient. Ask him to bend down and try to touch his toes (Fig. 14.16H). This highlights any abnormal spinal curvature or limited hip extension. If he can put his hands flat to the floor, he may have hypermobility.
- Stand behind the patient, hold the pelvis, and ask him to turn from side to side without moving his feet. This tests thoracolumbar rotation.

- Ask him to slide the hand down the lateral aspect of the leg towards the knee. This tests lateral lumbar flexion.
- Stand in front of the patient. Ask him to put his ear on his shoulder (Fig. 14.16I) to test lateral cervical flexion.
- Ask him to look up at the ceiling and then down at the floor to test cervical flexion and extension.
- Ask him to let the jaw drop open and move it from side to side. This tests both temporomandibular joints.

Stance phase (shaded leg)	Swing phase

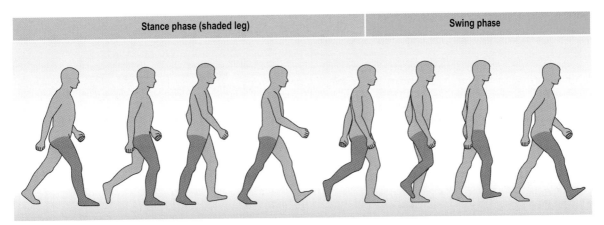

Fig. 14.17 Phases of the normal gait cycle.

14.13 The Beighton scoring system to assess hypermobility

Ask the patient to:	Score
Bring the thumb to touch the forearm, wrist flexed	1 point each side
Extend the little finger >90° with the hand in a neutral position	1 point each side
Extend the elbow >10°	1 point each side
Extend the knee >10°	1 point each side
Touch the floor with the palms of hands and the knees straight	1 point
A score of 4 or more indicates hypermobility	

Abnormal findings

Hypermobility Some patients have a greater than normal range of joint movement. They may present with recurrent dislocations or sensations of instability if this is severe, but frequently only complain of arthralgia. Mild hypermobility is normal but two inherited conditions affecting connective tissues – Marfan's syndrome and Ehlers–Danlos syndrome – cause hypermobility.

Assess hypermobility (Box 14.13).

Further examination

The GALS screen provides a rapid, but limited, assessment. This section describes the detailed examination required for better evaluation.

Gait

Gait is the cyclical pattern of musculoskeletal motion that carries the body forwards. Normal gait is smooth, symmetrical and ergonomically economical, with each leg 50% out of phase with the other.

For each leg, gait has two phases: stance and swing. The stance phase is from foot-strike to toe-off, when the foot is on the ground and load bearing (Fig. 14.17). The swing phase is from toe-off to foot-strike, when the foot clears the ground. When both feet are on the ground this is double stance.

A limp is an abnormal gait due to pain or structural change, e.g. lower limb length discrepancy, tone abnormality (including spasticity and co-contraction, in both of which there is inappropriate muscle contraction) or weakness.

Pain

An antalgic gait is one altered to reduce pain. Pain in a lower limb is usually aggravated by weight-bearing, so minimal time is spent in the stance phase on that side. This results in a 'dot–dash' mode of walking. If the source of pain is in the spine, axial rotatory movements are minimised, resulting in a slow gait with small paces. Patients with hip pain may lean towards the affected side as this decreases the compression force on the hip joint.

Structural change

Patients with limb-length discrepancy may walk on tiptoe on the shorter side, with compensatory hip and knee flexion on the longer side. Assess for limb-length discrepancy with block testing (p. 344). Other structural changes producing an abnormal gait include joint fusion, bone malunion and contracture.

Weakness

This may be due to nerve or muscle pathology or alteration in muscle tone. In a normal gait the hip abductors of the stance leg raise the contralateral hemipelvis. In Trendelenburg gait, abductor function is poor when weight bearing on the affected side, so the contralateral hemipelvis falls (Fig. 14.46).

Common causes of a Trendelenburg gait are:

- weakness of the hip abductors, e.g. in polio or paresis of the superior gluteal nerve after total hip replacement
- structural hip joint problems, e.g. congenital dislocation of the hip
- painful hip joint problems, e.g. osteoarthritis.

Foot drop occurs in common peroneal nerve palsy. The gait is high-stepping to allow clearance of the weak foot.

Increased tone

This occurs following an upper motor neurone lesion, e.g. cerebrovascular accident (stroke) or cerebral palsy.

14

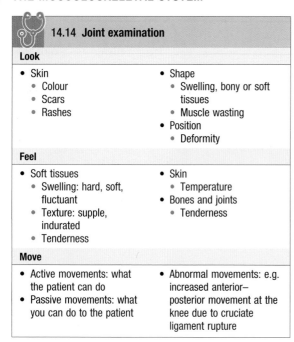

14.14 Joint examination

Look

- Skin
  - Colour
  - Scars
  - Rashes
- Shape
  - Swelling, bony or soft tissues
  - Muscle wasting
- Position
  - Deformity

Feel

- Soft tissues
  - Swelling: hard, soft, fluctuant
  - Texture: supple, indurated
  - Tenderness
- Skin
  - Temperature
- Bones and joints
  - Tenderness

Move

- Active movements: what the patient can do
- Passive movements: what you can do to the patient
- Abnormal movements: e.g. increased anterior–posterior movement at the knee due to cruciate ligament rupture

The gait depends on the specific lesion, contractures and compensatory mechanisms. A common pattern in cerebral palsy is the crouch gait, in which the hips and knees are always flexed.

Examination sequence

Gait

- Ask the patient to walk barefoot in a straight line; then repeat in shoes.
- Observe the patient from behind, in front and from the side.
- Evaluate what happens at each level (foot, ankle, knee, hip and pelvis, trunk and spine) during both stance and swing phases.
- Assess each joint (Box 14.14).

The spine

The spine is divided into the cervical, thoracic, lumbar and sacral segments. Most spinal diseases affect multiple segments, causing alteration in the posture or function of the whole spine. Spinal disease may occur without local symptoms and present with pain, neurological symptoms or signs in the trunk or limbs. Accurate diagnosis depends on knowing the underlying bony and neurological anatomy (Fig. 14.18), a careful history, and eliciting signs and symptoms to differentiate between mechanical (non-inflammatory) and inflammatory causes (Box 14.15).

Definitions

Scoliosis is lateral curvature of the spine (Fig. 14.19A).

Kyphosis is curvature of the spine in the sagittal (anterior–posterior) plane, with the apex posterior (Fig. 14.19B). The thoracic spine normally has a mild kyphosis.

Lordosis is curvature of the spine in the sagittal (anterior–posterior) plane, with the apex anterior (Fig. 14.19C).

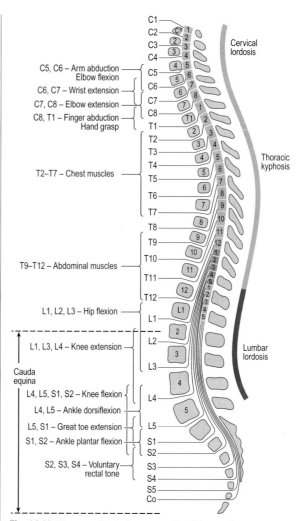

Fig. 14.18 The normal spinal curves and root innervations.

C5, C6 – Arm abduction Elbow flexion
C6, C7 – Wrist extension
C7, C8 – Elbow extension
C8, T1 – Finger abduction Hand grasp
T2–T7 – Chest muscles
T9–T12 – Abdominal muscles
L1, L2, L3 – Hip flexion
Cauda equina
L1, L3, L4 – Knee extension
L4, L5, S1, S2 – Knee flexion
L4, L5 – Ankle dorsiflexion
L5, S1 – Great toe extension
S1, S2 – Ankle plantar flexion
S2, S3, S4 – Voluntary rectal tone
Cervical lordosis
Thoracic kyphosis
Lumbar lordosis

14.15 Common spinal problems

- Mechanical back pain
- Prolapsed intervertebral disc
- Spinal stenosis
- Ankylosing spondylitis
- Compensatory scoliosis from leg length discrepancy
- Cervical myelopathy
- Pathological pain/deformity, e.g. osteomyelitis, tumour, myeloma
- Osteoporotic vertebral fracture resulting in kyphosis (or rarely lordosis), especially in the thoracic spine with loss of height
- Cervical rib
- Scoliosis
- Spinal instability, e.g. spondylolisthesis

Gibbus is a spinal deformity caused by an anterior wedge deformity localised to a single vertebra, producing an increase in forward flexion (Fig. 14.19D).

Spondylosis is degenerative change in the spine.

Spondylolysis is a defect in the pars interarticularis of a vertebral arch (Fig. 14.20A).

Spondylolisthesis is one vertebra slipping anteriorly on an inferior vertebra (Fig. 14.20B).

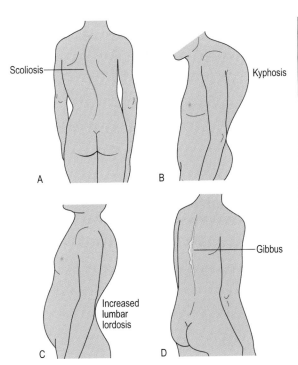

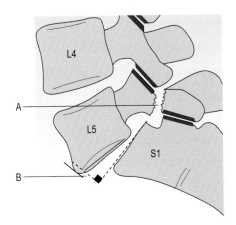

Fig. 14.19 Spinal deformities.

Fig. 14.20 Lumbosacral junction. (A) Defect in pars interarticularis (spondylolysis). **(B)** Anterior translation of L5 on S1 (spondylolisthesis).

Retrolisthesis is one vertebra slipping posteriorly on an inferior vertebra.

Cervical spine

Anatomy

Head nodding occurs at the atlanto-occipital joints, and rotational neck movements mainly at the atlantoaxial joint. Flexion, extension and lateral flexion occur mainly at the mid-cervical level. The neural canal contains the spinal cord and the emerging nerve roots, which pass through exit foramina bounded by the facet joints posteriorly and the intervertebral discs and neurocentral joints anteriorly. The nerve roots, particularly in the lower cervical spine, may be compressed or irritated by lateral disc protrusion or by osteophytes arising from the facet or neurocentral joints. Central disc protrusions may press directly on the cord (Fig. 11.34).

The history

The most common symptoms are pain and difficulty turning the head and neck. Patients find difficulty driving, especially when attempting to reverse. Neck pain is usually felt posteriorly but may be referred to the head, shoulder, arm or interscapular region. Cervical disc lesions cause radicular pain in one or other arm, roughly following the dermatomes of the affected nerve roots (Box 14.4). If the spinal cord is compromised (cervical myelopathy), then lower limb weakness, difficulty walking, loss of sensation and sphincter disturbance may occur.

Be particularly careful when examining patients with rheumatoid arthritis, as atlantoaxial instability can lead to spinal cord damage when the neck is flexed.

In patients with neck injury, never move the neck. Splint it and check for abnormal posture. Check neurological function in the limbs and X-ray to assess bony injury.

Examination sequence

Ask the patient to remove enough clothing for you to see the neck and upper thorax, then to sit on a chair.

Look

- Face the patient. Observe the posture of the head and neck. Note any abnormality or deformity, e.g. loss of lordosis (usually due to muscle spasm) (Box 14.16).

Feel

- Feel the midline spinous processes from the occiput to T1 (the T1 process is usually the most prominent).
- Feel the paraspinal soft tissues.
- Feel the supraclavicular fossae for cervical ribs or enlarged lymph nodes.
- Feel the anterior neck structures, including the thyroid.
- Note any tenderness in the spine, trapezius, interscapular and paraspinal muscles.

Move

- Assess active movements (Fig. 14.21).
- Ask the patient to put his chin on to the chest to assess forward flexion. The normal range is 0 (neutral) to 80°. Record a decreased range as the chin–chest distance.
- Ask him to look upwards at the ceiling as far back as possible, to assess extension. The normal range is 0 (neutral) to 50°. Thus the total flexion–extension arc is normally ~130°.
- Ask him to put his ear on to the shoulder, to assess lateral flexion. The normal range is 0 (neutral) to 45°.
- Ask the patient to look over his right/left shoulder. The normal range of lateral rotation is 0 (neutral) to 80°.
- If active movements are reduced, gently perform passive movements. Establish if the end of the range has a sudden or a gradual resistance and whether it is pain or stiffness that restricts movement. Pain or paraesthesiae in the arm on passive neck movement suggests nerve root involvement.
- Perform a neurological assessment of the upper and lower limbs (Figs 11.18 and 11.19).

Thoracic spine

Anatomy

This segment of the spine is the least mobile and maintains a physiological kyphosis throughout life.

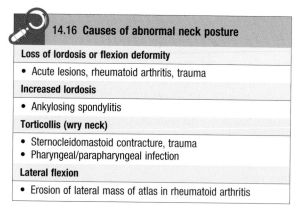

Loss of lordosis or flexion deformity
• Acute lesions, rheumatoid arthritis, trauma
Increased lordosis
• Ankylosing spondylitis
Torticollis (wry neck)
• Sternocleidomastoid contracture, trauma • Pharyngeal/parapharyngeal infection
Lateral flexion
• Erosion of lateral mass of atlas in rheumatoid arthritis

Adolescents and young adults	
• Scheuermann's disease • Ankylosing spondylitis	• Disc protrusion (rare)
Middle-aged and elderly	
• Degenerative change	• Osteoporotic fracture
Any age	
• Tumour	• Infection

Examination sequence

Ask the patient to undress to expose the neck, chest and back.

Look

■ With the patient standing, inspect the posture from behind, the side and the front, noting any deformity, e.g. rib hump or abnormal curvature.

Feel

■ Feel the midline spinous processes from T1 to T12. Feel for increased prominence of one or more posterior spinal processes, implying anterior wedge-shaped collapse of the vertebral body – often related to osteoporosis.

■ Feel the paraspinal soft tissues for tenderness.

Move

■ Ask the patient to sit with his arms crossed. Ask him to twist round both ways and look at you.

Lumbar spine

Anatomy

The surface markings are the spinous processes of L4/5, which are level with the pelvic brim, and the 'dimples of Venus', which overlie the sacroiliac joints. The normal lordosis may be lost in disorders such as ankylosing spondylitis and lumbar disc protrusion.

The principal movements are flexion, extension, lateral flexion and rotation. Most patients can bring the tips of their fingers at least to the level of the knees in forward and lateral flexion. Extension should be approximately 10–20°. In flexion, the upper segments move first, followed by the lower segments, to produce a smooth lumbar curve. However, even with a rigid lumbar spine, patients may be able to touch their toes if their hips are mobile.

In the adult, the spinal cord ends at L2. Below this, the spinal nerve roots may be injured or compressed by disc protrusion. Above this level the spinal cord itself may be involved.

The history

Low back pain is extremely common. Most is 'mechanical', and due to degenerative disease. Radicular back pain due to nerve root compression radiates down the posterior aspect of the leg to the lower leg or ankle. Pain due to inflammation of the sacroiliac joints is commonly felt in the buttocks, but may be referred down both legs to the knees. Groin and thigh pain in the absence of hip abnormality suggests referred pain from L1–2.

Red flag features suggest significant spinal pathology (Box 14.18). Consider abdominal and retroperitoneal

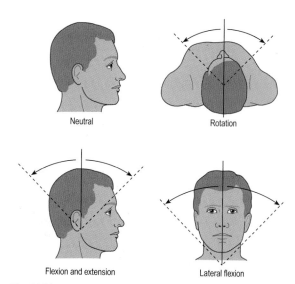

Neutral

Rotation

Flexion and extension

Lateral flexion

Fig. 14.21 Movements of the cervical spine.

Movement is mainly rotational with a very limited amount of flexion, extension and lateral flexion.

The history

Presenting symptoms in the thoracic spine are localised spinal pain (Box 14.17), pain radiating round the chest wall or, less frequently, symptoms of paraparesis, including sensory loss, leg weakness, and loss of bladder or bowel control. Disc lesions are rare but may be accompanied by pain radiating around the chest (girdle pain), mimicking cardiac or pleural disease. Patients with osteoporotic vertebral fractures may not complain of pain, but lose height and have deformity (increased kyphosis).

Patients with vertebral collapse due to malignancy may have associated spinal cord compression. Consider infection as a cause of acute pain, especially if systemic upset or fever is present. With poorly localised thoracic pain, consider intrathoracic causes, e.g. myocardial ischaemia or infarction, oesophageal or pleural pain and aortic aneurysm.

14.18 'Red flag' and 'yellow flag' features for acute low back pain

'Red flag' features

Red flags are features that may indicate serious pathology and require urgent referral

History

- Age <20 years or >55 years
- Recent significant trauma (fracture)
- Pain:
  - Thoracic (dissecting aneurysm)
  - Non-mechanical (infection/tumour/ pathological fracture)
- Fever (infection)
- Difficulty in micturition

- Faecal incontinence
- Motor weakness
- Sensory changes in the perineum (saddle anaesthesia)
- Sexual dysfunction, e.g. erectile/ejaculatory failure
- Gait change (cauda equina syndrome)
- Bilateral 'sciatica'

Past medical history

- Cancer (metastases)
- Previous steroid use (osteoporotic collapse)

System review

- Weight loss/malaise without obvious cause, e.g. cancer

'Yellow flag' features

These are psychosocial factors associated with greater likelihood of long-term chronicity and disability

- A history of anxiety, depression, chronic pain, irritable bowel syndrome, chronic fatigue, social withdrawal
- A belief that the diagnosis is severe, e.g. cancer. Faulty beliefs can lead to 'catastrophisation' and avoidance of activity
- Lack of belief that the patient can improve leads to an expectation that only passive, rather than active, treatment will be effective
- Ongoing litigation or compensation claims, e.g. work, road traffic accident

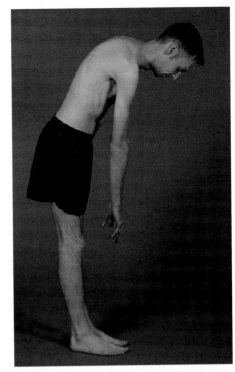

Fig. 14.22 Ankylosing spondylitis: patient trying to touch toes.

EBE 14.19 Ankylosing spondylitis

In a young man with gradual-onset chronic back pain, a positive family history for reactive arthritis, psoriasis or inflammatory bowel disease, and the presence of peripheral joint involvement or anterior uveitis all suggest a diagnosis of ankylosing spondylitis.

Rudwaleit M, Feldtkeller E, Sieper J. Easy assessment of axial spondyloarthritis (early ankylosing spondylitis) at the bedside. Ann Rheum Dis 2006;65:1251–1252.

pathology too, e.g. abdominal aortic aneurysm, pancreatitis, peptic ulcer and renal disorders.

Important spinal conditions are acute disc protrusion, spinal stenosis, ankylosing spondylitis (Fig. 14.22), osteoporotic fracture, infection and tumours. Infection and tumours are associated with fever or weight loss. In many patients, however, backache reflects age-related degenerative change in discs and facet joints (spondylosis).

Mechanical low back pain is common after standing for too long or sitting in a poor position. Symptoms worsen as the day progresses and improve after resting or on rising in the morning.

Insidious onset of backache and stiffness in an adolescent or young adult suggests inflammatory disease of the sacroiliac joints and lumbar spine, e.g. ankylosing spondylitis (Box 14.19). Symptoms are worse in the morning or after inactivity, and ease with movement. Morning stiffness is more marked than in osteoarthritis, lasting at least 30 minutes. Other clues to the diagnosis are peripheral joint involvement, extra-articular features or a positive family history.

Acute onset of low back pain in a young adult, often associated with bending or lifting, is typical of acute disc protrusion (slipped disc). The acute episode may be superimposed on a background of preceding episodic backache due to disc degeneration. Activities such as coughing or straining to open the bowels exacerbate the pain. There may be symptoms of lumbar or sacral nerve root compression. Cauda equina syndrome involves a central disc prolapse, or similar space-occupying lesion, impinging on the cauda equina. There are features of sensory and motor disturbances, including diminished perianal sensation and bladder function disturbance. The motor disturbance may be profound, e.g. paraplegia.

Acute back pain in the middle-aged, elderly or those with risk factors, e.g. steroid therapy, may be due to osteoporotic fracture. This is eased by lying, exacerbated by spinal flexion and not usually associated with neurological symptoms.

Acute onset of severe progressive pain, especially associated with malaise, weight loss or night sweats, may indicate pyogenic or tuberculous infection of the lumbar spine or sacroiliac joint. The patient may have a

14

past history of diabetes mellitus or immunosuppression, e.g. steroid therapy or HIV infection, and complain of pain and great difficulty in moving. The infection may involve the intervertebral discs and adjacent vertebrae and may track into the psoas muscle sheath, presenting as a painful flexed hip or a groin swelling.

Consider malignant disease involving a vertebral body in patients with unremitting spinal pain of recent onset, disturbing sleep. Other clues are a previous history of cancer, and systemic symptoms or weight loss. Tumours rarely affect intervertebral discs.

Cauda equina syndrome and spinal cord compression are neurosurgical emergencies. If suspected, refer the patient immediately for assessment and possible surgical decompression.

Intermittent discomfort or pain in the lumbar spine occurring over a long period of time is typical of degenerative disc disease. There is stiffness in the morning or after immobility. Pain and stiffness are relieved by gentle activity but recur with, or after, excessive activity. Over years there is gradual loss of lumbar spine mobility, sometimes with spontaneous improvement in pain as the facet joints increasingly stiffen.

Diffuse pain in the buttocks or thighs brought on by standing too long or walking is the presenting symptom of lumbosacral spinal stenosis. This can be difficult to distinguish from intermittent claudication (p. 128). The pain may be accompanied by tingling and numbness and difficult for the patient to describe. Typically, it is relieved by rest or spinal flexion. Stooping or holding on to a supermarket trolley may increase exercise tolerance. Narrowing of the spinal canal or neural exit foramina is caused by degenerative changes in the intervertebral discs and facet joints, and there is a long preceding history of discomfort typical of degenerative joint disease.

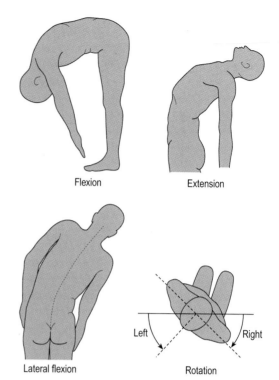

Fig. 14.23 Movements of the lumbar and dorsal spine.

Examination sequence

Ask the patient to stand with the back fully exposed.

Look
- Look for obvious deformity, such as decreased/increased lordosis, obvious scoliosis, soft-tissue abnormalities like a hairy patch or lipoma that might overlie a congenital abnormality, e.g. spina bifida.

Feel
- Palpate the spinous processes and paraspinal tissues. Note the overall alignment and focal tenderness (the L4/5 interspinous space is palpable at the level of the iliac crests).
- After warning the patient, lightly percuss the spine with your closed fist and note any tenderness.

Move
- Flexion: ask the patient to try to touch his toes with his legs straight. Record how far down his legs he can reach. Some of this movement depends on hip flexion. Usually the upper segments flex before the lower ones, and this progression should be smooth.
- Extension: ask the patient to straighten up and lean back as far as possible (normal 10–20° from neutral erect posture).
- Lateral flexion: ask him to reach down to each side, touching the outside of the leg as far down as possible while keeping the legs straight (Fig. 14.23).

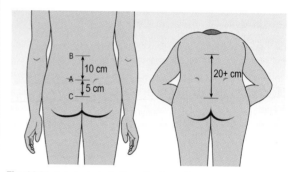

Fig. 14.24 Schober's test. Measuring forward flexion of the spine.

Special tests

Examination sequence

Schober's test for forward flexion
- Mark the skin in the midline at the level of the posterior iliac spines (L5), which overlie the sacroiliac joints (Fig. 14.24; mark A).
- Use a tape measure to draw two more marks: one 10 cm above (mark B) and one 5 cm below this (mark C).
- Place the end of the tape measure on the upper mark (B). Ask the patient to touch his toes. The distance from mark B to mark C should increase from 15 to more than 20 cm.

Root compression tests Intervertebral disc prolapse causing nerve root pressure occurs most often in the lower lumbar region, leading to compression of the corresponding nerve roots.

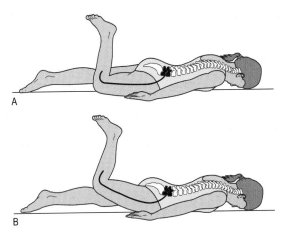

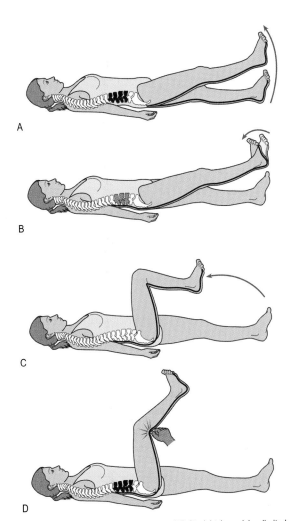

Fig. 14.26 Stretch test: femoral nerve. (A) Pain may be triggered by knee flexion alone. **(B)** Pain may be triggered by knee flexion in combination with hip extension.

- If a limit is reached, raise the leg to just less than this level, and dorsiflex the foot to test for nerve root tension (Fig. 14.25).

Tibial nerve stretch tests L4–5, S1–3

Examination sequence

- With the patient supine, flex the hip to 90°.
- Extend the knee. In this position the tibial nerve 'bowstrings' across the popliteal fossa.
- Press over either of the hamstring tendons, and then over the nerve in the middle of the fossa. The test is positive if pain occurs when the nerve is pressed, but not the hamstring tendons (Fig. 14.25D).

Femoral nerve stretch tests L2–4

Examination sequence

- With the patient lying on his front (prone), flex the knee and extend the hip (Fig. 14.26). This stretches the femoral nerve. A positive result is pain felt in the back, or the front of the thigh. This test can, if necessary, be performed with the patient lying on his side (with the test side uppermost).

Flip test for functional overlay

Examination sequence

- Ask the patient to sit on the end of the couch with the hips and knees flexed to 90° (Fig. 14.27A).
- Examine the knee reflexes.
- Extend the knee, as if to examine the ankle jerk. A patient with nerve root impingement will lie back ('flip'; Fig. 14.27B).

The sacroiliac joints

Examination sequence

Examination is unreliable, but compressing the pelvis or pressing down on the sacrum with the heel of your hand with the subject lying prone may produce pain if these joints are inflamed.

Fig. 14.25 Stretch tests: sciatic nerve. (A) Straight-leg raising limited by tension of root over prolapsed disc. **(B)** Tension increased by dorsiflexion of foot (Bragard's test). **(C)** Root tension relieved by flexion at the knee. **(D)** Pressure over centre of popliteal fossa bears on posterior tibial nerve, which is 'bowstringing' across the fossa, causing pain locally and radiation into the back.

The femoral nerve (L2–4) lies anterior to the pubic ramus, so straight-leg raising or other forms of hip flexion do not increase its root tension. Problems with the femoral nerve roots may cause quadriceps weakness and/or diminished knee jerk on that side.

The sciatic nerve (L4–5; S1–3) runs behind the pelvis, so manoeuvres to put tension on the lower nerve roots (L4 exiting the L4/5 foramen, L5 exiting the L5/S1 foramen) differ from those for the upper lumbar nerve roots (L2, L3).

Straight-leg raise tests L4, L5, S1 nerve root tension (L3/4, L4/5 and L5/S1 disc prolapse respectively).

Examination sequence

- With the patient lying supine, lift the foot to flex the hip passively, keeping the knee straight.
- Measure the angle between the couch and the flexed leg to determine any limitation (normal 80–90° hip flexion) caused by thigh or leg pain.

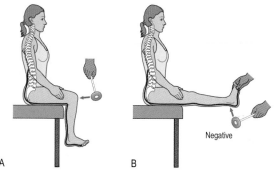

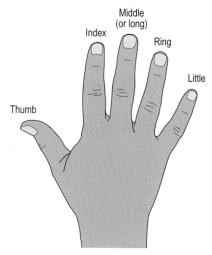

Fig. 14.27 Sciatic nerve. The 'flip' test. **(A)** Divert the patient's attention to the tendon reflexes. **(B)** The patient with physical nerve root compression cannot permit full extension of the leg.

14.20 Motor innervation of the hand	
Nerve	**Muscles supplied**
Median	Opponens and abductor muscles of the hand and most of the wrist and finger flexors
Ulnar	Adductor of thumb, most of lumbricals and interossei
Radial	Extensors of wrist and hand

THE UPPER LIMB

The prime function of the upper limb is to position the hand appropriately in space. This requires shoulder, elbow and wrist movements. The hand may function in both precision and power modes. The intrinsic muscles of the hand allow grip and fine manipulative movements, and the forearm muscles provide power and stability.

Distinguish between systemic and local conditions. Systemic conditions, e.g. rheumatoid arthritis, usually cause pathology at several sites. Differentiate local conditions from referred or radicular pain. Establish whether the condition is inflammatory or not on the pattern of diurnal stiffness and pain.

The hand and wrist

Motor innervation of the hand is shown in Box 14.20. The wrist joint has metacarpocarpal, intercarpal, ulnocarpal and radiocarpal components. There is a wide range of possible movements, including flexion, extension, adduction (deviation towards the ulnar side), abduction (deviation towards the radial side) and the composite movement of circumduction (the hand moves in a conical fashion on the wrist). When examining and documenting the fingers, use their names to avoid confusion (Fig. 14.28). The PIP and DIP joints are hinge joints and allow only flexion and extension. The metacarpophalangeal (MCP) joints allow flexion and extension, and some abduction/adduction that is greatest when the MCP joints are extended.

The history

The patient will often localise complaints of pain, stiffness, loss of function, contractures, disfigurement and

Fig. 14.28 Names of fingers used in documentation.

trauma. If symptoms are vague or diffuse, consider referred pain or a compressive neuropathy, e.g. median nerve compression as it traverses the carpal tunnel in the wrist, which leads to symptoms and signs of carpal tunnel syndrome (Fig. 14.29). If PIP or MCP joint swelling is prominent consider inflammatory arthritis.

Examination sequence

Seat the patient, facing you, with arms and shoulders exposed. Start examining the hand and fingers first, and move proximally.

Look

- Colour changes including palmar erythema.
- Swelling of MCP joints produces loss of interknuckle indentation on the dorsum of the hand, especially when the MCP and IP joints are fully flexed (loss of normal 'hill–valley–hill–valley' aspect; Fig. 14.30A). Swelling at the PIP joints produces 'spindling' (Fig. 14.30B).
- Deformity of phalangeal fractures may produce rotation. Ask the patient to flex the fingers together (Fig. 14.31) and then in turn. Normally, with the MCP and IP joints flexed, the fingers should not cross, and should point to the scaphoid tubercle in the wrist.

Extra-articular signs

- Small muscle wasting, especially of the interossei in inflammatory arthritis (T1 nerve root lesion or ulnar nerve palsy).
- Vasculitis of the fingers, most commonly detected in the nail folds (Fig. 4.15E).
- Nail changes, e.g. pitting (psoriasis) and onycholysis (loosening of the nail from its bed) in psoriatic arthritis (Fig. 4.15B).

Feel

- Hard swellings are bony; soft swelling suggests synovitis.
- Palpate above and below the IP joints with your thumb and index finger to detect sponginess.
- Test the MCP joints by examining for sponginess and squeeze gently across them for pain.
- Palpate the flexor tendon sheaths in the hand and fingers to detect local swellings or tenderness. If you detect any swelling (usually just proximal to the MCP joints), ask the patient to flex and then extend the finger and see if there is triggering or 'locking'.

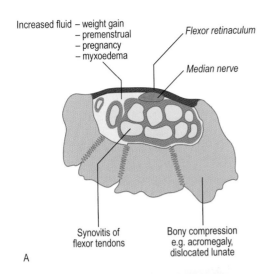

Increased fluid – weight gain
– premenstrual
– pregnancy
– myxoedema

Flexor retinaculum

Median nerve

Synovitis of flexor tendons

Bony compression e.g. acromegaly, dislocated lunate

A

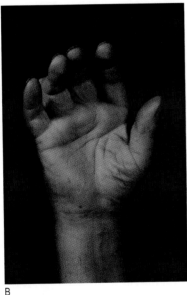

B

Fig. 14.29 Carpal tunnel syndrome. (A) Causes of median nerve compression. **(B)** Thenar muscle wasting.

- Feel for crepitus. Place your index finger across the fully extended fingers and ask the patient to open and close the fingers.

Move

Active movements
- Ask the patient to make a fist, and then extend his fingers fully.
- Insert your index and middle finger from the thumb side into the patient's palm and ask him to squeeze them as hard as possible to test grip.

Passive movements
- Move each finger through flexion and extension and notice any triggering.
- Ask the patient to put the palms of his hands together and extend the wrists fully – the 'prayer sign' (normal is 90° of extension) (Fig. 14.32A).
- Ask the patient to put the backs of his hands together and flex the wrists fully – the 'reverse prayer sign' (normal 90° of flexion) (Fig. 14.32B).

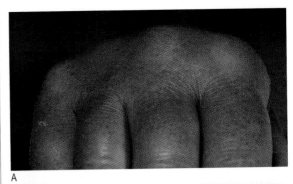

A

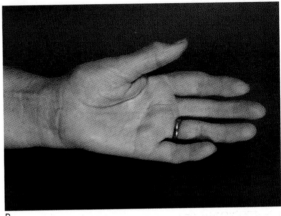

B

Fig. 14.30 Hand and wrist swelling. (A) Ask the patient to make a fist. Look at it straight on to detect any loss of 'hill and valley'. **(B)** Squaring of the wrist due to osteophytes at the carpometacarpal joint of the thumb.

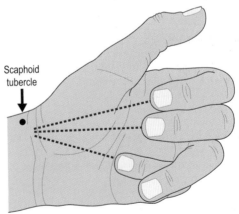

Scaphoid tubercle

Fig. 14.31 Flexion of the fingers showing rotational deformity of the ring finger.

Abnormal findings

Look Erythema suggests acute inflammation caused by soft-tissue infection, septic arthritis, tendon sheath infection or crystalopathy (gout and pseudogout). Swelling at the MCP and/or IP joints suggests synovitis. Spindling is typically seen in rheumatoid arthritis and collateral ligament injuries (Box 14.21).

The fingers are long in Marfan's syndrome (arachnodactyly; Fig. 3.28B).

14

14.21 Examples of visible abnormalities of the hands

Abnormality	Appearance and consistency	Typical site	Associated disease
Heberden's nodes	Small bony nodules	Distal interphalangeal joints	Osteoarthritis
Bouchard's nodes	Small bony nodules	Proximal interphalangeal joints	Osteoarthritis
Rheumatoid nodules	Fleshy and firm	Extensor surface of knuckles	Rheumatoid arthritis
Tophi	White subcutaneous	Juxta-articular	Gout
Calcific deposits	White subcutaneous	Finger pulp	Systemic sclerosis, dermatomyositis
Dilated capillaries	(Use magnifying glass)	Nail folds	Systemic sclerosis, dermatomyositis, systemic lupus erythematosus

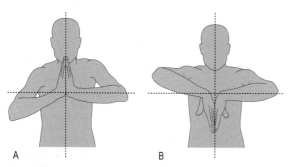

A   B

Fig. 14.32 Assessing the wrist. (A) Extension. **(B)** Flexion. Reduced range of movement at right wrist.

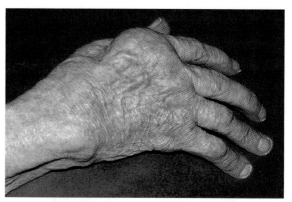

Fig. 14.34 Rheumatoid hand, showing ulnar deviation of the fingers, small-muscle wasting and synovial swelling at carpus, metacarpophalangeal and proximal interphalangeal joints.

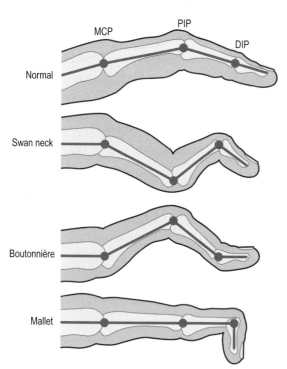

Fig. 14.33 Deformities of the finger in rheumatoid arthritis. MCP, metacarpophalangeal; PIP, proximal interphalangeal; DIP, distal interphalangeal.

At the DIP joints (Fig. 14.33), a 'mallet' finger is a flexion deformity which is passively correctable. This is usually caused by minor trauma disrupting the terminal extensor expansion at the base of the distal phalanx, with or without bony avulsion.

Boutonnière (or buttonhook) deformity is a flexion deformity at the PIP joint with hyperextension at the DIP joint and fixed flexion at the PIP joint (Fig. 14.33). 'Swan neck' deformity is hyperextension at the PIP joint with flexion at the DIP joint.

There may be subluxation and ulnar deviation of the MCP joints in rheumatoid arthritis (Fig. 14.34). Dupuytren's contracture affects the palmar fascia, resulting in the MCP and PIP joints of the little and ring fingers becoming fixed in flexion (Fig. 3.13). Anterior (or volar) displacement (partial dislocation) of the wrist may be seen in rheumatoid arthritis.

Feel Hard swellings may be due to osteophytes (characteristic of osteoarthritis), mucous cysts or, rarely, tumours. Heberden's and Bouchard's nodes occur at the DIP and PIP joints respectively.

Sponginess suggests synovitis. Swelling, tenderness and crepitus are found over the tendon sheaths of abductor pollicis longus and extensor pollicis brevis in De Quervain's tenosynovitis. Symptoms are aggravated by movements at the wrist and thumb. Crepitus at this site is often felt as a creaking sensation and may even be audible. Crepitus may also occur with movement of the radiocarpal joints in osteoarthritis, most commonly secondary to old scaphoid or distal radial fractures.

Move Lack of full extension of one or more fingers may indicate tendon rupture.

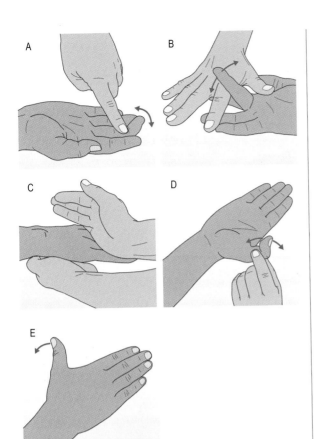

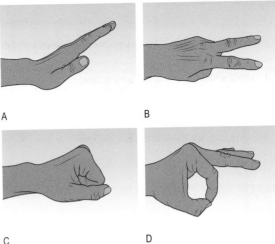

Fig. 14.36 Rapid assessment of the motor functions of the radial, ulnar and median nerves. (A) Paper (radial). **(B)** Scissors (ulnar). **(C)** Stone (median). **(D)** OK (median – anterior interosseus).

14

Fig. 14.35 Testing the flexors and extensors of the fingers and thumb. (A) Flexor digitorum profundus. **(B)** Flexor digitorum superficialis. **(C)** Extensor digitorum. **(D)** Flexor pollicis longus. **(E)** Extensor pollicis longus.

Examining the wrist and hand with a wound

Test the tendons, nerves and circulation in a patient with a wrist or hand wound. The wound site and the hand position at the time of injury can suggest the structures that are possibly damaged. However, normal movement may still be possible, even with 90% division of a tendon, so surgical exploration is needed for correct diagnosis and treatment. Sensory aspects of nerve injury are covered on page 269.

Examination sequence

Muscles and tendons

- Flexor digitorum profundus: ask the patient to flex the DIP joint while you hold the PIP joint in extension (Fig. 14.35A).
- Flexor digitorum superficialis: hold the other fingers fully extended (to eliminate the action of flexor digitorum profundus, as it can also flex the PIP joint) and ask the patient to flex the PIP joint in question (Fig. 14.35B).
- Extensor digitorum: ask the patient to extend the fingers with the wrist in the neutral position (Fig. 14.35C).
- Flexor and extensor pollicis longus: hold the proximal phalanx of the patient's thumb firmly and ask him to flex and extend the IP joint (Fig. 14.35D).

- Extensor pollicis longus: ask the patient to place his palm on a flat surface and to extend his thumb like a hitch-hiker (Fig. 14.35E). If the tendon is intact, the patient will be able to do this. Pain occurs in De Quervain's disease.

Nerves (radial, ulnar and median motor function only)

Use 'Paper – scissors – stone – OK' as an aide-mémoire.
Ask the patient to:

- Fully extend the wrist and fingers ('paper sign') (Fig. 14.36A). The radial nerve supplies the wrist and finger extensors.
- Make the 'scissors sign' (Fig. 14.36B).

The ulnar nerve supplies the hypothenar muscles, interossei, two medial lumbricals, adductor pollicis, flexor carpi ulnaris and the ulnar half of flexor digitorum profundus.

- Clench the fist fully ('stone sign') (Fig. 14.36C).

The median nerve supplies the thenar muscles that abduct and oppose the thumb, the lateral two lumbricals, the medial half of flexor digitorum profundus, flexor digitorum superficialis, flexor carpi radialis, palmaris longus and pronator teres. Because of inconstant cross-over in the nerve supply to the thenar eminence muscles other than abductor pollicis brevis, the best test of median nerve motor function is the ability to abduct the thumb away from the palm (Fig. 14.37). However, clenching a fist fully ('rock' sign) also depends on median function because of its flexor supply.

- Make the 'OK' sign (Fig. 14.36D).

The anterior interosseous nerve (commonly injured in supracondylar fractures) is a purely motor terminal branch of the median nerve. It supplies flexor pollicis longus, the index finger flexor digitorum profundus and pronator quadratus. Making the OK sign depends on both flexor pollicis longus and index finger flexor digitorum profundus functioning.

The elbow

Anatomy

The elbow joint has humero-ulnar, radio-capitellar and superior radio-ulnar articulations. The medial and lateral epicondyles are the flexor and extensor origins

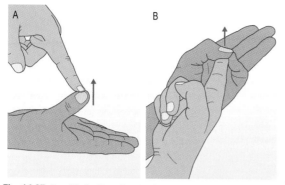

Fig. 14.37 Specific testing of motor function of the median nerve.

respectively for the forearm muscles. These two prominences and the tip of the olecranon are easily palpated. They normally form an equilateral triangle when the elbow is flexed to 90°, and lie in a straight line when the elbow is fully extended. A subcutaneous bursa overlies the olecranon and may become inflamed or infected (bursitis). Elbow pain may be localised or referred from the neck. Rheumatoid arthritis and epicondylitis commonly cause elbow pain.

Examination sequence

Look

- At the overall alignment of the extended elbow. There is normally a valgus angle of 11–13° when the elbow is fully extended (the 'carrying angle').
- For:
  - swelling, bruising and scars
  - swelling of synovitis between the lateral epicondyle and olecranon
  - rash, olecranon bursitis, tophi or nodules
  - rheumatoid nodules on the proximal extensor surface of the forearm.

Feel

- The bony contours of the lateral and medial epicondyles and olecranon tip, defining an equilateral triangle with the elbow flexed at 90°.
- For sponginess on either side of the olecranon and ask about tenderness. Synovitis feels spongy or boggy when the elbow is fully extended.
- Focal tenderness, over the lateral or medial epicondyle. When isolated to one site, this may indicate 'tennis' (lateral) or 'golfer's' (medial) elbow.
- For bursae, fluid-filled sacs which are usually soft, but if acutely inflamed or infected may be firm.
- For rheumatoid nodules on the proximal extensor surface of the forearm.

Move

- Assess the extension–flexion arc: ask the patient to touch his shoulder on the same side and then straighten the elbow as far as possible. The normal range of movement is 0–145°; a range less than 30–110° will cause functional problems.
- Assess supination and pronation: ask the patient to put his elbows by the side of the body and flex them to 90°. Now ask him to turn the hands upwards to face the ceiling (supination: normal range 0–90°) and then downwards to face the floor (pronation: normal range 0–85°).

14.22 Causes of shoulder girdle pain	
Rotator cuff	
• Degeneration • Tendon rupture	• Calcific tendonitis
Subacromial bursa	
• Calcific bursitis	• Polyarthritis
Capsule	
• Adhesive capsulitis	
Head of humerus	
• Tumour • Osteonecrosis	• Fracture/dislocation
Joints	

• Glenohumeral, sternoclavicular
  • Inflammatory arthritis, osteoarthritis, dislocation, infection
	• Acromioclavicular
	  • Subluxation, osteoarthritis

Special tests

Examination sequence

Tennis elbow (lateral epicondylitis)

- Ask the patient to flex the elbow to 90° and pronate and flex the hand/wrist fully.
- Support the patient's elbow. Ask him to extend the wrist against your resistance.
- Pain is produced at the lateral epicondyle and may be referred down the extensor aspect of the arm.

Golfer's elbow (medial epicondylitis)

- Ask the patient to flex the elbow to 90° and supinate the hand/wrist fully.
- Support the patient's elbow. Ask him to flex the wrist against your resistance.
- Pain is produced at the medial epicondyle and may be referred down the flexor aspect of the arm.

The shoulder

Anatomy

The shoulder joint consists of the glenohumeral joint and the acromioclavicular joint, but movement also occurs between the scapula and the posterior chest wall (see Fig. 14.42). Movements of the shoulder girdle, especially abduction and rotation, also produce movement at the sternoclavicular joint. The rotator cuff muscles are supraspinatus, subscapularis, teres minor and infraspinatus. They and their tendinous insertions help stability and movement (especially abduction; Fig. 14.7) at the glenohumeral joint.

Symptoms and definitions

Pain is common (Boxes 14.22 and 14.23) and frequently referred to the upper arm. Glenohumeral pain may occur over the anterolateral aspect of the upper arm. Pain felt at the shoulder may be referred from the

14.23 Common conditions affecting the shoulder

Non-trauma

- Rotator cuff syndromes, e.g. supraspinatus, infraspinatus tendonitis
- Impingement syndromes (involving the rotator cuff and subacromial bursa)
- Adhesive capsulitis ('frozen shoulder')
- Calcific tendonitis
- Bicipital tendonitis
- Inflammatory arthritis
  - Polymyalgia rheumatica

Trauma

- Rotator cuff tear
- Glenohumeral dislocation
- Acromioclavicular dislocation
- Fracture of the clavicle
- Fracture of the head or neck of the humerus

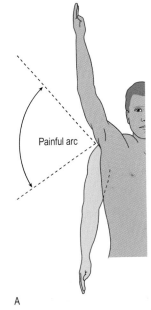

Painful arc

A

cervical spine, radicular pain caused by central nerve root compression, or diaphragm and subdiaphragmatic peritoneum via the phrenic nerve. The most common cause of referred pain is cervical spondylosis, where disc space narrowing and osteophytes cause nerve root impingement and inflammation.

Stiffness and limitation of movement around the shoulder, caused by adhesive capsulitis of the glenohumeral joint, are common after immobilisation or disuse following injury or stroke. This is a 'frozen shoulder'. However, movement can still occur between the scapula and chest wall.

Some rotator cuff disorders, especially impingement syndromes and tears, present with a painful arc where abduction of the arm between 60 and 120° causes discomfort (Fig. 14.38).

Examination sequence

Ask the patient to sit or stand and expose the shoulder completely.

Look

Examine from the front and the back and in the axilla for:

- deformity: the deformities of anterior glenohumeral and complete acromioclavicular joint dislocation are obvious (Figs 14.39 and 14.40), but the shoulder contour in posterior glenohumeral dislocation may only appear abnormal when you stand above the seated patient and look down on the shoulder
- swelling
- muscle wasting: especially of the deltoid, supraspinatus and infraspinatus. Wasting of supraspinatus or infraspinatus indicates a chronic tear of their tendons
- the size and position of the scapula, i.e. elevated, depressed or 'winged' (Fig. 14.41).

Feel

- Feel from the sternoclavicular joint along the clavicle to the acromioclavicular joint.
- Palpate the acromion and coracoid (2 cm inferior and medial to the clavicle tip) processes, the scapula spine and the biceps tendon in the bicipital groove.
- Extend the shoulder to bring supraspinatus anterior to the acromion process. Palpate the supraspinatus tendon.

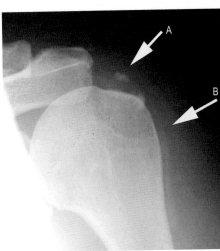

B

Fig. 14.38 (A) Painful arc. **(B)** Calcific deposits in supraspinatus (arrow A) and biceps tendons (arrow B).

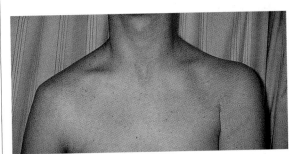

Fig. 14.39 Right anterior glenohumeral dislocation. Note loss of normal shoulder contour.

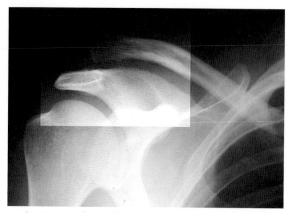

Fig. 14.40 X-ray of right acromioclavicular dislocation.

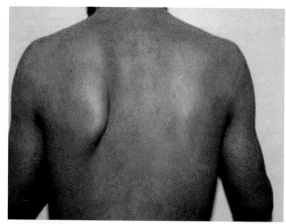

Fig. 14.41 'Winging' of the left scapula due to paralysis of the nerve to serratus anterior.

Move

To screen for shoulder dysfunction:

- Stand behind the patient.
- Ask the patient to put both hands behind the head.
- Then put the arms down and reach behind his back to touch the shoulder blades.

If there is pain, swelling or limitation of movement, proceed to examine the shoulder fully.

Range of movement

- First assess active movement, then passive.
- Ask the patient to flex and extend the shoulder as far as possible.
- Abduction: ask the patient to lift his arm away from his side.
  - Palpate the inferior pole of the scapula between your thumb and index finger to detect scapular rotation and determine how much movement occurs at the glenohumeral joint. In all, 50–70% of abduction occurs at the glenohumeral joint (the rest with movement of the scapula on the chest wall). This increases if the arm is externally rotated. Note the degree and smoothness of scapular movement. If the glenohumeral joint is excessively stiff, movement of the scapula over the chest wall will predominate. If there is any limitation or pain (painful arc) associated with abduction, test the rotator cuff (Fig. 14.42).

- Internal rotation: with the patient's arm by his side and the elbow flexed at 90°, ask him to put his hand behind his back and feel as high up the spine as possible. Document the highest spinous process that he can reach with the thumb.
- External rotation: in the same position with the elbow tucked against his side, ask him to rotate the hand out.
- Deltoid: ask the patient to abduct the arm out from his side, parallel to the floor, and resist while you push down on the humerus. Compare each side.

Rotator cuff

- Ask the patient to start abducting the arm from his side against your resistance. If abduction cannot be initiated or is painful, this suggests a rotator cuff problem.

Impingement (painful arc)

- Passively abduct the patient's arm fully
- Ask him to lower (adduct) it slowly (Fig. 14.38).

Pain occurring between 60 and 120° of abduction occurs in painful arc.

- If the patient cannot initiate abduction, place your hand over the scapula to confirm there is no scapular movement.
- Passively abduct the internally rotated arm to 30–45°
- Ask him to continue to abduct the arm.

Pain on active movement, especially against resistance, suggests impingement.

Ligamentous tears and injuries

Discrepancy between active and passive ranges suggests a tendinous tear – in particular subscapularis, where there may be an excessive range of passive internal rotation. To test the component muscles of the rotator cuff, it is necessary to neutralise the effect of other muscles crossing the shoulder.

- Subscapularis and pectoralis major (internal rotation of the shoulder):
  - To isolate subscapularis, test internal rotation with the patient's hand behind his back. Loss of power suggests a tear. Pain on forced internal rotation suggests tendonitis.
- Supraspinatus. With the arm by his side, test abduction. Loss of power suggests a tear. Pain on forced abduction at 60° suggests tendonitis.
- Infraspinatus and teres minor. Test external rotation with the arm in the neutral position, and 30° flexion to reduce the contribution of deltoid. Loss of power suggests a tear. Pain on forced external rotation suggests tendonitis.

Bicipital tendonitis

- Palpate the bicipital tendon in its groove, noting any tenderness.
- Ask the patient to supinate the forearm, and then flex the arm against resistance. Pain occurs in bicipital tendonitis.

THE LOWER LIMB

The hip

Anatomy

The hip is a ball-and-socket joint and allows flexion, extension, abduction, adduction, internal/external rotation and the combined movement of circumduction. With age, the most common restrictions in movement are extension and internal rotation, followed by abduction.

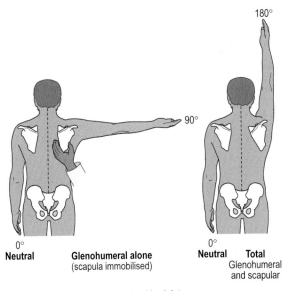

Fig. 14.42 Movements at the shoulder joint.

90°

180°

0°
Neutral

Glenohumeral alone
(scapula immobilised)

0°
Neutral

Total
Glenohumeral
and scapular

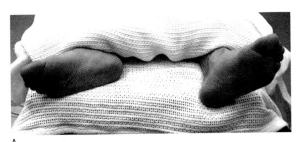

A

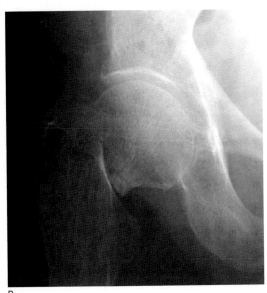

B

Fig. 14.43 Fracture of neck of right femur. **(A)** Shortening and external rotation of the leg. **(B)** X-ray showing translation and angulation.

Symptoms and definitions

Pain is usually felt in the groin, but can be referred to the anterior thigh, the knee or buttock. Hip pain is usually aggravated by activity, but osteonecrosis and tumours may be painful at rest and at night. Lateral hip or thigh pain, aggravated when lying on that side, suggests trochanteric bursitis.

Distinguish pain arising from the hip from:
- lumbar nerve root irritation (pp. 334-5)
- spinal or arterial claudication (p. 128)
- abdominal causes, e.g. hernias (p. 186).

Find out how the pain restricts activities. Ask about walking in terms of the time and distance the patient manages outside the house and up and down stairs, whether he does his own shopping and which walking aids he uses.

Fracture of the neck of femur is common following relatively minor trauma in postmenopausal women and those over 70 years. The fracture may be minimally displaced or impacted and need not have the classical appearance of a shortened, externally rotated leg (Fig. 14.43A). The patient may even be able to weight-bear.

14

Examination sequence

Patients should undress to their underwear and remove socks and shoes. You should be able to see the iliac crests.

Look
- Assess gait (p. 329).
- General inspection: ask the patient to stand.
- From the front, observe whether the:
  - stance is straight
  - shoulders are parallel to the ground and symmetrically over the pelvis (which may mask a hip deformity or true shortening of one leg)
  - hip, knee, ankle or foot are deformed
  - muscles are wasted (from polio or disuse secondary to arthritis).
- From the side, assess for a stoop or increased lumbar lordosis (both may result from a flexion contracture).
- From behind, assess whether:
  - the spine is straight or curved laterally (scoliosis)
  - there is scoliosis: note the relative positions of the shoulders and pelvis, and measure leg lengths
  - there is any gluteal atrophy.
- Look for scars, sinuses, dressings or skin changes around the hip.

Feel
- Tenderness over the greater trochanter suggests trochanteric bursitis.
- Tenderness over the lesser trochanter and ischial tuberosity is common in sporting injuries due to strains of the iliopsoas and hamstring insertions respectively.

Move
- With the patient face-up on the couch, check the pelvic brim is perpendicular to the spine.
- Flexion: place your left hand under the back (to detect any masking of hip movement by movement of the pelvis and lumbar spine, use Thomas's test) and check the range of flexion of each hip in turn (normal 0–120°).
- Abduction and adduction: stabilise the pelvis by placing your left hand on the opposite iliac crest. With your right hand abduct the leg until you feel the pelvis start to tilt

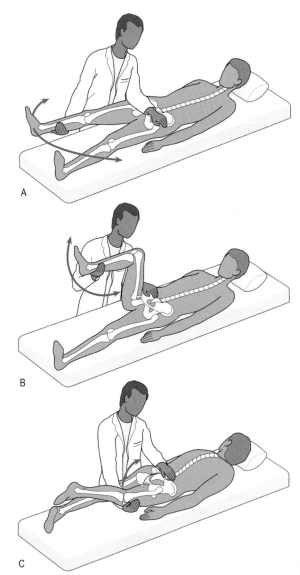

Fig. 14.44 Testing hip movement. (A) Abduction. (B) Flexion.
(C) Extension.

(normal 45°). Test adduction by crossing one of the patient's legs over the other and continuing to move it medially (normal 25°) (Fig. 14.44A).

■ Internal and external rotation: with the leg in full extension, roll it on the couch and watch the foot to indicate the range of rotation. Test with the knee (and hip) flexed at 90°. Move the foot medially to test external rotation and laterally to test internal rotation (normal 45° for each movement) (Fig. 14.44B).

■ Extension: ask the patient to lie face-down on the couch. Place your left hand on the pelvis to detect any movement. Lift each leg in turn to assess the range of extension (normal range 0–20°) (Fig. 14.44C).

Shortening

Shortening occurs in hip and other lower limb conditions (Box 14.24). Apparent shortening is present if the

14.24 Causes of true lower limb shortening

Hip

- Fractures, e.g. neck of femur
- Following total hip arthroplasty
- Slipped upper femoral epiphysis
- Perthes' disease (juvenile osteochondritis)
- Unreduced hip dislocation
- Septic arthritis
- Loss of articular cartilage (arthritis, joint infection)
- Congenital coxa vara
- Missed congenital dislocation of the hip

Femur and tibia

- Growth disturbance secondary to:
  - Poliomyelitis
  - Cerebral palsy
  - Fractures
  - Osteomyelitis
  - Septic arthritis
  - Growth plate injury
  - Congenital causes

affected limb appears shortened, usually because of an adduction or flexion deformity at the hip.

Examination sequence

■ Ask the patient to lie supine and stretch both legs out as far as possible equally to eliminate any soft-tissue contracture/abnormal posture.
■ Measure with a tape:
  ■ from umbilicus to medial malleolus: the apparent length
  ■ from anterior superior iliac spine to medial malleolus: the 'true length' (Fig. 14.45).
■ Confirm any limb length discrepancy by 'block testing':
  ■ Ask the patient to stand with both feet flat on the ground.
  ■ Raise the shorter leg using a series of blocks of graduated thickness until both iliac crests feel level.

Trendelenburg's sign

Examination sequence

■ Stand in front of the patient.
■ Palpate both iliac crests and ask him to stand on one leg for 30 seconds.
■ Repeat with the other leg.
■ Watch and feel the iliac crests to see which moves up or down.
■ Normally, the iliac crest on the side with the foot off the ground should rise. The test is abnormal if the hemipelvis falls below the horizontal (Fig. 14.46). It may be caused by gluteal weakness or inhibition from hip pain, e.g. osteoarthritis, or structural abnormality of the hip joint, e.g. coxa vara or developmental hip dysplasia.

Thomas's test

This measures fixed flexion deformity (incomplete extension), which may be masked by compensatory

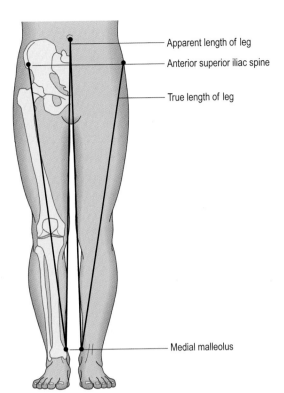

Fig. 14.45 **True and apparent lengths of the lower limbs.**

- Apparent length of leg
- Anterior superior iliac spine
- True length of leg
- Medial malleolus

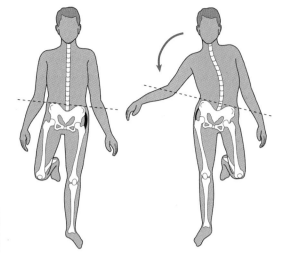

Fig. 14.46 **Trendelenburg's sign.** Powerful gluteal muscles maintain the position when standing on the left leg; weakness of the right gluteal muscles results in pelvic tilt when standing on the right leg.

14

movement at the lumbar spine or pelvis and increasing lumbar lordosis.

Do not perform the test if the patient has a hip replacement on the non-test side, as forced flexion may cause dislocation.

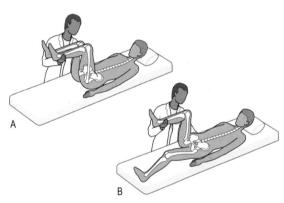

A

B

Fig. 14.47 **Thomas's test:** for examining the left hip.

Examination sequence 🎥

- Ask the patient to lie supine on the couch.
- Place your left hand palm upwards under the lumbar spine.
- Passively flex both legs (hips and knees) as far as possible.
- Keep the non-test hip maximally flexed and by feeling with your left hand confirm that the lordotic curve of the lumbar spine remains eliminated.
- Ask the patient to extend the test hip. Incomplete extension in this position indicates a fixed flexion deformity at the hip (Fig. 14.47).
- If the contralateral hip is not flexed enough, lumbar lordosis will not be eliminated and fixed flexion deformity of the ipsilateral knee confuses the issue. In this case, perform the test with the patient lying on his side.

The knee

Anatomy

The knee is a complex hinge joint with tibio-femoral and patello-femoral components. It has a synovial capsule that extends under the quadriceps (the suprapatellar pouch), reaching 5 cm above the superior edge of the patella. The joint is largely subcutaneous, allowing easy palpation of the patella, tibial tuberosity, patellar tendon,

tibial plateau margin and femoral condyles. The knee depends on its muscular and ligamentous structures for stability (Fig. 14.48).

The hamstring muscles flex the knee. Extension requires the quadriceps muscles, quadriceps tendon, patella, patellar tendon and tibial tuberosity. Any disruption of this 'extensor apparatus' prevents straight-leg raising or produces an extensor lag (a difference between active and passive ranges of extension).

The medial and lateral collateral ligaments resist valgus and varus stress respectively. The anterior cruciate ligament prevents anterior subluxation of the tibia on the femur, and the posterior cruciate ligament resists posterior translation. The medial and lateral menisci are crescentic fibrocartilaginous structures that lie between the tibial plateaus and the femoral condyles. There are several important bursae around the knee:

- anteriorly: the suprapatellar, prepatellar (between the patella and the overlying skin) and infrapatellar bursae (between the skin and the tibial tuberosity/ patellar ligament)
- posteriorly: several bursae lie in the popliteal fossa (Fig. 14.48D).

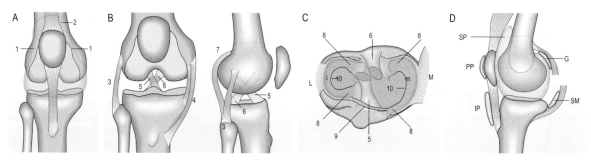

Key

L	Lateral tibiofemoral articulation	1	Extensions of synovial sheath on either side of the patella
M	Medial tibiofemoral articulation	2	Extension of synovial sheath at upper pole of patella
SP	Suprapatellar pouch (or bursa)		
PP	Prepatellar bursa	3	Lateral ligament
IP	Infrapatellar bursa	4	Medial ligament
G	Bursa under the medial head of gastrocnemius	5	Anterior cruciate ligament
		6	Posterior cruciate ligament
SM	Semimembranosus bursa	7	Posterior ligament
		8	Horns of lateral (l) and medial (m) menisci
		9	Connection of anterior horns
		10	Unattached margin of meniscus

Fig. 14.48 Structure of the right knee. (A) Anterior view, showing the common synovial sheath. **(B)** Anterior and lateral views, showing the ligaments. **(C)** Plan view of the menisci. **(D)** Bursae.

Symptoms and definitions

Pain

In trauma, take a detailed history of the injury mechanism. The direction of impact, load and deformation predict what structures are injured. Remember that pain in the knee may be referred from the hip. Anterior knee pain, particularly after prolonged sitting or going downstairs, suggests patellofemoral joint pathology.

Swelling

The normal volume of synovial fluid is 1–2 ml and is clinically undetectable. An effusion (collection of fluid within the joint space) indicates intra-articular pathology. It may be due to synovial fluid, blood, pus or a mixture of these fluids.

Haemarthrosis (bleeding into the knee) is caused by injury to a vascular structure within the joint, e.g. torn cruciate ligament or intra-articular fracture. Patients with a coagulation disorder, e.g. haemophilia or on anticoagulant therapy, are particularly prone to haemarthroses. The menisci are predominantly avascular, and unless torn at their periphery or in conjunction with some other internal derangement, do not cause a haemarthrosis.

In acute injury the speed of onset of swelling is a clue to the diagnosis.

- Rapid (<30 minutes), severe swelling suggests a haemarthrosis.
- Swelling of a lesser degree over 24 hours is more suggestive of traumatic effusion, e.g. meniscal tear.
- Septic arthritis develops over a few hours with pain, marked swelling, tenderness, redness and extreme reluctance to move the joint actively or passively. Concurrent oral steroid or non-steroidal anti-inflammatory drug therapy modifies these features.

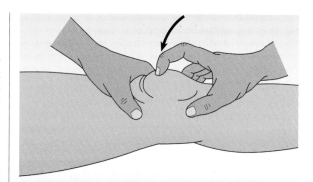

Fig. 14.49 Testing for effusion by the patellar tap.

- Crystal-induced arthritis (gout or pseudogout) can mimic septic arthritis. Confirm the diagnosis by looking at aspirated fluid under polarised light microscopy.

Locking

This is a block to full extension. It may be longstanding or intermittent. The two common causes are a loose body, e.g. from osteochondritis dissecans, osteoarthritis or synovial chondromatosis, and a meniscal tear. Bucket handle and anterior beak meniscal tears are especially associated with locking. Posterior horn tears commonly cause pain on extreme flexion and prevent the last few degrees of flexion. Meniscal tears also cause local joint line tenderness. Congenital discoid meniscus may present with locking and clunking.

Instability ('giving way')

Any of the four main ligaments may rupture from trauma or become incompetent with degenerative disease. Because the normal knee has a valgus angle the patella is prone to dislocate laterally.

Examination sequence

Observe the patient walking and standing, as for gait.

- Ask the patient to lie face up on the couch. Expose both legs fully.

Look

- Note scars, sinuses, erythema or rashes.
- Posture and common deformities, genu valgum (knock knee) or genu varum (bow legs).
- Muscle wasting: quadriceps wasting is almost invariable with inflammation or chronic pain and develops within days. Measure the thigh girth in both legs 20 cm above the tibial tuberosity.
- Leg length discrepancy (Fig. 14.45).
- Flexion deformity: if the patient lies with one knee flexed, this may be caused by a hip, knee or combined problem.
- Swelling: an enlarged prepatellar bursa (housemaid's knee) and any knee joint effusion. Large effusions form a horseshoe-shaped swelling above the knee. Swelling extending beyond the joint margins suggests infection, major injury or, rarely, tumour.
- Baker's cyst: bursa enlargement in the popliteal fossa.

Feel

- Warmth: feel the skin, comparing both sides.
- Effusion.
- The patellar tap:
  - With the patient's knee extended, empty the suprapatellar pouch by sliding your left hand down the thigh until you reach the upper edge of the patella.
  - Keep your hand there and, with the fingertips of your right hand, press down briskly and firmly over the patella (Fig. 14.49).
  - In a moderate-sized effusion you will feel a tapping sensation as the patella strikes the femur. You may feel a fluid impulse in your left hand.
- The 'bulge or ripple test' (Fig. 14.50):
  - Extend the patient's knee and with the quadriceps muscles relaxed, empty the suprapatellar bursa by sliding your hand down the thigh until you reach the upper edge of the patella (Fig. 14.50A).
  - Empty the medial compartment of the joint by firmly stroking the medial side of the knee caudally with the palm of your hand (Fig. 14.50B).

- Firmly stroke the lateral side of the knee joint with the back of your hand (Fig. 14.50C). The test is positive if a ripple or bulge of fluid appears on the medial side of the knee. It is useful for detecting small amounts of fluid but may be falsely negative if a tense effusion is present.
- Synovitis: with the knee extended and the quadriceps relaxed, feel for sponginess on both sides of the quadriceps tendon.
- Joint lines: feel the tibial and femoral joint lines. If there is tenderness, localise this as accurately as possible. In adolescents, localised tibial tuberosity tenderness suggests Osgood–Schlatter disease, a traction osteochondritis.

Move

- Active flexion and extension:
  - With the patient supine, ask him to flex his knee up to the chest and then extend the leg back down to lie on the couch (normal range 0–140°).
  - Feel for crepitus between the patella and femoral condyles, suggesting chondromalacia patellae (more common in younger female patients) or osteoarthritis.
  - Record the range of movement: if there is a fixed flexion deformity of 15° and flexion is possible to 110°, record this as a range of movement of 15–110°.
  - Ask the patient to lift the leg, keeping it straight. If the knee cannot be kept fully extended an extensor lag is present, indicating quadriceps weakness or other abnormality of the extensor apparatus.
- Passive flexion and extension:
  - Normally the knee can extend so that the femur and tibia are in longitudinal alignment. Record full extension as 0°. A restriction to full extension occurs with meniscal tears, osteoarthritis and inflammatory arthritis. To assess hyperextension, lift both legs by the feet. Hyperextension (genu recurvatum) is present if the knee extends beyond the neutral position. Up to 10° is normal (Box 14.25).

> **EBE 14.25 Osteoarthritis**
>
> Palpable bony enlargement, varus deformity, morning stiffness lasting <30 minutes and crepitus on passive movement in a patient with chronic knee pain suggest osteoarthritis.
>
> McGee S. Evidence based physical diagnosis. St Louis, MO: Saunders/Elsevier, 2007, p. 648.

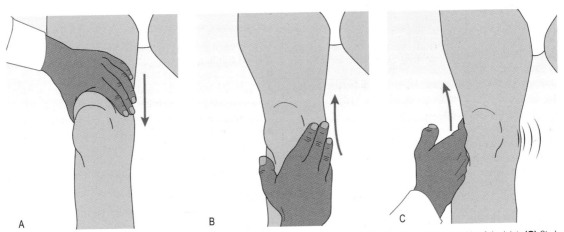

Fig. 14.50 The bulge or ripple test. (A) Empty the suprapatellar pouch, as for the patellar tap test. **(B)** Stroke the medial side of the joint. **(C)** Stroke the lateral side while watching the medial side closely for a bulge or ripple.

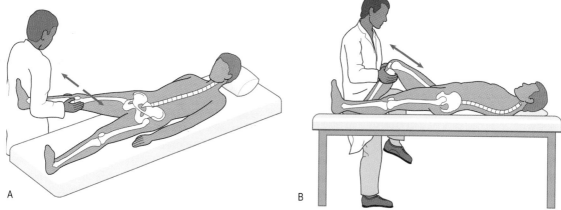

Fig. 14.51 Testing the ligaments of the knee. (A) Collateral ligaments. **(B)** Cruciate ligaments.

Ligament testing

Tests of stability

Collateral ligament With the knee fully extended, abduction or adduction should not be possible. If either ligament is lax or ruptured, movement can occur. If the ligament is strained (partially torn) but intact, pain will be produced but the joint will not open.

Examination sequence

- With the patient's knee fully extended, hold the ankle between your elbow and side. Use both hands to apply a valgus and then varus force to the knee.
- Use your thumbs to feel the joint line and assess the degree to which the joint space opens. Major opening of the joint indicates collateral and cruciate injury (Fig. 14.51A).
- If the knee is stable, repeat the process with the knee flexed to 30° to assess minor collateral laxity. In this position the cruciate ligaments are not taut.

Cruciate ligament

- Flex the patient's knee to 90° and maintain this position by sitting with your thigh trapping the patient's foot.
- Check that the hamstring muscles are relaxed and look for posterior sag (posterior subluxation of the tibia on the femur). This causes a false-positive anterior drawer sign which should not be interpreted as anterior collateral ligament laxity.

The anterior drawer sign

- With your hands behind the upper tibia and both thumbs over the tibial tuberosity, pull the tibia anteriorly (Fig. 14.51B). Significant movement (compare with the opposite knee) indicates that the anterior cruciate ligament is lax. Movement of >1.5 cm suggests anterior cruciate ligament rupture. There is often an associated medial ligament injury.

The posterior drawer sign

- Push backwards on the tibia. Posterior movement of the tibia suggests posterior cruciate ligament laxity.

Patella

Examination sequence

The patellar apprehension test

- With the patient's knee fully extended, push the patella laterally and flex the knee slowly. If the patient actively resists flexion, this suggests previous patellar dislocation or instability.

Tests for meniscal tears

Meniscal tears in younger sporty patients usually result from twisting injury to the flexed weight-bearing leg. In middle-aged patients, degenerative horizontal cleavage of the menisci is common, with no history of trauma. Meniscal injuries commonly cause small effusions, especially on weight bearing or after exercise. Associated localised joint line tenderness is common.

Meniscal provocation test

Examination sequence

Ask the patient to lie face-up on the couch. Test the medial and lateral menisci in turn.

Medial meniscus

- Passively flex the knee to its full extent.
- Externally rotate the foot and abduct the upper leg at the hip, keeping the foot towards the midline (i.e. creating a varus stress at the knee).
- Extend the knee smoothly. In medial meniscus tears a click or clunk may be felt or heard, accompanied by discomfort.

Lateral meniscus

- Passively flex the knee to its full extent.
- Internally rotate the foot and adduct the leg at the hip (i.e. creating a valgus stress at the knee).
- Extend the knee smoothly. In tears of the lateral meniscus, a click or clunk may be felt or heard, accompanied by discomfort.

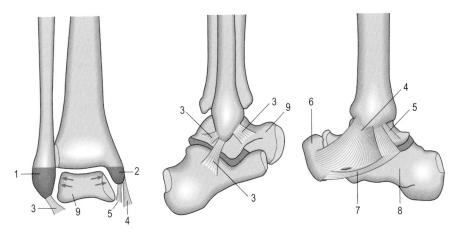

1 Lateral malleolus
2 Medial malleolus
3 Lateral (external) ligament
4 Medial ligament
5 Deep fibres of medial ligament
6 Navicular
7 Spring ligament
8 Calcaneus
9 Talus

Fig. 14.52 The ankle ligaments.

Squat test

- Ask the patient to squat, keeping his feet and heels flat on the ground. If he cannot do this, there is incomplete knee flexion on the affected side. This may be caused by a tear of the posterior horn of the menisci.
- Test the extreme range of knee flexion with the patient face-down on the couch, which makes comparison with the contralateral side easy.

The ankle and foot

Anatomy

The ankle is a hinge joint. The talus articulates with a three-sided mortise made up of the tibial plafond and the medial and lateral malleoli. This allows dorsiflexion and plantar flexion, although some axial rotation can occur at the plantar-flexed ankle. During dorsiflexion the trochlea of the talus rocks posteriorly in the mortise and the malleoli are forced apart because the superior articular surface of the talus is wider anteriorly than posteriorly. The bony mortise is the major factor contributing to stability but the lateral, medial (deltoid) and inferior tibiofibular ligaments are also important (Fig. 14.52).

Foot movements are inversion and eversion, and principally occur at the mid-tarsal (talo-navicular/calcaneo-cuboid) and subtalar (talo-calcaneal) joints. Toe movements are dorsiflexion and plantar flexion.

Symptoms and definitions

Trauma

A 'twisted' ankle is very common, and is usually related to a sporting injury or stepping off a kerb or stair awkwardly. Establish the exact mechanism of injury and the precise site of pain. Frequently there has been a forced inversion injury stressing the lateral ligament. A sprain occurs when some fibres are torn but the ligament remains structurally intact. A complete ligament tear allows excessive talar movement in the ankle mortise with instability.

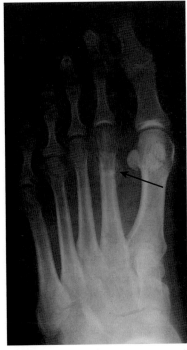

Fig. 14.53 Stress fracture of second metatarsal. Fracture site and callus are arrowed.

Achilles tendon rupture (see Fig. 14.55) is associated with attempted sudden plantar flexion at the ankle. It is common in middle-aged patients doing unaccustomed activity, e.g. badminton, squash or the fathers' race at sports day, and is associated with some drug therapy, e.g. oral steroids, fluoroquinolone antibiotics. Sudden pain occurs above the heel and there is often a sensation or noise of a crack. Patients may feel as if they have been kicked or even shot.

Forefoot pain, often localised to the second metatarsal, after excessive activity such as trekking, marching or dancing, suggests a stress fracture (Fig. 14.53). Symptoms are relieved by rest and aggravated by weight bearing. X-rays in the first week may be normal.

14

14

Non-traumatic conditions

Anterior metatarsalgia with forefoot pain is common, especially in middle-aged women. Acute joint pain with swelling suggests an inflammatory arthropathy such as rheumatoid arthritis or gout. The forefoot is commonly affected in rheumatoid arthritis. In severe cases the metatarsal heads become prominent and walking feels like 'walking on pebbles or broken glass'.

Plantar surface heel pain that is worse in the foot-strike phase of walking may be due to plantar fasciitis and tends to affect middle-aged patients and those with seronegative arthritides.

Posterior heel pain may be caused by Achilles tendonitis.

Spontaneous lancinating pain in the forefoot radiating to contiguous sides of adjacent toes occurs with Morton's neuroma. A common site is the interdigital cleft between the third and fourth toes. This occurs predominantly in women aged 25–45 years and is aggravated by wearing tight shoes.

Examination sequence

Ask patients to remove their socks and shoes.

Look
- Examine the soles of the shoes for abnormal patterns of wear.
- Gait: observe (p. 329). Look for:
  - increased height of step, indicating 'foot drop'
  - ankle movement (dorsi/plantar flexion)
  - position of the foot as it strikes the ground (supinated/pronated)
  - hallux rigidus – loss of movement at the MTP joints.
- With the patient standing, observe:
  - from behind: how the heel is aligned (valgus/varus).
- From the side:
  - The position of the midfoot, looking particularly at the longitudinal medial arch. This may be flattened (pes planus – flat foot) or exaggerated (pes cavus).
  - If the arch is flattened, ask the patient to stand on tiptoe. This restores the arch in a mobile deformity, but not in a structural one.
- A 'splay foot' has widening at the level of the metatarsal heads, often associated with MTP joint synovitis.
- Examine the ankle and foot for scars, sinuses, swelling, bruising, callosities (an area of thickened skin at a site of repeated pressure), nail changes, oedema, deformity and position, e.g. fixed plantar flexion or foot drop.
- The toes: look for deformities of the great and other toes.

Feel
- Feel for focal tenderness and heat. In an acute ankle injury, palpate the proximal fibula, both malleoli, the lateral ligament and base of the fifth metatarsal.
- Gently compress the forefoot.

Move
- Active:
  - Assess the range of plantar flexion and dorsiflexion at the ankle and inversion/eversion of the foot by asking the patient to perform these movements.
- Passive ankle dorsiflexion/plantar flexion:
  - Grip the heel with the cup of your left hand from below, with the thumb and index finger on the malleoli.

- Put the foot through its arc of movement (normal range 15° dorsiflexion to 45° plantar flexion).
- If dorsiflexion is restricted, assess the contribution of gastrocnemius (which functions across both knee and ankle joints) by measuring ankle dorsiflexion with the knee extended and flexed. If more dorsiflexion is possible with the knee flexed, this suggests a gastrocnemius contracture.
- Passive foot inversion/eversion:
  - Examine the subtalar joint in isolation by placing the foot into dorsiflexion to stabilise the talus in the ankle mortise.
  - Move the heel into inversion (normal 20°) and eversion (normal 10°).
  - Examine the combined mid-tarsal joints by fixing the heel with your left hand and moving the forefoot with your right hand into dorsiflexion, plantar flexion, adduction, abduction, supination and pronation.

Abnormal findings

Hallux valgus is common, familial and may be aggravated by footwear and activities such as ballet dancing (Fig. 14.54). A bunion (a soft-tissue bursal swelling) may develop over the protuberant first metatarsal head and become inflamed or infected. As the condition progresses, the hallux may adduct over the second toe.

Gout of the first MTP joint causes marked redness and soft-tissue swelling. This is followed by peeling of the superficial skin and pain on movement or touch.

Swelling of the entire digit, 'sausage toe' (dactylitis), is characteristic of psoriatic arthropathy.

Claw toes result from dorsiflexion (hyperextension) at MTP joints and plantar flexion at PIP and DIP joints. Hammer toes are due to dorsiflexion at MTP and DIP joints and plantar flexion at PIP joints.

Mallet toes describe plantar flexion at DIP joints.

Tenderness on metatarsal compression suggests Morton's neuroma or, if associated with sponginess, synovitis due to rheumatoid arthritis. If there is toe deformity, assess whether there is impingement on the other toes, e.g. overriding hallux valgus. Pain and stiffness at the first MTP joint suggest hallux rigidus.

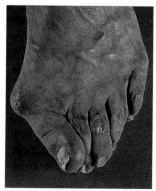

Fig. 14.54 Hallux valgus overriding the second toe.

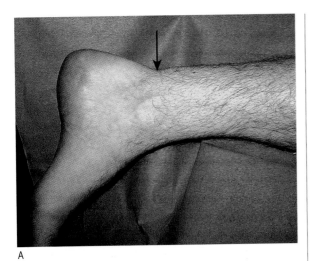

A

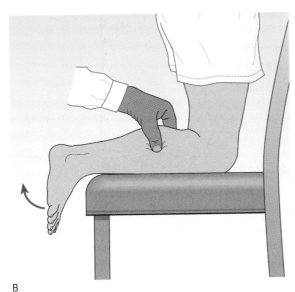

B

Fig. 14.55 Ruptured Achilles tendon. (A) The arrow indicates the site of a palpable defect in the Achilles tendon. **(B)** Thomson's test. Failure of the foot to plantar flex when the calf is squeezed is pathognomonic of an acute rupture of the Achilles tendon.

Achilles tendon

Examination sequence

■ Ask the patient to kneel with both knees on a chair.
■ Palpate the gastrocnemius and Achilles tendon for focal tenderness and soft-tissue swelling. Achilles tendon rupture is often palpable as a discrete gap in the tendon about 5 cm above the calcaneal insertion (Fig. 14.55A).

Thomson's (Simmond's) test

Squeeze the calf just distal to the level of maximum circumference. If the Achilles tendon is intact, plantar flexion of the foot will occur (Fig. 14.55B).

14.26 Bone conditions associated with pathological fracture

- Osteoporosis
- Osteomalacia
- Primary or secondary tumour
- Osteogenesis imperfecta
- Renal osteodystrophy
- Parathyroid bone disease
- Paget's disease

14.27 Risk factors for osteoporosis

- Age
- Sex
  - Female (lifetime risk of fracture over age of 50 years: 1 in 2 women and 1 in 5 men)
- Menstrual history
  - Decreased menstrual cycling, i.e. early menopause, amenorrhoea
- Past history
  - Previous fragility fracture
  - Rheumatoid arthritis
  - Malabsorption
  - Hypogonadism
- Drug history
  - Previous or current steroid therapy
- Family history
  - First-degree relative (risk increased × 2)
- Social history
  - Immobilisation, smoking, alcohol, low calcium/vitamin D in diet

14

FRACTURES, DISLOCATIONS AND TRAUMA

A fracture is a breach in the structural integrity of a bone. This may arise in:

- normal bone from excessive force
- normal bone from repetitive load-bearing activity (stress fracture)
- bone of abnormal structure (pathological fracture) (Box 14.26) with minimal or no trauma.

The epidemiology of fractures varies geographically. There is an epidemic of osteoporotic fractures because of increasing elderly populations. Fractures resulting from road traffic accidents and falls are decreasing because of legislative and preventive measures, e.g. seat belts, air bags and improved road engineering.

Osteoporosis is systemic skeletal loss of bone mineral density with associated microarchitectural deterioration. It is the most common cause of abnormal bone structure. The incidence increases with age, particularly in postmenopausal women (Box 14.27). In the absence of complications, osteoporosis is asymptomatic. Although any osteoporotic bone can fracture, common sites are the distal radius (Fig. 14.56), neck of femur (Fig. 14.43), proximal humerus and the spinal vertebrae. Caucasians in Europe have a lifetime risk of osteoporotic fracture of 50% in women and 20% in men.

A fracture may occur in the context of severe trauma (Ch. 19). Complications of fractures are shown in Box 14.28.

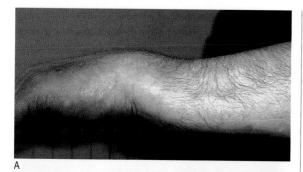

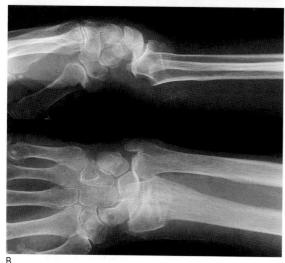

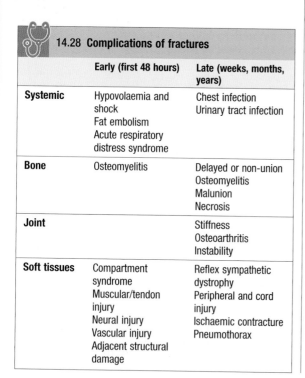

Fig. 14.56 Colles' fracture. **(A)** Clinical appearance of dinner fork deformity. **(B)** X-ray appearance.

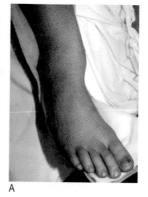

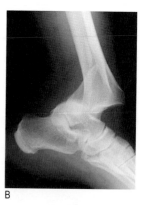

Fig. 14.57 Ankle deformity. **(A)** Clinical appearance. **(B)** Lateral X-ray view showing tibiotalar fracture dislocation.

History

Establish the mechanism of injury. For instance, a patient who has fallen from a height on to his heels may have obvious fractures of the calcaneal bones in his ankles but is also at risk of fractures of the proximal femur, pelvis and vertebral column.

Physical examination

Use the Look – Feel – Move approach. Observe patients closely to see if they move the affected part and are able to weight bear.

Examination sequence

Look
- See if the skin is intact. If there is a breach in the skin and the wound communicates with the fracture, the fracture is open or compound; otherwise it is closed.
- Look for associated bruising, deformity, swelling or wound infection (Fig. 14.57).

Feel
- Gently feel for local tenderness.
- Feel distal to the suspected fracture to establish if sensation and pulses are present.

Move
- Establish whether the patient can move joints distal and proximal to the fracture.
- Do not move a fracture site to see if crepitus is present; this causes additional pain and bleeding (Figs 14.58 and 14.59).

Putting it all together

Decide whether joints are affected and establish the mode of onset. If the problem was caused by a major injury follow the system in Chapter 19. Which joints, and are they affected symmetrically? How do the symptoms behave during the day? Ascertain any extra-articular

14.28 Complications of fractures

	Early (first 48 hours)	Late (weeks, months, years)
Systemic	Hypovolaemia and shock Fat embolism Acute respiratory distress syndrome	Chest infection Urinary tract infection
Bone	Osteomyelitis	Delayed or non-union Osteomyelitis Malunion Necrosis
Joint		Stiffness Osteoarthritis Instability
Soft tissues	Compartment syndrome Muscular/tendon injury Neural injury Vascular injury Adjacent structural damage	Reflex sympathetic dystrophy Peripheral and cord injury Ischaemic contracture Pneumothorax

symptoms. The problem may be focal, e.g. lateral epicondylitis of the elbow – 'tennis elbow' – medial meniscal tear of the knee, osteoarthritis at the hip, or systemic.

The history and examination direct your investigations and produce a confident diagnosis (Box 14.29).

If the joints are not involved, the problem may arise from the surrounding tissues or be referred from another site, e.g. in nerve root impingement. The process may be inflammatory (infective or non-infective) or non-inflammatory. Features of systemic illness, e.g. weight loss, rash, e.g. rheumatoid arthritis, psoriasis or SLE, suggest a systemic cause.

Investigations

For each suspected fracture, X-ray two views (at least) at perpendicular planes of the affected bone, and include the joints above and below.

INVESTIGATIONS

See Box 14.30.

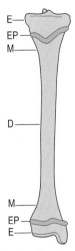

Fig. 14.58 Describing a fracture. The site of the fracture: anatomical divisions. D, diaphysis or shaft; E, epiphysis; EP, epiphyseal plate; M, metaphysis.

14.29 Describing a fracture

- What bone(s) is/are involved?
- Is the fracture open (compound) or closed?
- Is the fracture complete or incomplete?
- Where is the bone fractured (intra-articular/epiphysis/physis/metaphysis/diaphysis)?
- What is the fracture's configuration (transverse/oblique/spiral/comminuted/butterfly fragment)?
- What components of deformity are present?
  - Translation is the shift of the distal fragment in relation to the proximal bone. The direction is defined by the movement of the distal fragment, e.g. dorsal or volar, and is measured as a percentage
  - Angulation is defined by the movement of the distal fragment, measured in degrees
  - Rotation is measured in degrees along the longitudinal axis of the bone, e.g. for spiral fracture of the tibia or phalanges
  - Shortening: proximal migration of the distal fragment can cause shortening in an oblique fracture. Shortening may also occur if there has been impaction at the fracture site, e.g. Colles' fracture of the distal radius
- Is there distal nerve or vascular deficit?
- What is the state of the tissues associated with the fracture – soft tissues and joints, e.g. fracture blisters, dislocation?

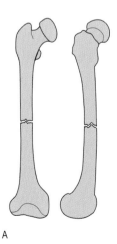
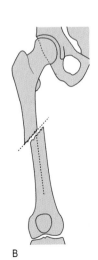
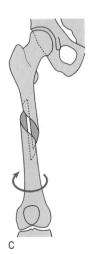
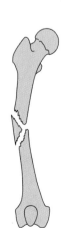
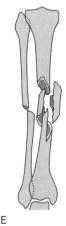

| A | B | C | D | E |

Fig. 14.59 The nature of the fracture. (A) If there is no deformity (no movement of the bone ends relative to one another), the fracture is in anatomical position. **(B)** Oblique fracture: the fracture runs at an oblique angle of 30° or more. **(C)** Spiral fracture: simple spiral fractures result from twisting forces. **(D)** Multifragmentary (comminuted) fracture: there are more than two fragments. **(E)** Multifragmentary complex fracture: there is no contact between the main fragments after reduction.

14.30 Common musculoskeletal investigations

Investigation	Indication/comment
Bedside	
Schirmer tear test: salivary flow test	Keratoconjunctivitis sicca (dry eyes), Sjögren's syndrome
Urinalysis	
Protein	Secondary amyloid in rheumatoid arthritis and other chronic arthropathies
	Drug adverse effects, e.g. myocrisin, penicillamine
Blood	Glomerular disease, e.g. SLE, vasculitis
Haematological	
Full blood count	Anaemia in inflammatory arthritis, blood loss after trauma
	Neutrophilia in sepsis and very acute inflammation, e.g. acute gout
	Leukopenia in SLE, Felty's syndrome and adverse effects of antirheumatic drug therapy
Erythrocyte sedimentation rate/plasma viscosity/C-reactive protein	Non-specific indicator of inflammation or sepsis
	Acute-phase protein
Biochemical	
Urea and creatinine	$\uparrow$ in renal impairment, e.g. secondary amyloid in rheumatoid arthritis or adverse drug effect
Uric acid	May be $\uparrow$ in gout. Levels may be normal during an acute attack
Calcium	$\downarrow$ in osteomalacia; normal in osteoporosis
Alkaline phosphatase	$\uparrow$ in Paget's disease, metastases, osteomalacia, and immediately after fractures
Angiotensin-converting enzyme	$\uparrow$ in sarcoidosis
Urinary albumin : creatinine ratio	Glomerular disease, e.g. vasculitis, SLE
Serological	
IgM rheumatoid factor	$\uparrow$ titres in 60–70% of cases of rheumatoid arthritis; occasionally low titres found in other connective diseases. Present in up to 15% of normal population
Anticyclic citrullinated peptides (ACPA)	Present in 60–70% of cases of rheumatoid arthritis and up to 10 years before onset of disease. Highly specific for rheumatoid arthritis. Occasionally found in Sjögren's syndrome
Antinuclear factors	$\uparrow$ titres in most cases of SLE; low titres in other connective tissue diseases and rheumatoid arthritis
Anti-Ro, Anti-La	Sjögren's syndrome
Anti-dsDNA	SLE
Anti-Sm	SLE
Anti-RNP	Mixed connective tissue disease
Antineutrophil cytoplasmic antibodies	Granulomatosis with polyangiitis, polyarteritis nodosa, Churg–Strauss vasculitis
Imaging	
Plain radiography (X-rays)	Fractures, erosions in rheumatoid arthritis and psoriatic arthritis, osteophytes and joint space loss in osteoarthritis, bone changes in Paget's disease, pseudofractures (Looser's zones) in osteomalacia
Ultrasonography	Detection of effusion, synovitis, cartilage breaks, enthesitis and erosions in inflammatory arthritis
	Detection of bursae, tendon pathology and osteophytes
Isotope bone scan	Increased uptake in Paget's disease, bone tumour
MR imaging	For joint structure and soft-tissue imaging
CT scanning	High-resolution scans of thorax for pulmonary fibrosis
Dual-energy X-ray absorptiometry (DXA)	Gold standard for determining osteoporosis. Usual scans are of lumbar spine and hip
Joint aspiration	
Polarised light microscopy	Positively birefringent rhomboidal crystals – calcium pyrophosphate
	Negatively birefringent needle-shaped crystals – monosodium urate monohydrate
Bacteriology	Raised white cell count in infection
	Organism may be isolated
Biopsy and histology	Synovitis – rheumatoid arthritis and other inflammatory arthritis

Ben Stenson
Steve Turner

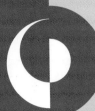

Babies and children

15

15

EXAMINATION OF BABIES

A baby is a neonate for the first 4 weeks of life and an infant for the whole of the first year. Neonates are classified by gestational age or birthweight (Box 15.1).

SYMPTOMS AND DEFINITIONS

Infants cannot report symptoms so you must recognise the signs of illness, which are non-specific in young infants. Always take seriously the concerns of parents as they describe symptoms.

Pallor

Always investigate pallor in a newborn as it implies anaemia or poor perfusion. Newborn infants have higher haemoglobin levels than older children and are therefore not normally pale. Haemoglobin levels <120g/dl in the perinatal period are low. Preterm infants look red because they lack subcutaneous fat.

Respiratory distress

Respiratory distress is tachypnoea (respiratory rate) >60 breaths/min with intercostal and subcostal indrawing, sternal recession, nasal flaring and the use of accessory muscles.

Cyanosis

The bluish discoloration of the lips and mucous membranes due to hypoxia is difficult to see unless oxygen saturation (SpO_2) is <80% (normal is >95%) because of the high haematocrit of newborn infants (Box 15.2). Causes include congenital heart disease and respiratory disease and it always needs investigation (p. 147).

Acrocyanosis

Acrocyanosis is a bluish-purple discoloration of the hands and feet and, when the newborn is centrally pink, is a normal finding.

Jaundice

Many newborns develop jaundice in the early days after birth. Inspect the sclerae in newborns with coloured skin or you may miss it (Box 15.3). Normal or physiological causes cannot be distinguished clinically from pathological ones.

Jitteriness

Jitteriness is high-frequency tremor of the limbs. It is common in term infants in the first few days. It is stilled by stimulating the infant and is not associated with other physiological disturbance. Exclude hypoglycaemia, polycythaemia and neonatal abstinence syndrome (due to withdrawal of drugs) if it is excessive. Infrequent jerks in light sleep are common and normal, but regular clonic jerks are abnormal.

Dysmorphism

Dysmorphism is an abnormality of body structure. Identifying dysmorphic features is subjective because of human variability. Individual features may be minor and isolated, or may signify a major problem requiring definitive investigation and management. When certain dysmorphic features occur together in a recognisable pattern, a 'dysmorphic syndrome' is present, e.g. Down's syndrome (p. 47). Discuss possible dysmorphic features with parents in the immediate newborn period with great caution and sensitivity.

Hypotonia

Hypotonia (reduced tone) may be obvious when you handle the infant or the infant may lack normal flexion at rest. Term infants' muscle tone normally produces a flexed posture at the hips, knees and elbows. Hypotonia occurs in systemic conditions such as hypoxia, hypoglycaemia or septicaemia or may be due to a specific problem of brain, nerve or muscle. Preterm infants have

---

EBE 15.2 Neonatal congenital heart disease screening

Measurement of oxygen saturation (SpO_2) by pulse oximetry is a simple, non-invasive method to assist clinical examination of the neonate in screening for congenital heart disease.

Ewer AK, Middleton LJ, Furmston AT et al. PulseOx Study Group. Pulse oximetry screening for congenital heart defects in newborn infants (PulseOx). Lancet 2011;378:785–794.

EBE 15.3 Jaundice in the newborn

When looking for jaundice in the newborn, examine the naked baby in bright, preferably natural light. Do not rely on visual inspection alone to estimate the bilirubin level in a baby with jaundice.

NICE. Neonatal jaundice. 2010. Available online at: www.nice.org.uk/CG98.

15.1 Classification of newborn infants

Birthweight	
Extremely low	<1000 grams
Very low	<1500 grams
Low	<2500 grams
Normal	≥2500 grams
Gestational age	
Extremely preterm	<28 weeks
Preterm	<37 weeks (<259th day)
Term	37–42 weeks
Post-term	>42 weeks (>294th day)

lower tone than term infants and are much less flexed at rest.

Apgar score

This first clinical assessment of a neonate is made immediately after birth. It describes the tone, colour, breathing, heart rate and response to stimulation. Each element is scored 0, 1 or 2 (Box 15.4), giving a total maximum of 10. Healthy neonates commonly score 8–10 at 1 and 5 minutes. The score provides feedback about the need for, and efficacy of, resuscitation. A low score should increase with time. A decreasing score is concerning. Persistently low scores at 10 minutes predict death or later disability. Neonates with scores of less than 8 at 5 minutes require continued evaluation until it is clear they are healthy.

THE HISTORY

Ask the mother and look in the maternal notes for the medical history (Box 15.5).

In later infancy, ask additional questions about specific signs and systems as well as obtaining information about developmental progress, depending on the presenting complaint (Box 15.6).

THE PHYSICAL EXAMINATION

Timing and efficacy of the routine neonatal examination

Examine a newborn with the parents present. There is no ideal time. If performed on day 1 some congenital heart disease may be missed because signs are not yet present. If delayed, some babies will present before this with illness that may have been detected earlier. Nine per cent of neonates have an identifiable congenital abnormality, but most are not serious. Always clearly record which elements of the examination you perform to avoid problems if symptoms and signs develop later. Explain clearly to the parents the limitation of the examination (Box 15.7).

15.4 Apgar score

Clinical score	0	1	2
Heart rate	Absent	<100 bpm	>100 bpm
Respiratory effort	Absent	Slow and irregular	Good: strong
Muscle tone	Flaccid	Some flexion of arms and legs	Active movement
Reflex irritability	No responses	Grimace	Crying vigorously, sneeze or cough
Colour	Blue, pale	Pink body, blue extremities	Pink all over

15.5 The medical history

Family history of illness
Outcome of previous pregnancies
Maternal health in the current pregnancy, including drug history
Issues identified by antenatal screening tests
Current gestation
Mode of delivery
Duration of membrane rupture
Pyrexia in labour
Meconium staining of the amniotic fluid
Non-reassuring fetal status during labour
Condition at birth, including cord blood gas results and Apgar scores
Passage of urine and meconium since birth

15.6 Developmental attainment of preschool children at different ages*

	4 months	6 months	10 months	1–2 years	2–3 years	3–5 years
Gross motor	Good head control on pull to sit Keeps back straight when held in sitting position	Supports weight on hands when laid prone Rolls front to back	Sits unsupported Pulls to stand	Walks without support	Runs Bounces on trampoline	Pedals a tricycle
Fine motor	Hands opening Holds objects placed in hand	Transfers objects from hand to hand and to mouth	Pincer grip bilaterally without hand preference	Holds a crayon and scribbles	Can draw a circle	Can draw a cross and square. Can draw a face/man
Personal social	Shows interest in toys Laughs, vocalises	Variety of speech noises. Plays peep-bo	Starting to understand some words Claps hands	Has 10–20 recognisable words	Can communicate verbally	500–1500 words Dry by day

*Development is extremely variable and failure to attain only one milestone is of little significance whereas failure to attain several milestones is cause for concern.

EBE 15.7 **Structural heart lesions in the newborn**

Two per cent of babies have a cardiac murmur, but only half of these have structural heart disease. More than half of the infants with important structural heart lesions have no murmur in the immediate newborn period.

Ainsworth S, Wyllie JP, Wren C. Prevalence and significance of cardiac murmurs in neonates. Arch Dis Child 1999;80:F43–F45.

15.8 **Skin characteristics**

Colour

- Jaundice
- Pallor
- Plethora

Rash

- Distribution
- Size
- Colour
- Macules or papules
- Pus
- Bleeding
- Exudation

General examination

Examine babies and infants in a warm place. Have a system to avoid omitting anything, but refrain from an overly rigid approach as you may be unable to perform key elements if you unsettle the baby. Examine newborn infants on a bed or examination table but older infants on their parent's lap.

Examination sequence

- Carefully observe whether the baby looks well and is well grown.
- Look for
  - cyanosis
  - respiratory distress
  - pallor
  - plethora (suggesting polycythaemia).
- Note the posture and behaviour.
- Note any dysmorphic features.
- Auscultate the heart and palpate the abdomen if the baby is quiet.
- If the baby cries, does the cry sound normal?

Leave things that may disturb the baby until later.

Skin

Normal findings

The skin may look normal, dry, wrinkled or vernix-covered in healthy babies. There may be meconium staining of the skin and nails.

Prominent capillaries commonly cause pink areas called 'stork's beak marks' at the nape of the neck, the eyelids and the glabella (Fig. 15.1). The facial ones fade without treatment over subsequent months. Marks on the neck often persist. Milia (fine white spots) and acne neonatorum (larger cream-coloured spots) are due to collected glandular secretions and disappear within 2–4 weeks.

Abnormal findings

Document any trauma, e.g. scalp cuts, bruising.

Dense capillary haemangiomas (port wine stains) will not fade. Laser treatment may help. Around the eye they may indicate Sturge–Weber syndrome (a facial port wine stain with an underlying brain lesion associated with risk of later seizures, cerebral calcification and reduced cognitive function). Melanocytic naevi require

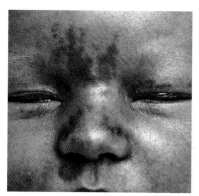

Fig. 15.1 Stork's beak mark.

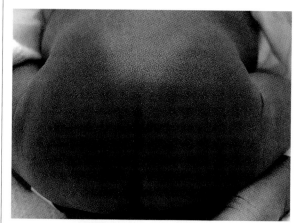

Fig. 15.2 Mongolian blue spot.

follow-up and treatment by a plastic surgeon or dermatologist. A mongolian blue spot (Fig. 15.2) is an area of bluish discoloration over the buttocks, back and thighs. Easily mistaken for bruising, it usually fades in the first year. Erythema toxicum is a common fleeting blanching idiopathic maculopapular rash of no consequence, seen on the trunk and face.

Subcutaneous fat necrosis causes palpable firm plaques, often with some erythema under the skin, over the body. If extensive, there can be associated hypercalcaemia that may require treatment. Blisters or bullae are usually pathological; causes include infection and significant skin disease (Box 15.8).

15.9 Neonatal head shapes

Head shape	Description
Microcephalic (small-headed)	Small cranial vault
Megalencephalic (large-headed)	Large cranial vault
Hydrocephalic (water-headed)	Large cranial vault due to enlarged ventricles
Brachycephalic (short-headed)	
Dolichocephalic (long-headed)	
Plagiocephalic (oblique-headed)	Asymmetrical skull

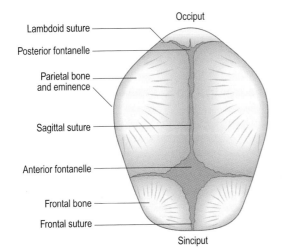

Fig. 15.3 The fetal skull from above.

Labels: Occiput, Lambdoid suture, Posterior fontanelle, Parietal bone and eminence, Sagittal suture, Anterior fontanelle, Frontal bone, Frontal suture, Sinciput

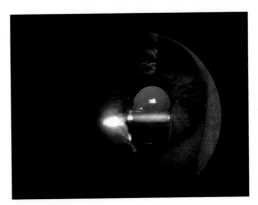

Fig. 15.4 Coloboma.

In rare cases the cranial sutures are prematurely fused (synostosis), producing ridging, and the head shape is usually abnormal.

Head

Examination sequence

- Note the baby's head shape (Box 15.9) and any swellings.
- Feel the anterior fontanelle (Fig. 15.3) and whether it is sunken, flat or bulging.
- Palpate the cranial sutures.

Normal findings

Head moulding is common after birth. Caput succedaneum is soft-tissue swelling over the vertex due to pressure in labour. The cranial sutures may be overriding, giving a palpable step.

Abnormal findings

Cephalhaematoma is a firm, usually parietal swelling due to a collection of blood under the periosteum of a skull bone. It may be bilateral and is not mobile. Periosteal reaction at the margins gives the feeling of a raised edge. No treatment is required. Do not confuse this with the boggy, mobile, poorly localised swelling of subgaleal (beneath the flat sheet of fibrous tissue that caps the skull) haemorrhage which can conceal a large blood loss capable of causing life-threatening shock if unrecognised.

Separated cranial sutures with an obvious gap are due to raised intracranial pressure.

Eyes

Examination sequence

- Look at the eyebrows, lashes, lids and eyeballs.
- Gently retract the lower eyelid and look at the sclera for jaundice or any discoloration.
- Test ocular movements and vestibular function:
  - Turn the newborn's head to one side; watch as the eyes move in the opposite direction. This is called doll's-eye movements and disappears in infancy (Fig. 12.25).
  - Hold the infant upright at arm's length and move him in a horizontal arc. The infant should look in the direction of movement and have optokinetic nystagmus. This response becomes damped by 3 months.

Normal findings

Harmless yellow crusting without inflammation is common after birth in infants with narrow lacrimal ducts.

Term infants usually fix visually.

Abnormal findings

Eye infection gives a red eye and purulent secretions. An abnormal pupil shape is usually due to coloboma (a defect in the iris inferiorly that gives the pupil a keyhole appearance: Fig. 15.4). This can affect deeper structures in the eyeball, including the optic nerve, leading to visual impairment. It can be associated with various syndromes, as can microphthalmia (small eyeballs). Large eyeballs that feel hard when palpated through the lids suggest buphthalmos (congenital glaucoma).

Ophthalmoscopy

Examination sequence

- Hold the baby in your arms. Gently rotate your upper body from side to side so that the baby will open his eyes.
- Keep your eye close to the ophthalmoscope and look through it at each pupil from about 20 cm. You should see the red reflex of reflected light from the retina (like 'red eye' in a photo).

15

Normal findings

Puffy eyes in the first days after birth impede the examination. If this is the case, always repeat the examination later as, if missed, failure to detect and treat a cataract will cause permanent amblyopia.

Abnormal findings

No red reflex suggests a cataract; refer to an ophthalmologist.

Nose

Examination sequence

- Check that the nostrils are patent by blocking each one with your finger in turn to show that the infant breathes easily through the other.

Mouth

Examination sequence

- Gently press down on the lower jaw so that the baby will open his mouth. Do not use a wooden tongue depressor as this may cause trauma or infection.
- Shine a torch into the mouth and look at the tongue and the palate.
- Palpate the palate using your fingertip.

Normal findings

Epstein's pearls are small white mucosal cysts on the palate that disappear spontaneously.

White coating on the tongue which is easily scraped off with a swab is due to curdled milk.

Abnormal findings

Macroglossia (a large protruding tongue) occurs in Beckwith–Wiedemann syndrome. A normal-sized tongue protrudes through a small mouth in Down's syndrome (glossoptosis). Ankyloglossia (tongue tie) is when the lingual frenulum which joins the midline of the tongue to the floor of the mouth is abnormally short. Consequently the tongue cannot move freely, interfering with feeding. A white coating on the tongue, not easily removed and which may bleed when scraped, is due to the fungus, Candida albicans (thrush).

Cleft palate may involve the soft palate or both hard and soft palates. It can be midline, unilateral or bilateral and may involve the gum (alveolus). Cleft lip can appear in isolation or in association with it. Refer affected infants early to a specialist multidisciplinary team. Micrognathia (a small jaw) is sometimes associated with cleft palate in the Pierre Robin syndrome with posterior displacement of the tongue (glossoptosis) and upperairway obstruction.

A ranula is a mucous cyst on the floor of the mouth related to the sublingual or submandibular salivary ducts. Congenital ranulas may resolve spontaneously but sometimes require surgery.

Teeth usually begin to erupt at around 6 months but can be present at birth.

Ears

Examination sequence

- Note the size, shape and position.
- The helix should join the cranium above an imaginary line through the inner corners of the eyes.
- Check that the external auditory meatus looks normal.
- Otoscopic examination is not required for the newborn but is indicated in young infants to exclude otitis. A carer should hold the child to keep the head still (Fig. 15.22).
- Choose the smallest earpiece available that fits the child's meatus.
- Gently pull the earlobe down and back to straighten the external auditory canal.
- Insert the otoscope to approximately 0.5 cm. Adjust the angle gently until you see the tympanic membrane.

Normal findings

The helix can be temporarily folded due to local pressure in utero.

Preauricular skin tags do not require investigation.

Abnormal findings

See Chapter 13.

Neck

Examination sequence

- Inspect the neck for asymmetry, sinuses and swellings.
- Palpate any masses. Use SPACESPIT to decide their likely origin (Box 3.11).
- Transilluminate swellings to see if they are cystic. Cystic swellings glow, as the light is easily transmitted through clear liquid. Solid or blood-filled swellings do not.

Normal findings

One-third of normal neonates have palpable cervical, inguinal or axillary lymph nodes. Neck asymmetry is often due to fetal posture and usually resolves.

Abnormal findings

A lump in the sternocleidomastoid muscle (sternomastoid 'tumour') is caused by a fibrosed haematoma with resultant muscle shortening. This may produce torticollis, with the head turned in the contralateral direction.

Cardiovascular examination

Examination sequence

- Observe the baby for pallor, cyanosis and sweating.
- Count the respiratory rate.
- Look for the apex beat in the mid-clavicular line in the fourth or fifth intercostal space.
- Palpate it with your palm.
- Note if the heart beat moves your hand up and down (parasternal heave) or if you feel a vibration (thrill).

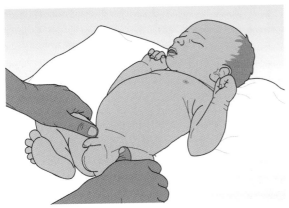

Fig. 15.5 Palpating the femoral pulses. The pulse can be difficult to feel at first; use a point halfway between the pubic tubercle and the anterior superior iliac spine as a guide.

- Count the heart rate for 15 seconds and multiply by 4. Record the heart rate.
- Feel the femoral pulses by placing your thumbs or fingertips over the mid-inguinal points while abducting the hips (Fig. 15.5).
- Auscultate the heart. Start at the apex using the stethoscope bell (best for low-pitched sounds). Then use the diaphragm in all positions for high-pitched sounds and murmurs (Fig. 15.6).
- Describe the heart sounds S_1 and S_2, splitting of S_2, any additional heart sounds and the presence of murmurs. The fast heart rate of a newborn makes it difficult to time additional sounds. Take time to tune into the different rate of the harsh breath sounds of a newborn as they are easily confused with a murmur.
- Do not measure the blood pressure of healthy babies. In ill babies, cuff measurements overestimate the values when compared with invasive measurements. The cuff width should be at least two-thirds of the distance from the elbow to the shoulder tip.
- Palpate the abdomen for hepatomegaly (p. 362).

Normal findings

In the early newborn period the femoral pulses may feel normal in an infant who later presents with coarctation because an open ductus arteriosus can maintain flow to the descending aorta. Routine measurement of postductal saturation is increasingly popular as an additional newborn screening test to avoid missing this. The liver edge is often palpable in healthy infants.

Heart rates between 80 and 160 bpm can be normal in the newborn, depending on the arousal state (Box 15.10).

Abnormal findings

Infants with heart failure typically look pale and sweaty and often present with respiratory distress (p. 356).

If the apex beat is displaced laterally there may be cardiomegaly, or mediastinal shift due to contralateral pneumothorax or pleural effusion.

Weak or absent femoral pulses suggest coarctation of the aorta. In older children and adults coarctation causes

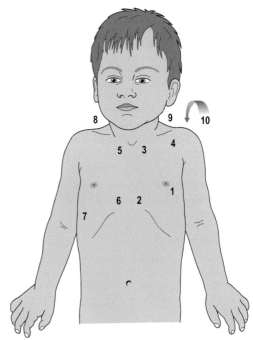

Fig. 15.6 Auscultation positions. Recommended order of auscultation: **1**, apex; **2**, left lower sternal edge; **3**, left upper sternal edge; **4**, left infraclavicular; **5**, right upper sternal edge; **6**, right lower sternal edge; **7**, right mid-axillary line; **8**, right side of neck; **9**, left side of neck; **10**, posteriorly.

15.10 Normal ranges or values for heart and respiratory rate in the newborn		
Sign	**Preterm neonate**	**Term neonate**
Heart rate (bpm)	120–160	100–140
Respiratory rate (breaths/min)	40–60	30–50

radiofemoral delay but this is not identifiable in the newborn.

Patent ductus arteriosus may cause a short systolic murmur in the early days of life because the pulmonary and systemic blood pressures are similar and this limits shunting through the duct. The murmur progressively lengthens over subsequent weeks or months to become the continuous 'machinery' murmur recognised later in childhood.

Murmurs are heard in up to 2% of neonates but only a minority have a structural heart problem. Many murmurs are transient. An echocardiogram is needed to make a structural diagnosis and this should be performed before discharge from hospital. If this is not possible and the infant is clinically well, with no respiratory distress and has normal femoral pulses and postductal oxygen saturation >95%, it may be reasonable to arrange outpatient review at 4–6 weeks, with advice to the parents to consult a doctor if they are concerned about breathlessness, poor feeding or cyanosis.

Respiratory examination

Examination sequence

- Note chest shape and symmetry of chest movement.
- Count the respiratory rate and listen for additional noises with breathing.
- Look for signs of respiratory distress: tachypnoea, suprasternal, intercostal and subcostal recession, flaring of the alar nasae.
- Percussion of the newborn's chest is not helpful.
- Use the diaphragm to auscultate anteriorly, laterally and posteriorly. Assess the air entry on each side and note any crackles and wheeze. Breath sounds in the healthy newborn have a bronchial quality compared with older individuals (p. 154).

Normal findings

Male and female newborn infants at term have small buds of palpable breast tissue. Small amounts of fluid are sometimes discharged from the nipple in the early days after birth.

Abnormal findings

Stridor is a large-airway sound and is predominantly inspiratory (pp. 140 and 310). Stridor and indrawing beginning on day 2–3 of life in an otherwise well baby may be due to laryngomalacia (softness of the larynx). Causes of respiratory distress include retained lung fluid, infection, immaturity, aspiration, congenital anomaly, pneumothorax, heart failure and metabolic acidosis.

Abdominal examination

Examination sequence

- Remove the nappy.
- Inspect the abdomen, including the umbilicus and groins, noting any swellings.
- From the infant's right side, gently palpate with the flat of your warm right hand. Palpate superficially before feeling for deeper structures.
- Palpate for the spleen. In the neonate it enlarges down the left flank rather than towards the right iliac fossa.
- Palpate for hepatomegaly:
  - Place your right hand flat across the abdomen beneath the right costal margin.
  - Feel the liver edge against the side of your index finger.
  - If you feel more than the liver edge, measure the distance in the mid-clavicular line from the costal margin to the liver's edge. Describe it in fingerbreadths or measure it with a tape in centimetres.
- Look at the anus to confirm that it is present, patent and in a normal position.
- Digital rectal examination is usually unnecessary and could cause an anal fissure. Indications include suspected rectal atresia or stenosis and delayed passage of meconium. Put on gloves and lubricate your little finger. Gently press your fingertip against the anus until you feel the muscle resistance relax and insert your finger up to your distal interphalangeal joint.

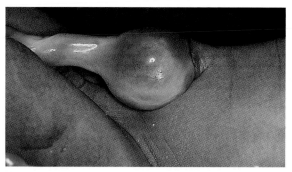

Fig. 15.7 Small exomphalos with loops of bowel in the umbilicus.

Normal findings

Distension from a feed or swallowed air is common.

You may see the contour of individual bowel loops through the thin anterior abdominal wall in the newborn, particularly with intestinal obstruction.

The umbilical cord stump usually separates after 4–5 days. A granuloma may appear later as a moist, pink lump in the base of the umbilicus. A small amount of bleeding from the umbilicus is common in the neonate.

The liver edge is often palpable in healthy infants.

In the neonate the kidneys are often palpable, especially if balloted (Fig. 9.8).

Abnormal findings

In excessive bleeding from the umbilicus, check that the infant received vitamin K, and consider clotting factor XIII deficiency. Spreading erythema around the umbilicus suggests infective omphalitis, and requires urgent treatment.

Umbilical hernias are common, easily reduced, have very low risk of complication and close spontaneously in infancy. An omphalocoele, or exomphalos (Fig. 15.7), is a herniation through the umbilicus containing intestines and other viscera covered by a membrane that includes the umbilical cord. It may be associated with other malformations or a chromosomal abnormality. Gastroschisis is a defect in the anterior abdominal wall with intestines herniated through it. There is no covering membrane. The commonest site is above and to the right of the umbilicus.

A hydrocoele is a collection of fluid beneath the tunica vaginalis of the testis and/or the spermatic cord (p. 236). Most resolve spontaneously in infancy. Inguinal hernias are common in the newborn, especially in boys and preterm infants (Fig. 15.8).

Meconium in the nappy does not guarantee that the baby has a patent anus because meconium can be passed through a rectovaginal fistula.

Perineum

Examination sequence

Female

- Abduct the legs and gently separate the labia.
- In preterm infants the labia minora appear prominent, giving a masculinised appearance, which resolves spontaneously over the next few weeks. Milky secretions in the vagina are normal.

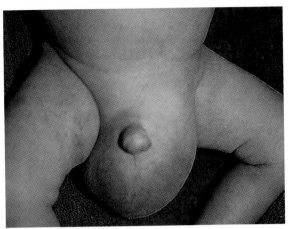

Fig. 15.8 Bilateral inguinal hernias in a preterm infant. An inguinal hernia is primarily a groin swelling; only when it is large does it extend into the scrotum.

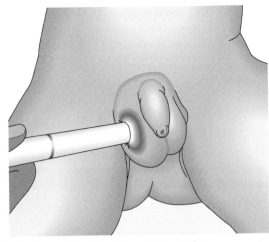

Fig. 15.9 How to transilluminate a scrotal swelling.

Later in the first week there is sometimes slight vaginal bleeding (pseudomenses) as the infant uterus 'withdraws' from maternal hormones. Vaginal skin tags are common and do not require investigation or treatment.

Male

- Do not attempt to retract the foreskin. It is normal for it to be adherent in babies.
- Check that the urethral meatus is at the tip of the penis.
- Note the shape of the penis.
- Palpate the testes.
- If you cannot feel the testes in the scrotum, assess for undescended, ectopic or retractile testes. Palpate the abdomen for smooth lumps, moving your fingers down from over the inguinal canal to the scrotum and perineum.
- A retractile testis just below the inguinal canal may be gently milked into the scrotum. Re-examine at 6 weeks if there is any doubt about the position of the testes.
- Transilluminate any large scrotal swelling by placing a torch against it to see if the light is transmitted through the skin. This suggests a hydrocoele but can be misleading, because a hernia of thin-walled bowel may transilluminate (Fig. 15.9).
- An inguinal hernia usually produces a groin swelling but if large this may extend into the scrotum. Try to reduce it by gently pushing the contents upwards from the scrotum through the inguinal canal into the abdomen. If this is possible it is an indirect inguinal hernia (Fig. 15.8).

Normal findings

The testes are smooth, soft and 0.7×1 cm across. The right testis usually descends later than the left and sits higher in the scrotum.

Abnormal findings

In hypospadias the meatal opening is on the ventral aspect of the glans, the ventral shaft of the penis, the scrotum or more posteriorly on the perineum (Figs 15.10 and 15.11A). In epispadias it is on the dorsum of the penis – this is rare. Chordee is curvature of the penis and is commonly associated with hypospadias and tethering of the foreskin (Fig. 15.11B).

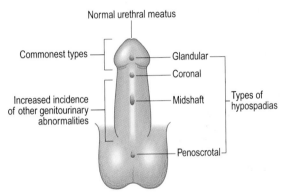

Fig. 15.10 Varieties of hypospadias.

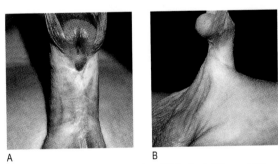

A   B

Fig. 15.11 Hypospadias and chordee. (A) Penile shaft hypospadias. **(B)** In this lateral view, the ventral curvature of the penis (chordee) can be seen.

Spine and sacrum

Examination sequence

- Turn the baby over and inspect the back from the neck to the sacrum.
- Palpate the entire vertebral column to check for neural tube defects.

Normal findings

Sacral dimples are common. They are not important provided the base of the dimple has normal skin.

15

Abnormal findings

Pigmented patches may indicate spina bifida occulta. Dimples above the natal cleft, away from the midline, or hairy or pigmented patches with a base that cannot be visualised require further investigation.

Neurological examination

This includes tone, posture, movement and primitive reflexes.

Examination sequence

- Look for asymmetry in posture and movement and for muscle wasting.
- To assess tone, pick the baby up and note if he is stiff or floppy. Note any difference between each side.
- Power is difficult to assess and depends on the state of arousal. Look for strong symmetrical limb and trunk movements and grasp.
- Tendon reflexes are only of value in assessing infants with neurological or muscular abnormalities.
- Check sensation by seeing whether the baby withdraws from gentle stimuli. Do not inflict painful stimuli or use a pin or needle.
- Check eyesight by carrying the alert baby to a dark corner where she may open her eyes wide. If moved to a bright area she will then screw up her eyes.
- Test hearing by noting the startle response to a sound. Ideally electronic audiological screening should be performed in the newborn period.

Normal findings

Movements should be equal on both sides.

Tone varies and may be floppy after a feed.

Reflexes are brisk in term infants, often with a few beats of clonus.

The plantar reflex is normally extensor in the newborn.

Abnormal findings

Hypotonic infants may have a 'frog-like' posture with abducted hips and extended elbows. Causes include Down's syndrome, meningitis and sepsis.

Increased tone may cause back and neck arching and limb extension; the baby feels stiff when picked up. Causes include meningitis, asphyxia and intracranial haemorrhage.

Erb's palsy affects brachial plexus roots C5 and C6, producing reduced movement of the arm at the shoulder and elbow, medial rotation of the forearm and failure to extend the wrist (Fig. 15.12).

Klumpke's palsy may be seen after breech delivery due to damage to roots C8 and T1, with weakness of the forearm and hand.

Brachial plexus injuries can be associated with ipsilateral Horner's syndrome and/or diaphragmatic weakness in severe cases. Most perinatal brachial plexus injuries do not involve complete disruption of the nerve roots and recover over subsequent weeks.

Facial nerve palsy causes reduced movement of the cheek muscles, and the side of the mouth does not turn down when the baby cries. Most cases are transient.

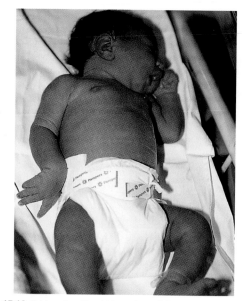

Fig. 15.12 Erb's palsy. The right arm is medially rotated and the wrist is flexed.

Primitive reflexes

The primitive reflexes are lower motor neurone responses present at birth but which disappear by 4–6 months as they become suppressed by higher centres. They may be absent in infants with neurological depression or asymmetrical in infants with nerve injuries. Persistence into later infancy may indicate neuro-developmental abnormality (Ch. 11). There are many examples and there is no need to elicit them all because their individual value is limited.

Examination sequence

Grasp responses
- Gently stimulate the palm or sole with your finger to produce a palmar or plantar grasp.

Ventral suspension/pelvic response to back stimulation
- Hold the baby prone and look for neck extension. Stroke the skin over the vertebral column to produce an extensor response with pelvic elevation.

Place and step reflexes
- Hold the baby upright and touch the dorsum of his foot against the edge of the table. The baby will flex the knee and hip, placing the foot on the table (Fig. 15.13A).
- Lower the upright baby towards the surface of the table. When the feet touch the surface, a walking movement occurs.

Moro reflex
- Support the supine baby's trunk and head in a semi-upright position. Let his head fall backwards slightly. The baby will quickly throw out both arms and spread his fingers (Fig. 15.13B).

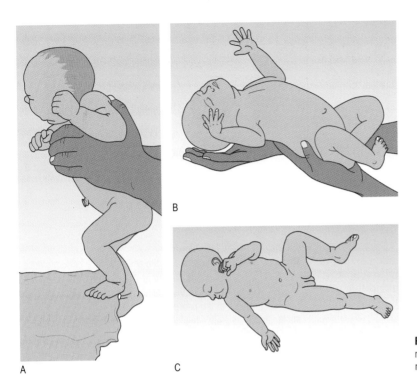

Fig. 15.13 Primitive reflexes. (A) Placing reflex. **(B)** The Moro reflex. **(C)** Tonic neck reflex.

Root and suck responses

- Gently stroke the baby's cheek. The baby turns to that side and opens his mouth, as though looking for a nipple. This is 'rooting'. If you place your finger in a healthy infant's mouth, he will suck it vigorously.

Asymmetric tonic neck reflex

- Turn the supine infant's head to the side. The arm and leg on the same side will extend and the arm and leg on the opposite side will flex. This reflex is present at term and maximal at 1 month (Fig. 15.13C).

Limbs

- Look at the limbs and count the digits.
- Try to place the foot in a normal position without significant force if it is abnormally positioned. If the position is at all fixed, then refer to a specialist.

Normal findings

A small percentage of normal babies have single palmar creases but this is also associated with Down's syndrome (Fig. 3.12B) and other chromosomal abnormalities. Tibial bowing is common in the newborn.

Abnormal findings

Oligodactyly (too few digits), polydactyly (too many) or syndactyly (joined digitis) may occur. In talipes equinovarus the foot is plantar flexed and rotated, so that the sole faces medially. In talipes calcaneovalgus the foot is dorsiflexed so that the heel is prominent and the sole faces laterally.

Hips

Check for developmental dysplasia of the hip (DDH). Many cases have associated risk factors, including a family history of DDH, breech delivery, positional talipes (especially calcaneovalgus) or oligohydramnios.

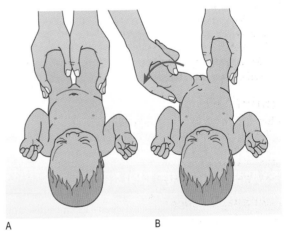

Fig. 15.14 Examination for developmental dysplasia of the hip. (A) The hip is dislocated posteriorly out of the acetabulum (Barlow manoeuvre). **(B)** The dislocated hip is relocated back into the acetabulum (Ortolani manoeuvre).

Examination sequence

- Lay the baby supine on a firm surface.
- Look at the thighs for symmetry of the skin creases.
- Examine each hip separately. Hold the thigh with the knee and hip flexed and your thumb on the medial aspect of the thigh.
- Move the proximal end of the thigh laterally and then push down towards the examining table (Barlow manoeuvre) (Fig. 15.14A); a clunk indicates that the hip is dislocatable.
- Now abduct the thigh; if you feel a clunk, this is the head of the femur returning into the acetabulum (Ortolani manoeuvre) (Fig. 15.14B). If the femoral head feels lax and you feel a clunk with an Ortolani manoeuvre without first performing the Barlow manoeuvre, then the hip is already dislocated.

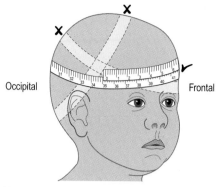

Fig. 15.15 Measurement of head circumference.

Occipital   Frontal

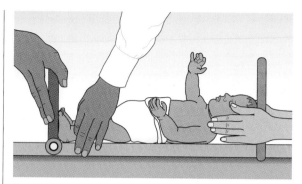

Fig. 15.16 Measuring length accurately in infants.

Never use the term 'clicky hips'. It is common to hear or feel minor ligamentous clicks during hip examination. These are of no consequence and feel quite different to the dislocation and relocation of DDH. If in any doubt, obtain an expert opinion. Some centres have an ultrasound screening programme.

Check the hips whenever you examine an infant until he is walking normally. After the first few months the Ortolani and Barlow manoeuvres cannot be performed and the most important signs are limitation of abduction in the hip and thigh skin crease asymmetry.

Weighing and measuring

Examination sequence

- Weigh the infant fully undressed using electronic scales that are accurate to 5 grams.

- Use a paper tape to measure the occipitofrontal circumference round the forehead and occiput at the largest part (Fig. 15.15). Take the measurement three times. Note the largest measurement to the nearest millimetre.
- Measure the crown–heel length using a neonatal stadiometer (Fig. 15.16). Ask a parent or assistant to hold the baby's head still and stretch out the legs so that the baby is fully extended (the least reproducible of the three measurements).
- Record the results on a centile chart appropriate to the infant's population.

Final inspection

Perform a final top to toe inspection to ensure that you do not miss anything and allow the parents a further opportunity to ask questions.

EXAMINATION OF CHILDREN

Children are individuals between 12 months and 16 years and are known by non-specific terms, including toddlers, preschoolers, school children, students, adolescents, teenagers or youths.

SYMPTOMS AND DEFINITIONS

Growth and development

Growth

Growth after infancy is extremely variable. Use gender- and ethnic-specific growth charts (Fig. 15.17). These compare the individual to the general population and with his own previous measurements. Failure to thrive is failure to attain the expected growth trajectory. An individual child should grow along a centile line for height and weight throughout childhood. A child on the 0.4th centile for height may be thriving if this has always been his growth trajectory, while a child on the 50th centile for height can have failure to thrive if previously he was on the 99.6th centile.

A child's height is related to the average of his parent's height centile ± 2 standard deviations above and below this average. Parents whose average height centile is the 50th will have children whose height will normally lie between the 2nd and 98th centile (approximately 10 cm above and below the 50th centile).

Neurological development

Normal development is heterogeneous within the population. The major determinant is the child's environment. The second is the child's genetic potential. This variability makes identifying abnormalities difficult. Developmental assessment requires patience, familiarity with children and an understanding of the range of normality for a given age.

The preschool child (1–5 years)

At the younger end of this age range, questions relating to gross motor skills are most sensitive; as the child becomes older, questions relating to fine motor and personal social skills are more meaningful. Delayed speech

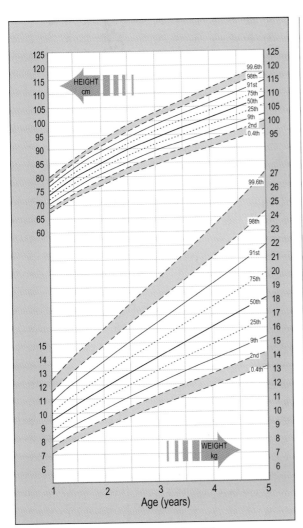

Fig. 15.17 Growth chart. © Child Growth Foundation.

EBE **15.11 Development of the premature infant**

Infants born prematurely without neurological complications tend to catch up in growth and developmental milestones after going home. At 1 year, they may demonstrate some subtle growth and developmental delay but by their second birthday their growth and development should be the same as that of a term infant.

Wilson SL, Cradock MM. Review: Accounting for prematurity in developmental assessment and the use of age-adjusted scores. J Pediatr Psychol 2004;29:641–649.

---

with normal attainment of motor milestones is not uncommon, particularly in boys, but needs hearing assessment (Box 15.6).

The school-age child (5+ years)

By this age, any developmental problems are usually known to parents and relevant agencies may already be engaged, e.g. education. However, more subtle developmental problems such as dyslexia (a learning disability affecting the individual's fluency and comprehension in reading) may be unrecognised and can be a major

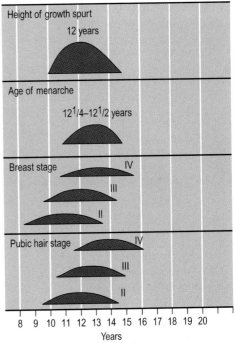

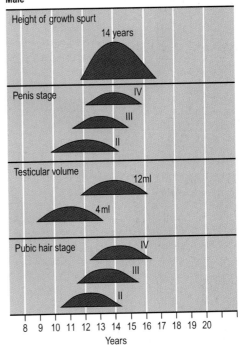

Fig. 15.18 Timing of puberty in males and females.

handicap. Ask general questions, such as: 'How is your child getting on at school?' and follow up by enquiring specifically about academic and social activity.

Growth and developmental assessment of the child born prematurely

Infants born prematurely are small and transiently demonstrate developmental delay in early life, partly due to

15

A Female breast changes

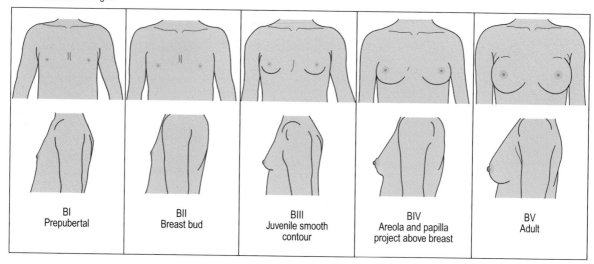

| BI
Prepubertal | BII
Breast bud | BIII
Juvenile smooth
contour | BIV
Areola and papilla
project above breast | BV
Adult |

B Pubic hair changes — female and male

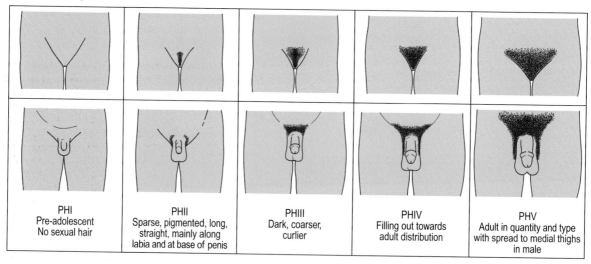

| PHI
Pre-adolescent
No sexual hair | PHII
Sparse, pigmented, long,
straight, mainly along
labia and at base of penis | PHIII
Dark, coarser,
curlier | PHIV
Filling out towards
adult distribution | PHV
Adult in quantity and type
with spread to medial thighs
in male |

C Male genital stages

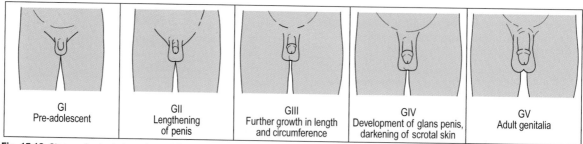

| GI
Pre-adolescent | GII
Lengthening
of penis | GIII
Further growth in length
and circumference | GIV
Development of glans penis,
darkening of scrotal skin | GV
Adult genitalia |

Fig. 15.19 Stages of puberty in males and females. Pubertal changes are shown according to the Tanner stages of puberty.

their immaturity and partly to them being in a hospital environment for long periods after delivery (Box 15.11).

Puberty

This stage of adolescence, when an individual becomes physiologically capable of sexual reproduction, is a time of rapid physical and emotional development. The age at onset and end of puberty varies hugely but is generally 10–14 years for girls and 12–16 years in boys (Fig. 15.18). The average child grows 30 cm during puberty and gains 40–50% in weight.

If required, a chart to stage puberty (Fig. 15.19). Pubertal staging has a wide normal range, with abnormalities only apparent on follow-up. Delayed or precocious puberty is not uncommon.

15.12 Pain assessment tool: FLACC* scale

0	1	2
No particular expression or smile	Occasional grimace or frown, withdrawn, uninterested	Frequently or constantly quivering chin, clenched jaw
Normal position or relaxed	Uneasy, restless, tense	Kicking or legs drawn up
Lying quietly, normal position, moves easily	Squirming, shifting back and forth, tense	Arched, rigid or jerking
No cry (awake or asleep)	Moans or whimpers, occasional complaint	Crying steadily, screams or sobs, frequent complaints
Content, relaxed	Reassured by occasional touching, hugging or being talked to, distractible	Difficult to console or comfort

Each category is scored on a 0–2 scale to give a total score of 0–10: 0 = no pain; 1–3 = mild pain; 4–7 = moderate pain; 8–10 = severe pain.
*FLACC, face, legs, activity, cry, consolability.

EBE 15.13 Consultation and children

The child is the focus of the consultation and examination, but recognise that the parents often provide the most clinical information.

van Dulmen AM. Children's contributions to paediatric outpatient encounters. Pediatrics 1998;102:563–568.

15

Pain

Pain and the need for analgesia can be difficult to assess in young children. Use an objective scoring system (Box 15.12).

THE HISTORY

Introduce yourself to the child and accompanying adult. Establish who the adult is, e.g. parent, grandparent, and decide whether the child will be prepared to give a useful history. You should already be observing the child.

Similarities in history taking between children and adults

There are many similarities in taking a history from a child and an adult. Start with open-ended questions, encouraging the parent or child to respond. During this you should be considering the differential diagnosis while informally inspecting the patient. The differential diagnosis determines which closed questions you ask and also focuses your examination. The closed questions are similar to those used in adults, although the conditions may be different. Good communication skills are equally relevant in paediatrics and adult practice, e.g. listening carefully, prompts such as 'yes' to encourage the historian to continue, and internal summarisation, e.g. 'so what you are saying is that…'.

Differences in history taking from adults

The considerable differences in physical, emotional and social attributes of children mean there is no single approach to history taking and examination. Be flexible and adapt your approach for every clinical encounter with children. The history may not be provided by the patient (Box 15.13). Children <6 years cannot give a history and children 6–11 years often have difficulty in expressing themselves clearly and are reluctant historians. If appropriate, ask the child about the problem, although in many cases the parent will volunteer the history. Direct your questions to children >11 years. Always acknowledge the younger child (say hello) even if the parent is providing the history. A paediatric history includes components not in the adult history (obstetric, developmental, immunisation histories) and the systematic enquiry is different from that for adults (Box 15.14). Some conditions affect only children, some only adults and some affect both.

Symptoms and signs

First make a differential diagnosis by identifying the part or system of the body involved; then use closed questions to identify the most likely diagnosis. Diagnosis is built upon patterns of symptoms. Rarely will any one symptom or sign lead to a 'spot diagnosis'. Pattern recognition is an art which requires regular practice.

Boxes 15.15–15.18 describe symptoms in the context of:

- duration (acute, <1 week; chronic, >3 weeks)
- frequency in primary and secondary care (***very common; **seen frequently; *rarely seen)
- diagnostic significance (with/without other symptoms)
- the likely differential diagnosis.

15.14 Common chronic/recurrent conditions in children and/ or adults

	Limited to children	Affects children and adults	Limited to adults
Cardiac		Supraventricular tachycardia Congenital cardiac defects	Coronary artery disease
Dermatological		Eczema Psoriasis (seen in teenagers)	Malignancy
Gastrointestinal	Abdominal migraine Toddler's diarrhoea	Coeliac disease Constipation Gastroenteritis Gastro-oesophageal reflux Inflammatory bowel disease Non-specific abdominal pain Food allergy/intolerance	Diverticulitis Malignancy
Respiratory	Croup Viral wheeze	Asthma Pneumonia	COPD Malignancy
Musculoskeletal		Septic arthritis Reactive arthropathy	
Neurological	Febrile convulsion	Meningitis Migraine Non-specific headache Malignancy	
Urinary	Vesico-ureteric reflux	Urinary tract infection	Malignancy

15.15 Respiratory system

Symptom		Frequency	Diagnostic significance	Significance heightened if associated with…	Differential diagnosis
Acute	Shortness of breath at rest (SOBar)	***	High (indicates loss of all respiratory reserve)		Lower respiratory tract infection, asthma, acute episodic wheeze, inhaled foreign body. Rarely heart failure or weakness
	Cough	***	Low	SOBar, wheeze, fever	Lower respiratory tract infection, asthma, acute episodic wheeze, foreign body
	Wheeze	***	Moderate	SOBar, wheeze, fever	Lower respiratory tract infection, asthma, acute episodic wheeze, foreign body
	Chest pain	*	High	Exercise Fever	Musculoskeletal pain, empyema, reflux oesophagitis, cardiac ischaemia
Chronic	Shortness of breath on exercise (SOBoe)	**	Low	Cough, wheeze, failure to thrive	Lack of fitness, respiratory pathology, cardiac pathology, neurological weakness
	Cough	***	Low	Wheeze, SOBoe, failure to thrive	Isolated cough with sputum production suggestive of infection, commonly bronchitis, rarely bronchiectasis, cystic fibrosis, inhaled foreign body. In combination with wheeze, asthma or viral-induced wheeze
	Wheeze	***	Moderate	Wheeze, SOBoe, failure to thrive	Isolated and persistent 'wheeze' usually arises from the nose (stertor, e.g. adenoidal hypertrophy) or from the very largest airways (stridor, e.g. laryngomalacia). Episodic genuine wheeze in combination with cough is suggestive of asthma or viral-induced wheeze
	Chest pain	*	High	Exercise	Non-specific chest pain, musculoskeletal chest pain, very rarely cardiac ischaemia

Respiratory sounds: clarify what noise the parent or child is describing. The historian can sometimes identify where the sound is coming from, e.g. nose (stertor), throat (stridor) or chest (rattle or wheeze). A constant respiratory sound is more likely to be stertor, stridor or rattle. A sound associated with vibration of the chest is a rattle. A very loud sound, e.g. heard in the next room, is not genuine wheeze.
Coexistent failure to thrive or weight loss always increases the significance of any symptom.

15.16 Gastrointestinal system

Symptom		Frequency	Diagnostic significance	Significance heightened if associated with…	Differential diagnosis
Acute	Vomiting	***	Low: a very non-specific symptom in children	Fever, drowsiness, dehydration	Acute gastritis/gastroenteritis, any infection (otitis media, pneumonia, urinary tract infection, meningitis), head injury, encephalitis
	Diarrhoea	***	Moderate	Fever, dehydration	Acute gastroenteritis/colitis, appendicitis
	Abdominal pain	**	Moderate	Fever, bloody stools	Acute gastroenteritis or colitis. Acute surgical causes, e.g. appendicitis, intussusception
Chronic	Vomiting	***	Moderate	Failure to thrive Headache	Gastro-oesophageal reflux (rare in older children compared with infants). Raised intracranial pressure
	Diarrhoea	***	Moderate	Failure to thrive	Commonly toddler's diarrhoea, also lactose intolerance. If failure to thrive, consider coeliac disease, inflammatory bowel disease
	Abdominal pain	***	Low	Pain not periumbilical Headaches Diarrhoea and vomiting Failure to thrive	If isolated and periumbilical, non-specific abdominal pain is common and other diagnoses include abdominal migraine, renal colic. If associated with other symptoms and/or failure to thrive, consider coeliac disease, inflammatory bowel disease

Symptoms of dehydration include dry mouth, foul-smelling breath, anuria and lethargy.
Coexisting failure to thrive or weight loss always increases the significance of any symptom.
Abdominal pain can be difficult to identify in young children who are not able to express themselves.

15.17 Nervous system

Symptom		Frequency	Diagnostic significance	Significance heightened if associated with…	Differential diagnosis
Acute	Headache	**	Low	Vomiting, fever, neck stiffness, photophobia	Acute (simple) headache Migraine Meningitis/encephalitis
	Unsteady gait	*	High		Varicella encephalomeningitis Vestibular neuronitis
	Seizure	*	High		Febrile seizure, meningitis/encephalitis Epilepsy, metabolic disorder
	Disturbed level of consciousness	*	High		Encephalitis, intoxication/drug ingestion (accidental/deliberate)
Chronic	Headache	**	Low	Vomiting Abdominal pain	Brain tumour, migraine, chronic headache
	Failure to pass developmental milestones	*	Moderate	Widening gap between age and age at which 'normal' milestone should have been passed	Cerebral palsy, neglect
	Developmental regression	*	High		Muscular dystrophy, inborn error of metabolism, neurodegenerative conditions
	Seizure	*	High		Epilepsy; rarely, long QT syndrome or inborn error of metabolism

Chronic headache can also arise from the mouth, e.g. dental abscess, or face.
An acute seizure can be confused with a rigor in a febrile child. A seizure involves slow (1 beat/second) coarse, jerking which cannot be stopped, loss of consciousness and postictal drowsiness. A rigor is characterised by rapid (5 beats/second) fine jerking which can be stopped by a cuddle and no loss of consciousness.

15

15.18 Skin

Symptom		Frequency	Diagnostic significance	Significance heightened if associated with...	Differential diagnosis
Acute	Itch	**	Low	Stridor, shortness of breath, urticarial lesions	Insect bite, can be feature of type I hypersensitivity
	Blister	**	Moderate	Stridor, shortness of breath Yellow crust (Staphylococcal infection)	Urticaria, bullous impetigo
	Rash	**	Low	Fever Petechial rash Present over trunk/flexor surfaces of legs Red annular lesions with pink centres	Petechial rash associated with meningococcal septicaemia, petechial rash (often truncal) associated with idiopathic thrombocytopenic purpura Erythema multiforme
Chronic	Plaques	***	High	Flexural distribution and itch Present over elbow/knees	Eczema Psoriasis
	Hair loss	*	High	Itch Systemic illness 2–4 months previously	Tinea capitis Telogen effluvium Alopecia

Presenting complaint

What is the primary symptom? What is its duration? Knowing the child's age, symptom and its duration provides an initial differential diagnosis.

For chronic conditions, establish how symptoms affect the quality of life and activities of daily living of the child and family.

Past medical history

Does the child have other health problems and medication? Has he been in hospital before and if so, why?

Birth history

This is more relevant to a 3-week-old baby than a 14-year-old.

- Were there any pregnancy complications?
- At what gestation was the baby born?
- Method of delivery, e.g. normal vaginal, caesarean section?
- What was the birthweight?
- Was the neonatal period normal, e.g. did the baby need to go to a special care baby unit?

Vaccination history

Vaccination schedules vary over time and between countries. Are the child's immunisations up to date and if the child is not immunised, why not?

Developmental history

See above and Box 15.6.

Family history

Do any of the child's first- or second-degree relatives have similar symptoms? This information may not be available for adopted children and when a parent is not known. Consider parental consanguinity, which is not uncommon among some ethnic groups.

Social history

Children's families may include step siblings and several adults who share responsibility for raising them. Establish who is responsible for the child and find out how the child perceives his family. Children at risk for neglect often have complex domestic arrangements, e.g. several caregivers.

Ask about exposure to tobacco smoke and offer parents who smoke cessation advice. Asking about the presence of cats and dogs is usually unhelpful as no interventions are proven to benefit (unless there is a very clear relation between symptoms and exposure, in which case hopefully parents will have removed the pet from the household).

Some chronic symptoms are associated with anxiety or potential gain for the child, e.g. chronic cough, abdominal pain and headache in a well-looking 8–12-year-old with normal examination. A psychological history helps determine the degree of associated anxiety and potential gain for the child. Look carefully for the child's facial expression, eye contact and body language. Ask specifically about school (avoidance and bullying), social interactions (does the child have many friends?) and out-of-school activities.

Open-ended questions showing empathy, such as 'That sounds difficult. How did it make you feel?' are useful. Symptoms in a child who misses a lot of school but is never unwell during summer holidays are likely to be less severe than those which stop a keen footballer from playing.

Dietary history

This is not routinely needed except in situations such as poor weight gain, obesity or food-related symptoms, e.g. anaphylaxis.

Drug history

Prescribing errors often arise from a poorly documented drug history. Transcribe the medication, dose and frequency direct from the medication package or referral letter if possible. Find out about any difficulties in taking medication to establish concordance. Clarify any adverse reactions to medications, especially antibiotics.

Psychiatric history

Psychiatric disorders are uncommon, and often atypical, in primary school children. Take a full adult psychiatric history from adolescents with a potential psychiatric diagnosis (p. 21).

Systematic enquiry

This screens for illnesses or symptoms not recognised as important by the child or parents. Use the adult questions, excluding irrelevant ones for the age group (Box 15.19).

THE PHYSICAL EXAMINATION

Children usually present with a symptom. Children with acute symptoms often have physical signs such as wheeze (Box 15.20) but examination is normal in the majority of children with chronic symptoms. Routine screening examination after infancy is unhelpful as most paediatric diseases only produce signs late in the illness.

Similarities in examination between children and adults

The techniques used when examining children are the same as those in adults, with some exceptions. Examining a child is a skill which takes time to learn. Usually the history suggests the diagnosis; the examination confirms it and its severity.

Differences in examination between children and adults

Consider children in three age ranges: 1–3, 3–5 and >5 years.

1–3 years

Carefully inspect the child while taking the history since formal examination may not be feasible. All children pass through a stage when they can be reluctant to be examined, commonly known as the 'terrible twos'. This developmental stage begins in mid-infancy and carries on to ~3 years. During this time children are anxious in the presence of strangers and become upset when parents leave them (separation anxiety). Carefully observe the child's general condition, colour, respiratory rate and effort, and state of hydration while taking the history and the child is oblivious to your close attention. For the formal examination, ask the parent to sit the child on her knees. Examine the cardiorespiratory system and the abdomen with the young child sitting upright on the parent's knee. With patience, abdominal

15.19 The paediatric systematic enquiry		
	Child aged 1–3	**Child aged 4–11**
Cardiac	No 'routine' question	
Ear, nose and throat	Do you think your child hears well? (Chronic otitis media is a common cause of hearing loss and can be managed easily)	Do you think your child hears well and can speak clearly? (Chronic otitis media commonly reduces hearing) Does your child snore and briefly stop breathing at night? (Primary snoring is present in 10% of children and can be a feature of obstructive sleep apnoea)
Gastrointestinal	Is your child thriving? (Failure to thrive is not common but indicates serious underlying pathology) Does your child open his bowels at least once a day? (Constipation is common) Is your child regularly vomiting? (Gastro-oesophageal reflux may persist beyond infancy)	Is your child thriving? (Failure to thrive is not common but indicates serious underlying pathology) Does your child open his bowels at least once a day? (Constipation is common)
Respiratory	In the last year has your child regularly coughed and/or wheezed? (Asthma/viral-induced wheeze and respiratory infections are common)	In the last year has your child regularly coughed or wheezed? (Mild asthma is underdiagnosed)
Neurological	No routine questions, see development	
Urinary		Is your child dry by day and night? (Primary nocturnal enuresis is present in 15% of 5-year-olds)

EBE 15.20 **Wheeze**

Parents and children often call wheeze, stridor, stertor or rattle, 'wheeze'.

Saglani S, McKenzie SA, Bush A et al. A video questionnaire identifies upper airway abnormalities in preschool children with reported wheeze. Arch Dis Child 2005;90:961–964.

15.21 **Common non-specific signs in children**

- Fever
- Pallor
- Lethargy
- Vomiting
- Blanching rash
- Irritability
- Runny nose

15.22 **Serious signs requiring immediate attention**

- Poor perfusion (indicating shock)
- Reduced capillary refill (indicating shock)
- Cool peripheries (indicating shock)
- Petechial rash over the trunk (suggesting meningococcal septicaemia)
- Headache, photophobia or neck stiffness (suggesting meningitis)
- Dyspnoea at rest (indicating loss of respiratory reserve due to pneumonia, asthma)

examination can be done with the child lying supine on the bed next to a parent or on the parent's lap. Removing your stethoscope from around your neck can trigger the child to become upset. If the child starts crying, chest auscultation and abdominal palpation become almost impossible; persevering will provoke more crying.

3–5 years

Some children in this age range have the confidence and maturity to comply with some components of the adult examination. Others remain apprehensive with strangers. Children's social skills regress when they are unwell.

5+ years

The child may comply with a full adult style of examination. Although children <11 years are often not able to express themselves well, children >5 years are able to understand and comply with requests, e.g. finger-to-nose pointing, heel-to-toe walking, 'sit forward' and 'take a deep breath in and hold it'.

Remember that a normal examination does not exclude pathology.

The acutely unwell child

There are many non-specific signs that are not diagnostic and common to a range of conditions from a simple cold to meningitis (Box 15.21). However, some signs are serious, requiring immediate investigation and management (Box 15.22).

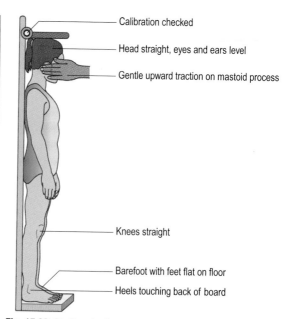

Calibration checked

Head straight, eyes and ears level

Gentle upward traction on mastoid process

Knees straight

Barefoot with feet flat on floor

Heels touching back of board

Fig. 15.20 Stadiometer for measuring height accurately in children.

Children become ill quickly. A child unwell for <24 hours where the initial examination reveals only non-specific signs should ideally be reassessed in 1–2 hours.

Leave throat and ears examination until the end and be opportunistic and flexible in the order of examination.

General examination

Height

Use a stadiometer (Fig. 15.20).

Vital signs

Normal values for vital signs vary according to age (Box 15.23).

Ears, nose and throat

Children are often reluctant to be examined.

Preschool child

Examination sequence

Throat
- Ask the parent to:
  - sit the child on her knees, both facing you
  - place one arm over the child's upper arms and chest (to stop the child pushing you away) (Fig. 15.21)
  - hold the child's forehead with the other hand (to stop the child pulling his chin down to his chest).
- Hold the torch in your non-dominant hand to illuminate his throat.
- Slide a tongue depressor inside the child's cheek with your dominant hand. He should open his clenched teeth (perhaps with a shout), showing his tonsils and pharynx.

15.23 Upper limit of normal values (97.5th or 98th centile) for physiological measurements in children of different ages			
	Pulse (bpm)	Respiratory rate (breaths/min)	Blood pressure (mmHg)
Age 2–5 years	120	25	120/70
Age 5–10 years	110–120	22–25	120–130/70–75
Age 10–16 years	100–110	18–22	120–130/70–75

Abnormal findings

Healthy tonsils and pharynx look pink; when inflamed they are crimson red.

Inspecting the throat reveals the presence, but not the cause, of the infection; pus on the tonsils and pharynx does not differentiate a bacterial from viral infection (p. 310).

Examination sequence

Ears

- Ask the parent to
  - sit the child across her knees with the child's ear facing you
  - place one arm around the child's shoulder and upper arm facing you (to stop him pushing you away) (Fig. 15.22)
  - place the other hand over the parietal area above his ear facing you (to keep the child's head still).
- Use an otoscope with the largest speculum that will comfortably fit the child's external auditory meatus.
- To straighten the ear canal and visualise the canal and tympanic membrane, hold the pinna gently and pull it out and down in a baby or toddler with no mastoid development and up and back in a child whose mastoid process has formed. Mastoid development causes the canal to elongate forwards and medially, changing the direction of pull required to straighten it (p. 301).

Lymphadenopathy

Normal findings

Palpable neck and groin nodes are extremely common in children <5 years old. They are typically bilateral, <1 cm in diameter, hard, mobile and with no overlying redness and can persist for many weeks. In the absence of systemic symptoms, e.g. weight loss, fevers, night sweats, these are invariably a normal, healthy immune response to infection. Only very rarely are they due to malignancy (Box 15.24).

Respiratory system

Abnormal findings

The child <3 years has a soft chest wall and relatively small stiff lungs. In respiratory distress the diaphragm

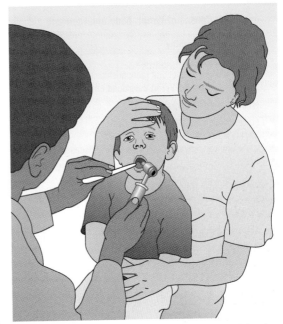

Fig. 15.21 How to hold a child to examine the mouth and throat.

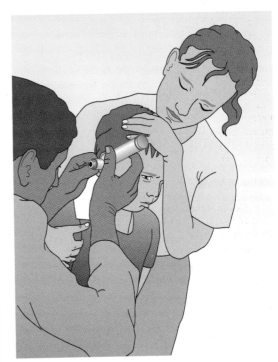

Fig. 15.22 How to hold a child to examine the ear.

contracts vigorously to reduce intrathoracic pressure and draw air into the airways. This produces chest wall recession (ribs 'sucking in') and extrusion of the abdomen (wrongly called 'abdominal breathing').

Children's thinner chests transmit noises easily and their smaller airways are more prone to turbulence and added sounds. Auscultation may reveal a variety of sounds, including a fine expiratory polyphonic wheeze, fine end-expiratory crackles (similar to the noise made by

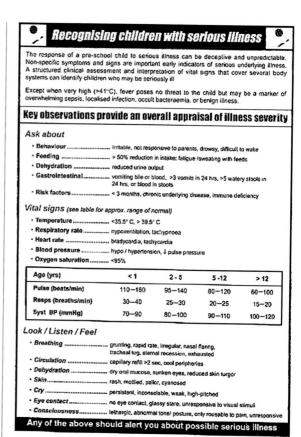

15.24 Causes of lymph node enlargement

Cervical lymphadenopathy

- Tonsillitis, pharyngitis, sinusitis
- 'Glandular fever' (infectious mononucleosis/cytomegalovirus)
- Tuberculosis (uncommon in developed countries)

Generalised lymphadenopathy

- Febrile illness with a generalised rash
- 'Glandular fever'
- Systemic juvenile chronic arthritis (Still's disease)
- Acute lymphatic leukaemia
- Drug reaction
- Mucocutaneous lymph node syndrome (Kawasaki syndrome)

Recognising children with serious illness

The response of a pre-school child to serious illness can be deceptive and unpredictable. Non-specific symptoms and signs are important early indicators of serious underlying illness. A structured clinical assessment and interpretation of vital signs that cover several body systems can identify children who may be seriously ill

Except when very high (>41°C). fever poses no threat to the child but may be a marker of overwhelming sepsis, localised infection, occult bacteraemia, or benign illness.

Key observations provide an overall appraisal of illness severity

Ask about

- Behaviour .... Irritable, not responsive to parents, drowsy, difficult to wake
- Feeding .... > 50% reduction in intake; fatigue /sweating with feeds
- Dehydration .... reduced urine output
- Gastrointestinal.......................... vomiting bile or blood, >3 vomits in 24 hrs, >5 watery stools in 24 hrs, or blood in stools
- Risk factors.......................... < 3 months, chronic underlying disease, immune deficiency

Vital signs (see table for approx. range of normal)

- Temperature .... <35.5° C, > 39.5° C
- Respiratory rate.............. hypoventilation, tachypnoea
- Heart rate .... bradycardia, tachycardia
- Blood pressure.............. hypo / hypertension, ↓ pulse pressure
- Oxygen saturation .... <95%

Age (yrs)	< 1	2 - 5	5 -12	> 12
Pulse (beats/min)	110—160	95—140	80—120	60—100
Resps (breaths/min)	30—40	25—30	20—25	15—20
Syst BP (mmHg)	70—90	80—100	90—110	100—120

Look / Listen / Feel

- Breathing .... grunting, rapid rate, irregular, nasal flaring, tracheal tug, sternal recession, exhausted
- Circulation .... capillary refill >2 sec, cool peripheries
- Dehydration .... dry oral mucosa, sunken eyes, reduced skin turgor
- Skin.......................... rash, mottled, pallor, cyanosed
- Cry .... persistent, inconsolable, weak, high-pitched
- Eye contact.......................... no eye contact, glassy stare, unresponsive to visual stimuli
- Consciousness.......................... lethargic, abnormal tone/ posture, only rousable to pain, unresponsive

Any of the above should alert you about possible serious illness

Fig. 15.23 Rapid cardiopulmonary evaluation.

rubbing hairs between your fingers by your ear), coarse louder crackles transmitted from the larger airways and other sounds described as pops and squeaks (typically in the chest of recovering asthmatics). Loud added sounds without dyspnoea or recession are unlikely to be clinically relevant. Dyspnoea with or without recession is a more important sign than added sounds. What you see is more important than what you hear.

Cardiovascular system

Feel the brachial pulse in the antecubital fossa in children <2–3 years. Do not palpate the carotid or radial pulses in young children. Measure blood pressure using a cuff sized two-thirds the distance from elbow to shoulder tip. Repeat with a larger cuff if the reading is elevated. If in doubt, use a larger cuff as smaller cuffs yield falsely high values.

Gastrointestinal system

In children 6 months to 3 years, examine the abdomen with the child sitting upright on his parent's knee. In the young child, splenic enlargement causes the spleen to move down into the left iliac fossa. In older children the enlarged spleen moves towards the right iliac fossa. Rectal examination is rarely indicated in children.

Nervous system

You are stronger than the child so test power by watching the child demonstrate his strength against gravity. Ask him to lift his arms above his head; raise his leg from the bed whilst lying; stand from a squatting position.

Neck stiffness is usually apparent in a child when you are talking to him or the parents. If in doubt, ask the child to move his head from side to side or test as for adults (Fig. 11.2). With a young child, move a toy to catch his attention and see if he moves his head.

Spotting the sick child

It can be difficult to identify a child with severe illness. With experience you will learn to identify whether a child is just miserable or really ill (Fig. 15.23). Early-warning scores can help (Box 15.25).

EBE 15.25 Early-warning scores in children

Early-warning scores, involving the measurement of temperature, pulse, respiratory rate and blood pressure, can help identify children at risk for severe illness.

Akre M, Finkelstein M, Erickson M et al. Sensitivity of the pediatric early warning score to identify patient deterioration. Pediatrics 2010;125:e763–e769.

Certain features correlate with severe illness (Box 15.26).

Child protection

Children who experience neglect or physical and/or emotional abuse are at increased risk of health problems. At-risk children are often already known to other agencies but this information may not be known to you in the acute setting. Injuries from physical abuse can be detected visually. Consider non-accidental injury if the history is not consistent with the injury or the injury is present in unusual places, e.g. over the back. It is difficult to detect neglect during a brief encounter but think of it if the child appears dirty and wearing dirty or torn clothes which are too small or too large. The parent–child relationship gives insight into neglect; the child is apparently scared of the parent ('frozen watchfulness') or the parent is apparently oblivious of the child's attention (Box 15.27).

15.26 Clinical signs associated with severe illness in children

- Fever >38°C
- Drowsiness
- Cold hands and feet
- Petechial rash
- Neck stiffness
- Shortness of breath at rest
- Tachycardia
- Hypotension (a late sign in shocked children where blood pressure is initially maintained by tachycardia and increased peripheral vascular resistance)

PUTTING IT ALL TOGETHER

Children are not small adults. They need assessment in age-appropriate surroundings. The history is the key to diagnosis and rarely will an examination finding change the diagnosis.

15.27 Signs that may suggest child neglect or abuse

Behavioural signs

- 'Frozen watchfulness'
- Passivity
- Over-friendliness
- Sexualised behaviour
- Inappropriate dress
- Hunger, stealing food

Physical signs

- Identifiable bruises, e.g. fingertips, handprints, belt buckle, bites
- Circular (cigarette) burns or submersion burns with no splash marks
- Injuries of differing ages
- Eye or mouth injuries
- Long bone fractures or bruises in non-mobile infants
- Posterior rib fracture
- Subconjunctival or retinal haemorrhage
- Dirty, smelly, unkempt child
- Bad nappy rash

15

Andrew Elder
Elizabeth MacDonald

The frail elderly

16

EXAMINATION OF THE FRAIL ELDERLY

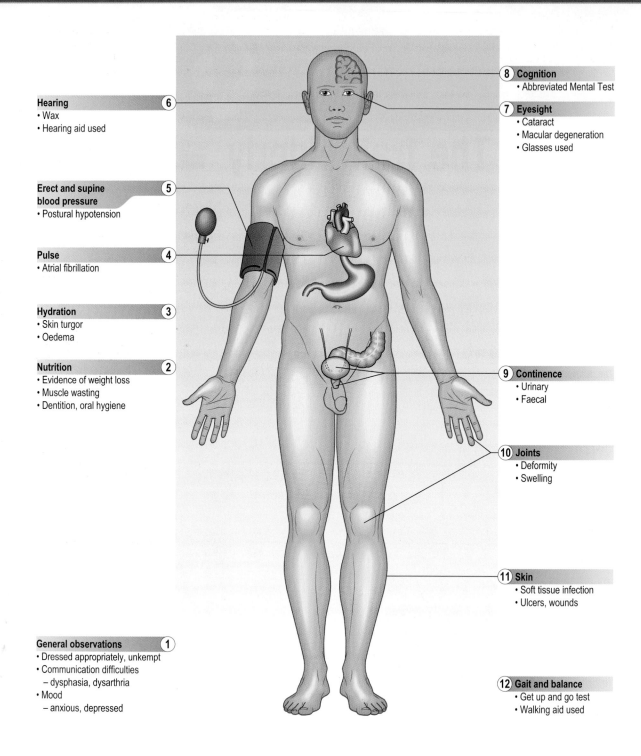

Hearing 6
• Wax
• Hearing aid used

Erect and supine blood pressure 5
• Postural hypotension

Pulse 4
• Atrial fibrillation

Hydration 3
• Skin turgor
• Oedema

Nutrition 2
• Evidence of weight loss
• Muscle wasting
• Dentition, oral hygiene

General observations 1
• Dressed appropriately, unkempt
• Communication difficulties
  – dysphasia, dysarthria
• Mood
  – anxious, depressed

8 **Cognition**
• Abbreviated Mental Test

7 **Eyesight**
• Cataract
• Macular degeneration
• Glasses used

9 **Continence**
• Urinary
• Faecal

10 **Joints**
• Deformity
• Swelling

11 **Skin**
• Soft tissue infection
• Ulcers, wounds

12 **Gait and balance**
• Get up and go test
• Walking aid used

ASSESSMENT OF THE FRAIL ELDERLY

Comprehensive geriatric assessment is an evidence-based process which improves outcomes. It involves taking the history from the patient and, with the patient's consent, that of a carer or relative, and is followed by a systematic examination, including assessment of:

- Cognitive function and mood
- Nutrition and hydration
- Skin
- Pain
- Continence
- Hearing and vision
- Functional status.

Ideally the multiprofessional team (Box 16.1) work together to create a comprehensive assessment and individualised management plan.

The extent and focus of the assessment required depend on the clinical presentation. In non-acute settings, e.g. GP/outpatient clinic or day hospital, do not focus only on establishing what diseases are present, but also which functional impairments and problems most affect the patient's life.

In acute settings, e.g. following acute hospital referral, primarily focus on what has changed; detect any new symptoms or signs of illness and any changes from baseline physical or cognitive function.

The complexity of problems presented, and need for comprehensive and systematic analysis, means that assessment is divided into components undertaken at different times, by different members of the multiprofessional team.

Definitions

Elderly

There is no specific age when a patient is 'elderly' and although >65 years is commonly used as the definition, there is no biological basis for this. There is considerable variation in ageing with many chronologically elderly patients appearing biologically and functionally younger and vice versa.

16.1 The multiprofessional team

Professional	Key roles in assessment of:
Physician	Physical state, including diagnosis and therapeutic intervention
Psychiatrist	Cognition, mood and capacity
Physiotherapist	Mobility, balance, gait and falls risk
Occupational therapist	Practical functional activities (self-care and domestic)
Nurse	Skin health, nutrition and continence
Dietician	Nutrition
Speech and language therapist	Speech and swallowing
Social worker	Social care needs

Frailty

Frailty becomes more common with advancing age and is a response to chronic disease and ageing itself. A frail elderly person typically suffers multimorbidity, often with cognitive impairment, visual and hearing loss, and may be on multiple medications. His general functional reserve and the capacity of individual organs and physiological systems are impaired, making the individual vulnerable to the effects of minor illness.

Multimorbidity

Multimorbidity (multiple illnesses) and disability (impaired capacity to undertake specific functions) are defining features of frailty (Box 16.2).

Presentation of disease

Classical patterns of symptoms and signs do occur in the frail elderly, but modified or non-specific presentations are common due to the effects of co-morbidity, drug treatment and the ageing process itself. As the combination of these factors is unique for each individual, the presentation of disease is distinct in each patient. In the frail elderly the first sign of new illness may not be a specific new symptom but a change in their functional status; typically, reduced mobility, altered cognition or impairment of balance leading to falls. Common precipitants are infections, changes in drug treatment and metabolic derangements but almost any acute insult can produce this response (Fig. 16.1).

Communication difficulties, cognition and mood

Communication can be challenging (Box 16.3). The history can be incomplete, difficult to interpret or

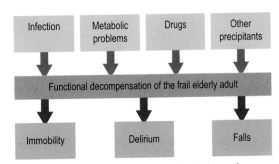

Fig. 16.1 Functional decompensation in frail elderly people.

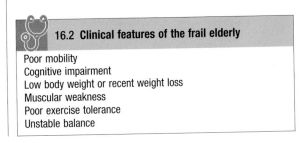

16.2 Clinical features of the frail elderly

Poor mobility
Cognitive impairment
Low body weight or recent weight loss
Muscular weakness
Poor exercise tolerance
Unstable balance

16.3 Communication difficulties – the seven Ds	
Problem	**Comment/causes**
Deafness	Nerve or conductive
Dysphasia	Most commonly due to stroke disease but sometimes a feature of dementia
Dysarthria	Cerebrovascular disease, motor neurone disease, Parkinson's disease
Dysphonia	Parkinson's disease
Dementia	Global impairment of cognitive function
Delirium	Impaired attention, disturbance of arousal and perceptual disturbances
Depression	May mimic dementia or delirium

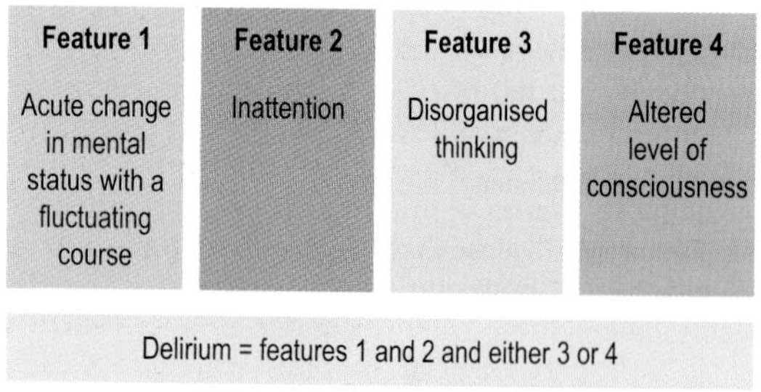

16.4 Decision-making capacity	
Capacity	**Comment**
Task-specific	Patients with dementia may be able to make a decision about treatment they do or do not wish for a new medical problem but be unable to make decisions about their financial affairs
Depends on demonstrating the ability to: • make a decision • retain memory of a decision • understand a decision • communicate a decision	Ask patients to explain their understanding of the decision they are making. Can they recall the decision when asked later? Can they reason their way through the decision? Do they understand the consequences of the decision? Can they effectively communicate their decision to a third party?
Changes over time	Patients can regain capacity or lose capacity over relatively short periods, particularly during intercurrent illness. Always reassess at times important decisions are made

Feature 1	Feature 2	Feature 3	Feature 4
Acute change in mental status with a fluctuating course	Inattention	Disorganised thinking	Altered level of consciousness

Delirium = features 1 and 2 and either 3 or 4

Fig. 16.2 The Confusion Assessment Method (CAM) score.

misleading and the whole assessment, including physical examination, time-consuming.

Whenever possible, assess the patient somewhere quiet with few distractions. Make your patient comfortable, with access to a drink of water. Patients should wear any glasses, hearing aids or dentures they need. Help them to switch on and adjust their hearing aid if necessary. If they still cannot hear you clearly, use an electronic communicator. If communication remains difficult and they can read, write down simple questions and instructions.

Cognitive function includes the processes of perception, attention, memory, reasoning, decision making and problem solving. Cognitive impairment increases with age and has implications for assessment, treatment, consent and prognosis. Be alert to cognitive impairment with evidence of poor recall or limited ability to co-operate. Patients may not recall their medical history or may deny all symptoms, even when they are clearly unwell. Consider the possibility of cognitive impairment early, and tailor your assessment appropriately. Dementia and delirium commonly cause cognitive impairment and are underrecognised in community and hospital settings (p. 24).

Use the Mini Mental State Examination (MMSE) or Abbreviated Mental Test (AMT) or Addenbrooke's Cognitive Examination (p. 26) to help detect cognitive impairment, but recognise that these should not be used alone to diagnose dementia or delirium.

In acute presentations, consider delirium and use a validated screening tool, e.g. the Confusion Assessment Method (CAM) score to distinguish between delirium and dementia (Fig. 16.2). Remember that patients with delirium need not be agitated and are frequently quiet and withdrawn (hypoactive). Assessing capacity to make decisions is part of assessing cognitive function but specialised psychiatric assessment may be required (Box 16.4).

Coexisting problems, including impaired hearing, low mood or bradykinesia, can mimic cognitive impairment. Some patients present with apparently good social skills or 'façade' and cover their impaired memory by diverting the conversation to another topic. Do not ascribe changes in cognition to age alone without excluding dementia or delirium. Never use terms such as 'vague' or 'poor historian'.

Depression is common in frail elderly people and may be difficult to diagnose. A formal psychiatric assessment and corroborating history from a carer or friend may be valuable. Standardised rating scales are available, e.g. the Geriatric Depression Scale. Consider using these for all patients >80 years.

Patients are often fearful that they will not return home after admission to hospital, and accordingly play down their symptoms or functional limitations. Always try to corroborate the history from a carer, relative or friend, with the patient's consent.

THE HISTORY

Presenting complaint

Frail elderly patients often have multiple symptoms. Take time to detail each symptom, and separate those arising from new acute illness from those due to background disabilities. Ask the patient:

- How long have you had a particular symptom?
- Has it changed recently?
- When were you last totally free of the symptom?

If the patient focuses on a functional change such as difficulty walking, find out what the patient feels is the specific cause. Is there pain when moving? Is balance difficult or is there weakness, and if so, in one limb or both?

Try and gauge baseline health status. Find out what the patient's symptoms, functional abilities and mental status were before the new presenting problem. This helps set realistic goals.

The patient's perspective may vary from yours, particularly when you are assessing an acute episode. For example, a patient referred following sudden loss of consciousness may be unconcerned by this but anxious about long standing back pain. These symptoms are not coincidental; if it is important to your patient, it should be important to you.

Past history

Detail the past history and known comorbidities using all sources, including any previous records. Comorbidity may not relate directly to the current problem but may influence new problems and the feasibility and appropriateness of potential treatments (Box 16.5).

16.5 How comorbidities or drugs can influence symptoms

Comorbidity/ drug	Effect of comorbidity or drug	Effect on presentation of new disease
Osteoarthritis of weight-bearing joint	Limited mobility	Patient does not experience exertional dyspnoea, resulting in late presentation of heart disease
Cognitive impairment	Poor recall or no recognition of symptoms	Patient does not describe symptoms of disease and diagnosis is not recognised
Anticholinergics Diuretics Some calcium antagonists	Dry mouth Urinary frequency Ankle swelling	A symptom is caused by drug treatment rather than disease
Vasodilators, diuretics Beta-blockers L-dopa (usually long-term)	Postural hypotension Bradycardia Dyskinetic limb movements	A sign is caused by drug treatment rather than disease
Beta-blocker	No tachycardia in gastrointestinal bleeding	An expected sign does not occur because of drug treatment

Drug history

Polypharmacy, drug interactions, adverse events and difficulties with compliance are common. Take a detailed drug history (p. 14), supplemented by additional information.

- Identify all medications, including over-the-counter preparations.
- Ask about any drugs that have been started or stopped recently, and if doses of regular medications have been altered.
- Explore ability to self-administer drugs; ask if the patient uses a dosette box or if a carer helps with administration.
- Explore ability to read labels, open bottles or use inhalers correctly.
- If patients have their drugs with them, go through them together. Ask patients what they believe each one is for, how it affects them and how often they take it.
- Ask if there are any drugs that they sometimes omit, e.g. diuretics on days that they are going out.
- Ask carers if there are partially used supplies of drugs in the house.
- Clarify any 'allergies' or previous adverse events; if in doubt, regard the allergy as significant.
- Explore which symptoms patients believe are caused by their drugs.
- Contact the prescriber, if necessary, to confirm details of drug history.

Some patients describe multiple drug intolerances, often imprecisely or inconsistently. Clarify what symptoms the patient believes to be adverse effects of drug treatment, as some may be unrelated. Failure to do so may deny the use of potentially useful treatment.

Family history

New presentation of disease with a strong genetic predisposition is unlikely, but family history may be important to patients who have lost siblings or their own children to specific conditions. They may think their own symptoms relate to the same problem.

Social and functional history

Complement a comprehensive social history with information about the patient's functional capability as this affects their ability to cope at home, and what assistance they need to support their function there. Establish the patient's current level of function, what it was before the onset of any new problem, and the time course of any functional deterioration. Abrupt functional decline suggests a more acute underlying precipitant or disease. Insidious decline suggests alternate pathologies or progression of underlying chronic disease. Get corroboration from a friend, relative or carer, but interpret all information obtained in association with objective functional assessment by yourself and other members of the multiprofessional team (Box 16.1).

16

Mobility and transfers

Can the person transfer from chair to bed or toilet and walk alone? Does he use a walking aid and can he manage stairs?

Home environment

Find out who is at home with the patient. If the patient lives alone, he may require additional support. Has the patient lived there long? A recent move may cause problems. What is access like to the house/bedroom/toilets? Does the patient need to use stairs, inside or outside? If the patient lives in sheltered accommodation, are meals provided, and is there an on-site warden or personal safety alarms? How does the patient feel about living there?

Daily activities

Can patients wash and dress themselves? Do they do their own shopping and prepare their own meals? Patients may need a carer to help them with these tasks.

Support

Find out what formal carer support the patient has, e.g. home help. Establish how often any carer visits and what that person does for the patient. Do family or friends help? If so, how much and how often?

Social interaction

Social isolation can contribute to mood disorders. Can patients still get out of the house by themselves or accompanied, or are they house-bound? How many visitors do they have?

Occupation

Do they still have a job and if so, what? If retired, find out about what they did as it may be relevant to current disease as well as allow you to see another side to them.

Smoking and alcohol

The elderly may be sensitive to even small amounts of alcohol and there may be many pack years of cigarette use.

Driving

Patients may still be driving and there will be safety issues if there are visual or cognitive defects.

Systematic enquiry

The systematic enquiry forms part of a screening process and is important because many diseases present with non-specific functional deterioration, e.g. immobility, and you need clues to specific underlying precipitants. Because comorbidity is common, many conditions are underdiagnosed.

Use standard framework questions to concentrate on certain areas.

Cognitive impairment

Have patients noticed any memory problems or has anyone else commented on their memory? Does anyone help them with letters and bills?

Mood

Ask about how they sleep at night. How would they describe their mood and appetite? Are they still interested in previous pursuits, such as reading or following favourite television programmes?

Nutrition

Has their weight been steady over the past few months? Ask the patient whether they have noticed their clothes getting loose; this helps establish weight loss. How many meals do they have in the day and do they eat meat, fish, vegetables and fruit? Who prepares their meals?

Oral health

Do they have any problems with their teeth or gums? If they wear dentures, do they fit well? Ask if their mouth is dry.

Pain

Ask specifically about pain as this may affect moving around the home and disturb sleep.

Continence

Sensitively ask whether patients ever notice incontinence or leakage from their bladder or bowels. Are they aware when they are about to pass urine or a stool? Do they ever find it hard to get to the toilet in time? Do these problems stop them doing activities?

Sensory impairment

Ask about any problems with vision and whether they wear glasses. Ask directly whether they can see the television and read a newspaper. If they wear a hearing aid, find out if it is working and whether they brought it and are wearing it.

Falls and balance

Do they ever feel unsteady on their feet? Ask about any falls in the past year and whether they could get up off the floor if it happened. Find out how they would call for help if they did fall and could not get up in the house.

THE PHYSICAL EXAMINATION

Physical examination is easiest when your patient can comply with your instructions. All patients benefit from clear, careful instruction and this is particularly important for the frail elderly who may have communication problems or find the examination routine demanding. Many have low levels of stamina and movement may be limited by physical disability. Integrate your physical examination to minimise movement for patients and maximise their understanding and cooperation. Help them to move around the room, to get on and off the examination couch and recognise that they will take longer to undress and dress. Some patients feel more comfortable if a family member, carer or friend is present, but always check that this is what they wish.

It may be challenging to examine a frail elderly person comprehensively because of communication barriers, the patient's reduced physical stamina and functional impairment. Often the patient, doctor and carer have different goals or concerns. This means there are additional elements in the physical examination and an altered emphasis. It takes time and patience to perform a detailed assessment of a frail elderly patient.

Some elderly people have difficulty maintaining personal hygiene, grooming or appearance. Their hair and clothes may be unclean, nails unkempt and facial hair longer than in younger life. These findings may reflect underlying functional or cognitive impairment, social isolation or low mood, and are relevant to the patient's overall functional status, condition and outlook, or need for social support.

Be aware of the common clinical signs found in frail elderly patients. Just as the history elicits multiple diverse and unexpected symptoms, a careful examination will often reveal many clinical signs in different clinical systems. In acute presentations, be alert to those signs that may, misleadingly, be absent (Box 16.6).

Document all signs. Try to determine their relevance to the presentation and care of each individual patient. Your history and subsequent targeted investigations will help determine the significance of examination findings. Assume that a physical sign is due to disease, which may be treatable, rather than ageing, which is not.

General examination

Hydration and nutrition

Disorders of hydration are common in frail elderly patients but accurate clinical assessment is difficult and classical signs less reliable (Box 16.7).

Undernutrition and low body weight are common features of frailty that may develop rapidly in hospitalised patients. They are frequently multifactorial so seek reversible factors. Consider chronic disease, e.g. COPD, new serious disease, e.g. cancer, poor social support or isolation and depression or dementia as these may present with low body weight. Other factors that contribute are poor oral health, poor function (being unable to obtain/prepare food) and cognitive impairment (being unable to prepare food or remember to eat it) (Fig. 16.3).

The skin

Bruising may suggest past or present steroid use, but is often simply age-related due to the reduction in subcutaneous supporting tissue. Rarely, it is due to scurvy (p. 56). Soft-tissue infections often cause functional decompensation and consequent confusion, immobility and falls (Fig. 16.1). Leg ulcers are common and frequently have multifactorial causes (p. 135). Pain from ulcers may reduce mobility. On admission to hospital many frail elderly patients have skin wounds that have been dressed in the community. Always remove these dressings, with the help of a nurse when possible, and assess the underlying lesion.

Frail elderly patients with limited mobility are vulnerable to the rapid development of pressure sores, particularly at times of intercurrent acute illness. Standardised

16

16.6 Modified signs in acutely unwell frail elderly patients

Feature	Clinical context	Modification
Temperature	Possible sepsis	Systemic inflammatory response obtunded, may not mount pyrexia (or may become hypothermic) Core temperature normally lower and diurnal variation lost – ↑ temperature may occur, but not > 37°C
Pulse rate	Volume status, response to sepsis or pain	Altered baroreceptor function may attenuate the rise in heart rate typically associated with these stressors
Blood pressure	Volume status, response to sepsis or pain	Altered baroreceptor function may modify BP response to acute illness
Postural blood pressure	Volume status	May be found in volume-replete patients due to primary autonomic dysfunction. Less reliable indicator of volume depletion
Skin turgor	Hydration	↓ but less specific because of reduction in subcutaneous fat

16.7 Assessment of dehydration

Classical feature of dehydration	Interpretation in frail elderly
Postural hypotension	Less specific than in younger patients; may be caused by drugs, disease or age-related abnormal autonomic responses to postural change
Decreased skin turgor	Decreased collagen elasticity and reduced subcutaneous fat can mimic reduced turgor. Best assessed at the sternum
Impaired capillary refill time	Less reliable in the frail elderly because less specific
Dry mouth	A non-specific finding caused by other problems such as anticholinergic drugs or mouth breathing
Tachycardia in hypovolaemia	Less sensitive due to drug- or age-related abnormal autonomic responses

16

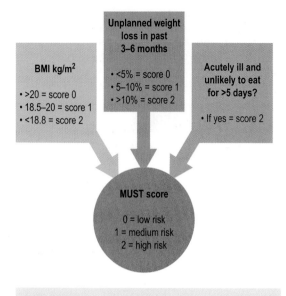

Fig. 16.3 The Malnutrition Universal Screening Tool (MUST) score for assessment of risk of malnutrition.

assessment scores, e.g. the Waterlow Score, help identify patients at risk of skin breakdown.

Pain

In patients with impairment of communication or cognitive impairment, look for pain-related behaviour (Box 16.8).

Continence

Urinary incontinence is common. The acute onset of incontinence can be caused by specific disease (p. 200), but can also be a non-specific feature of any acute illness or insult. It is common with advanced cognitive impairment. Faecal incontinence is less common, but has a major impact on care needs.

Vision and hearing

Hearing loss and visual symptoms, including impairment of visual acuity, are common (Box 16.9). They are often not noted and this will adversely affect communication, interaction and function. Hearing loss may be misinterpreted as cognitive impairment and vice versa. Use a Snellen chart (Fig. 12.17) or ask the patient to read from a newspaper to assess vision.

Make sure the external auditory meatus is not blocked with wax. Ensure patients wear their hearing aids with a functioning battery so you do not incorrectly diagnose cognitive impairment simply because they could not hear you properly. Assess hearing using the whispered voice test if they do not have hearing aids (p. 302).

16.8 Signs and behaviours associated with pain

Type	Description
Autonomic changes	Pallor, sweating, tachypnoea, altered breathing patterns, tachycardia, hypertension
Facial expressions	Grimacing, wincing, frowning, rapid blinking, brow raising, brow lowering, cheek raising, eyelid tightening, nose wrinkling, lip corner pulling, chin raising, lip puckering
Body movements	Altered gait, pacing, rocking, hand wringing, repetitive movements, increased tone, guarding,* bracing[†]
Verbalisation/vocalisation	Sighing, grunting, groaning, moaning, screaming, calling out, aggressive/offensive speech
Interpersonal interactions	Aggression, withdrawal, resisting
Changes in activity patterns	Wandering, altered sleep, altered rest patterns
Mental status changes	Confusion, crying, distress, irritability

*Guarding = abnormal stiff, rigid or interrupted movement while changing position.
[†]Bracing = a stationary position in which a fully extended limb maintains and supports an abnormal weight distribution for at least 3 seconds.

16.9 Sensory problems

Visual	Underlying disease process
Loss of near vision (presbyopia)	Common in elderly because lens less pliable
Loss of central vision	Macular degeneration
Loss of peripheral vision	Glaucoma Stroke disease (homonymous hemianopia)
Glare from lights at night	Cataracts
Eye pain	Glaucoma
Auditory	
High-frequency loss	Presbyacusis Conductive deafness commoner due to otosclerosis
Generalised loss	Conductive – otosclerosis; wax Nerve – Paget's disease, drug-induced ototoxicity; acoustic neuroma

Systems examination

Fully examine each system, but particularly note the differences that may occur in the frail elderly.

Cardiovascular system

Corneal arcus increases in prevalence in the elderly but is a poor sign of dyslipidaemia (Fig. 6.8C).

Blood pressure

A widened pulse pressure occurs because there is decreased arterial compliance. Isolated systolic hypertension and postural hypotension occur more frequently. The latter may result from age-related baroreceptor reflex change, disease or drugs. It may not be symptomatic but increases the risk of a fall.

Pulse

Medial sclerosis and arterial calcification can make it difficult to feel peripheral pulses but without signs of impaired perfusion and circulation. The carotid artery may become more tortuous and its pulsations more easily visible. This can create a false impression of arterial dilation.

Heart sounds

Atrial contribution to left ventricular filling increases with age, partly due to diastolic dysfunction of the heart and a fourth heart sound (S_4) is more commonly heard.

Respiratory system

The significance of localised crackles is uncertain and they may not represent acute disease. Always exclude new respiratory disease.

Gastrointestinal system

Dry mouth and tongue are common side-effects of drugs and may affect taste and swallowing. Abnormal dentition or oral thrush or mouth ulcers may reduce oral intake and nutrition.

Nervous system

Cognitive impairment may reduce the accuracy of the history and affect consent for investigation and treatment. It will reduce the person's awareness of safety and compliance. Impaired vibration and position sense occur in old age but always exclude correctable causes, e.g. vitamin B_{12} deficiency. They may impair balance and increase the risk of falls. Bilateral absent ankle reflexes may be normal, but unilateral loss is likely to indicate pathology.

Musculoskeletal system

Osteoarthritic changes in the hands and weight-bearing joints may predispose to falls or unsteadiness even if relatively asymptomatic or painless. Gouty tophi may be asymptomatic and reflect underlying renal dysfunction and influence the choice of drug therapy. Kyphosis occurs frequently from painless osteoporotic vertebral collapse. It may affect postural stability and even respiratory function. Low muscle mass is a frailty indicator and a risk factor for falls.

Gait

Gait abnormalities are risk factors for falls or exacerbate joint problems. They may indicate undiagnosed neurological disease, such as Parkinson's disease. Sometimes gait problems may be helped by orthoses or mobility supports (Fig. 3.2).

16.10 Key components of physical function
Personal activities of daily living (PADL)
Washing Dressing Feeding Toileting
Domestic activities of daily living (DADL)
Preparing food Laundering clothes Cleaning the house

EBE 16.11 Mobility
The Timed Get-Up and Go test is a simple measurement of mobility. Perform it in all patients presenting in non-acute settings.
Podsiadlo D, Richardson S. The timed 'Up & Go': a test of basic functional mobility for frail elderly patients. J Am Geriatr Soc 1991;39:142–148.

16

Feet

Bunions, onychomycosis with or without nail overgrowth and foot ulcers are common. All can compromise mobility and stability, be a source of sepsis or pain and affect gait.

Functional assessment

Functional assessment is divided into assessment of:
- Mobility
- The ability to undertake activities of daily living (ADLs), those activities required for self-care and domestic tasks:
  - personal activities of daily living (PADL)
  - domestic activities of daily living (DADL) (Box 16.10).

Mobility is a key determinant of physical function (Box 16.11). A wide variety of pathologies can impair mobility and produce distinctive abnormalities of gait (Box 11.13). Other diseases may affect mobility by causing decreased muscle strength or joint function. Frailty causes generally impaired muscle strength, function and poor mobility but no specific clinical findings on examination of muscle, nerves, joints or gait (Fig. 16.4).

Standardised rating scales are used for different components of function, e.g. the modified Barthel Index for activities of daily living and the Elderly Mobility Score for mobility. Use these scales to describe the patient's abilities succinctly and, using sequential recording over time, objectively assess improvement or deterioration.

Common presentations

The frail elderly person with immobility

Establish patients' normal mobility, when it changed and if the change was abrupt. Have they fallen? Is there

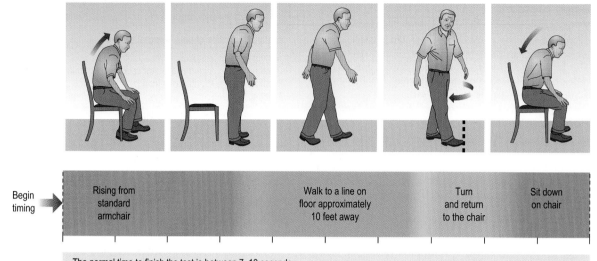

| Begin timing | Rising from standard armchair | Walk to a line on floor approximately 10 feet away | Turn and return to the chair | Sit down on chair |

The normal time to finish the test is between 7–10 seconds.
Patients who cannot complete the task in that time, probably have some mobility problems, especially if they take more than 20 seconds.

Fig. 16.4 The Timed Get Up and Go Test.

any history of recent head injury, fevers or rigors, dizziness or poor balance? Have they noticed lower limb weakness, numbness or paraesthesia? Ask about joint pain, especially in the back, neck or lower limbs, and if there are any bladder or bowel symptoms. What is their current drug treatment and has this changed recently?

Examination sequence

- General examination: look particularly for signs of acute illness (Box 16.6). If they are able to walk, assess the posture and gait and any inappropriate footwear. Are they visually impaired? (Box 16.9). Are there signs of sepsis, or a distended bladder?
- Cardiovascular system: check for postural hypotension.
- Nervous system: note any neurological signs, particularly in the lower limbs, and look for evidence of Parkinson's disease (p. 247).
- Locomotor system: look for muscle wasting or fasciculation, joint abnormality and foot deformity.
- Consider specific investigations (Box 16.12).

The acutely confused frail elderly person

Always take a collateral history. Establish the person's normal cognitive state and whether the change has been abrupt or gradual. Ask about symptoms of common acute illness, particularly infection, such as urinary frequency, productive cough, fever or rigors. Has the person complained of pain and if so, where? What is the current drug treatment and compliance? In particular, have there been any recent changes to drug treatment?

Examination sequence

- Look for signs of acute illness (Box 16.6) and pain (Box 16.8).
- Examine the skin, large joints, heart valves, prostheses and abdomen, e.g. biliary tract, colonic diverticulae, meninges, bladder and lungs.

16.12 Specific investigations in the frail elderly

Presentation	Investigations
Immobility and/or Falls	Timed Get Up and Go test Mental state: AMT or MMSE CT head* MR spine**
Confusion	Mental state assessment: AMT or MMSE Confusion Assessment Method (CAM) Score CT head*
Urinary incontinence	Urinalysis, urine culture Voiding chart (frequency & volume) Bladder ultrasound (post-residual volume) Prostatic specific antigen in men
Faecal incontinence	Stool culture if diarrhoea Abdominal X-ray if high impaction suspected

*if new neurological signs or head injury suspected.
**if cord pathology suspected.

- Measure the pulse oximetry (SpO$_2$).
- Feel for a distended bladder.
- Do a rectal examination (p. 187) to check for faecal impaction.
- If patients have problems with vision or hearing, ensure they wear their glasses or working hearing aid.
- Consider specific investigations (Box 16.12).

The frail elderly person with falls

What is patients' normal mobility and have they had any blackouts? Find out how many falls they have had, over what timescale and if they have ever had any injury – in particular, a head injury. If they complain of dizziness, is this true vertigo (p. 243)? Ask systematically about

16.13 The problem-based approach: examples of how this might be used in a patient with falls and confusion

Problem	Potential contributory factors	Management plan
Urinary incontinence	Urinary tract infection Faecal impaction	Urinalysis Send midstream specimen of urine to confirm Rectal examination
Hyponatraemia	Bendroflumethiazide	Withhold bendroflumethiazide Monitor serum sodium
Confusion with features of delirium	Urinary infection Hyponatraemia Underlying dementia	As above plus: Check MMSE Collateral history from carer Thyroid function Occupational therapy review
Foot ulcer	Absent pedal pulses	Check ankle brachial pressure index Discuss dressing with nurse
Poor mobility	Urinary infection Hyponatraemia Pain from foot ulcer Underlying cerebrovascular disease	As above plus: Prescribe simple analgesia Full neurological/gait examination Assess vascular risk factors Physiotherapy review

16

palpitation, limb weakness, numbness or paraesthesia and any joint pain, especially in the back, neck or lower limbs. How is their vision? Have they had symptoms of infection recently, such as rigors or urinary symptoms? Ask about current drug treatment and any recent changes in drugs. A collateral history of a witnessed fall is helpful.

Examination sequence

- Look for signs of bony or soft-tissue injury and acute illness, e.g. sepsis (Box 16.6).
- Cardiovascular system: check for postural hypotension, arrhythmias and aortic stenosis.
- Nervous system: are there neurological signs in lower limbs or evidence of Parkinson's disease (p. 247)? Is there visual impairment?
- Musculoskeletal system: look for joint or muscle abnormality and foot deformity. Do they have appropriate footwear? Note any posture or gait abnormality (Fig. 3.2).
- Consider specific investigations (Box 16.12).

The incontinent frail elderly person

This may be either urinary or faecal incontinence or both.

Ask if patients can transfer and mobilise from a chair to toilet or commode?

Are they aware of the need to pass urine or defecate? Are they incontinent all the time or only intermittently? Is the stool formed or unformed?

Examination sequence

- Nervous system: are they cognitively impaired? Is there other evidence of neurological disease? Palpate for the bladder and check that perianal sensation is normal.

- Gastrointestinal: palpate for any abnormal abdominal masses. Examine the perineal skin and see if it is intact. Perform a rectal examination looking for anal fissure, haemorrhoids or other local disease. Note if the rectum is empty or impacted with faeces and assess anal tone. In a man, assess prostate enlargement; in a woman look for vaginal prolapse or atrophy.

PUTTING IT ALL TOGETHER

Comprehensive geriatric assessment requires excellent communication between members of the multiprofessional team. A problem-based approach helps to pull all this information together and formulate a clear individualised management plan.

Start by creating a problem list to summarise all the problems identified. Generate a provisional list after speaking with the patient and refine it after interviewing carers, undertaking the physical examination and hearing the outcome of functional assessments. Do not confine the list to medical diagnoses, but include symptoms, laboratory results and presenting features (Box 16.13).

The problem list builds a complete picture of the patient and alerts you to how the different problems may interact. If a problem has several contributing factors, list them all. Use the list to develop a management plan addressing each problem and contributing factor. Include actions such as diagnostic investigations, treatment of identified disease, alteration of drug therapy and rehabilitation. Tailor your management plan specifically to the individual patient, considering the outcome goals you have agreed with the patient. Explain the proposed management plan to your patient and ensure that he understands and agrees.

Dilip Nathwani
Kum Ying Tham

The febrile adult 17

EXAMINATION OF THE FEBRILE ADULT

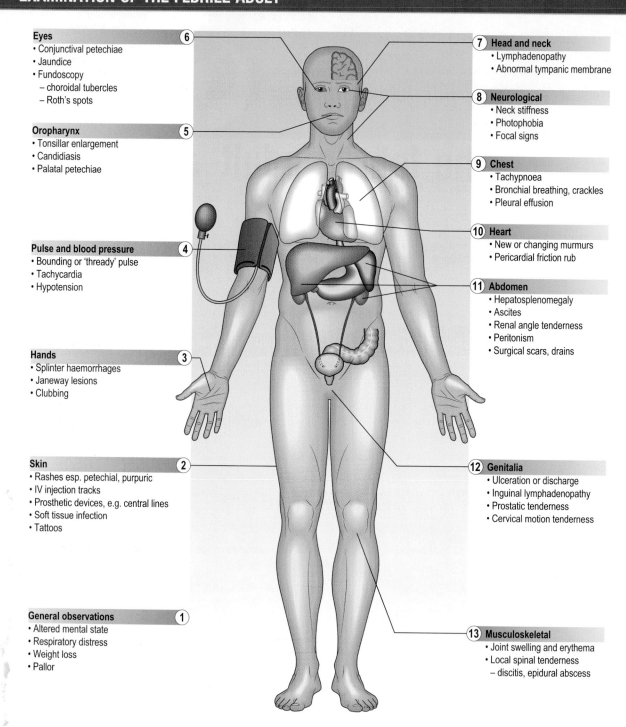

Eyes (6)
- Conjunctival petechiae
- Jaundice
- Fundoscopy
  - choroidal tubercles
  - Roth's spots

Oropharynx (5)
- Tonsillar enlargement
- Candidiasis
- Palatal petechiae

Pulse and blood pressure (4)
- Bounding or 'thready' pulse
- Tachycardia
- Hypotension

Hands (3)
- Splinter haemorrhages
- Janeway lesions
- Clubbing

Skin (2)
- Rashes esp. petechial, purpuric
- IV injection tracks
- Prosthetic devices, e.g. central lines
- Soft tissue infection
- Tattoos

General observations (1)
- Altered mental state
- Respiratory distress
- Weight loss
- Pallor

(7) **Head and neck**
- Lymphadenopathy
- Abnormal tympanic membrane

(8) **Neurological**
- Neck stiffness
- Photophobia
- Focal signs

(9) **Chest**
- Tachypnoea
- Bronchial breathing, crackles
- Pleural effusion

(10) **Heart**
- New or changing murmurs
- Pericardial friction rub

(11) **Abdomen**
- Hepatosplenomegaly
- Ascites
- Renal angle tenderness
- Peritonism
- Surgical scars, drains

(12) **Genitalia**
- Ulceration or discharge
- Inguinal lymphadenopathy
- Prostatic tenderness
- Cervical motion tenderness

(13) **Musculoskeletal**
- Joint swelling and erythema
- Local spinal tenderness
  - discitis, epidural abscess

SYMPTOMS AND DEFINITIONS

Fever (pyrexia) is a body temperature >99th percentile of the healthy adult maximum (p. 61). Fever is present if the oral temperature is >37.7°C, or tympanic temperature >37.5°C. In immunodeficient or neutropenic patients, fever is a single temperature >38.3°C, or a temperature >38°C sustained for >1 hour.

Body temperature is tightly controlled to maintain normal metabolic processes. The set point is controlled by the hypothalamus and modified by infection, inflammation and, rarely, other conditions, e.g. hypothyroidism, lymphoma. Infection is the most common cause but in very young or elderly patients and those with impaired immune function (due to primary disease, e.g. human immunodeficiency virus (HIV), or following treatment, e.g. oral steroids, immunosuppressants) it may not produce fever.

Body temperature depends upon the balance between heat generation and loss, and the ambient environment. Heat-related illness occurs with exercise in high temperatures and humidity. It is more common at the extremes of age and may be precipitated or aggravated by drugs which affect thermoregulation, e.g. phenothiazines, alcohol, or which are associated with excessive exercise, e.g. 'rave' drugs, including ecstasy, amphetamines (Boxes 17.1 and 17.2).

Fictitious fever is produced artificially by the patient or an attendant. It may form part of a Munchausen or Munchausen-by-proxy syndrome (Box 17.3).

Extreme fever (>41°C) is life-threatening and is usually associated with:

- Gram-negative bacteraemia
- central problems with temperature regulation, e.g. following intracranial haemorrhage or head injury
- drug reactions, e.g. to anaesthetic agents, or drugs associated with the neuroleptic malignant syndrome
- severe environmental conditions often with strenuous unaccustomed exertion (heatstroke)

Fever (pyrexia) of unknown origin (FUO or PUO) is documented fever which remains unexplained after 2–3 weeks' investigation. Healthcare-acquired PUO is fever in patients hospitalised for >48 hours with no infection evident at admission, and in whom the diagnosis remains uncertain after ≥3 days of appropriate evaluation (Box 17.4).

Rigors (chills) are bouts of uncontrollable muscular shaking, often with 'chattering' teeth, lasting for minutes. They are associated with rapid temperature rises and may be caused by cytokines and acute-phase proteins resetting the hypothalamic temperature set point.

17

EBE 17.2 Fever

A patient who reports fever or whose forehead feels abnormally warm is highly likely to have a fever.

Buckley RG, Conine M. Reliability of subjective fever in triage of adult patients. Ann Emerg Med 1996;27:693–695.
Hung OL, Kwan NS, Cole AE et al. Evaluation of the physician's ability to recognize the presence or absence of anaemia, fever and jaundice. Acad Emerg Med 2000;7:146–156.

17.3 Clues to fictitious fever

- Patient looks well
- Temperature is normal when taken by an independent, supervised observer
- Bizarre temperature chart with temperatures >41°C, absence of diurnal variation
- No correlation between temperature and pulse rate
- No sweating during resolution of fever
- Evidence of self-harm, injection
- Normal erythrocyte sedimentation rate/C-reactive protein

17.1 Common causes of immunocompromise

Lifestyle-related and social factors

- Chronic alcohol consumption
- Injecting, IV drug use
- Malnutrition

Disease-related

- Malignancy, e.g. solid organ cancer, lymphoproliferative disorders
- Diabetes mellitus
- HIV infection
- Liver cirrhosis
- Renal failure
- Severe or debilitating illness resulting in immobility and malnutrition
- Splenectomy, hyposplenia and functional asplenia

Treatment-related

- Indwelling catheters and tubes
- Corticosteroids
- Chemotherapy/immunosuppressants/immunomodulators for cancer, rheumatoid arthritis, post-transplant
- Post-radiotherapy
- Solid organ transplantation

17.4 Causes of pyrexia of unknown origin

Infection (~30%)	Non-infectious causes (~70%)

• Tuberculosis (extrapulmonary and disseminated)
• Endocarditis
• Abdominal abscess
• Bone and joint infection
• Urinary and prostatic infection
• HIV-related
• Travel-related, e.g.
  ◦ Malaria
  ◦ Typhoid
  ◦ Dengue
  ◦ Rickettsial infections
• Healthcare-acquired infection
	• Malignancy
	• Connective tissue disorders

1 Are any 2 of the following present and new to the patient?
   • Temperature > 38°C or < 36°C
   • Heart rate > 90/min
   • Respiratory rate > 20/min
   • White cells < 4 or > 12 × 10^9/l
   • PaCO$_2$ < 32 mmHg (4.3kPa)

IF YES, PATIENT HAS SIRS
(Systemic Inflammatory Response Syndrome)

2 Is the history suggestive of a new infection?
   • Pneumonia
   • Diarrhoea
   • Meningitis
   • Soft tissue infection/cellulitis/fasciitis
   • Septic arthritis
   • Indwelling urinary catheter, central line etc
   • Urinary infection
   • Peritonitis
   • Endocarditis
   • Wound infection

IF YES, PATIENT HAS SEPSIS

3 Are any of the following present and new to the patient?
   • BP: systolic < 90 or a fall of > 40 mmHg
   • New or increased O$_2$ requirements to maintain SpO$_2$ > 90%
   • Acutely altered mental state
   • Creatinine >177 μmol/l or urine output < 0.5 ml/kg/hr for 2 hrs
   • Bilirubin > 34 μmol/litre
   • Platelets < 100 × 10^9/l
   • Coagulopathy: INR > 1.5 or APTT > 60 sec

IF YES, PATIENT HAS SEVERE SEPSIS

Fig. 17.1 Sepsis assessment.

Subjectively the patient feels cold and unwell and the episode may be followed by sweating. A rigor may be associated with bacteraemia or malaria and is of poor diagnostic value.

The terms systemic inflammatory response syndrome (SIRS), sepsis, severe sepsis and septic shock reflect progressively increasing morbidity and mortality in response to infection. Multiple organ failure and death ensue if recognition or treatment is delayed (Fig. 17.1). The term SIRS is not specific to infection.

THE HISTORY

Presenting complaint

How has the fever been documented? What is its severity and time course? Have there been rigors or sweating?

Has there been a rash or skin changes? If yes, ask about its timing in relation to the fever, the distribution and direction of any progression and associated symptoms, e.g. pruritus, local lymphadenopathy.

Systematically ask about localising symptoms, e.g. cough, pleuritic chest pain, purulent sputum, vomiting, abdominal pain, jaundice, diarrhoea, dysuria, urinary frequency, headache, photophobia, neck stiffness, altered consciousness, joint pain, muscle aches, throat or ear discomfort and nasal discharge.

Are there constitutional symptoms, including easy fatigability, anorexia, weight loss, falls, change in daily activities or behaviour? Such symptoms may indicate infection in the elderly or immunocompromised.

Past medical history

Have there been previous or recurrent infections, illnesses, surgical operations or dental treatment?

Has there been contact or residence in a healthcare facility (including long-term care facility)?

Ask about a history of immunosuppression, e.g. HIV infection, chemotherapy, steroid therapy, transplantation, diabetes mellitus. Ask about indwelling catheters, e.g. urethral, intravenous (IV) or implants, e.g. pacemakers, joint replacements.

Drug history

Find out about all prescribed and non-prescribed medications, e.g. herbal remedies taken and ask specifically about immunosuppressants (including oral steroids), antibiotics, antipyretics. Have any 'recreational' drugs been taken; if so, have they ever been injected?

Note any history of adverse reactions, allergies or hypersensitivity to any drugs, particularly antibiotics.

Family and social history

Has the patient had contact with anyone with a similar illness? Find out about exposure to animals, birds or pets and if so, is the animal unwell? Note the patient's occupation and hobbies. Are there clusters of similar symptoms or infections among family, friends or workmates?

Travel history

Has there been recent (in the past year) travel abroad? If so, take a detailed travel history including:

• travel destinations: dates, duration, mode of travel, stop-overs (Box 2.18)
• environment abroad: accommodation, altitude, climate, activities
• lifestyle: including diet, e.g. raw or unpasteurised products, sexual contact (who, when, how many partners), water sports, healthcare, piercings, tattoos
• medical history: including vaccination status, pre-existing conditions, antimalarial measures, particularly type, duration and compliance (Boxes 17.5 and 17.6).

17.5 Common causes of fever in travellers

Developing countries	Worldwide
Malaria	Influenza
Schistosomiasis	Pneumonia
Dengue	Upper respiratory tract infection
Typhoid	Urinary infection
Tick typhus	Traveller's diarrhoea
Tuberculosis	
Dysentery	
Hepatitis A	
Amoebiasis	

17.6 Specific exposures and causes of fever in the tropics

Exposure	Infection or disease
Mosquito bite	Malaria, dengue fever, chikungunya, filariasis, tularaemia
Tsetse fly bite	African trypanosomiasis
Tick bite	Rickettsial infections, including typhus, Lyme disease, tularaemia, Crimean–Congo haemorrhagic fever, Kyasanur forest disease, babesiosis, tick-borne encephalitis
Louse bite	Typhus
Flea bite	Plague
Sandfly bite	Leishmaniasis, arbovirus infection
Reduviid bug	Chagas' disease
Animal contact	Q fever, brucellosis, anthrax, plague, tularaemia, viral haemorrhagic fevers, rabies
Fresh-water swimming	Schistosomiasis, leptospirosis, *Naegleria fowleri*
Exposure to soil	Inhalation: dimorphic fungi Inhalation or inoculation: *Burkholderia pseudomallei* Inoculation (most often when barefoot): hookworms, *Strongyloides stercoralis*
Raw or undercooked fruit and vegetables	Enteric bacterial infections, hepatitis A or E virus, *Fasciola hepatica, Toxocara* spp., *Echinococcus granulosus* (hydatid disease), *Entamoeba histolytica*
Undercooked pork	*Taenia solium* (cysticercosis)
Crustaceans or molluscs	Paragonimiasis, gnathostomiasis, *Angiostrongylus cantonensis* infection, hepatitis A virus, cholera
Unpasteurised dairy products	Brucellosis, salmonellosis, abdominal tuberculosis, listeriosis
Untreated water	Enteric bacterial infections, giardiasis, *Cryptosporidium* spp. (chronic in immunocompromised), hepatitis A or E virus

EBE 17.7 Typhoid

In tropical countries, a 'stepladder' pattern of remittent fever is highly specific for typhoid.

Haq SA, Alam MN, Hossain SM et al. Value of clinical features in the diagnosis of enteric fever. Bangladesh Med Res Council Bull 1997;23:42–46.

17.8 'Red flag' features

- Altered mental state
- Headache and/or stiff neck
- Petechial/purpuric skin rash
- Hypotension – systolic blood pressure <90 mmHg
- Tachycardia – heart rate >90 bpm –with narrowed pulse pressure and 'thready' pulse
- Tachypnoea – respiratory rate >20 breaths/min
- Recent travel to or recent arrival from malaria or tuberculosis endemic area
- Recent use of immunosuppressant drugs
- Significant active comorbidities (cancer, HIV, organ transplantation)
- Temperature > 38°C or < 36°C
- Rigors (chills)

THE PHYSICAL EXAMINATION

General

Examination sequence

- Record the temperature and the site of measurement (p. 61). Fever may be intermittent or be suppressed or modified by antipyretic or antimicrobial drugs. With one exception (Box 17.7), fever 'patterns', e.g. sustained, intermittent, relapsing, are of little diagnostic value.
- Look for 'red flag' features indicating serious infection (Box 17.8).
- Assess the general appearance: look for any weakness, lethargy, cachexia, distress or altered conscious state (use the Abbreviated Mental Test and the Mini-Mental State Examination: p. 26).
- Inspect the entire body for rashes, particularly petechial or haemorrhagic (Fig. 17.2). If a rash is present, characterise the lesions (Box 17.9) and note any change in morphology, e.g. papules to vesicles or petechiae, and whether the rashes are coalescing or denuding.
- Look for areas of erythema, swelling or blistering, suggesting skin or soft-tissue infection (Fig. 17.2).
- Examine the neck, axillae, epitrochlear and groin areas for lymphadenopathy and feel for the spleen (p. 184).
- In hospitalised patients, look for evidence of inflammation at the site of IV lines or devices (Fig. 17.2) or urinary catheters.
- Carefully inspect recent surgical wound sites for signs of infection.
- Look at hands and feet for splinter haemorrhages (Fig. 4.15A) and Janeway lesions (non-tender haemorrhagic macules on the palms or soles) (Fig. 6.8B).

17

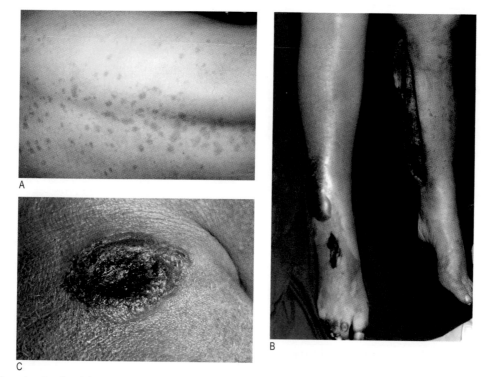

Fig. 17.2 Examples of serious infections. (A) Meningococcal rash. **(B)** Necrotising fasciitis with fasciotomy. **(C)** Anthrax eschar.

17.9 Some infections associated with rash and fever	
Macular/maculopapular	**Vesicular**
Measles	Chickenpox (varicella virus)
Rubella	Shingles (zoster virus)
Enterovirus	Herpes simplex virus
Human herpes virus 6	Herpangina (Coxsackie virus)
Epstein–Barr virus	Hand, foot and mouth disease (Coxsackie virus)
Cytomegalovirus	**Erythematous**
Human parvovirus B19	Scarlet fever
HIV	Toxic shock syndrome
Typhoid	Lyme disease (erythema chronica migrans)
Dengue	Human parvovirus B19
Secondary syphilis	**Petechial/haemorrhage**
Rickettsial spotted fevers	Meningococcal septicaemia
Urticarial (worm infestations)	Septicaemia with disseminated intravascular coagulation
Toxocara	Rickettsiae
Schistosomiasis	Yellow fever
Strongyloides	Ebola and Marburg virus
Cutaneous larva migrans	Lassa fever
Other	Dengue
Primary syphilis (chancre)	Rift valley fever
Tick typhus (eschar)	

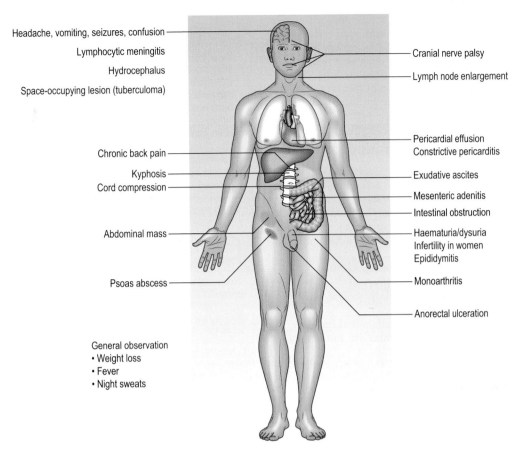

Headache, vomiting, seizures, confusion

Lymphocytic meningitis

Hydrocephalus

Space-occupying lesion (tuberculoma)

Cranial nerve palsy

Lymph node enlargement

Chronic back pain

Kyphosis

Cord compression

Pericardial effusion
Constrictive pericarditis

Exudative ascites

Mesenteric adenitis

Intestinal obstruction

Abdominal mass

Haematuria/dysuria
Infertility in women
Epididymitis

Psoas abscess

Monoarthritis

Anorectal ulceration

General observation
• Weight loss
• Fever
• Night sweats

Fig. 17.3 Systemic presentation of extrapulmonary tuberculosis.

Systemic examination

Examination sequence

If a febrile patient looks unwell, rapidly assess the mental state, pulse rate, respiratory rate, blood pressure and pulse oximetry (SpO_2). If the history and general examination suggest severe sepsis or septic shock, begin resuscitation immediately (Ch. 19).

Most patients with bacterial infection have localising symptoms or signs, e.g. tender swelling of an abscess or murmurs of bacterial endocarditis, but it is essential to examine the patient from head to toe because clues may be in any system.

Examine the head and neck:

- Look at the tympanic membranes with an otoscope for middle-ear infection.
- Percuss the frontal and maxillary sinuses for tenderness (sinusitis).
- Palpate the temporal arteries for tenderness (giant cell arteritis).
- Examine the nose for congestion and discharge (clear or purulent).
- Look in the mouth at the oropharynx and gums for inflammation (Fig. 13.21), oral candidiasis (Fig. 13.25A), immunodeficiency, e.g. HIV, or recent broad-spectrum antibiotic use.
- Examine the sclerae for conjunctivitis or jaundice.

- Use an ophthalmoscope to examine the retinae for Roth's spots (endocarditis) (Fig. 6.6).
- Gently flex the neck to detect discomfort, stiffness, or both, indicating meningism.
- Palpate for neck lymphadenopathy (Fig. 17.3).
- Percuss and auscultate the lungs for crackles, signs of consolidation (pneumonia) or effusion (empyema).
- Listen to the heart for murmurs (endocarditis).
- Examine the abdomen for enlargement and tenderness of the liver and spleen.
- Percuss the flanks for renal tenderness (pyelonephritis).
- In women, pelvic examination (p. 222) may reveal cervical motion or adnexal tenderness; in men, look for urethral discharge or local genital tenderness (p. 235).
- Perform a rectal examination (p. 187) looking for tenderness and swelling, suggesting perirectal abscess (which may be occult in immunocompromised patients) and prostatic enlargement or tenderness (urinary or prostate infection).
- Examine the major joints for swelling, erythema and tenderness (joint infection or rheumatologic disorder).

Specific situations

Injecting drug users

Injecting drug users are at particular risk of serious bacterial infection as well as viral diseases, e.g. HIV, hepatitis B and C. The commonest infections are of skin and soft tissue with bacteraemia leading to endocarditis (especially involving the tricuspid valve) and bone and joint infections. In an injecting drug user with fever, examine injection sites for discharge or signs of infection, listen to the chest for crackles or pleural rub (septic pulmonary emboli) and auscultate the heart for murmurs (right-sided valve endocarditis),

The immunocompromised patient

Although immunocompromised patients have less fever with infection, it is still the main presenting complaint. Because they are less able to mount an inflammatory response at the site of infection, the usual signs and symptoms may be absent, e.g. pneumonia without purulent sputum, tenderness without visible inflammation in a perirectal abscess.

In a febrile immunocompromised patient:

- symptoms are diminished or atypical
- obtain a detailed history for possible sources of infection
- expect atypical clinical and radiological findings
- expect the infection to be advanced at the time of presentation
- use computed tomography (CT) and magnetic resonance imaging (MR) scanning early for anatomic delineation of infection
- obtain tissue for histopathology and microbiology early for specific microbiologic diagnosis.

Use the examination sequence above, but additionally look for:

- cushingoid features (Fig. 5.18) suggestive of oral corticosteroid use
- malnourished or wasted appearance
- features of chronic alcohol consumption and liver cirrhosis (Fig. 8.11)
- changes related to renal failure and replacement therapy (Fig. 9.5)
- changes associated with diabetes mellitus (Ch. 5)
- subtle signs of infection around indwelling catheters and tubes
- poor wound healing
- radiotherapy skin markings
- constellations of lesions commonly seen in neutropenic patients, e.g. erythema, rash, erythema nodosum, soft-tissue infection, ulcers, furuncles, herpetic eruptions, paronychia, mucositis, dental or peritonsillar abscesses, perirectal infection
- constellations of lesions commonly seen in HIV infection – carefully examine the skin, mouth, genitalia and perianal area. In a severely immunocompromised patient avoid rectal examination as this may breach the rectal mucosa and cause iatrogenic infection (Boxes 17.10 and 17.11).

Healthcare-acquired infection (HAI)

HAIs affect up to 10% of all hospital admissions. The close proximity of ill patients, coupled with the concentrated use of antimicrobial drugs and ease of transmission by healthcare workers, has led to multidrug-resistant organisms, e.g. meticillin-resistant *Staphylococcus aureus*

17.10 Features suggesting immunocompromise

- Recurrent infections
- Severe infections that progress rapidly, or are associated with many complications
- Infections last longer, or are slower to respond to standard treatment
- Infections caused by a wider variety of microorganisms and/or unusual organisms
- Concurrent or close temporal proximity of infectious, autoimmune and malignant diseases
- Chronic diarrhoea, malabsorption
- Poor wound healing

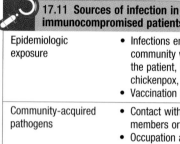

17.11 Sources of infection in immunocompromised patients

Epidemiologic exposure	• Infections endemic in the patient's community which may be latent in the patient, e.g. tuberculosis, chickenpox, worm infestation • Vaccination history
Community-acquired pathogens	• Contact with unwell family members or colleagues • Occupation and hobbies • Pets • Recent travel history, especially to unusual destinations or unusual activities, e.g. rural areas or farm stays in developing countries, river water sports
Reactivation of infection	• Infections that occurred many years prior to onset of immunocompromised state may be reactivated, e.g. herpes simplex/zoster, cytomegalovirus, tuberculosis • Use of prophylactic therapy, e.g. post-transplant, during chemotherapy-induced neutropenia

Healthcare-acquired infections (HAI): nosocomial infections	• All hospitalised patients are susceptible to HAI, but immunocompromised patients are at even higher risk, especially:
	  • Cancer or other patients with neutropenia
	  • Transplant recipients during early post-transplant and post-surgical stage
	  • HIV patients with low CD4 cell count
	  • High-dose or long-term steroid therapy
	  • Bone marrow irradiation

Donor-derived infections	• Any concern about inadequate screening of donor

(MRSA), *Clostridium difficile*. These infections are transmitted by many routes – contact, droplet spread, medication-related, transfusion, needlestick and airborne. The commonest HAIs relate to indwelling urinary catheters and invasive devices, e.g. IV cannulae, and procedures. In a patient with fever and any invasive device find out how long the cannula, prosthesis or catheter has been present and look for redness or discharge at the entry site (Box 17.12).

INVESTIGATIONS

See Box 17.13.

17.12 Infections associated with invasive procedures and devices

Procedure/device	Type of infection
Intravascular cannula	Bacteraemia, catheter site infection
Bladder catheter	Urinary tract infection, bacteraemia
Mechanical ventilation	Pneumonia, sinusitis
Stents, prosthesis, devices, grafts	Bacteraemia, subacute or chronic focal infection of device
Surgery	Surgical site infections, pneumonia
Endoscopy	Bacteraemia, pneumonia, cholangitis, gastroenteritis
Blood transfusion	Viral infection, bacteraemia, fungaemia

17.13 Investigations in the febrile adult

Investigations	Indication/comment
Bedside	
Urinalysis and urine microscopy	Haematuria, white blood cells, bacteria or proteinuria in urinary infection Microscopic haematuria and proteinuria in endocarditis
Blood tests	
Full blood count*	White cell count $>12 \times 10^9/l$ or $<4 \times 10^9/l$ in septic shock CD4 lymphocyte count to assess HIV infection ↑ Eosinophil count in worm infestation and drug allergy
Blood film	Malarial parasites
Renal/liver function	Abnormal in bacteraemia with severe sepsis syndrome ↑ Transaminases in acute hepatitis
C-reactive protein	↑ in bacterial infection
Serology	Less helpful in the immunocompromised: IgM in acute viral infection: IgG in previous viral infection, bacterial infection, e.g. syphilis; protozoal infection, e.g. amoebiasis, toxoplasmosis; worm infection, e.g. schistosomiasis
Culture	
Blood*	Bacteraemia, e.g. typhoid, endocarditis. Particularly useful during rigors
Sputum	e.g. Pneumococcal pneumonia, tuberculosis
Urine*	Urinary infection
Stool culture and microscopy + toxin	Culture: diarrhoea, e.g. *Campylobacter*, *Salmonella*. Microscopy for ova, cysts and parasites, e.g. giardiasis, amoebiasis. Toxin test: *Clostridium difficile*
Cerebrospinal fluid	Bacterial, viral and fungal meningitis
Joint fluid	Septic arthritis
Tissue biopsy	e.g. Tuberculosis lymph node
Polymerase chain reaction	
Cerebrospinal fluid	Viral meningitis, e.g. Herpes simplex Bacterial meningitis for pneumococcus and meningococcus
Throat swab	Viral infections, e.g. Influenza

17

17.13 Investigations in the febrile adult – *cont'd*

Investigations	Indication/comment
Imaging	
Chest X-ray*	Pneumonia, tuberculosis. Perform in immunocompromised even if no apparent respiratory features
Ultrasound	Localising abscesses, empyema, gallstones
CT scan*	Intra-abdominal or intracranial abscesses, lymphadenopathy
MR scan*	Intracranial infections, bone and joint infections
Positron emission tomography/CT	Localising infections and pyrexia of unknown origin
Others	
Mantoux skin test and interferon-γ release assay Induced sputum or bronchoscopic lavage	Latent tuberculosis Useful for *Pneumocystis jirovecii* pneumonia in HIV or ventilator-associated pneumonia

*Investigations most often required in immunocompromised patients.

Laura Robertson
Andrew Longmate

Assessment for anaesthesia and sedation

EXAMINATION FOR ANAESTHESIA AND SEDATION

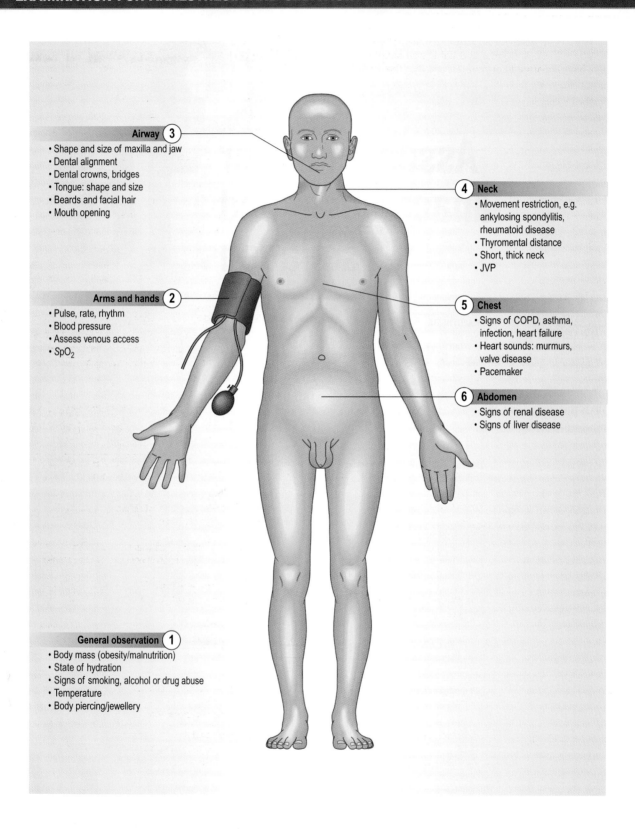

Airway ③
- Shape and size of maxilla and jaw
- Dental alignment
- Dental crowns, bridges
- Tongue: shape and size
- Beards and facial hair
- Mouth opening

Arms and hands ②
- Pulse, rate, rhythm
- Blood pressure
- Assess venous access
- SpO_2

Neck ④
- Movement restriction, e.g. ankylosing spondylitis, rheumatoid disease
- Thyromental distance
- Short, thick neck
- JVP

Chest ⑤
- Signs of COPD, asthma, infection, heart failure
- Heart sounds: murmurs, valve disease
- Pacemaker

Abdomen ⑥
- Signs of renal disease
- Signs of liver disease

General observation ①
- Body mass (obesity/malnutrition)
- State of hydration
- Signs of smoking, alcohol or drug abuse
- Temperature
- Body piercing/jewellery

Many clinical, investigative and therapeutic procedures are performed under anaesthesia or sedation. Prior patient evaluation is important to:

- identify risk factors: estimate absolute risk and ensure the patient and team recognise these
- modify risk: mitigate modifiable risk factors
- obtain informed consent: ensure that the patient understands the risks and benefits of the procedure and anaesthetic and can discuss and question the proposed plan.

PRE-ANAESTHESIA AND SEDATION CONSULTATION

Aims to:
- establish rapport and discuss the patient's anxieties
- obtain relevant information about:
  - medical history
  - medications
  - family
  - social history
- undertake relevant systematic enquiry and elicit clinical conditions or abnormalities that could influence anaesthesia
- inform/discuss options and preferences, e.g. regional versus general anaesthetic techniques

- provide information and specific advice that could decrease risk
- obtain and document consent.

THE HISTORY

Presenting complaint

Why and when is sedation/anaesthesia required?
- emergency situations, e.g. fracture manipulation, cardioversion
- planned events, e.g. endoscopy, elective surgery.

Could the presenting complaint affect this process, e.g. deranged fluid/electrolyte status, altered conscious state, alcohol/drug intoxication?

Could a pre-existing condition affect the process, e.g. pregnancy or steroid/immunosuppressive therapy?

Past history

18

Document previous relevant illnesses and chronic conditions (Box 18.1). Ask specifically about cardiovascular and respiratory conditions, including congenital, rheumatic or ischaemic heart disease, pacemakers, chronic obstructive pulmonary disease (COPD), asthma. Many less common conditions can be relevant (Box 18.2).

18.1 Features of the history particularly relevant to anaesthesia assessment

Condition	Key features relevant to anaesthesia	Reason
Angina	What is the frequency? What brings it on? Has there been a change in symptoms? What is the response to treatment?	Poorly controlled angina: ↑ risk of perioperative cardiovascular complications. Aim to optimise medical conditions preoperatively if there is time
Myocardial infarction (MI)	Past history of MI(s)? How long ago? Post-MI angina and exercise tolerance? Was treatment with indwelling coronary artery stents performed? What kind of stents (bare metal or drug-eluting)? Is the patient taking one or more antiplatelet agents, e.g. aspirin or clopidogrel?	Risk factor for postoperative death or serious complications Risk of perioperative cardiac events ↑↑ if within past 3–6 months Effective treatment of angina or MI with medical treatment or invasive treatments (surgery or coronary stenting) may modify risk Surgery shortly after stenting is associated with increased risks Withdrawing antiplatelet agents is associated with stent occlusion Antiplatelet drugs are associated with increased bleeding risks Balance risk of bleeding against risk of stent occlusion
Hypertension	How well is it controlled?	Poor control may mean greater blood pressure lability perioperatively
Heart failure/valve disease	How severe are the symptoms (exercise tolerance, breathlessness, oedema)?	Heart failure is an important adverse risk factor for perioperative risk Optimise heart failure preoperatively
Cardiac arrhythmia	Is arrhythmia present? Is the patient taking warfarin or other anticoagulants for atrial fibrillation or other conditions? Is pacemaker or implantable cardiac defibrillator (ICD) present?	Optimise arrhythmia control Some anaesthetic drugs may exacerbate arrhythmias Anticoagulation requires management perioperatively Pacemakers may need checking and/or reprogramming preoperatively. There are important implications for the use of diathermy and the underlying condition requiring a pacemaker or ICD

Continued

18.1 Features of the history particularly relevant to anaesthesia assessment – *cont'd*

Condition	Key features relevant to anaesthesia	Reason
Chronic obstructive pulmonary disease and asthma	How severe are the symptoms (exercise tolerance, breathlessness, steroid requirement, frequency of hospital admissions, lung function)?	Severe disease ↑ perioperative risk and influences choice of anaesthetic technique
Obstructive sleep apnoea	May be undiagnosed – ask about symptoms (snoring, apnoeic spells, daytime hypersomnolence) Use of continuous positive airway pressure (CPAP) machine at night?	↑ Risk of perioperative airway obstruction and respiratory failure with sedative drugs, influences choice of anaesthetic technique May require postoperative CPAP. Ask the patient to bring the CPAP machine into hospital
Renal failure	What was the underlying cause? Is it dialysis-dependent? What volume of urine is still passed? Recent complications, e.g. hyperkalaemia, fluid overload?	Influences fluid management, choice of technique and drugs
Liver conditions Diabetes mellitus	Any condition affecting hepatic function, e.g. cirrhosis, hepatitis, chronic liver disease? Is glycaemic control achieved? Look at chronic control preoperatively (patient history, note books, measurement of HbA1c)	Influences fluid management, glycaemic control, coagulation, drug metabolism Optimise glucose control preoperatively and also perioperatively Aim to control blood glucose between 6 and 10 mmol/L Avoid hypo- or hyperglycaemia which have serious and severe consequences. Managing the change between omission of hypoglycaemic agents, interruption of oral feeding and the stress response to injury requires careful assessment planning and observation
	Any complications? If so, how severe?	Complications ↑ anaesthetic and surgical risk, e.g. postoperative infections, cardiac disease, cerebrovascular disease, neuropathy, delayed gastric emptying

18.2 Some conditions with special relevance

Condition	Considerations
Rheumatoid arthritis	Neck may be unstable and mouth opening impaired; comorbidity, e.g. reduced functional capability, immobility, respiratory and renal impairment; thin skin and poor wound healing, poor vascular access; complex drug therapy, including the consequences of immunosuppressive treatments such as steroids and antitumour necrosis factor agents. Need for careful evaluation of airway and neck preoperatively and careful positioning under anaesthesia
Epilepsy	Drug treatment can interact with anaesthetics; surgical stress and some anaesthetics can ↑ seizure risk. Ensure that usual antiepileptic medication is given as normal
Scoliosis and spinal abnormalities	Can ↓ respiratory reserve; tracheal intubation can be difficult; regional anaesthesia difficult
Myasthenia gravis and other chronic neuromuscular disorders	Risk of respiratory failure; sensitivity to anaesthetic drugs; surgical and anaesthetic stress can cause acute exacerbations, e.g. multiple sclerosis
Sickle cell disease	Stress of surgery, hypoxia, hypothermia or dehydration can precipitate sickle cell crisis
Porphyria	Some anaesthetic agents, e.g. barbiturates, etomidate may trigger a porphyric attack; acute porphyria may mimic a 'surgical' acute abdomen

Drug history

Record all current drugs, including over-the-counter medications and herbal preparations. You may need to stop, start or modify drug therapy prior to surgery (Box 18.3), e.g. patients taking steroids may require perioperative supplementation.

Document all allergies, and the nature of the reaction. Some may be a side-effect rather than true allergy, e.g. nausea. Record any reactions to skin preparation agents, e.g. iodine, or to skin dressings, and to specific foods as these may result in cross-sensitivity. Ask about latex allergy.

Previous anaesthetic history

Ask about past anaesthetics and examine the charts from previous procedures. Record any problems, particularly

18.3 Perioperative drugs

Some drugs that may need to be stopped or have their dose adjusted before surgery

Drug	Reason
Antiplatelet agents, e.g. aspirin, clopidogrel	Evaluate why the person takes this medication Balance the risks of continued antiplatelet drugs (bleeding) against the risks of cessation, e.g. coronary artery stent occlusion
Oral anticoagulants, e.g. warfarin	Evaluate why the person takes this medication Balance the risks of continued oral anticoagulation (bleeding) against the risk of stopping (thromboembolism) – consider bridging therapy with heparin if appropriate Recommence anticoagulation postoperatively when appropriate
Angiotensin-converting enzyme (ACE) inhibitors and antihypertensives	Usually continue antihypertensives for elective surgery. In emergencies or when shock is present, stop antihypertensives because of the risk of hypotension or renal impairment (ACE inhibitors)
Diabetic treatment	Aim to control blood glucose between 6-10 mmol/L Avoid hypoglycaemia, which has serious and severe potential consequences. Avoid hyperglycaemia. Managing the change between omission of hypoglycaemic agents, interruption of oral feeding (preoperative fasting then postoperative delays to enteral nutrition) and the stress response to injury requires careful assessment, planning and observation

Some drugs that should normally be continued perioperatively

Drug	Reason
Beta-blockers	↓ Perioperative cardiac risk
Steroids	Adrenocortical suppression may require perioperative supplementation
Immunosuppressants	Patients with transplants require lifelong continuous immunosuppression

18

difficult intubation/airway control and any complications or distressing side-effects, e.g. postoperative nausea/vomiting. If major complications have occurred, or there is a family history of anaesthetic reactions, consider rare inherited abnormalities. The two most important are:

- Pseudocholinesterase deficiency: this causes prolonged apnoea following the administration of some neuromuscular blocking agents, e.g. suxamethonium chloride, necessitating unexpected/prolonged mechanical ventilation.
- Malignant hyperpyrexia: an autosomal dominant abnormality of skeletal muscle metabolism. Certain anaesthetic agents trigger life-threatening abnormal muscle activity with rigidity, rhabdomyolysis and hyperpyrexia. These patients, or those with a family history, require specialist investigation.

Family and social history

Have any family members suffered problems related to anaesthesia? This may reveal important familial conditions (see above) or bad experiences, e.g. nausea or pain. Patients often worry that they will experience similar problems and benefit from explanation and reassurance.

Take a smoking and alcohol history (Box 18.4 and p. 16). Ask specifically about recreational or illicit drugs, their frequency and route(s) of use.

Find out any religious, cultural or ethnic aspects that affect the procedure, e.g. non-acceptance of blood/animal products.

18.4 Importance of the smoking and alcohol history

History	Relevance
Smoking	↑ Risk of smoking-related diseases, e.g. COPD, ischaemic heart disease, peripheral vascular disease, cancer – and will affect risk stratification ↑ Risk of intraoperative bronchospasm ↑ Risk of chest infection ↓ Oxygen-carrying capacity of blood (COHb) ↑ Sympathetic stimulation (tachycardia, hypertension)
Alcohol	Risk of alcohol-related chronic disease (especially liver) ↓ Sensitivity to many anaesthetic drugs Risk of alcohol withdrawal in perioperative period

The systematic enquiry

Take a detailed cardiovascular and respiratory history to assess the status of known disease and detect undiagnosed conditions. Ask specifically about exercise tolerance and functional limitations (Boxes 18.5 and 18.6).

Symptoms of recent upper or lower respiratory tract infection may increase perioperative complications and require surgery to be postponed.

Reflux, e.g. heartburn, waterbrash, may need prophylactic drug treatment and airway protection to minimise the risks of aspiration.

When did the patient last eat or drink? In emergency cases relate this time to symptom onset because pain, trauma, opioids and some metabolic conditions, e.g. diabetes mellitus and renal failure, delay gastric emptying.

18.5 Metabolic equivalents of task (MET) scoring

MET score	Activity level
1	Dress, walk indoors
2	Light housework, slow walking
4	Climb one flight of stairs, run a short distance
6	Moderate sport, e.g. golf, dancing
10	Strenuous sport or exercise

1 MET = O₂ consumption ~3.5 ml/kg/min.
MET score assesses cardiorespiratory capacity and ability to respond to perioperative stress.

EBE 18.6 Risk of perioperative cardiac events

Patients who can achieve >4 Metabolic Equivalents of Task (METs) of activity without significant symptoms have a low risk of perioperative cardiac events.

ACC/AHA. Guidelines on perioperative cardiovascular evaluation and care for noncardiac surgery. Am J Coll Cardiol 2007;50:e159–e241.

Enquire about any relevant musculoskeletal conditions, e.g. rheumatoid disease which may be associated with cervical spine instability, other medical problems or functional impairment or back problems which may be relevant if epidural/spinal anaesthesia is planned. Assess neurological conditions such as epilepsy or conditions with pre-existing sensorimotor or autonomic abnormalities (Box 18.2).

THE PHYSICAL EXAMINATION

General

Examination sequence

- Measure the patient's weight and height and calculate the body mass index (BMI: p. 55) to guide drug dosage and stratify risk. Obesity and malnutrition increase risks.
- Measure the temperature. Pyrexia may indicate intercurrent infection (p. 61).
- Look for anaemia, central cyanosis and jaundice and assess hydration (p. 58).
- Assess the veins (for intravenous access) and other anatomy relevant to planned techniques, e.g. wrist pulses (if intra-arterial catheter planned), thoracic/lumbar spine flexion (epidural catheter placement).
- Body jewellery may need removal or protection to prevent it being caught, causing pressure/heat injury or infection.

The airway

- Assess potential airway difficulties, including those which may occur if using a face mask, laryngeal mask or tracheal tube:
  - Ask about and look for loose or false teeth, dental caps and crowns.
  - Remove tongue, mouth and facial jewellery as this may compromise the airway.

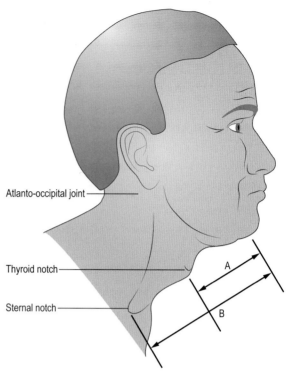

Fig. 18.1 Assessing thyromental distance. (A) Thyromental distance < 6.5 cm may predict difficult intubation. **(B)** Sternomental distance < 12.5 cm may predict difficult intubation.

- Inspect the face, head and neck from the front and side. Assess the shape of the maxilla and jaw.
- Ask the patient to breathe through his nose. Occlude each nostril in turn to assess patency.
- Look at the neck for length, scars, e.g. tracheostomy and goitre and measure the thyromental and sternomental distance (Fig. 18.1).
- Ask the patient to:
  - 'Put your chin on your chest; now tilt your head to look as far back as possible' (assess head/neck movement).
  - 'Open your mouth as wide as you can' (measure interincisor distance).
  - 'Now stick out your tongue fully' (determine Mallampati score: Fig. 18.2).
  - 'Protrude your jaw so your bottom teeth are in front of the top ones' (to assess jaw movement: Fig. 18.3).

Abnormal findings

These can predict a 'difficult' airway:

Predictors of difficult face mask ventilation

- age >55 years
- BMI >26
- edentulous
- history of snoring
- beard.

Predictors of difficult tracheal intubation

- limited head/neck movement
- short, thick neck
- thyromental distance < 6.5 cm and/or sternomental distance < 12.5 cm

Relevance

Inspect the patient's face, head and neck from the front and side Note the shape of the maxilla and jaw, and alignment of teeth

Facial hair — makes face–mask seal more difficult.
Difficult intubation is associated with:
- Protruding maxilla (overbite) and/or receding chin
- A short thick neck
- Obesity
- A short thyromental or sternomental distance

Examine the range of neck movement Assess the patient's ability to extend their head on the neck (atlanto-occipital joint function) and flex the cervical spine on the body

Airway control is more difficult in: patients who cannot achieve the "sniffing the morning air" position — with head extended and neck flexed forward on the body

Ask the patient to open the mouth fully Document the completeness and state of the teeth, especially the position of loose teeth and those at higher risk of damage (crowns, bridges) Assess size of mouth and degree of mouth opening possible (temporomandibular joint function) Note size of tongue and presence of tongue or oral jewellery

Poor dentition increases risk of dental damage

More difficult to obtain a seal between mask and face in edentulous patients

Reduced mouth opening makes airway access difficult

Large tongue associated with more difficult airway. Oral jewellery should be removed

Ask patient to stick out the tongue with mouth fully open and tongue pointing at chin Examine the view of the mouth and throat

Assess airway using Mallampati risk classification. Classes III and IV are associated with increased likelihood of difficult intubation

Class 1 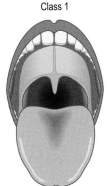 Class 2 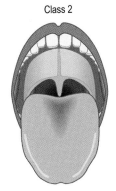 Class 3 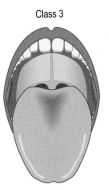 Class 4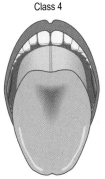

Fig. 18.2 Assessing the airway. The modified Mallampati test: class 1, pharyngeal pillars, soft palate and uvula visible; class 2, only soft palate and uvula visible; class 3, only soft palate visible; class 4, soft palate not visible.

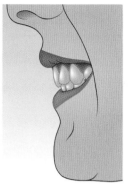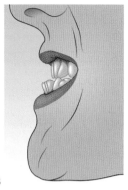

A   B

Fig. 18.3 Assess jaw movement from the side. Can the patient protrude the lower incisors in front of the upper incisors?

- interincisor gap <3 cm
- inability to protrude lower in front of upper incisors
- Mallampati class 3 or 4.

Cardiorespiratory and other systems

Examination sequence

- Examine specifically for arrhythmias, heart murmurs and signs of heart failure (Ch. 6).
- Auscultate the chest for crackles or wheezes that could indicate poorly controlled chronic lung disease or acute infection.
- Document any pre-existing neurological deficits, especially if regional anaesthetic techniques may be used.
- Briefly examine the remaining systems to identify abnormalities and exclude occult disease.

Use the American Society of Anesthesiologists (ASA) grading system to summarise anaesthetic and perioperative risk. Anaesthetic mortality in adult ASA grade I/II patients is ~1:100 000. Risk increases markedly in ASA grade III–V patients (Boxes 18.7 and 18.8).

PREOPERATIVE INVESTIGATIONS

Preoperative investigations depend on the type of surgery, the patient's condition and local policies. Only perform these if the results will influence patient treatment and/or outcome (Box 18.9).

Consent and advice

Consent for anaesthesia is often linked to surgical consent. Consent is only valid if the patient:
- has capacity to give consent
- has sufficient information to make a balanced decision
- can make a voluntary decision.

This requires careful explanation of procedures and their risks. Discuss more frequent or serious side-effects or complications, e.g. in relation to cannula insertion or epidural anaesthesia.

18.7 The American Society of Anesthesiologists (ASA) risk-grading system

ASA class	Description of patient
I	Normally healthy individual
II	Patient with mild systemic disease
III	A patient with severe systemic disease that is not incapacitating
IV	A patient with incapacitating systemic disease that is a constant threat to life
V	A moribund patient who is not expected to survive 24 hours with or without an operation
VI	A declared brain-dead patient whose organs are being removed for donor purposes
E	Added as a suffix for emergency operations (which carry greater risk)

18.8 Factors associated with significantly increased risk during anaesthesia

Type of surgery
- Emergency procedures
- Major thoracic, abdominal or cardiovascular surgery
- Perforated bowel
- Acute pancreatitis
- Palliative surgery

Patient factors
- Older age (>70 years)
- Cardiac:
  - Myocardial infarction within last 6 months
  - Heart failure (especially if poorly controlled)
  - Aortic stenosis
- Respiratory:
  - Productive cough
  - Breathlessness at rest or minimal exertion
  - Smoker
- Gastrointestinal:
  - Jaundice
  - Chronic liver disease
  - Malnutrition (low weight and/or low albumin)
- Renal:
  - Acute or chronic kidney disease
- Haematological:
  - Ongoing haemorrhage
  - Anaemia (<100 g/L)
  - Polycythaemia
- Neurological:
  - Confusion
- Metabolic:
  - Poorly controlled diabetes mellitus
  - Steroid therapy

Advise smokers to stop smoking. Give clear advice about which medications should be stopped or continued to the day of surgery, particularly for cardiac, antihypertensive and diabetic treatments. This is especially important for patients who will attend on the day of surgery.

Ensure the patient knows how long to fast, referring to local policies. Usually, centres fast patients for solids for 6 hours before elective surgery, and allow clear fluids up to 2 hours before.

18.9 Preoperative investigations

Investigation	Indication
Full blood count*	Patients with known abnormalities, e.g. anaemia, thrombocytopenia, suspected infection
Urea and electrolytes*	Pre-existing disease affecting biochemistry, e.g. renal failure or liver disease Drugs that could affect electrolytes, e.g. diuretics, ACE inhibitors
Coagulation	Known states that can alter coagulation, e.g. warfarin therapy, liver disease Prior to major surgery that may affect coagulation, e.g. cardiac surgery, hepatobiliary surgery
Blood cross-matching*	Use local surgical blood-ordering schedule to guide requests
12-lead electrocardiogram*	Known or suspected heart disease
Chest X-ray	Selected patients with known respiratory disease
Respiratory function tests (FEV/FVC)	Prior to major thoracic surgery Selected patients with chronic respiratory disease
Echocardiography	Selected patients with heart disease (especially heart murmurs)

*Required as a minimum for patients undergoing major surgery.
FEV, forced expiratory volume; FVC, forced vital capacity.

18

Gareth Clegg
Colin Robertson

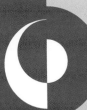

The critically ill

19

EXAMINATION OF THE CRITICALLY ILL

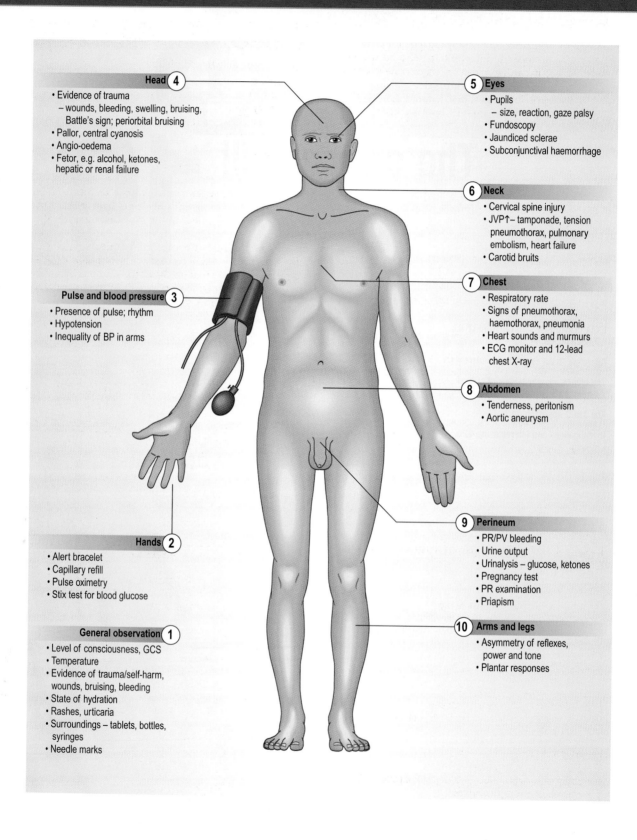

Head (4)
- Evidence of trauma
  - wounds, bleeding, swelling, bruising, Battle's sign; periorbital bruising
- Pallor, central cyanosis
- Angio-oedema
- Fetor, e.g. alcohol, ketones, hepatic or renal failure

(5) **Eyes**
- Pupils
  - size, reaction, gaze palsy
- Fundoscopy
- Jaundiced sclerae
- Subconjunctival haemorrhage

(6) **Neck**
- Cervical spine injury
- JVP↑– tamponade, tension pneumothorax, pulmonary embolism, heart failure
- Carotid bruits

(7) **Chest**
- Respiratory rate
- Signs of pneumothorax, haemothorax, pneumonia
- Heart sounds and murmurs
- ECG monitor and 12-lead chest X-ray

Pulse and blood pressure (3)
- Presence of pulse; rhythm
- Hypotension
- Inequality of BP in arms

(8) **Abdomen**
- Tenderness, peritonism
- Aortic aneurysm

(9) **Perineum**
- PR/PV bleeding
- Urine output
- Urinalysis – glucose, ketones
- Pregnancy test
- PR examination
- Priapism

Hands (2)
- Alert bracelet
- Capillary refill
- Pulse oximetry
- Stix test for blood glucose

(10) **Arms and legs**
- Asymmetry of reflexes, power and tone
- Plantar responses

General observation (1)
- Level of consciousness, GCS
- Temperature
- Evidence of trauma/self-harm, wounds, bruising, bleeding
- State of hydration
- Rashes, urticaria
- Surroundings – tablets, bottles, syringes
- Needle marks

APPROACH TO THE CRITICALLY ILL PATIENT

Systematic examination is inappropriate for critically ill patients as immediate intervention may be needed to save life, e.g. in cardiac arrest or tension pneumothorax, or to halt processes which untreated, would lead to death, e.g. hypovolaemic shock. Examination and interventions are often performed simultaneously.

Rapidly identify the main problems affecting the patient and use the resources available to gain control of the situation. Your aim is to stabilise the patient's condition and address life-threatening problems. This temporary phase should always be followed by a full history and clinical examination when the patient is 'stable' to make a full diagnosis, perform specialist investigations and institute definitive therapy.

THE CLINICAL MANIFESTATIONS OF CRITICAL ILLNESS (BOX 19.1)

Critical illness can present as:

- acute respiratory compromise affecting **A**irway or **B**reathing (Box 19.2)
- acute cardiovascular compromise, detectable as reduced **C**irculation (Box 19.3)
- altered conscious state manifest as neurological **D**isability (Box 19.4).

Initially, you may not be aware of events or the timeframe preceding the current state. Concentrating on the system which appears most likely to be causing the problem may be misleading, wastes time and further compromises the patient. Use a simple and safe ABCD approach to address and correct conditions using a logical framework.

THE ABCD APPROACH

This has four interlinked phases:

- preparation before you see the patient (where possible)
- primary survey
- secondary survey
- definitive care intervention.

Seek senior, experienced help immediately. If you have to work alone, only proceed to the next item once you have adequately completed the preceding one. A team can deal with the separate elements simultaneously, but the leader should ensure that all components are covered and if a patient's condition deteriorates, should immediately review the ABCD sequence.

Communicating with others in order to get help requires careful, concise delivery of information that can be difficult in an emotionally charged resuscitation. A useful and widely used format with which to structure your thoughts is SBAR (situation, background, assessment, recommendation: Box 19.5).

19

19.1 Clinical features of the critically ill patient

Airway and Breathing

- Respiratory arrest
- Obstructed or compromised airway
- Respiratory rate <8 or >35 breaths/min
- Respiratory distress: stridor, inability to speak in complete sentences, use of accessory muscles, intercostal indrawing

Circulation

- Cardiac arrest
- Pulse rate <40 or >140 bpm
- Systolic blood pressure <100 mmHg
- Features of shock: altered conscious level, peripheral perfusion, urine output <0.5 ml/kg/h

(Neurological) Disability

- Failure to obey commands
- Glasgow Coma Scale (GCS) <9, or fall of 2 points in GCS
- Frequent or prolonged seizures

Other

- Temperature
- Any patient you are seriously concerned about, even if he does not fulfil any of the above criteria

---

19.2 Common causes of acute respiratory compromise

Airway obstruction

- Altered conscious state (Box 19.4)
- Upper-airway/maxillofacial injury
- Tracheolaryngeal injury
- Foreign body
- Infections, e.g. epiglottitis, quinsy
- Angio-oedema
- Tumours

Pulmonary conditions

- Pneumothorax (especially if bilateral or if tension is present)
- Chest injury
  - Blunt: rib fractures, flail segment, lung contusion
  - Penetrating: pneumothorax, open chest wound, major vessel injury with haemothorax
- Severe acute asthma
- Pulmonary embolism
- Pneumonia
- Acute pulmonary oedema
  - Cardiogenic: acute left heart failure
  - Non-cardiogenic: smoke, toxic fume inhalation
- Acute respiratory distress syndrome (ARDS)
- Exacerbation of chronic obstructive pulmonary disease (COPD)
- Massive pleural effusion

Non-pulmonary conditions

- Metabolic acidosis
  - Diabetic ketoacidosis
  - Severe renal or hepatic failure
  - Lactic acidosis
  - Overdose: methanol, ethylene glycol, (late) salicylate
- Severe anaemia
- Psychogenic hyperventilation

19.3 Common causes of acute cardiovascular compromise

Cardiac

- Cardiac arrest
- Acute myocardial infarction or ischaemia
- Acute valve dysfunction, e.g. endocarditis, mechanical valve failure or obstruction
- Arrhythmia
- Pericardial tamponade
- Cardiomyopathy: viral, alcohol-related, postpartum

Vascular

- Dissection, or rupture, of abdominal or thoracic aortic aneurysm
- Mesenteric infarction

Massive pulmonary embolus

Blood loss

- Gastrointestinal
  - Upper: varices, peptic ulcer, tumour, Mallory–Weiss tear, non-steroidal anti-inflammatory drugs (NSAIDs)
  - Lower: diverticular disease, angiodysplasia, ischaemic bowel, Meckel's diverticulum, tumour
- Trauma
  - Overt: wounds, especially to scalp, face; long bone or pelvic fractures
  - Concealed: chest – haemothorax; abdomen – splenic and/or hepatic injury, retroperitoneal
- Obstetric/gynaecological: placenta praevia, miscarriage, ectopic pregnancy, trauma, tumour
- Anticoagulant use or bleeding diathesis

Miscellaneous

- Anaphylaxis
- Hypothermia
- Hyperthermia
- Electric shock/lightning injury
- Envenomation (bites or stings from snakes, insects, jellyfish)
- Toxicological

19.4 Common causes of altered conscious state

Non-central nervous system causes

- Hypoxia
- Hypovolaemia
- Hypoglycaemia
- Drugs and poisons, e.g. opioids, alcohol, carbon monoxide, benzodiazepines, tricyclic antidepressants
- Metabolic
  - Type II respiratory failure ($\uparrow PaCO_2$), hepatic or renal failure
  - Thyrotoxicosis/myxoedema/addisonian crisis, non-ketotic hyperosmolar states
- Hypothermia or hyperthermia

Central nervous system causes

- Intracranial haemorrhage, e.g. subarachnoid haemorrhage
- Ischaemia: thrombosis, embolism
- Trauma: concussion, white-matter shearing (diffuse axonal injury), haemorrhage (extradural, subdural and/or intracerebral)
- Infections: meningitis, encephalitis, cerebral malaria
- Seizures
- Primary or secondary tumour
- Hypertensive encephalopathy

19.5 SBAR framework for communication

Situation

Identify yourself, identify the patient and give the reason for your concern – what is the problem?

Background

What is this patient's background? What is the recent history of events?

Assessment

Your observations and evaluation of patient's current state. What are the current issues?

Recommendation

What should be done to respond to the current situation? (This may even be a simple request for assistance)

See: http://www.institute.nhs.uk/quality_and_service_improvement_tools/quality_and_service_improvement_tools/sbar_-_situation_-_background_-_assessment_-_recommendation.html.

19.6 Key preliminary data

A	Allergies
M	Medication
P	Past medical history
L	Last meal
E	Events leading up to presentation and environment

Preparation

Information gathering

The patient may be unable to give a history, so use all possible sources of information (Box 19.6). Include previous primary care or hospital records, relatives, friends, bystanders and emergency or ambulance personnel. Look for diabetic/steroid/anticoagulant cards and medications, and Alert bracelets/necklaces (Fig. 3.3). If possible, contact the patient's GP, who is often a key source of current and background information.

Managing your resources

Identify your available resources: which staff can help? What is their level of seniority and experience and what can they do? If you have others to help you, identify roles and responsibilities. If you are team leader, communicate your thinking to the whole team clearly and frequently.

Primary survey

The primary survey, investigations and interventions should take 5–10 minutes, unless you have to undertake a life-saving intervention such as tracheal intubation. The patient may be unable to sit up. If this is the case examine him supine throughout.

Examination sequence

A: Airway

- Approach the patient so that he can see you if conscious.
- Speak slowly and clearly and assess his response.
- If the patient talks to you normally, the airway is clear and there is perfusion of the brain; if his speech is lucid, cerebral function is adequate.
- Give a high inspired concentration of oxygen by mask, and move on to B (breathing).
- If there is no response to speech, usually because the patient has altered consciousness, perform a more detailed assessment of the airway. Look, listen and feel. Open his mouth and remove secretions, blood, vomit or foreign material by gentle suction with a Yankauer catheter (Fig. 19.1) under direct vision. Leave well-fitting dentures or dental plates in place to maintain the normal airway anatomy. If they are loose or poorly fitting, remove them.
- Listen for upper airway noises (Box 19.7). Gurgling, snoring or stridor suggests partial airway obstruction. Grunting respiration may be a sign of respiratory muscle fatigue, or an attempt to slow expiration in a patient with a flail segment (see below). Absent breath sounds indicates either complete airway obstruction or absence of breathing.
- Open the airway by tilting the patient's head and lifting his chin (Fig. 19.2). If you suspect neck injury, do not move the neck. Control the head and neck by manual in-line control and open the airway using the jaw lift technique (Fig. 19.3). Appropriately

19.7 Airway noises

No noise (the 'silent airway')

- Implies complete airway obstruction and/or absence of, or minimal, respiratory effort

Snoring

- Caused by partial upper airway obstruction from soft tissues of the mouth and oropharynx

Gurgling

- Caused by fluids (secretions, blood or vomit) in the oropharynx

Grunting

- A grunt during expiration is a sign of respiratory muscle fatigue. It may be present after chest wall trauma with a flail segment. Grunting improves gas exchange by slowing expiration and preventing alveolar collapse by ↑ positive end-expiratory pressure.

Hoarseness

- Caused by partial laryngeal obstruction associated with oedema

Wheeze

- A 'musical' noise, best heard on auscultation
- When loudest in expiration, relates to obstruction in the small bronchi and bronchioles, most often in asthma and COPD

Stridor

- A harsh noise, usually loudest in inspiration, caused by partial obstruction around the larynx or main bronchi
- In febrile patients, consider epiglottitis or retropharyngeal abscess
- Other causes are foreign bodies, laryngeal trauma, burns or tumours

19

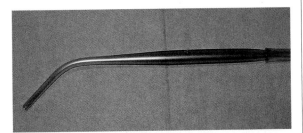

Fig. 19.1 Yankauer suction catheter. This may have a small hole to control airflow – if present, occlude this with your thumb to generate suction.

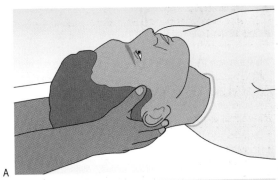

A

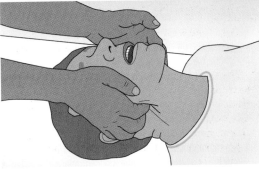

B

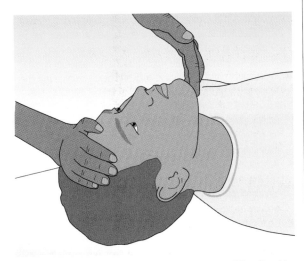

Fig. 19.2 Opening the airway by tilting the head and lifting the chin.

Fig. 19.3 Manoeuvres in patients with suspected neck injury.
(A) Control the head and neck manually. **(B)** Open the airway using the jaw thrust technique. N.B. A rigid cervical collar will normally then be applied.

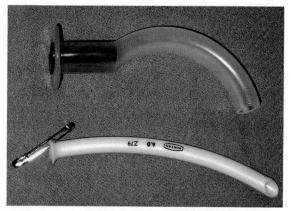

Fig. 19.4 Airway adjuncts. Guedel airway (top); nasopharyngeal airway (bottom). Note the 'safety pin' is to prevent migration of the proximal end of the airway beyond the nasal orifice.

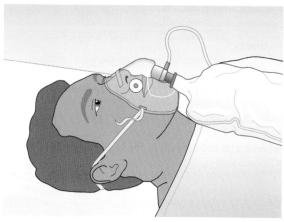

Fig. 19.5 Administering oxygen using a mask with reservoir bag.

19.8 Principal indications for emergency advanced airway and ventilation techniques

- Apnoea
- Airway obstruction
  - Inability to maintain airway with simple manoeuvres/ adjuncts
  - Facial trauma, uncontrolled vomiting/bleeding
  - Glasgow Coma Scale <9
  - Potential for subsequent clinical deterioration, e.g. facial/ airway burns
- Oxygenation and ventilation
  - Raised intracranial pressure
  - Potential environmental risk, e.g. ambulance transfer, CT/MR imaging scan

19.9 Situations in which SpO$_2$ may give misleading values

- Shock
- Hypotension/poor peripheral perfusion
- Hypothermia
- Excessive movement
- Nail varnish, false fingernails
- Severe anaemia
- Abnormal haemoglobins, e.g. carboxyhaemoglobin, methaemoglobin or sulphaemoglobin
- Skin pigmentation or excessively dirty fingers

sized airway adjuncts, such as nasopharyngeal or oropharyngeal (Guedel) airways, can maintain the airway in patients with altered consciousness (Fig. 19.4). Do not use a nasopharyngeal airway if you suspect a skull base fracture, if epistaxis, nasal trauma or deformity is present, or if the patient is taking anticoagulants. Tracheal intubation may be needed if the patient cannot maintain a patent airway. This should only be performed by an experienced clinician (Box 19.8).

B: Breathing

Hypoxia hastens and causes death. Central cyanosis is a late, unreliable sign of hypoxia. Even in critical hypoxia, cyanosis may be absent because of severe anaemia or massive blood loss.

- Attach a pulse oximeter probe to a fingertip (Fig. 7.25) or earlobe. Pulse oximetry (SpO$_2$) can non-invasively assess peripheral oxygenation simply (Box 19.9). Use an oxygen mask with reservoir bag and adjust the oxygen flow rate to maintain an SpO$_2$ of 94–98% (Fig. 19.5). If the oxygen mask 'mists' on exhalation, the patient has (some) respiratory effort. The only exception to this initial treatment is if you know the patient has chronic obstructive pulmonary disease with CO$_2$ retention (type II respiratory failure). These patients may lose the hypoxic stimulus to breathe if given high concentrations of oxygen. In these patients aim to maintain an SpO$_2$ of 88-92%.
- Look for movements of the chest, the accessory muscles and the abdomen. Paradoxical respiration is movement of the abdomen exactly out of phase with that of the chest and

indicates respiratory compromise. It is most often due to fatigue of the diaphragm and/or airway obstruction. In patients with chronic airflow obstruction a breathing pattern with abnormal abdominal movements is associated with a much poorer prognosis. Look for other abnormal breathing patterns (Box 19.10).

- Seek signs of injury (bruising, pattern imprinting, wounds) and of flail segment in trauma patients. In a flail segment the affected area moves paradoxically: it moves outwards from the chest wall during expiration and inwards during inspiration.
  - Kneel at the patient's side and look tangentially across the chest. A flail segment is often well localised and, if present, implies that at least three ribs are broken in at least two places (Fig. 19.6). Underlying lung injury is common.
- Assess the position of the trachea in the suprasternal notch.
- In a trauma patient, systematically and gently palpate the chest to identify any areas of injury. Rib and sternal fractures are associated with localised discomfort. Subcutaneous emphysema feels like 'crackling' under your fingers. Examine for consolidation, pneumothorax, pleural effusion and haemothorax (Ch. 7).
- Auscultate for breath sounds and added sounds. Critically ill patients may not have the signs you expect. For example, a patient with life-threatening asthma may have little or no wheeze (a silent chest) because airflow into the lungs is poor.
- Expose the chest, back, axillae and abdomen. Look for wounds (usually gunshot or stab) producing an open defect in the chest wall (Fig. 19.7). Recognise and treat open pneumothorax or a pneumothorax under tension. An open chest wound equalises

19.10 Respiratory patterns: common causes

Tachypnoea

- Anxiety
- Pain
- Asthma
- Metabolic acidosis
- Chest injury
- Pneumothorax
- Pulmonary embolus
- Brainstem stroke

Bradypnoea/apnoea

- Cardiac arrest
- Opioids
- Central neurological causes (stroke, head injury)

Cheyne–Stokes respiration

- Left ventricular failure
- Central neurological causes (stroke, head injury)
- Overdose (barbiturates, γ-hydroxybutyrate, opioids)

Küssmaul respiration

- Metabolic acidosis
  – diabetic ketoacidosis
- Uraemia
- Hepatic failure
- Shock (lactic acidosis)
- Overdose (methanol, ethylene glycol, salicylate)

Paradoxical respiration

- Respiratory failure
- Guillain–Barré syndrome
- High spinal cord lesions

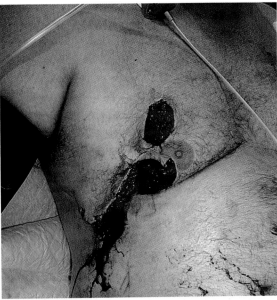

Fig. 19.7 Wound producing an open defect in the chest wall.

19

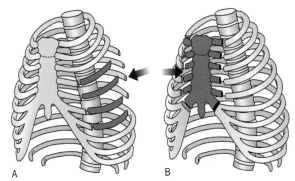

A   B

Fig. 19.6 Flail chest. (A) A direct blow (arrowed) that fractures several ribs at two points will result in a flail segment. **(B)** A severe blow to the sternum (arrowed) may cause multiple bilateral costochondral fractures, resulting in a flail chest.

pressure between the pleural space and atmosphere, and the affected lung is unable to expand or contract normally with respiration. During inspiration and expiration, you may hear air movement and see a spray of blood at the wound. Cover the wound with a sterile occlusive dressing secured on three sides. A formal tube thoracostomy with underwater seal drainage is then needed.

- Suspect tension pneumothorax in any patient who rapidly develops severe respiratory and cardiovascular distress. It occurs when lung injury produces a one-way valve effect (Fig. 19.8). On inspiration air escapes from the lung and accumulates in the pleural space. As the pleural pressure increases, the ipsilateral lung progressively collapses and the increased intrathoracic pressure reduces venous return to the heart, eventually causing cardiac arrest.

It occurs most commonly in chest injury, during positive-pressure ventilation or in underlying lung disease (especially when

ventilated). The diagnosis is clinical. The patient appears acutely breathless and agitated, has tachycardia and may be cyanosed. Hypotension, bradycardia and altered consciousness are preterminal features. Quickly examine for jugular venous distension, tachycardia and absent breath sounds on the affected side. If the patient is in extremis, insert a large-bore intravenous (IV) cannula through the second intercostal space in the mid-clavicular line on the affected side. Remove the needle from the cannula. A hiss of air, with rapid clinical improvement, confirms the diagnosis. Tube thoracostomy with underwater seal drainage is then required.

C: Circulation

- Feel for a central (carotid or femoral) pulse for 10 seconds. If you cannot feel a pulse and the patient is unresponsive, treat as for cardiac arrest (for current guidelines from the International Liaison Committee on Resuscitation on how to manage cardiac arrest, see www.ilcor.org) (Fig. 19.9).
- In responsive patients, feel for a peripheral (radial or brachial) pulse. If you cannot palpate a peripheral pulse, this suggests that the patient is significantly hypotensive.
- Note the pulse rate, rhythm, volume and character.
- Assess peripheral perfusion; press on the fingertip pulp for a few seconds, remove your finger and estimate the capillary refill time (normal <2 seconds).
- Attach an ECG monitor to the patient. Note the ventricular rate and the rhythm.
- Control external blood losses from wounds or open fractures by direct firm pressure with a sterile dressing placed over the site. Minimise blood loss from long bone fractures (femur, tibia/fibula, humerus and forearm) by splintage.
- Insert a large-bore (16 FG, 1.7 mm internal diameter or bigger) IV cannula and tape it securely to the skin. In trauma patients and when you suspect hypovolaemia, insert and secure two large-bore cannulae. Take initial blood samples (Box 19.11) from the cannula and then attach an IV fluid-giving set. Commence volume replacement, if needed, with warmed 0.9% saline or Ringer's solution.

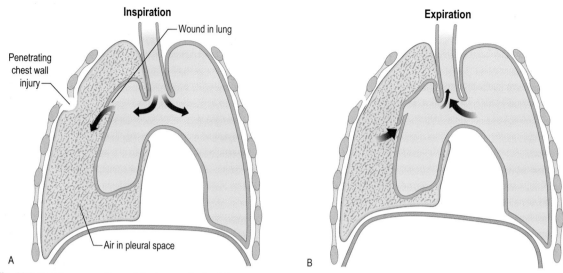

Inspiration — Wound in lung

Penetrating chest wall injury

Air in pleural space

A

Expiration

B

Fig. 19.8 Tension pneumothorax following penetrating injury. Air enters the pleural cavity via the punctured lung during inspiration. The chest wall and lung defects act as one-way valves. Air cannot escape from the pleural cavity during expiration. The right intrapleural pressure increases, collapsing the right lung, impeding venous return to the heart and occasionally shifting mediastinal structures to the contralateral side.

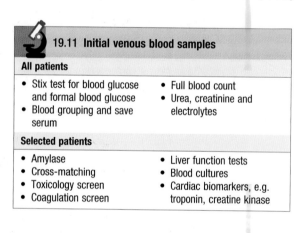

19.11 Initial venous blood samples

All patients

- Stix test for blood glucose and formal blood glucose
- Blood grouping and save serum
- Full blood count
- Urea, creatinine and electrolytes

Selected patients

- Amylase
- Cross-matching
- Toxicology screen
- Coagulation screen
- Liver function tests
- Blood cultures
- Cardiac biomarkers, e.g. troponin, creatine kinase

■ Examine the jugular venous pressure (JVP) (Fig. 6.19). In a sitting or semirecumbent patient, elevation of the JVP in the presence of shock suggests a major problem with the heart's pumping ability, such as acute heart failure, cardiac tamponade, massive pulmonary embolus, tension pneumothorax or an acute valvular problem.
■ Check the blood pressure (p. 113).
■ Examine the precordium and heart, identifying the presence of added heart sounds or murmurs.
■ Insert a urinary catheter (unless there is evidence of urethral or prostatic injury – blood at the urethral meatus and/or a high-riding, 'boggy' prostate on rectal examination) to monitor urine output.

Shock implies that the oxygen and blood supply to an organ or tissue is inadequate for its metabolic requirements. It is recognised clinically by a combination of features (Box 19.12). The extent to which each feature is present depends upon the cause (Box 19.13) and the time course. Signs of shock may be delayed or obscured in athletes, pregnant women, those on vasoactive drugs (beta-blockers, calcium channel blockers, angiotensin-converting enzyme inhibitors), those with pacemakers and the very young and old.

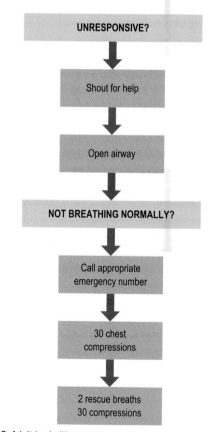

UNRESPONSIVE?

↓

Shout for help

↓

Open airway

↓

NOT BREATHING NORMALLY?

↓

Call appropriate emergency number

↓

30 chest compressions

↓

2 rescue breaths 30 compressions

Fig. 19.9 Adult basic life support algorithm.

Tachycardia (heart rate >100 bpm) and hypotension (systolic blood pressure <100 mmHg) are not required to diagnose shock: the heart rate may be normal or low in hypoxic shocked patients or those on drugs such as beta-blockers. Blood pressure may be temporarily maintained by sympathetic activity and peripheral vasoconstriction. In critically ill patients non-invasive cuff blood pressure measurements are often inaccurate.

19.12 Clinical features of shock

- Altered consciousness, confusion, irritability
- Pallor, cool skin, sweating
- Heart rate >100 bpm
- Hypotension (systolic blood pressure <100 mmHg):
  N.B. Hypotension is a late sign
- Respiratory rate >30 breaths/min
- Oliguria (urine output <0.5–1 ml/kg/h)

19.13 Classification of shock

Hypovolaemic

- Blood loss: trauma, gastrointestinal or obstetric haemorrhage, abdominal aortic aneurysm rupture
- Fluid loss: burns, gastrointestinal loss (diarrhoea, vomiting), severe dehydration, diabetic ketoacidosis, 'third space' losses, e.g. sepsis, pancreatitis, ischaemic bowel

Cardiogenic

- Arrhythmia, myocardial infarction, myocarditis, acute valve failure, overdose of negatively inotropic drugs, e.g. calcium channel blocker or beta-blocker

Obstructive

- Major pulmonary embolism, tension pneumothorax, cardiac tamponade, acute valve obstruction

Neurogenic

- Major cerebral or spinal injury

Others

- Toxic causes: carbon monoxide, cyanide, hydrogen sulphide, poisons causing methaemoglobinaemia
- Anaphylaxis

19.14 Glasgow Coma Scale

Eye opening	
Spontaneous	4
To speech	3
To pain	2
No response	1

Verbal response	
Orientated	5
Confused: talks in sentences but disorientated	4
Verbalises: words, not sentences	3
Vocalises: sounds (groans or grunts), not words	2
No vocalisation	1

Motor response	
Obeys commands	6
Localises to pain, e.g. brings hand up beyond chin to supraorbital pain	5
Flexion withdrawal to pain: no localisation to supraorbital pain but flexes elbow to nail bed pressure	4
Abnormal flexion to pain	3
Extension to pain: extends elbow to nail bed pressure	2
No response	1

Record the GCS as a total and its three separate components: e.g. GCS 9/15: E3, V2, M4

19

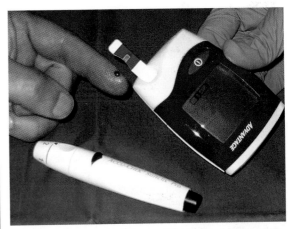

Fig. 19.10 Monitoring blood glucose with a testing strip and meter.

Do not concentrate on absolute figures of systolic or diastolic blood pressure. Readings of 90/50 mmHg are normal in many healthy young women, while 120/70 mmHg indicates significant hypotension in a patient whose pressures are usually 195/115 mmHg. Trends in pulse and blood pressure give far more information than initial or isolated readings. If the patient has a rising pulse rate, with a falling blood pressure and reduced urine output, this strongly implies continuing volume loss and inadequate replacement.

In trauma the most likely cause of shock is blood loss. External blood loss from wounds and compound fractures is usually apparent, but haemorrhage into the abdomen and chest, or from closed long bone or pelvic fractures, is often missed.

D: Disability

- Assess the patient's Glasgow Coma Scale (GCS). Separately record the three components: eye opening, verbal response and motor response (Box 19.14).
- Examine the limbs for localising signs or paraplegia.
- Check the pupils for size, reactivity and equal reaction to light. In structural causes of coma (intracranial haemorrhage, infarction) the light reflex is usually absent; in metabolic causes (poisoning, hypoglycaemia, sepsis) it is usually present. A difference in pupil diameters >1 mm suggests a structural cause. The GCS can be misleading in some types of non-traumatic brain injury, for example stroke.

- Hypoglycaemia:
  - Check the blood glucose using a Stix test (Fig. 19.10). Hypoglycaemia usually causes a global neurological deficit with reduced consciousness, but may present with irritability, erratic or violent behaviour (sometimes mistaken for alcohol or drug intoxication), seizures or focal neurological deficits, e.g. hemiplegia.
  - If the stix test reading is <3 mmol/l, take a venous sample for formal blood glucose measurement, but treat before you get the result. Give 25–50 ml of 50% dextrose IV. If you cannot obtain venous access rapidly, give 1 mg glucagon by intramuscular (IM) injection. The conscious level should start to improve in 10–20 minutes if hypoglycaemia is the cause of the altered mental state. Repeat the stix test to confirm correction of hypoglycaemia.

Persistent altered consciousness where hypoglycaemia has been adequately corrected implies coexistent pathology, e.g.

stroke, or cerebral oedema from prolonged neuroglycopenia. In patients with hypoglycaemia where you suspect chronic alcohol use or withdrawal, or malnutrition, give 100 mg IV thiamine to prevent and treat Wernicke's encephalopathy (confusion, ataxia and eye signs – nystagmus and conjugate gaze palsies).

Overdose

If you cannot clearly identify a cause for the patient's altered conscious state, consider drug overdose. The most common acutely life-threatening drugs are opioids, which cause altered consciousness, respiratory depression (reduced respiratory rate and volume) and small pupils.

- Titrate 0.8–2 mg IV naloxone (a specific opioid antagonist) as a diagnostic aid and definitive treatment to any patient with no clear cause for altered consciousness. In opioid intoxication, the patient responds within 30–60 seconds of IV administration. If IV access is difficult, give naloxone IM. If the patient responds, give further doses, as naloxone has a short duration (minutes), while the half-life of most opioids and their active metabolites is hours/days.

Seizures (fits)

- Give immediate treatment to stop active focal or generalised seizures. First-line therapy is IV lorazepam (0.5–1 mg/min up to 4 mg) or diazepam (1–2 mg/min up to 10–20 mg). If seizures continue despite this, other agents may be required, e.g. phenytoin.
- Manage seizures in pregnancy using the ABCDE approach but consider the fetus as well. Seek senior obstetric and neonatal support immediately. Place women >20 weeks' gestation in the left lateral position by placing one or two pillows under the right hip. This prevents the gravid uterus from obstructing venous return to the heart with consequent hypotension. Eclamptic seizures in pregnant and postpartum patients are associated with hypertension (diastolic blood pressure >100 mmHg), oedema (usually generalised and often affecting hands and face) and proteinuria. IV magnesium sulphate is a first-line treatment.

E: Exposure and environment

- If the patient is not already fully undressed, remove remaining clothing. Cover the patient with a gown and warm blankets to prevent hypothermia and maintain dignity. Critically ill patients lose heat rapidly and cannot maintain normal body temperature.
- Trauma patients may arrive on a rigid spinal board with neck immobilisation. Remove them from the board to reduce pressure sores and facilitate radiological examination. If the patient is conscious, explain what you are going to do before the patient is 'log-rolled' and lifted (Fig. 19.11). The process needs five people. One holds the head/neck and directs the procedure; one removes the spinal board and other debris, and examines the back and spine; the remaining three roll and hold the patient.
- While the patient is rolled, perform a rectal examination, assess anal tone and perianal sensation, and check the core temperature (p. 187).
- Examine the patient's skin surface rapidly but comprehensively. Look for bruises and wounds. In particular, examine the scalp, perineum and axillae. Note open fractures and rashes, e.g. the non-blanching purpuric rash of meningococcal septicaemia (Fig. 17.1) and hyperpigmentation (hypoadrenalism).

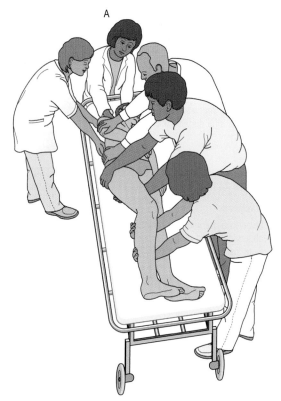

Fig. 19.11 Deployment of personnel and hand positions used when 'log-rolling' a patient from the supine to the lateral position. The person (A) controlling the cervical spine should direct the manoeuvre.

INVESTIGATIONS

See Box 19.15.

19.15 The primary survey: investigations and interventions	
ABCDE	
A	Administer high-flow oxygen
B	Measure respiratory rate and SpO_2
C	Monitor the electrocardiogram (ECG) continuously and measure blood pressure every 5 minutes Insert and secure large-bore intravenous cannula(e) and take blood samples
D	Record Glasgow Coma Scale Record pupil size and reactivity Stix test for blood glucose
E	Measure temperature (rectal or tympanic membrane)
Others	
• Arterial blood gas measurement • 12-lead ECG • Chest X-ray (+ pelvic and cervical spine views in multiply injured) • Urinary catheter* (and measure urine output hourly) • Urinalysis (stix test) for blood, protein, glucose, ketones, nitrite, bilirubin and urobilinogen • Urine pregnancy test in females • Nasogastric tube†	

*Contraindicated if urethral injury is suspected.
†Contraindicated if skull base fracture is suspected.

Secondary survey

The secondary survey reassesses the patient after the primary survey is complete. This is a systematic, detailed top-to-toe examination that fully documents additional signs and identifies injuries in the trauma patient. Only start the secondary survey once you are confident that there is no immediate need for further resuscitation and the patient does not require immediate transfer for definitive care, e.g. to theatre for a patient with a ruptured abdominal aortic aneurysm. Continually re-evaluate to assess the response to treatment. If the patient deteriorates or you are unsure about clinical status, return to the primary survey.

Give adequate analgesia to all patients in pain. There is no 'standard' dose. Slowly titrate an opioid drug, e.g. morphine IV in 1–2 mg aliquots to achieve pain relief. The amount needed varies according to the patient's response and adverse effects, e.g. respiratory depression, hypotension.

Examination sequence

- Examine the entire body surface. The skin appearance may suggest an underlying diagnosis, e.g. pallor (blood loss or anaemia), jaundice (hepatic failure), vitiligo or pigmentation in sun-exposed areas, recent scars and skin creases (Addison's disease).
- Look for rashes (in particular, the non-blanching purpuric rash of meningococcal disease) (Fig. 17.1), foci of infection (cellulitis, abscesses, erysipelas), bruising and wounds.
- Perform a systematic top-to-toe examination, starting with the head. In a trauma patient palpate the scalp for swelling, and look for wounds which may be hidden in thick or tangled hair.

- Look for signs of skull base fracture. These include periorbital bruising ('raccoon' or 'panda' eyes; Fig. 19.12A), subconjunctival haemorrhage (usually without a posterior margin; Fig. 19.12B), otorrhoea or rhinorrhoea, and most commonly bleeding from the ear or behind the tympanic membrane (haemotympanum). Battle's sign (bruising over the mastoid process; Fig. 19.12C) may take 1–3 days to develop.
- Examine the eyes for foreign bodies, including retained contact lenses (remove them at this stage), and signs of chronic disease, such as jaundice or anaemia. If you suspect corneal abrasions, stain the eye with fluorescein to identify them (Ch. 12).
- Assess the pupils for size, shape, reactivity to light and accommodation.
- Examine the eye movements, visual acuity and optic fundi. Urgently refer any patient with penetrating injury, disruption of the globe or loss of vision to a specialist ophthalmologist.
- Smell the patient's breath. The sweet odour of ketones in diabetic ketoacidosis is characteristic, but not everyone can detect it. Severe uraemia causes a 'fishy' smell, and hepatic failure a 'mousy' smell (fetor hepaticus) due to dimethyl sulphide. Note whether a patient smells of alcohol, but never attribute altered conscious level to alcohol alone.
- Look in the mouth for injury to the palate, tongue and teeth.
- Check the ears and throat for potential sources of infection.
- Assume that the spine and/or spinal cord is injured in all trauma patients, especially those with altered consciousness. Conscious patients may complain of localised neck or back pain, but may be distracted by pain from other injuries. Maintain spinal immobilisation until you can exclude underlying injury. This is rarely possible in the initial assessment period, and many cases require imaging to exclude cord or bony injury.
- If there is no history of trauma, ask the patient to flex his neck to touch his chin on his chest. If this causes discomfort, gently

19

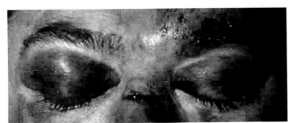

A

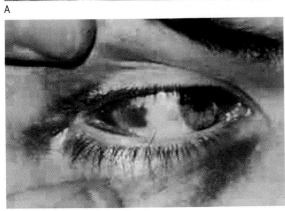

B

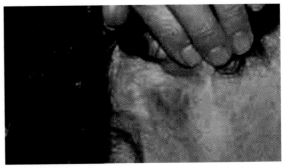

C

Fig. 19.12 Signs of skull base fracture. (A) Periorbital bruising ('raccoon' or 'panda' eyes). **(B)** Subconjunctival haemorrhage. **(C)** Battle's sign.

flex his neck passively. Meningeal irritation causes spasm of the paraspinal neck muscles with neck stiffness. Meningitis and subarachnoid haemorrhage are common causes and may be associated with photophobia and a positive Kernig's sign (p. 246). Neck stiffness may be absent early in these conditions or with altered consciousness.

- Re-examine the chest and precordium in detail (Chs 6 and 7).
- Examine the abdomen, including the pelvis and perineum. Perform a rectal and vaginal examination if necessary. Remove any tampon in a menstruating female and consider toxic shock syndrome as a cause of her symptoms. Rectal examination is mandatory in patients presenting with signs of hypovolaemia, to help identify gastrointestinal bleeding. In trauma patients examine the perineum, rectum and urethral orifice before inserting a urinary catheter.
- Check perianal sensation and rectal sphincter tone to assess potential spinal cord injury.
- Clinical assessment of pelvis injury is often misleading. Palpation may identify fractures, but do not 'spring' the pelvis to assess stability, as this may precipitate further bleeding.
- Examine each limb in turn. Look for wounds, swelling and bruising; palpate all bones and joints for tenderness and crepitus, and assess passive and active joint movements. Undisplaced long-bone fractures are easily missed in trauma patients. Always examine the neurovascular integrity of the limb distal to any injury.
- Perform a full neurological examination. This is particularly important in patients with altered conscious level or possible spinal injury.
- Examine joints for swelling suggesting septic or reactive arthritis (Box 19.16).

Investigations

Specific investigations will depend upon the presentation involved, e.g. CT for head injury. A 12-lead ECG and chest X-ray are standard and in patients with blunt trauma the initial X-rays should, as a minimum, include views of the cervical spine, chest and pelvis.

EBE	19.16 **Pupil changes and structural intracranial lesions**

A dilated pupil (>1 mm in size between the pupils, anisocoria) in a patient with coma strongly suggests a structural intracranial lesion.

Touda Y, Nakazato N, Stein GH. Pupillary evaluation for differential diagnosis of coma. Postgrad Med 2003;79:49–51.

Perform a urinary pregnancy test in all women of child-bearing age.

Ensure tetanus prophylaxis for all trauma patients who are non-immune. Give IV antibiotic therapy to patients with presumed meningococcal disease, septic shock and open fractures.

Document all investigations, therapy and response to treatment. Stop the assessment process if the patient needs immediate definitive care or investigation. Let the receiving team know exactly which stage of the assessment process you have reached when you hand over care of the patient.

Definitive treatment

Once stable, the patient is moved to a critical care area, theatre, scanning room or another hospital. This is high-risk and there must be sufficiently trained staff accompanying the patient. The critically ill patient needs to be adequately monitored and as 'stable' as possible. All relevant documentation and investigation results should accompany the patient, with clear lines of communication between clinicians.

If you discover that the patient is terminally ill and that this crisis is not unexpected, it may not be appropriate for the patient to be given aggressive or 'heroic' treatment. It may be difficult to recognise and prepare for a patient's death but it is essential and humane. Communicate with the family, the GP and the senior clinician previously involved in the patient's care. Care for the patient in a dignified manner, with the emphasis on analgesia, relief of distressing symptoms and the highest quality of nursing care.

Jamie Douglas
Graham Douglas

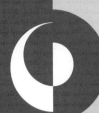

Confirming death

20

EXAMINATION TO CONFIRM DEATH

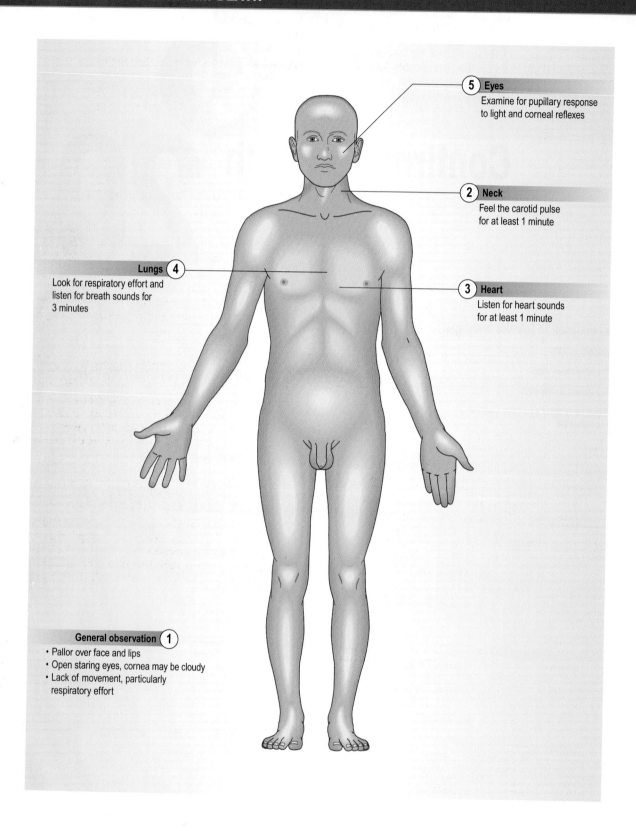

5 Eyes
Examine for pupillary response
to light and corneal reflexes

2 Neck
Feel the carotid pulse
for at least 1 minute

Lungs 4
Look for respiratory effort and
listen for breath sounds for
3 minutes

3 Heart
Listen for heart sounds
for at least 1 minute

General observation 1
• Pallor over face and lips
• Open staring eyes, cornea may be cloudy
• Lack of movement, particularly
  respiratory effort

DEFINITION

In the UK there is no legal definition of death. It is the clinician's responsibility to declare when a patient has died. Death is defined by the UK Academy of Medical Royal Colleges as: 'the irreversible loss of the capacity for consciousness, combined with irreversible loss of the capacity to breathe'. For practical purposes, death has occurred if there is absence of spontaneous cardiac function, respiratory effort and central nervous system activity.

Death used to be synonymous with the sudden and unexpected loss of spontaneous cardiac activity and respiration (cardiopulmonary arrest). Appropriate and prompt treatment can, however, successfully resuscitate some people in this category (Ch. 19).

Timing

The exact timing of death is rarely predictable, but is sometimes anticipated and accepted, e.g. in a patient with advanced metastatic cancer. Some patients with very severe chronic or terminal illness do not wish to have resuscitative efforts performed. In some countries, including the UK, the applicability of a 'do not attempt resuscitation' (DNAR) directive may be discussed with the patient and close relatives. The outcome of this discussion should be clearly recorded in the notes, made known to relevant medical and nursing staff and reviewed regularly. The presence of a DNAR order does not in any way imply withdrawal of treatment: it should focus attention on the general care of the patient, including adequate analgesia.

Confirmation

Confirming death has major medicolegal implications and obligations. Your approach and manner should always be professional. Although death may appear obvious, carefully and systematically examine the body. Misdiagnosis is especially likely in situations where vital functions and general metabolism are greatly reduced (Box 20.1).

Examination sequence

- Feel for a major (carotid or femoral) pulse for at least 1 minute.
- Listen for heart sounds over the cardiac apex for at least 1 minute.
- While you are doing this, watch the chest wall for any movement.
- Listen to the chest for breath sounds for 3 minutes.
- Watch for any spontaneous movement during your examination.
- Press over the supraorbital notch and check there is no response to supraorbital pressure.
- Simultaneously retract both eyelids, shine a bright light into each eye in turn and check that both pupils are unreactive.
- Check for absence of the corneal reflexes (Fig. 11.6).

Other clinical features associated with death include unnatural pallor, particularly of the face and lips, relaxation of the facial muscles with drooping of the lower jaw and open staring eyes. Eye changes include cloudiness of the cornea, reduced eyeball tension and, on fundoscopy, segmentation of blood within the retinal veins. This is known as 'cattle-trucking', 'railroading' or 'boxcars' (Fig. 20.1). None of these changes, however, should be used in isolation as a marker of death. Other postmortem changes gradually develop (Box 20.2).

INVESTIGATIONS

In certain situations, additional investigations may be available and confirmatory: for example, an electrocardiograph monitor trace showing asystole, absence of pulsatile flow from an intra-arterial line, or of contractile motion on echocardiography.

BRAINSTEM DEATH

Modern resuscitative devices and techniques can maintain the function of the heart, lungs and visceral organs, even when brainstem function has stopped. Patients receiving mechanical ventilation require additional tests to confirm brainstem death, which should be carried out

20

20.1 Situations that can 'mimic' death

- Hypothermia
- Drug overdose
- Opioids
- Tricyclic antidepressants
- Barbiturates
- Alcohol
- Anaesthetic agents
- Near drowning, cold water immersion
- Severe hypoglycaemia
- Severe hepatic encephalopathy
- Myxoedema coma
- Severe catatonic state

Fig. 20.1 Optic fundus after death, showing segmentation of blood within retinal vessels (arrowed).

20.2 Postmortem changes

Body cooling

Varies according to:
- Temperature before death: fever, hypothermia
- Clothing/coverings
- Environmental temperature and air movement
- Body surface area

Postmortem lividity

Dark red/purple skin discoloration in gravity-dependent parts of the body develops within 20–30 minutes of death and becomes 'fixed' after about 12 hours

Rigor mortis

Generalised muscular stiffening of voluntary and involuntary muscles of variable onset (up to 12 hours) and duration

Putrefaction

- Soft-tissue breakdown caused by commensal bacteria and enzymes
- Rate of putrefaction depends upon the body type, disease processes before death and environmental conditions, including temperature and humidity
- In conditions of dehydration and dry heat, mummification can occur

20.3 Deaths that may require further enquiry

Death
- caused by an accident arising from use of a vehicle, e.g. aircraft, ship, train or car
- of a person while at work
- due to an industrial disease, e.g. mesothelioma
- due to poisoning
- where the circumstances suggest suicide
- following abortion or attempted abortion
- thought to be due to sudden infant death syndrome
- of a child in the care of a local authority or on an 'at risk' register
- in legal custody
- by drowning
- due to a disease, infectious disease or syndrome which poses a serious public health risk, e.g. hepatitis A, B, C or E, food poisoning, legionnaire's disease, any hospital-acquired infection
- by burning or scalding or as a result of fire or explosion which might have arisen from medical mishap
- related to drugs
- occurring in a general practitioner's surgery or health centre
- where a complaint has been received at the health board about the medical treatment given to the deceased
- with a violent, suspicious or unexplained cause

by two experienced doctors on two occasions 24 hours apart. Prior to such testing establish that the patient has irreversible brain injury of known cause producing deep coma and apnoea requiring artificial ventilation and that excludes potentially reversible causes (Box 20.1).

Examination sequence

There should be no response to any test below to confirm brainstem death.

- Apply a painful stimulus, e.g. supraorbital pressure or pinch an earlobe.
- Check the corneal reflexes (p. 252).
- Apply suction to the trachea to check for a cough or gag reflex. Note any response to the tracheal tube.
- Inject 20 ml of ice-cold water into the external auditory meatus and look for eye movements (oculovestibular reflexes/nystagmus).
- Stop ventilation long enough to allow $PaCO_2$ to rise to >6.7 kPa. Continue 100% oxygenation, by a cannula in the tracheal tube. Look for any respiratory effort: its absence indicates medullary brainstem failure.

WHAT TO DO AFTER YOU HAVE CONFIRMED DEATH

Record the death in the patient's medical notes, with the date and time at which you pronounced life extinct. If

possible, state what you believe to be the cause of death. Sign the notes legibly; include your designation.

Inform the close family or next of kin about the death as soon as possible. Wherever possible, do this in person rather than by telephone. Breaking bad news is difficult: always speak to the bereaved in a quiet and private environment, avoid interruption (ask someone to take your telephone and pager) and, wherever possible, involve a nurse or counsellor to act as a witness and provide future support if required. Relatives need time to understand and accept the situation. Use great care and sensitivity to try to support them. Inform the family doctor as soon as is reasonable. The followers of some faiths have procedures and rituals that should be followed after a death and which require the involvement of an appropriate religious leader.

If appropriate, ask about the deceased's wishes for organ donation. Some people carry an organ donor card stating their wishes. In the UK there is an organ donor register, which allows people to indicate their wishes for organ donation after death. You can check this register to confirm the deceased's wishes.

Where the circumstances of death are unexpected or where death has occurred in suspicious or prescribed circumstances, the legal authorities must be informed. Examples include suspected overdose, deaths related to alcohol or after surgery or if there is to be a post mortem examination. Do not give a death certificate until the coroner, procurator fiscal or other authority has agreed that you should do so (Box 20.3).

Paul O'Neill

OSCEs and other examination formats

21

21

INTRODUCTION

Formal assessments are designed to allow you to demonstrate your clinical skills. You must show the examiners that you are competent at undertaking a focused history and examination and can integrate these smoothly. Clinical assessments include:

- OSCE – Objective, Structured, Clinical Examination. The format varies in length, number and complexity of the stations and how the score is calculated.
- OSLER – Objective, Structured, Long Examination Record. Similar to OSCEs but with more time for a complete patient assessment.
- Mini-CEX – Mini-Clinical Evaluation eXercise. Individual, short (15 minutes) observed doctor–patient interactions assessing clinical skills, attitudes and behaviour.

You must demonstrate what you know, so consider how best to show your clinical technique. Exams make people nervous and being watched compounds this, so practise in similar situations. Take every opportunity to see and examine as many patients as possible and ask more senior staff to observe you. Involve your colleagues in role play and practise being the patient, examinee and examiner to give you each perspective. The more automatic and honed your examination technique is, the more likely you are to do yourself justice in the real assessment as well as to be a competent doctor with good technique.

Find out exactly what the exam will entail (coverage, format, timings) and check the fine details (time, place) well in advance of the actual day. Listen to the briefing before the OSCE as it contains important information. There is often a pause between stations to change over and allow you to read any briefing. This pause is vital. Forget the station you have just done – your mark is fixed, so concentrate on the next one.

Do not be put off by the examiner's manner: apparent 'hawks' may mark leniently and vice versa. Sometimes the simulated patient will mark you on communication or professionalism. Station formats and mark sheets vary but they are linked to the set task and have criteria covering various aspects of what is expected in the assessment.

This chapter provides a revision framework for a clinical assessment and highlights important things that must be done well, summarises common topics and details common mistakes. Review the details in each chapter and use the clinical videos. In each system, there is one illustrative common OSCE topic and examples of other topics.

An overall grade of pass, borderline or fail is widely used. This, together with the mark awarded, determines the overall pass score of the station. To pass overall, often you must achieve above the pass score as well as pass a minimum number of stations.

You should be able to demonstrate skills and attitudes that are common to most stations.

HISTORY TAKING AND GENERAL COMMUNICATION

Approach to the patient

Always dress professionally, introduce yourself, show respect, maintain confidentiality and obtain consent. Show good communication skills and awareness of patient safety, e.g. hand washing.

History taking

Have a clear beginning, listen actively, find out the patient's context, e.g. social situation, work, share information with the patient and agree goals, clarify and summarise. Have a clear structure and order; gather information, past history, drug/allergy history, family and social details and systems enquiry.

Demonstrate competence in communication

This is particularly required in sensitive or stressful scenarios, e.g. breaking bad news, or with a confused patient.

Have an appropriate communication framework

Find out the patient's ICE (ideas, concerns and expectations) (p. 8).

GENERAL EXAMINATION

Comment on your first impressions

For example, the patient's clothing (neat, unkempt), demeanour (withdrawn, agitated), complexion (jaundice, pigmentation), odours (ketones, uraemic).

Spot diagnosis or focus for further assessment

This might be linked to the face, hands, tongue, lymph nodes, obvious swelling or deformity and nutritional status. Look at any charts for temperature, blood pressure, pulse and oxygen saturation.

THE COMMUNICATION STATION

Good communication is essential for patient care and integral to OSCEs. Most OSCEs include specific 'communication stations'. Practise with your colleagues; take every opportunity to be videoed or recorded to reduce any anxiety and recognise your potential deficiencies.

Example

Task	Comment
Explain to this patient that she has multiple sclerosis (or cancer or human immunodeficiency virus (HIV))	Use a structure, e.g. SPIKES (Box 2.7), and know about the condition
Criteria	
Appropriate setting	Ensure privacy, comfort, seating at eye level, any accompanying person
Elicits patient's perceptions	Does the patient understand why she is there? What does she currently understand?
Invites the patient to discuss the situation	Ask if the patient consents to talk about the details of her medical condition and the results of her tests
Was the knowledge of the condition sufficient and given appropriately to the patient?	Know about multiple sclerosis (diagnosis, investigations, management, prognosis). Explain this to the patient in small chunks, avoid jargon and check understanding
Show appropriate empathy	Acknowledge and explore the patient's reactions or emotions
At the conclusion, were a summary and a strategy outlined?	Provide a summary; check the patient's understanding, that she knows the next steps and when these will happen

Other examples of communication stations

Possible scenarios include:
- A patient/relative unhappy with his care or talking with bereaved family members: you should manage the patient's emotions by remaining calm, acknowledging appropriate annoyance or upset.

Give the person time to explain in his own words what happened (in detail). Summarise and reflect back the patient's main concerns. Ensure that the patient knows what you will do about it and when he will get a response.
- Patients with impaired senses: Deafness (face the patient and speak clearly; use of sign language and written communication), blindness (touch and voice to show empathy).
- Patients whose first language is not English: How to use an interpreter (professional or other), 'chunking' what you say (wait for response), cultural competence (fasting in patients with diabetes).
- Talking to carers, partners or significant others: Ensure confidentiality, maintain patient autonomy, check the patient's competence to make decisions.
- Discussion of 'do not attempt resuscitation'.
- A distressed patient.

21

Omissions and difficulties	
Task or focus	Avoid common problems
Grasp all the important information	Read and think about the information given in the station briefing. Pause and recall what you know and decide on your strategy
Listen well	Make sure you listen and do not speak too much because you are anxious. Practise allowing patients to speak without interrupting. Ask rather than tell
Questioning	Use open questions ('Tell me about your weight', not 'Have you lost weight?') Do not lapse into a series of yes/no answers. Record yourself taking a history.
Ask about the patient's expectations	Often simulated patients are told not to volunteer information unless asked. Remember to ask about their ICE – ideas, concerns, expectations
Respond appropriately to patient's emotion	Look for verbal or non-verbal clues. Listen and observe carefully. Reflect back, e.g. 'You seem angry (or upset)'
Structure communication	Make sure you open, explore, summarise and close. Demonstrate a clear structure ('So can I just summarise what you have told me?')

21 THE ENDOCRINE STATION

This station requires you to think and focus your history taking and examination while maintaining good communication.

Thyroid

Example

Task	Comment
Examine this patient with weight loss and heat intolerance	Consider hyperthyroidism, and focus your examination on this
Criteria	
Weight loss and agitation	Comment on their presence or absence
Excessive warmth and sweating (hands)	Comment on the skin to demonstrate that you know what is required
Fine tremor of outstretched hands and acropachy of the fingers (hyperthyroidism)	Acropachy – clubbing and swelling of the end of the fingers; rare, but shows detailed knowledge (Fig. 5.4C)
The radial pulse	Usually rapid and high-volume in hyperthyroidism unless on a beta-blocker. An irregularly irregular pulse suggests atrial fibrillation
The size, surface and consistency of the thyroid	Use SPACESPIT (Box 3.11) to describe any mass or swelling
Auscultation for a thyroid bruit	Uncommon, but shows your awareness
Evidence of thyroid eye disease	Comment on exophthalmos; demonstrate lid lag, chemosis (conjunctival swelling) and any strabismus (severe)
Pretibial myxoedema	Uncommon, but extra marks for good students

Acromegaly

The commonest pituitary problem. 'Examine this patient with excessive sweating and snoring' (snoring because of soft tissues and jaw overgrowth). Note the large hands ('Have you changed much in your photographs?'), coarse facial features with prognathism. Check for carpal tunnel syndrome (extra marks), visual fields (bitemporal hemianopia). State you would measure blood pressure (hypertension in one-third) and test the urine for glycosuria (diabetes in one-third).

Diabetes mellitus

Very common; consider the classification (type 1 or 2). Insulin usage is increasing in type 2 diabetes so do not use it to differentiate between the two types. Ask about treatment (remember home monitoring). Complications affect eyes, peripheral nerves, large vessels (heart, stroke, claudication), kidney (dialysis, transplant), treatment (blood pressure, cholesterol). Hypoglycaemia is very unusual in non-diabetics. Ask about precipitating factors (exercise) and treatment changes. Find out what the patient understands and how he manages the condition (a good communication station).

Other metabolic disturbances

Relating to electrolyte disturbances, e.g. hyponatraemia, hypercalcaemia, diabetes insipidus.

A person with general tiredness and thirst

Tiredness is a non-specific symptom, e.g. liver disease, chronic kidney disease, malignancy but, if associated with thirst, think of diabetes mellitus and hypercalcaemia.

Omissions and difficulties	
Task or focus	**Avoid common problems**
Hypothyoidism	Be able to demonstrate delayed tendon reflexes; look for delayed relaxation after contraction
Hyperthyroidism	Do not confuse lid lag (demonstrate on eye movement) and exophthalmos (protrusion); look for this from above the patient
Diabetes/acromegaly	Ask to measure BP or examine vision
Diabetes mellitus	Cover all complications and details of treatment
Hypoglycaemia	Obtain details about the circumstances and patient's understanding.
Tiredness	Pick up clues to know where to focus your questions

THE CARDIOVASCULAR STATION

Cardiac symptoms and the peripheral vascular system may be connected, e.g. valvular heart disease and atrial fibrillation causing a peripheral embolus.

Peripheral vascular disease

Example

Task	Comment
Examine the peripheral vascular system in this patient with leg pain on walking	Symptoms could be due to other problems, e.g. arthritis
Criteria	
Inspection	Look at abdomen (scar from aneurysm repair) and legs – any discoloration, loss of toes, ulcers, scars, loss of hair?
Temperature difference between the legs	Compare the warmth of feet and legs with the back of your hand
Capillary refill time	Apply firm pressure with a finger or thumb on dorsum of foot – blanches then refills in <2 seconds
Palpation for femoral and popliteal arteries in both legs	Palpate the femoral and popliteal pulses. Comment on popliteal aneurysms
Palpation for foot pulses and comments on equality	Palpate for the dorsalis pedis and posterior tibial pulses
Measure blood pressure	Note hypertension
Ausculation of femoral arteries	Comment on any bruits
Abdominal examination	Palpate for aortic aneurysm. Listen for bruits of renal or aortoiliac disease
Buerger's test	p. 132
Ankle brachial pressure index (ABPI)	p. 133
Palpation of pulse and asks to examine heart	Comment on regularity of pulse (atrial fibrillation) and ask to examine heart (valvular disease)

Other examples of OSCEs

Examine this patient with a leg ulcer

Describe the site(s) of previous ulcers, e.g. skin discoloration, scarring. If an ulcer is present, describe it in detail (shape, size, base, edge). Consider arterial and venous ulcers.

Examine this patient with varicose veins

Inspect with the patient standing and lying. Do the cough impulse test and state you would perform the Trendelenburg test (p. 136).

Examine this patient with high blood pressure

Demonstrate good technique. Say that the patient should rest for 5 minutes (p. 113). Check blood pressure in both arms, consider coarctation (radiofemoral delay), examine optic fundi (hypertensive retinopathy). Examine for left ventricular hypertrophy and listen for renal artery bruits. Ask for urinalysis results.

The heart

Cardiac OSCE stations commonly include history (chest pain, breathlessness) and examination (murmurs).

Take a history from this person with chest pain

Differentiate between ischaemic, pericarditic (positional, sharp), dissection (radiating to back, severe), pleuritic (sharp, relationship with coughing/breathing, lateralised), oesophageal (heartburn) and musculoskeletal (movement). Once you are confident that it is ischaemic, focus on onset, worsening, associated symptoms, risk factors and treatment (including interventional cardiology).

Examine this person's heart

Use the routine: inspect (scars), palpate (apex beat, thrills, heaves) and auscultate. When auscultating, use a mental checklist: heart sounds, added sounds (third, fourth, opening snap) and murmurs. Consciously listen to systole and diastole (time using the carotid pulse). Characterise loud murmurs (site, radiation, systolic, diastolic, character), then listen for other murmurs.

Omissions and difficulties	
Task or focus	**Avoid common problems**
Diagnose and justify this	Ask all the questions, e.g. radiation or additional symptoms, and establish the severity of the problem ('on walking' – a mile or 100 metres?) and duration ('recent' – days, weeks or months?)
Describe an ulcer	Have a system to report findings and do not miss elements, e.g. peripheral staining of skin, or base of ulcer
Palpate the popliteal pulse	Practise your technique (Fig. 6.40B). The patient may have an aneurysm
Auscultate the heart	Use the diaphragm for high-pitched murmurs, e.g. aortic incompetence; use the bell for low-pitched murmurs, e.g. mitral stenosis
Comment on heart sounds	Focus on them; e.g. S_2 is quiet in aortic stenosis, loud in hypertension
Hear both murmurs	Do not be distracted by one dominant murmur, e.g. aortic stenosis or mitral incompetence; listen for a second murmur, e.g. aortic incompetence

21 THE RESPIRATORY STATION

This may cover history taking ('Take a history from this patient who has been coughing up blood'), examination ('Examine this patient with left-sided chest pain'), communication ('Explain to this patient about a pleural aspiration') or a procedure ('Check the peak expiratory flow rate in this patient with asthma').

Example

Task	Comment
Examine the respiratory system in this woman with acute breathlessness	
Criteria	
General state and respiratory rate	Is the patient comfortable at rest? Expose the chest (leave a woman's bra on; explain to the examiner why). Count respiratory rate
Peripheral and central cyanosis	Look at the tongue and lips (central) and fingers (peripheral)
Finger clubbing and asterixis	pp. 49 and 149
Comments on tracheal position and apex beat	Assesses for mediastinal shift, e.g. collapse of lung
Chest expansion	Unilateral reduction (large pleural effusion)
Chest percussion	Most consistent signs are 'stony' dull (effusion), others are dull (consolidation), hyperresonant (emphysema or pneumothorax)
Chest auscultation	Breath sounds: Bronchial (consolidation) Vesicular ($\downarrow$ in consolidation, effusion) Crackles – (unilateral – infection), (bilateral – oedema or pneumonia). Bilateral fine late inspiratory crackles + clubbing = pulmonary fibrosis Wheeze (asthma, chronic obstructive pulmonary disease (COPD), occasionally in pulmonary oedema). If unilateral – obstruction
Vocal resonance	$\downarrow$ = pleural effusion, $\uparrow$ = consolidation

Other examples of OSCEs

Take a history from this patient with breathlessness

Quantify severity, change with time, variability; wheeze (morning dipping, post-exercise), pleuritic pain (localised, sharp, worse on inspiration and coughing);

cough (when?), sputum (colour, amount) and haemoptysis. Detail smoking history as 'pack years'. Occupational history including previous asbestos exposure and important allergens. Note relationship of symptoms to work. History of any allergies, including hayfever and eczema. Detailed drug history, including inhalers.

Take a history from this patient with haemoptysis

Distinguish from haematemesis. Ask how much (streaked in sputum, egg cupful), how long and circumstances (severe bout of coughing). Take a detailed history, e.g. bronchiectasis, as well as other symptoms, e.g. weight loss.

Take a history from this patient with chest pain

Characterise the pain (non-cardiac, probably pleuritic) and distinguish pleuritic from musculoskeletal (movement, trauma). Then consider possible causes: infective – recent productive cough, fever, rigors, general malaise. Pulmonary infarction – risk factors for thromboembolic disease, e.g. recent surgery or significant illness, immobility, cancer, family history. Ask about deep vein thrombosis symptoms. Tumour – lung, mesothelioma, breast.

Examine this patient who complains of wheeze

Think of COPD or asthma (bronchiectasis can complicate either, so look for clubbing). Comment on general examination, e.g. using accessory muscles, and signs of cor pulmonale (raised jugular venous pressure, peripheral oedema, loud P_2 – pulmonary hypertension).

Omissions and difficulties	
Task or focus	**Avoid common problems**
Take a full respiratory history	Do not omit important elements e.g. occupational history
Assess breathlessness	Quantify this. Get an idea of level of exertion, duration, change with time and variability, e.g. how far can the person walk?
Distinguish cause of chest pain	Do not take too long to focus on the correct area and therefore miss out large chunks of history or exam
Comment on general examination	Closely observe the patient rather than simply doing it to be noticed by the examiner, e.g. is the patient comfortable at rest or tachypnoeic?
Chest expansion	Practise demonstrating this
Central trachea	p. 150

THE GASTROINTESTINAL STATION

This includes the upper and lower gastrointestinal tract, liver and pancreas. Structure your revision into segments and think about it in different ways, e.g. 'Examine this patient who might have an acute abdomen'.

Example

Task	Comment
Examine this patient with jaundice	Often chronic liver disease (including primary biliary cirrhosis)
Criteria	
Jaundice	Conjunctiva, colour very dark in longstanding jaundice with skin excoriation from pruritus (bile salt deposition)
Signs of chronic liver disease	Comment on presence / absence of clubbing, palmar erythema, leukonychia, spider naevi (upper trunk, head, neck and arms) and gynaecomastia and know the causes of each
Needle tracks, tattoos or body piercing	Needle track marks: evidence of intravenous drug use, hepatitis B and C and HIV Tattoos and body piercing: hepatitis B and C
Signs of liver failure	Flapping tremor of outstretched hands, fetor hepaticus, confusion, altered mental state, bruising, jaundice
Inspection of the abdomen	Scars, swelling (localised, or generalised in ascites), caput medusa (portal hypertension)
Palpation of the abdomen	Examine all areas and comment on pain, guarding and rigidity. Assess hepatosplenomegaly
Ascites	Percussion for shifting dullness
Peripheral oedema	Examine ankles and sacrum for oedema (hypoalbuminaemia)
Ask to do urinalysis	Dark urine in hepatic or post-hepatic jaundice

Other examples of OSCEs

Take a history from this patient with difficulty swallowing

Is this progressive or sudden? Differential diagnosis of malignancy or benign stricture.

Take a history from this patient with upper abdominal pain

Distinguish between dyspepsia and heartburn. Consider peptic ulcer disease and malignancy. 'Red flag'

symptoms include recent onset of pain in a person <50 years, particularly if associated with weight loss, vomiting or anaemia. In chronic pancreatitis symptoms include chronic pain and pancreatic insufficiency (malabsorption, steatorrhoea, diabetes). Ask about alcohol and history of gallstones.

Take a history from this patient with altered bowel habit

Consider malignancy in an older patient, positive family history (genetic) or inflammatory bowel disease. Ask about onset, progression, alternating constipation/diarrhoea. Inflammatory bowel disease in younger patients: flares of illness with painful diarrhoea, mucus, blood and weight loss. Take careful management history, including drugs and surgery. Consider coeliac disease in younger patients with bloating and chronic diarrhoea: ask about food (gluten sensitivity) and weight loss (malabsorption).

Examine this patient with abdominal swelling

Commonly hepatomegaly (and/or splenomegaly), adult polycystic kidneys or a hernia (inguinal or incisional).

21

Omissions and difficulties	
Task or focus	**Avoid common problems**
Alcohol history	Take a detailed history quantified over time. Ask about drugs (intravenous), travel, tattoos and sexual history (HIV), e.g. diarrhoea
'Red flag' symptoms	These are likely to be a focus for discussion and further investigation
Communication skills	Be able to ask about alcohol and lifestyle without being embarrassed or judgemental
Inflammatory bowel disease	Know how to differentiate Crohn's disease and ulcerative colitis
Abdominal examination	Have a systematic approach to different segments, superficial and deep palpation. Keep your arm horizontal to abdominal surface (kneel down). Palpate for organomegaly
Examine for ascites	Demonstrate shifting dullness (Box 8.19)
Complete the examination	Examine groins, hernial orifices

21 THE RENAL STATION

This includes the whole genitourinary tract and its common problems: kidney (polycystic, chronic kidney disease, acute kidney injury, infection, tumour), the calyces and ureter (stones), bladder (infection, cancer) and urethra (micturition – incontinence, retention).

Example

Task	Comment
Please take a history from this patient who has been passing blood in his urine	Consider causes from generalised to local along the genitourinary tract
Criteria	
Clarifiy haematuria	Onset, change with time, pain, clots. Differentiate from menstrual blood
Explore pain	Use SOCRATES (Box 2.10)
Micturition	Incontinence, prostatic symptoms in men
Family history	Adult polycystic kidney disease
Occupational history	Bladder cancer and chemical exposure, e.g. dyes
Sexual history	Infection, trauma
Consider general causes	Ask about bruising and purpura. Ask about warfarin and antiplatelet drugs
Explore systemic features	Infection (general malaise, rigor, antibiotics). Chronic kidney disease (kidney failure, hypertension, dialysis)
Palpation of kidneys	Bilateral palpable kidneys = adult polycystic kidney disease, renal transplant in groin

Other examples of OSCEs

Examine this patient with loin pain

Focused abdominal examination. Consider general features (temperature, infection), blood pressure (renal disease), abdominal tenderness (particularly in loins, renal angle), abdominal masses (bilateral = polycystic kidneys; unilateral = tumour). Consider other causes, e.g. spinal disease. Ask before examining the genitals and carrying out a rectal examination. Ask to examine the urine (infection, haematuria, proteinuria).

Examine this patient with newly diagnosed kidney failure

Think general and specific features. Comment on pallor, uraemic complexion, excoriation, bruising, uraemic fetor, asterixis (features of renal failure). Look for hyperventilation (Küssmaul respiration) suggesting metabolic acidosis. Examine skin for vasculitis, or purpura (Henoch–Schönlein disease). Look for the nail bed pigmentation of chronic kidney disease. Ask to examine optic fundi for hypertensive or diabetic retinopathy, or retinal infarcts in systemic vasculitis or systemic lupus erythematosus. Measure BP (elevated in chronic kidney disease; postural drop if fluid-depleted). Examine the abdomen for enlarged, smooth kidneys or bladder (obstructive uropathy) and polycystic kidney disease. Listen for epigastric, renal and femoral bruits, and assess peripheral pulses (generalised vasculopathy with renal artery stenosis). Look for generalised (nephritic) and peripheral oedema. Assess peripheral nerve function (peripheral neuropathy of chronic kidney disease or diabetic neuropathy). Ask to examine urine for haematuria, proteinuria, casts, crystals, white cells and bacteria.

Examine this patient with oedema

Assess the extent, site and severity of oedema, e.g. facial (nephrotic syndrome), flanks, abdominal wall, sacral, genitalia, thighs, ankles and pedal. Assess JVP (elevated in vascular overload and heart failure). Look for nail changes associated with hypoproteinaemia (leukonychia, Beau's lines). Examine the optic fundi and measure BP. Listen for heart murmurs, especially a pansystolic mitral murmur indicating left ventricle dilatation. Listen for extra heart sounds indicating fluid overload and/or heart failure. In the lungs, examine for pleural effusions (nephrotic syndrome) or crackles indicating pulmonary oedema. Examine the abdomen for enlarged, smooth kidneys (renal amyloidosis causing nephrotic syndrome) and for ascites (nephrotic syndrome). Ask to examine the urine.

Examine this patient with prostatism

Ask about nocturia, frequency, dribbling. Tell the examiner you would assess the prostate.

Examine this patient with urinary incontinence

Consider stress (sphincter incompetence), urge (detrusor instability) and overflow (obstruction or neuropathic).

Omissions and difficulties	
Task or focus	**Avoid common problems**
History	Do not miss out any history. Ask about occupational history in a patient with possible bladder cancer
Continence history	Do not ignore because of social embarrassment. Use a scheme to consider causes
Have a multisystem approach	Keep an open mind and think of other systems. Practise focused examination or history around a symptom or sign (cross-systems).
Abdominal examination	Practise
Look at the optic fundi	Practise (p.291)
Urinalysis	Often done poorly, practise it in the skills labs

THE VISUAL STATION

The patient with a visual problem may be a normal volunteer. In the early clinical years the task is likely to be: 'Examine this person's vision'. Later, the task will be more complicated: 'This patient has had an episode of redness and pain in her eye; please examine her'. Usually you will have to examine the eyes and possibly focus on one aspect, e.g. 'Use the ophthalmoscope'.

Example

Task	Comment
Examine this man with sudden loss of vision in one eye	Likely to be retinal vessel (artery) occlusion. Consider platelet emboli or (temporal) arteritis. Possible vitreous haemorrhage or retinal detachment
Criteria	
Which eye is causing problems?	Focuses and asks for permission
Inspection	Glasses, magnifying lens, lid or eye abnormalities (swelling, ptosis). Iris and pupil shape, clarity and colour. Any defects, e.g drainage procedure in glaucoma
Visual acuity in both eyes (corrected and uncorrected)	Assess the severity of the problem with and without glasses
Both peripheral visual fields	Homonymous hemianopia (stroke) and the affected eye's visual field for a horizontal or arcuate field defect – scotoma (optic nerve disease)
Light and accommodation reflexes	Check both direct and indirect light reflex and accommodation
Colour vision	Impaired in optic nerve disease, e.g. multiple sclerosis
Eye movements	Uses 'H' pattern of eye movement (VI, abduction; IV depresses eye when adducted, III, all other muscles). Ask about double vision and pain on movement (optic neuritis)
Ophthalmoscopy with good technique	Optic nerve: white and swollen (temporal arteritis), pink and swollen (non-arteritic anterior ischaemic optic neuropathy). Fundus: numerous retinal haemorrhages (venous occlusion). Unable to visualise (severe haemorrhage). Pallor (arterial occlusion). Retinal embolism at arterial bifurcations (thromboembolic disease). Retinal detachment (grey sheet)
Examine the pulse	Arrhythmia (atrial fibrillation)
Listen to the heart	Listen for cardiac murmurs (valvular heart disease)
Listen to the neck	Carotid bruits (Doppler ultrasound required)

Other examples of OSCEs

Examine the eyes in this patient with acute redness and pain in one eye

Distribution, diffuse redness (conjunctivitis, episcleritis or scleritis), red lower inner eyelid (conjunctivitis), circumciliary (keratitis, iritis or angle closure glaucoma). Comment on ocular discharge (conjunctivitis). Look at the clarity of the iris. A hazy iris suggests corneal oedema (acute angle closure glaucoma) and aqueous chamber inflammatory cells (acute iritis). Comment on the pupil. Small, irregularly shaped pupil (acute iritis), oval, mid-dilated, poorly reactive pupil (acute angle closure glaucoma). Pain on eye movement (scleritis). Examine the red reflex. Corneal ulceration appears black (confirm with fluorescein). Assess visual acuity.

Examine the eyes in this patient with diabetes mellitus

This is a common scenario. Comment on background (non-proliferative) retinopathy with soft and hard exudates and microaneurysms (dot/blot haemorrhages). This progresses to proliferative retinopathy with new vessel formation near the optic disc and haemorrhage with fibrovascular retinal detachments.

Examine the eyes in this patient with cataract

Look for central or peripheral lens opacities.

Examine the eyes in this patient with glaucoma

Common cause of blindness. Ask about episodes of pain and blurred vision (acute angle); insidious visual loss (chronic simple or open-angle); and family history. Test visual acuity; look for drainage procedures (small peripheral black hole in iris).

21

Omissions and difficulties	
Task or focus	**Avoid common problems**
Visual acuity	Test each eye separately either formally or using a newspaper or book. Test the patient with and without glasses
Eye movements	Be able to interpret these. Have good neuroanatomical knowledge
Ophthalmoscopy	Practise this repeatedly (p. 290)
Report ophthalmoscope findings	Use a system: think through the different chambers, optic nerve head, vessels, retina
Interpret findings	Have good knowledge and link it to other information, e.g. diabetes

21 THE EAR, NOSE AND THROAT STATION

Revise your ear, nose and throat examination. This scenario is common as a history or examination station.

Example

Task	Comment
Examine this patient who complains of earache	Examine the ears and hearing, and consider referred pain, e.g. temporomandibular joint
Criteria	
General patient demeanour	Is the patient in pain or does the patient have systemic upset (acute otitis media)? Note hearing aids
Inspection and palpation of the pinna and surrounding area	Look for evidence of acute mastoiditis, acute otitis externa, trauma (haematoma) or previous surgery
Inspection of both external auditory meati	Comment on signs of discharge, crusting (acute otitis media, acute otitis externa)
Palpate the tragus	Tenderness – acute otitis externa
Use the otoscope with good technique	Examine both external auditory meati
Visualise the tympanic membranes for surface appearance and integrity	If the view is obscured with wax/debris, suggest manual removal or microsuction
Hearing in each ear	Remember to mask the other ear
Rinne's test with correct interpretation	Air conduction and bone conduction
Weber's test with correct interpretation	Lateralising. Combine Rinne's and Weber's tests to determine if there is conduction or nerve deafness

Task	Comment
Palpate the temporomandibular joints while the patient opens and closes his mouth	Note pain and feel for a click (temporomandibular joint dysfunction)
Palpate cervical lymph nodes	Pre- and postauricular, anterior and posterior triangle
Examine the throat	Referred pain from the oropharynx
Suggest other investigations such as audiology	Formal hearing test

Other examples of OSCEs

Examine this patient who complains of being dizzy and lightheaded

Examine the pulse, lying and standing blood pressure, look for facial palsy, examine the ears. Examine for nystagmus, Dix–Hallpike test, Romberg's test, Unterberger's stepping test, check gait for ataxia.

Omissions and difficulties	
Task or focus	**Avoid common problems**
Distinguish between upper and lower motor neurone facial palsy	Know that the upper part of the face has bilateral innervation, so is spared in an upper motor neurone lesion
Interpret hearing tests	Understand Rinne's and Weber's test and the need to mask the opposite ear in a basic hearing test
Perform special tests of vestibular function	Know how to perform and interpret Dix–Hallpike, Romberg's and Unterberger's tests
Use the otoscope	Practise and use with an appropriate speculum

THE MUSCULOSKELETAL STATION

Many patients have chronic joint problems and are frequently used in clinical exams. Use GALS (gait, arms, legs, spine) as an initial screen and then move on to more detailed examination. The patient may have painful joints, so ask about this and take great care to avoid upsetting the patient.

Example

Task	Comment
Examine this patient with back pain	Cover the spine and general locomotor aspects
Criteria	
Observe the patient standing. Comment on any spinal deformity	Note decreased lordosis, scoliosis, scars, skin abnormality, e.g. hairy patch in spina bifida
Palpate gently for any focal tenderness	Gently feel the spinous processes and paraspinal tissues
Percuss along the vertebral column (warn the patient first)	Gently percuss using your closed fist; comment on any tenderness
Assess spinal movements	Describe any limitation
Straight-leg raise	Note limitation in degrees and which side (sciatic nerve L5, S1)
Femoral nerve stretch test	Traction on femoral nerve L3–4
Examination of other joints	e.g. seronegative arthropathy
Check lower limb reflexes, power and sensation (including the perineum) and anal tone	Describe any changes and link these with possible diagnoses

Other examples of OSCEs

Take great care not to exacerbate any pain.

Examine this patient with pain in the hands

Common scenarios are:
- Rheumatoid arthritis (symmetrical and metacarpophalangeal and proximal interphalangeal joints affected)
- Osteoarthritis (distal interphalangeal joints, first carpometacarpal joints)
- Psoriatic arthritis (asymmetrical, deformity, nail changes, rash).

Expose the arms to above the elbow. Comment on the finger positions and any deviation. Look at the skin and nails, and turn the patient's hands over gently to see both sides. Describe any small muscle wasting, swelling, nodules and deformity. Feel each joint in turn for warmth and swelling. Note the character of any swelling and decide whether it is bony, soft tissue or an effusion. Assess passive and active movements of each affected joint and note any limitation of movement. Feel the ulnar border of the forearm for nodules (seropositive rheumatoid arthritis) and look for scaling of the skin (psoriasis). Ask to conduct a general locomotor examination.

Examine this patient with pain in the hip

Expose the hips and legs. Comment on any muscle wasting. Examine hip movements in all directions. Compare the two hips. Measure leg lengths and do Thomas's test (p. 344) for fixed flexion deformity. With the patient standing, look for Trendelenburg's sign (p. 344). Ask the patient to walk; observe his gait from the front and side. Ask to perform a general locomotor examination.

Examine this patient with pain in the knee (worse on walking)

Likely to be osteoarthritis but remember crystal arthritis and rheumatoid arthritis. Note patient's age. Comment on erythema, scars, muscle wasting, deformity, swollen bursae. Feel both knees for temperature difference (septic arthritis, haemarthrosis and inflammatory arthritis). Examine for knee effusion (septic arthritis, trauma, haemarthrosis) and for tenderness over joint lines and soft tissues. Assess active and passive movements at both knees. Examine for collateral and cruciate ligament stability and menisci. Observe gait and knee movements from the front and side.

Take a history from this patient with joint pain

Ask about joints affected, pattern, duration, degree of pain, limitations in activity, variability and onset. Find out about features of inflammation: swelling, pain, early-morning stiffness and any systemic features (malaise, fever, weight loss and other systems involved). Note previous medical and family history, previous management and relief. Summarise and interpret your findings.

Omissions and difficulties	
Task or focus	**Avoid common problems**
Joint examination	Know the steps, and practise them enough for the examination to be integrated. Avoid lots of pauses and thinking time
Measuring leg lengths	Get a tape measure and practise
Specific tests	Know these and be able to demonstrate them, e.g. femoral stretch test
Differentiate between arthritides	Know that the pattern of joint involvement is key (large, small, distal, spine, symmetrical) and evidence of inflammation
Examine other systems	Demonstrate your knowledge by looking at the forearm for nodules in rheumatoid arthritis and skin for psoriasis

21 THE NERVOUS STATION

Neurological examination is daunting. The history usually gives the diagnosis. Ask about: onset (acute, subacute, chronic symptoms), changes with time (worsening, relapsing and remitting, improving), involvement of one or more sites in the nervous system (demyelination), symmetrical involvement or not (the latter implies a structural problem).

Break down the examination into visual, cranial nerve, motor and sensory. Examine co-ordination and gait last. Practise your technique on patients with and without neurological problems.

A neurology station will have an explicit focus as the system is too complex to examine completely.

Example

Task	Comment
This patient is complaining of weakness and numbness. Examine his legs	Examine both the motor and sensory systems. Think of peripheral neuropathy, cord compression, demyelination and Guillain–Barré syndrome. Ask him to walk and check Romberg's test
Criteria	
Inspection, looking for muscle wasting or fasciculation	Wasting implies chronicity. Describe its distribution and symmetry. Fasciculation (lower motor lesion with ongoing denervation, no sensory symptoms in motor neurone disease)
Tone, including clonus	Increased tone (upper motor neurone lesions above the cauda equina), reduced in lower motor neurone lesions
Knee, ankle and plantar reflexes	Reflexes lost early in Guillain–Barré syndrome and peripheral neuropathy. Elicit plantar responses. Hyperreflexia (upper motor neurone lesion)
Power at hip, knee and ankle	Test movement across each joint (hip – flexion, extension, adduction, abduction) and grade (0–5/5)
The sensory system for nerve, dermatomal (root) or level (cord)	Think about how sensation is conveyed back to the brain. Nerve – e.g. lateral cutaneous nerve to the thigh, root, e.g. L5, and level, e.g. T10 umbilicus
All sensory modalities	Break down into pinprick, vibration, joint position, heat and light touch. Dissociative sensory loss – anterior or central cord lesion
Coordination	Heel-to-shin and truncal ataxia. Remember spinocerebellar syndromes, e.g. Friedreich's ataxia.
Gait	If patient can manage – asymmetry, wide-based, parkinsonian
Asked to examine upper limbs and rest of nervous system	Glove loss in peripheral neuropathy and to determine level of cord compression
Asked to examine the spine	Comment on deformity and local tenderness (malignancy, infection)

Other examples of OSCEs

Take a history in a patient with sudden loss of consciousness

Establish that the patient did lose consciousness as opposed to a drop attack. Clarify the circumstances, how the patient was before and after, any witnesses and previous episodes. Ask about driving. Consider vasovagal syncope (young person, hot crowded environment, feeling sick, quick recovery), Stokes–Adams or cardiac syncope (brief or no warning, palpitation, looks pale then flushed, rapid recovery), seizure (aura, witness seeing limb shaking, drowsy after), hypoglycaemia (diabetes mellitus).

Take a history in a patient with headaches

Consider an acute neurological problem: subarachnoid haemorrhage, meningitis (associated systemic disturbance), temporal arteritis (uncommon <50 years, onset over weeks, severe with unilateral scalp tenderness, jaw claudication, visual disturbance and general malaise), migraine (unilateral, throbbing headache, visual symptoms, photophobia, nausea, may have aura and a family history), tension headache (generalised, often around neck and occiput, no aura, recurrent, explore personal and social history).

Take a history in a patient with transient ischaemic attack (TIA) or stroke

TIA is common in history stations. Stroke is common as an examination station. Ensure that the patient describes focal neurology, e.g. loss of speech, which came on suddenly and was most likely vascular. Make sure you can localise the lesion anatomically in the brain. In stroke, ask about activities of daily living and ongoing problems. Identify vascular risk factors (including atrial fibrillation). Remember amaurosis fugax for a TIA.

Take a history in a patient with brain tumour

This will be a simulated patient. Progressive focal neurology, no clear onset, can be associated with headaches (early morning) and sometimes cognitive changes.

Examine this patient with diplopia

The direction of maximal double vision indicates direction of affected muscle and the potential nerve affected. VI, lateral rectus; IV, superior oblique, depresses eye when adducted, rotates when abducted and tilts false image; III, all other muscles, so complete palsy is present with ptosis and eye turned down by superior oblique and out by lateral rectus. Remember myasthenia gravis as a cause.

Examine this patient with facial palsy

Bell's palsy (complete) and stroke (sparing upper face – bilateral innervation). Examine upper and lower parts of the face. Comment on any conjunctival changes (can the patient close the eye? exposed cornea) and flattening of the nasolabial fold on affected side.

Examine this patient with peripheral nerve lesion on the hand

Radial (wrist drop test, wrist extension), median (thenar eminence wasting ± fasciculation, test abductor pollicis brevis and opponens pollicis) and ulnar (adductor pollicis, test abduction and adduction of fingers). Sensory testing; ulnar (affects palmar surface of little and half of ring finger), median (palmar surface of thumb, index and middle finger plus possibly lateral half of ring finger), radial (none or anatomical snuffbox). Carpal tunnel syndrome affects the median nerve and causes pain radiating up the arm, particularly at night.

Omissions and difficulties	
Task or focus	**Avoid common problems**
Take a history	Clarify the course, including onset, duration, worsening and fluctuation
Link findings to anatomical site	Have good neuroanatomical knowledge. Locate lesion to one site if possible
Differential diagnosis	Know and link, diagnoses to symptoms or signs
Demonstrate tone	Test tone before power to avoid the patient continuing to move
Demonstrate the reflexes	Practise. Don't forget reinforcement
Assess different systems smoothly	Examine in the order: cranial nerves, motor, sensation, co-ordination and gait

21

Index

Page numbers in **bold** indicate figures and boxes.